Advances in Pain Research and Therapy
Volume 2

INTERNATIONAL SYMPOSIUM ON
PAIN OF ADVANCED CANCER

Advances in Pain Research and Therapy
Volume 2

International Symposium on Pain of Advanced Cancer

Editors

John J. Bonica, M.D.,
D.Sc., F.F.A.R.C.S.
*President of the International Association for the Study of Pain
Professor of Anesthesiology
Director of Pain Center
University of Washington
Seattle, Washington*

Vittorio Ventafridda, M.D.
*Director
Division of Pain Therapy
and Rehabilitation
Istituto Nazionale per lo
Studio e la Cura dei Tumori
Milano, Italy*

Associate Editors

B. Raymond Fink, M.D.
*Secretary of the International Association for the Study of Pain
Professor of Anesthesiology
University of Washington
Seattle, Washington*

Louisa E. Jones, B.S.
*Executive Secretary and Treasurer,
International Association for the
Study of Pain
Editor, Research Publications
Department of Anesthesiology
University of Washington
Seattle, Washington*

John D. Loeser, M.D.
*Associate Professor of Neurological Surgery
Member of Pain Clinic
University of Washington
Seattle, Washington*

Raven Press ▪ New York

**Raven Press, 1140 Avenue of the Americas, New York,
New York   10036**

© 1979 by Raven Press Books, Ltd. All rights reserved. This book is protected by copyright. No part of it may be reproduced, stored in a retrieval system, or transmitted, in any form or by any means, electronic, mechanical, photocopying, recording, or otherwise, without the prior written permission of the publisher.

Made in the United States of America

International Standard Book Number 0–89004–2705
Library of Congress Catalog Card Number 78–55811

This Volume is Dedicated to

Dr. Ing. Virgilio Floriani
and
Signora Loredana Floriani

Two wonderful human beings whose magnificent personal attributes and extraordinary sense of humanitarianism are a constant source of admiration and inspiration.

Preface

This monograph contains the scientific papers presented and discussions held at the International Symposium on Pain of Advanced Cancer held in Venice, Italy on May 24–27, 1978. This symposium, sponsored by the Floriani Foundation of Milan, Italy and under the auspices of the International Association for the Study of Pain, L'Union International Contre Le Cancer, and the three most important Italian agencies against cancer, was attended by nearly 500 scientists, physicians, and other health professionals representing several dozen disciplines from 22 countries. This was, without doubt, the largest gathering of people interested in cancer pain ever held anywhere.

The primary goal of this symposium was to help rectify the serious deficiencies that exist in the current management of pain of advanced cancer by bringing together outstanding authorities from different disciplines to discuss virtually every aspect of the topic. The objectives of the symposium were: (1) to discuss the importance and magnitude of cancer pain, its mechanisms, and the physiologic, psychologic, and sociologic impact it has on the patient, the family, and society; (2) to evaluate all of the methods that may be used to relieve cancer pain within the framework of our current knowledge and human resources; (3) to critically analyze deficiencies that exist and to suggest how they may be eliminated; (4) to suggest some future directions that research might take to improve current methods and develop new methods of cancer pain therapy. These objectives were achieved and the results are presented in this monograph.

The reader's attention is called to the introductory remarks by Albino Cardinal Luciani, then Patriarch of Venice, who 3 months later was elected Pope John Paul I.

Part I of the volume contains a discussion of the importance and magnitude of cancer pain as a serious national and world health problem and a comprehensive overview of the anatomic, neurophysiologic, biochemical, psychologic, and behavioral aspects of nociception and pain in general. This serves as a background for the material in Part II, which includes discussion of etiology and mechanisms of cancer pain and its psychologic, emotional, psychosocial, sociologic, and nursing aspects.

The subsequent five sections contain reports intended to evaluate all of the methods currently being used to relieve cancer pain including various anticancer modalities, psychologic techniques, and sociologic strategies, systemic analgesics and related drugs, nerve blocks, ablative neurosurgical procedures, and neurostimulating techniques. Each of these sections contains a number of reports dealing with different agents or techniques. Each report was written by a person who is nationally or internationally recognized as an expert in the specific field. Most of these reports contain an evaluation of the efficacy, advantages, limitations, side effects, and complications of each particular technique or method based upon the personal experience of the author and review of the recent literature.

The contents of the next three sections are intended to integrate the preceding material into discussions of the clinical management of patients with pain due to cancer in one of several body regions which are among the most frequent and most difficult problems to deal with: head and neck; brachial plexus and chest; abdominal viscera and perineum. Each of these three sections includes a brief description of the incidence of pain in that particular part of the body and a summary of the efficacy and limitations of the most important modalities used for its relief. These are followed by a section that contains discussions of the basic principles of continuing and terminal care of cancer patients with special emphasis on the management of pain and a description of the organization and function of St. Christopher's Hospice by two highly qualified and experienced individuals: Dr. R. Twycross and Dr. C. Saunders. Also in the same section, Dr. G. Ford presents important facts about the incidence of cancer and cancer pain and its treatment within the framework of the British National Health Service. The last section contains prepared and spontaneous comments on future needs, goals, and directions regarding the research, teaching, and patient-care in the field of cancer pain. Most of the comments in this section were based on the information presented during the preceding 4 days.

We believe that the contents of this volume will be of significant interest to many health professionals, but especially to surgical, medical, and radiation oncologists, algologists (dolorologists), psychologists, psychiatrists, clinical pharmacologists, neurosurgeons, anesthesiologists, social workers, nurses, theologians, and all others who have the serious responsibility of managing patients with cancer pain. The information contained herein should give basic scientists and clinical investigators an insight into the great voids in our knowledge about basic mechanisms and, it is hoped, should stimulate further research efforts in this area. In view of the great paucity of information on the basic principles of managing cancer pain in oncology textbooks or other sources of information, the book should prove useful to teachers and students alike. Finally, proper application of the information about the various therapeutic modalities should markedly enhance the capability of physicians and other health professionals to provide most, if not all, patients with cancer pain with optimal pain relief. We hope that in this and other ways the book will help to improve and sustain the quality of life in patients with cancer—a responsibility that remains one of the most important obligations and laudable objectives of all health professionals involved in the care of these patients.

John J. Bonica
Vittorio Ventafridda
October 1978

Acknowledgments

On behalf of all of the speakers and participants of the symposium and all of the millions of patients suffering from cancer pain, the editors wish to express sincerest thanks, great appreciation and, indeed, gratitude to Mr. and Mrs. Virgilio Floriani of the Floriani Foundation for their generous support of the symposium on which this volume is based. Mr. and Mrs. Floriani and the Board of Directors of the Foundation deserve warmest congratulations and commendation for their foresight and perspicacity for proposing the development of a major international meeting to discuss the pain of advanced cancer. As is emphasized throughout the book, effective pain relief and the prompt management of the patient with advanced cancer related thereto is one of the most urgent problems of modern society.

On behalf of the Floriani Foundation and the speakers and registrants of the symposium, we express appreciation to His Excellency Giovanni Leone, then President of the Republic of Italy, for the High Patronage and the moral support provided the symposium and to Albino Cardinal Luciani for taking time out of his extremely busy schedule to attend and give the opening remarks. We also wish to express appreciation to other members of the Honorary Committee. The senior editor is especially delighted to acknowledge the presence of a dear friend, Princess Yana Alliata di Montereale, at the opening ceremonies. Having had that important meeting held on the beautiful island of St. Giorgio was a fitting tribute to her late father, Count Vittorio Cini, a magnificent human being, great philanthropist, and a truly Renaissance man.

The auspices of five professional societies or institutions helped to assure the success of the symposium, and for this the editors thank them most sincerely.

L'Union International Contre le Cancer
The International Association for the Study of Pain
L'Associazione Italiana per lo Studio del Dolore
Lega Italiana per la Lotta Contro i Tumori
L'Istituto Nazionale per lo Studio e la Cura dei Tumori

The development and running of such a large, comprehensive, scientific program and the highly successful outcome of the symposium were made possible only by the contributions of many, many individuals to whom we wish to acknowledge our indebtedness. The senior editor wishes to express sincere thanks and appreciation to members of the Scientific Program Committee for the help given in the development of a scientific program which made the symposium highly successful and productive. We also wish to express great appreciation and indebtedness to the members of the Organizing Committee for their time and effort in taking care of the hundreds of details

ACKNOWLEDGMENTS

required for the arrangements of the facilities needed for the scientific program on the island of St. Giorgio and the social activities for the speakers, their spouses, and the participants. These made it possible for us to run the impressively full and very comprehensive program on time and without a single flaw or problem. Among the members of the Organizing Committee several people deserve special recognition for their contributions.

First and foremost is Signora Loredana Floriani, not only for her enthusiastic support of the symposium, but equally important for her extremely active participation in the planning of the conference, in the development of the local arrangements, and in providing valuable help during the meeting. It is virtuously admirable that, considering her position in the Floriani Foundation, she put aside national tradition and worked long hours alongside the staff managing the registration desk and taking care of every need mentioned by speakers and participants alike. Signora Floriani's personal touch and involvement made the social events memorable experiences. Her infectious smile, warm personality, her unusual ability to exude friendship and other attributes that make her a magnificent human being greatly facilitated the onerous tasks of both editors.

In a similar fashion, Mr. Virgilio Floriani worked long hours during the development and running of the program and for several weeks after the symposium. The reader's attention is called to his introductory remarks because they reveal some of the unusual characteristics of this man and his unusual interest in the welfare of people and his compassion for patients with cancer pain. It is worth noting that through his brilliant mind, his interest and expertise as an electronics engineer, and through his own personal herculean efforts, Mr. Floriani rose from virtual poverty after World War II to head one of the most important industrial complexes dealing with electronics in the world. In addition to the financial support which made the symposium possible, his personal involvement, planning, and running of the 4-day meeting, and taking care of the most menial tasks and his unremitting enthusiastic support were critical to the success of the conference and to the publication of this monograph.

We also express very special thanks to Ms. Wanda Segre, secretary of the Floriani Foundation, for coordinating all of the activities of the Organizing Committee and for personally taking care of many of the details during the development and running of the symposium. She also coordinated the translation of a number of papers into English and carried out innumerable other tasks in an extremely efficient and very cooperative manner.

Ms. Louisa Jones, Executive Secretary and Treasurer of the International Association for the Study of Pain and editor of the Department of Anesthesiology of the University of Washington, helped the senior editor coordinate the development of the scientific program, was responsible for the editing and printing of the program and book of abstracts, and also helped the members of the Organizing Committee during the symposium. During the

ACKNOWLEDGMENTS

past several months, she has expended an unusual amount of time and effort in collating and editing all of the typed manuscripts and galley and page proofs for this volume. For these and other efforts on this project, we express our thanks and gratitude, Ms. Jones.

The editors also wish to acknowledge their appreciation and thanks to Drs. B. R. Fink and John Loeser for their editorial assistance; to Ms. Rosita Walsh, administrative secretary to the senior editor, for her invaluable help during the long and arduous process of planning the scientific program and editing this volume; to Ms. Linda Hipps and Juanita Cooke for typing of the edited manuscripts; and to Ms. Virginia Martin of Raven Press for her invaluable help in the publication of the volume.

Contents

PART 1. BASIC CONSIDERATIONS

1   Importance of the Problem
John J. Bonica

13   Neurophysiology of Nociception, Pain, and Pain Therapy
Manfred Zimmermann

31   Neuroanatomy and Biochemistry of Antinociception
Costantino Benedetti

45   Psychologic and Behavioral Aspects of Cancer Pain
C. Richard Chapman

59   Pain Syndromes in Patients with Cancer
Kathleen M. Foley

77   The Role of Cerebral Cortex in the Pain of Advanced Cancer
C. V. Morpurgo

81   Psychologic and Emotional Aspects of Cancer Pain
M. R. Bond

89   Pain in Children with Cancer
J. Gerald Beales

99   Sociologic Effects of Cancer Pain
Margo McCaffery

103   Sociologic and Nursing Aspects of Cancer Pain
Ada G. Rogers

PART 2. MANAGEMENT OF PAIN OF ADVANCED CANCER

115 Introduction
     John J. Bonica

Role and Limits of Oncologic Treatment of Pain of Advanced Cancer (Anti-Cancer Modalities)

131 Role and Limits of Anticancer Drugs in the Treatment of Advanced Cancer Pain
     Gianni Bonadonna and Roberto Molinari

139 Role and Limits of Oncologic Chemotherapy of Advanced Cancer Pain
     Georges Brulé

145 The Role of Endocrine Therapy for Relief of Pain due to Advanced Cancer
     F. Pannuti, A. Martoni, A. P. Rossi, and E. Piana

167 Radiation Therapy
     S. Basso Ricci

175 Palliative Surgery
     Leandro Gennari

185 Hyperthermic Perfusion with Sympathectomy for the Treatment of Advanced Painful Limb Tumors
     R. Cavaliere, G. Moricca, G. Stradone, and F. di Filippo

195 Combined Whole-Body Treatment Hyperthermia and Chemotherapy in the Treatment of Advanced Cancer with Diffuse Pain
     G. Moricca, R. Cavaliere, M. Lopez, and A. Caputo

Psychologic and Sociologic Methods for the Relief of Pain of Advanced Cancer

215 Psychologic and Psychiatric Techniques
     M. R. Bond

223 Hypnotherapy in Pain of Advanced Cancer
     Basil Finer

231 Psychophysiologic Control of Cancer Pain
     Sophia S. Fotopoulos, Charles Graham, and Mary R. Cook

245 Psychosocial and Nursing Technique
     Ada G. Rogers

Systemic Analgesics and Related Drugs

255 Nonnarcotic Analgesics
     H. U. Gerbershagen

263 Systemic Analgesics and Related Drugs: Narcotic Analgesics
     Raymond W. Houde

275 Psychotropics, Ataractics, and Related Drugs
     Lawrence M. Halpern

285 The Use of Psychotropic Drugs in the Treatment of Cancer Pain
     R. Kocher

291 The Brompton Cocktail
     Robert G. Twycross

Nerve Blocks

303 Introduction to Nerve Blocks
     John J. Bonica

311 Blocks with Local Anesthetics in the Treatment of Cancer Pain
     H. U. Gerbershagen

325 Subarachnoid and Extradural Neurolytic Blocks
     M. Swerdlow

339 Phenol Subarachnoid Rhizotomy for the Treatment of Cancer Pain: A Personal Account on 290 Cases
I. Papo and A. Visca

347 Cranial Nerve Blocks
Jose L. Madrid and John J. Bonica

357 Celiac (Splanchnic) Plexus Block with Alcohol for Cancer Pain of the Upper Intra-abdominal Viscera
Daniel C. Moore

373 Chemical Hypophysectomy
John Miles

381 Chemical Hypophysectomy
Jose L. Madrid

393 Hypophysectomy for Relief of Pain of Disseminated Carcinoma of the Prostate
Charles R. West, Anthony M. Avellanosa, Alfonso M. Bremer, and Kazuo Yamada

Ablative Neurosurgical Procedures

405 General Comments on Ablative Neurosurgical Procedures
Carlo A. Pagni

425 Percutaneous Cervical Cordotomy
Sampson Lipton

439 Spinal Posterior Rhizotomy and Commissural Myelotomy in the Treatment of Cancer Pain
I. Papo

449 Open Cordotomy in the Treatment of Cancer Pain
I. Papo

453 Medullary Tractotomy for Cephalic Pain of Malignant Diseases
Albino Bricolo

463	Percutaneous Thermocoagulation of the Gasserian Ganglion in the Treatment of Pain in Advanced Cancer *Jean Siegfried and Giovanni Broggi*
469	Percutaneous Differential Radiofrequency Rhizotomy of Glossopharyngeal Nerve in Facial Pain Due to Cancer *Giovanni Broggi and Jean Siegfried*
475	Stereotaxic Thalamolaminotomy and Posteromedial Hypothalamotomy for the Relief of Intractable Pain *Keiji Sano*

Augmentative (Stimulating) Neurosurgical Procedures

487	Central Gray Stimulation for Control of Cancer Pain *Donald E. Richardson*
493	Thalamic and Hypothalamic Stimulation *David Fairman*
499	Dorsal Column and Peripheral Nerve Stimulation for Relief of Cancer Pain *John D. Loeser*
509	Transcutaneous Nerve Stimulation in Cancer Pain *Vittorio Ventafridda, E. P. Sganzerla, C. Fochi, G. Pozzi, and G. Cordini*

Therapy of Cancer Pain in the Head and Neck

519	Problems of Cancer Pain in the Head and Neck *Roberto Molinari*
523	Oncologic Therapy of Pain in Cancer of the Head and Neck *Roberto Molinari*
533	Cancer Pain in the Head and Neck: Role of Analgesics and Related Drugs *Raymond W. Houde*

537 Cancer Pain in the Head and Neck: Role of Nerve Blocks
John J. Bonica and Jose L. Madrid

543 Cancer Pain in the Head and Neck: Role of Neurosurgery
Carlo A. Pagni

Pain Involving the Chest and Brachial Plexus

555 Role of Oncologic Therapy in Pain Involving the Chest and Brachial Plexus
Georges Brulé

563 Role of Analgesics and Related Drugs in Pain Involving the Chest and Brachial Plexus
H. U. Gerbershagen

567 Role of Nerve Blocks in Pain Involving the Chest and Brachial Plexus
M. Swerdlow

577 Role of Neurosurgery in Pain Involving the Chest and Brachial Plexus
Donald E. Richardson

Visceral and Perineal Pain

589 Role of Analgesics and Related Drugs in Visceral and Perineal Pain
Raymond W. Houde

593 Role of Nerve Block with Neurolytic Solutions in Visceral and Perineal Pain
Daniel C. Moore

597 Neurolytic Blocks in Perineal Pain
V. Ventafridda

607 Role of Neurosurgery in Visceral and Perineal Pain
John D. Loeser

Continuing and Terminal Care

617 Overview of Analgesia
Robert W. Twycross

635	The Nature and Management of Terminal Pain and the Hospice Concept *Cicely Saunders*
653	Terminal Care from the Viewpoint of the National Health Service *Gillian Ford*
667	Panel: Future Needs, Goals, and Directions *J. Bonica and V. Ventafridda* (Moderators)
685	*Subject Index*

Contributors

A

A. M. Avellanosa, 393

B

S. Basso Ricci, 167
J. G. Beales, 89
C. Benedetti, 31
G. Bonadonna, 131
M. R. Bond, 81, 215, 676
J. J. Bonica, 1, 115, 303, 347, 537, 682
A. M. Bremer, 393
A. Bricolo, 453
G. Broggi, 463, 469
G. Brulé 139, 555
P. Bucalossi, 670

C

A. Caputo, 195
R. Cavaliere, 185, 195
C. R. Chapman, 45
M. R. Cook, 231
G. Cordini, 509

D

F. Di Filippo, 185

F

D. Fairman, 493
B. Finer, 223
D. Fink, 673
C. Fochi, 509
K. M. Foley, 59
G. Ford, 653
S. S. Fotopoulos, 231

G

L. Gennari, 175, 681
H. U. Gerbershagen, 245, 311, 563
C. Graham, 231

H

L. M. Halpern, 275
R. W. Houde, 263, 553, 589, 677

K

R. Kocher, 285

L

S. Lipton, 425
J. D. Loeser, 499, 607, 675
M. Lopez, 195

M

J. Madrid, 347, 381, 537
A. Martoni, 145
M. McCaffery, 99
J. Miles, 373
R. Molinari, 131, 519, 523
D. C. Moore, 357, 593
G. Moricca, 185, 195, 680
C. V. Morpurgo, 77

P

C. A. Pagni, 405, 543
F. Pannuti, 145, 679
I. Papo, 339, 439, 449
E. Piana, 145
G. Pozzi, 509

R

D. E. Richardson, 487, 577
A. G. Rogers, 103, 245
A. P. Rossi, 145

S

K. Sano, 475
C. Saunders, 635
E. P. Sganzerla, 509
J. Siegfried, 463, 469
G. Stradone, 185
M. Swerdlow, 325, 567

T

R. G. Twycross, 291, 617, 678

V

V. Ventafridda, 509, 597, 681
A. Visca, 339

W

C. R. West, 393

Y

K. Yamada, 393

Z

M. Zimmermann, 13

Page numbers refer to chapter opening page, or panel discussion page.

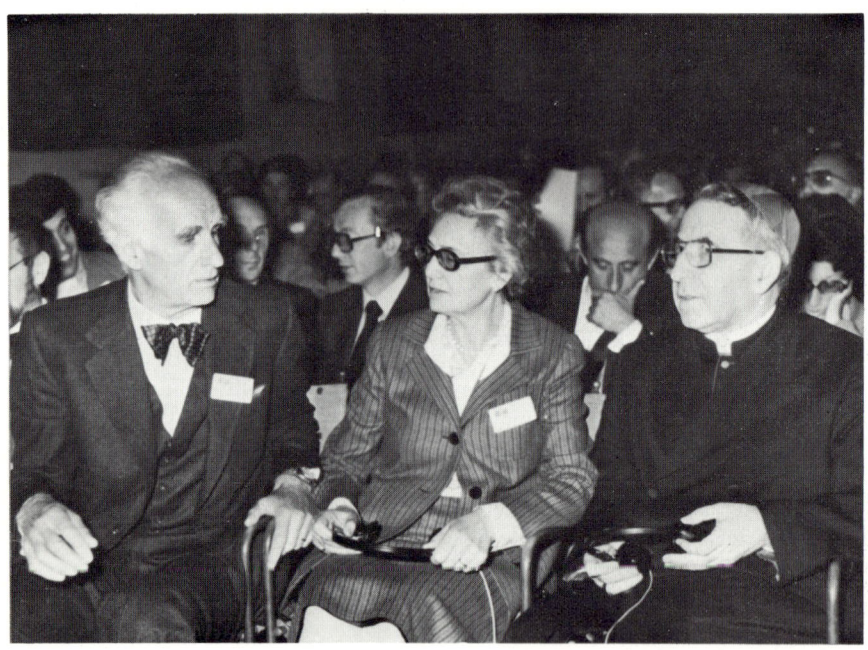

FIG. 1. *Left to right:* Ing. Virgilio Floriani, Mrs. Loredana Floriani, Albino Cardinal Luciani.

Introduction to Venice Symposium

Dr. Ing. Virgilio Floriani

One evening in the spring of 1977, Professors Maggi, Ventafridda, and Barbi, Dr. Motta, my son Marco, my wife, and myself met in Milano. We had recently formed the FONDAZIONE FLORIANI and we were examining the possible activities needed to fulfill the aims defined in the bylaws of the Foundation. The topic of pain, especially in the cancer patient, appeared not to have attracted sufficient attention in the past. Doctors tend to consider pain a secondary factor. The primary aim, the fundamental one in which they spent all their energy, is the cure and elimination of the disease. But the statistics tell us that in Italy alone there are more than 250,000 patients suffering from cancer and nearly 110,000 die annually from this disease. Of this latter group about 65 to 80% suffer such severe pain that it gravely affects both their quality of life and their relationship with their family and society.

We asked ourselves: Couldn't this be the subject of an international symposium? The answer was positive. But to have success, we had to stimulate the interest of a certain number of scientists of international renown from different disciplines with interest and expertise in this neglected field of medicine. In order to ensure that this would occur, it was necessary that the task be undertaken by a leading exponent in this field who was well-known and respected by other world scientists and clinicians. Professor Ventafridda suggested Professor John J. Bonica of Seattle.

In May 1977, while my wife and myself traveled in the United States, we went to Seattle and met Professor Bonica. We described to him our intention. We had no problem in convincing him to undertake such a task. I believe that we were favored in obtaining a positive response by the good reasons mentioned above, by Professor Bonica's long and intense interest in cancer pain, and also by the fact that he is of Italian origin and the symposium would be taking place in Venice—on the beautiful island of St. Giorgio. The symposium took place in May 1978, and this volume includes all the proceedings. The speakers were, in their essence, scientists: For them Nature is objective, its laws are unchangeable. The truth (or knowledge) obtains its origins from the systematic comparison between logic and experience, and this ensures a progressive character to knowledge itself.

The presentations, together with the discussions, took place before nearly 500 doctors and scientists from many countries; the publication of the proceedings and their diffusion constitute a further milestone in the fight against cancer pain. This was the aim that we had looked for. As it was foreseeable, such a symposium placed us face-to-face with a subject which is so complex that we were able to deal with it only in broad terms. Medicine as a true science—the study, the knowledge of the human body, the cure of its diseases—is a conquest of modern western civilization. Although its beginnings go back several millenia, it has been only since the time of Galileo that medicine has had a truly scientific basis. In the relatively short period of 300 years it has made many advances, especially during the past three or four decades, when more biomedical knowledge has been acquired than in all of the preceding period of human history. This has instilled great faith and confidence in the generations of our time, for many diseases which heretofore killed or disabled millions of people throughout the world have been eliminated or sufficiently controlled.

Although we still have not understood all of the mysteries of cancer, significant progress has been made in its therapy and some forms of this disease, if properly treated, in time can be cured. Since it is likely that the impressive momentum of biomedical research and new discoveries consequent thereto will continue at an even greater pace, we should have great faith that eventually this dreadful group of disorders given the generic term of *cancer* will be conquered. In the meantime, we must continue and indeed increase our efforts to assure patients with cancer that they will continue to enjoy the quality of life. To achieve this, we must effectively relieve the pain that is often associated with cancer, especially in the late phases of the disease. We may affirm that with the means we have today 70 to 80% of the patients with cancer pain could be relieved of the pain completely or it could be reduced to a tolerable level. Although progress has been made in this field, as attested by the papers presented in this volume, unfortunately it appears that heretofore the knowledge we already have has not been applied in the most effective way and often not at all. Consequently, innumerable patients with cancer continue to suffer and die with their pain unrelieved.

The presentations and discussions made during the 4-day symposium make it impressively clear, even to me as a layman, that we must mount a multi-pronged program suggested by Professor Bonica and emphasized by many others. We must disseminate the information already available and encourage all physicians and health professionals who assume the serious responsibility of caring for patients with cancer pain to apply it promptly and correctly. It is also clear that there must be a marked increase in research on all aspects of cancer pain in order to eliminate the voids of knowledge that currently exist. Only with new knowledge can we develop new drugs and modalities that will relieve pain more effectively without side effects and complications so that *all* patients with recurrent or inoperable cancer will enjoy a quality of life until their death.

To achieve the "total" answer to the problem of pain, to the doubts and apprehensions and suffering that it provokes, and to the fear of knowing that death is rapidly approaching requires many, many changes. For one thing, persons from many different disciplines must participate in this total effort of patient-care, research, and teaching. In addition to basic scientists, physicians, and other health professionals, there must be involvement of philosophers, theologians, and other men of culture. From this type of team effort will come the knowledge, the expertise, the hope, and the faith which will help patients with cancer, not only by relieving their pain, but also by giving them faith and hope that they will live the rest of their life in comfort and in the company of their family and friends.

Finally, and most importantly, the scientists, physicians, and other health professionals must have the moral and financial support from society, and the national, provincial, and municipal governments, as well as from the private sector. One of the most important reasons for organizing and supporting this symposium by the FLORIANI FOUNDATION has been to make the people more aware and appreciative of the serious nature of cancer pain as a major national and world health problem and to generate greater interest and support by various governmental and private agencies within and without Italy. The Board of Directors of the FLORIANI FOUNDATION hopes that this objective has been achieved. We will await with great anticipation for greater and more active involvement by all concerned in this noble cause.

Editor's Note

Almost exactly 3 months after Albino Cardinal Luciani, then Patriarch of Venice, made the following remarks as the first speaker at the official opening ceremony of the International Symposium on Pain of Advanced Cancer, he was elected Pope John Paul I. The feeling of extreme pride and pleasure by all those concerned with the symposium to have had such a great personality participate in the meeting was abruptly replaced 33 days later by immense grief and a sense of great loss. Mr. and Mrs. Floriani and other members of the Board of the Floriani Foundation, and members of the Scientific Program Committee, and the editors of this monograph take this opportunity to express great grief and distress at this tragically premature death of a man who in 34 days captured the imagination of the world and won the affection of millions—Catholic and non-Catholic alike—with his unprecedented humility, great humor, and winning smile.

On the basis of the remarks summarized here and his performance throughout his priestly life, it is apparent that he was intensely interested in the welfare and the rights of the individual, particularly those who were poor or ill—characteristics that caused him to be called "the Pastoral Pope." Moreover, in private conversation with the senior author at the time of the symposium, Cardinal Luciani expressed intense interest in patients with cancer pain and other chronic pain syndromes and his willingness to vigorously support future efforts by all those individuals involved in pain research and therapy and all those agencies interested in this field. We are confident that, had he lived, he would have lent his inestimably valued support and influence as Pope to "the cause of pain"—the current worldwide movement to markedly increase pain research and teaching and thus improve the lot of those who suffer cancer pain and other painful syndromes. In view of this and his many other attributes, the death of Pope John Paul I must be viewed as an immeasurable loss, not only to Catholics but all of the people of the world.

Remarks by Cardinal Albino Luciani

We are on the island of St. Giorgio, but thanks to its owner, the late, great philanthropist Count Cini, its name has been changed to "the Island of Hope." I sincerely wish that the results of this symposium will give great hope to patients affected with pain of advanced cancer.

I have been asked to say a few words on human suffering and its relief. In this world people ask you professors of medical research: "Please ease my pain, heal me with your expert knowledge and skill, help medicine take further steps forward toward the cure of cancer." In this same world people ask me other kinds of questions: "Why these pains that destroy the best part of the human being? Why must children and innocents suffer? If it is true that God exists, God our Father, how can we reconcile his Divine Providence with so many things that seem so out of place?" These questions hurt the heart of those who ask them and mine also because I have no clear, definite, and convincing answer to give, but only elements, bits and pieces of answers. I usually say: "I understand you, it is only human to have such problems." Christ on the cross cried: "God, why have you abandoned me?" And Christ said "no" to those who wanted to solve the problem of pain with "religious mathematics." He encountered the blind man and immediately His disciples asked him: "Master, who has sinned? He or his parents, that he was born blind?" And Jesus answered: "He has not sinned, nor have his parents."

Pilatus had ordered some Galileans killed; a tower fell in the same day killing 18 people. The disciples were tempted to apply "religious mathematics," but Jesus said: "Do you think that those Galileans were more sinners to have suffered such a fate? No, I tell you. Or do you think that the 18 killed were more guilty than all the inhabitants of Jerusalem? No, I tell you." The Bible thus shows us that the good are not always rewarded in this world, nor the bad punished. So? So we must remember that human life, to quote Cronin, is an adventure in two worlds. We begin here, but the conclusions are in the other world.

The Bible says: "The souls of the just are in God's hands. The foolish thought them dead, their end was considered a disaster, their departure from us a downfall; but they are in peace, their hope is full of immortality." Hope and faith in a future life are the first element for my answer.

When we think of Paradise we can understand a little about suffering that is not directly wanted but only permitted by the Lord, who wishes only well for His children. This even if He does not want to interfere with miracles, to modify the course of nature that He himself has created with its own laws.

Even Christ in the Gethsemane Garden at the beginning prayed the Father to remove the "chalice of pain," and only after having prayed and received courage was He able to add: "Thy will, not mine, be done." And it is not Christ's pain, as such, that saved us, but the patience, the love, the obedience with which He accepted pain. And here we have another element to answer our question on human suffering. If pain is accepted and mastered, it can help to teach us the way to become better persons.

I repeat these are only "bits and pieces" of answers, and I want to underline the fact that Christ has taught us more about how to endure our pain and other people's pain than why we must suffer, and He has shown us that he loves those who suffer.

When Jesus tells the story of the Good Samaritan who helped the man who had been robbed and beaten by the thieves, He ended saying: "Go and do the same." He even made Himself and the sick man one, saying: "I was sick and you visited me, you have done it to me." Many have taken these words seriously.

But Christ's pains give us precious indications toward understanding the behavior of sick people during their illness. In the Gethsemane Garden He wanted to try to undergo the horrors of suffering as if to tell us: "I shall open the way; I will not be so surprised if also you will be afraid of pain; only try to imitate me."

"The Lord our Father," Jesus once said, "knows what you need even before you ask Him." And when Jesus is afraid He calls to his Father, asks, and obtains the necessary force and faith.

Many sick Christians, taking example from Christ, pray to have the strength to accept and bear pain with courage and resignation. Sometimes passive resignation of pain becomes an active offering of sufferings to God.

But Christ did not overlook even the smallest remedies. In the Gethsemane

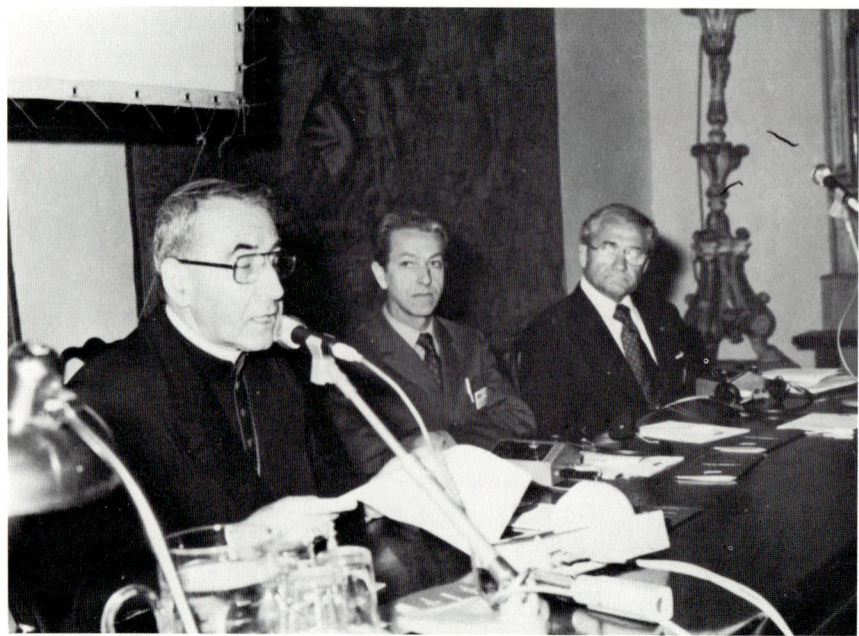

FIG. 1. *Left to right:* Albino Cardinal Luciani, Prof. Carlo Morpurgo, Prof. John Bonica.

Garden He looked for comfort from His disciples, and He was very sad when He found them sleeping because they were tired. This goes to prove that when people suffer they need their dear ones near; they don't want to be left alone, but they need understanding and love; they must be able to talk to people who can encourage them and comfort them.

Patients must be allowed to have visitors and to keep each other company. Hospitals must be technically and clinically well equipped, but they must also favor visits to patients and train their personnel to be kind and helpful with the ailing. Charles Fleury wrote that the way men are treated when sick and dying is a clear indication of the degree of civilization of an age and government.

The few things I have said are only "crumbs" of a Christian philosophy that can be found in the works of Seneca, St. Augustine, Boezio, Pascal, and Peguy and others. Our great writer Alessandro Manzoni exemplified very well this philosophy when he wrote: "Sufferings do often come because of our mistakes, but even the most innocent conduct cannot keep them away and when they do come, with or without our fault, faith in God makes them less unbearable or makes them useful for a better life."

Finally, as emphasized 21 years ago by His Holiness Pope Pius XII, the patient is not required by Christian or moral law "to will suffering for its own sake."[1] Physicians should use all their knowledge, skills, and energies to apply the best means at their disposal to relieve the pain of advanced cancer.

---

[1] *Editor's Note:* The following are excerpts of the address His Holiness Pope Pius XII made on February 24, 1957 (and alluded to by Cardinal Luciani and Professor Bucalossi (p. 670)) in reply to three questions concerning the religious and moral aspects of pain therapy which were submitted by the President of the Italian Society of Anesthesiologists at the time of the IX National Congress held in Rome, Italy, October 15–17, 1956. In response to the first question, "Is there a universal moral obligation to refuse analgesia and to accept physical pain in a spirit of faith?" Pope Pius stated, ". . . there is no obligation of this kind. Man, even after the Fall, retains the right of control over the forces of Nature, of employing them for his own use, and consequently of deriving benefit from all the resources which it offers him either to suppress or avoid physical pain." Although Pope Pius acknowledged the value of physical pain and suffering to help persons grow to maturity and rise "to the highest point of Christian heroism" and that under certain circumstances it must be accepted, he also stated that "the Christian, then, is never obliged to will suffering for its own sake." Indeed, he emphasized that pain is one of the forces that produces "harmful effects and prevents a greater good." In discussing the use of pain-relieving therapy for those who are dying from incurable cancer, he stated, "To declare that the dying have a greater moral obligation than others—whether from Natural Law or from Christian teaching—to accept suffering or to refuse its alleviation, is in keeping neither with the nature of things nor with the source of Revelation. . . . The growth in the love of God—does not come from the sufferings themselves which are accepted, but from the intention in the will supported by grace. This intention, in many of the dying, can be strengthened and become more active if their sufferings are eased, for these sufferings increase the state of weakness, physical exhaustion, check the ardour of the soul and sap the moral powers instead of sustaining them. On the other hand, the suppression of pain removes any tension in the body and mind, renders prayers easy and makes possible a more generous gift of self." He emphasized the responsibility of the doctor to provide pain-relief by stating, "The doctor who accepts (the responsibility of providing analgesia) . . . is seeking in accordance with the Creator to bring suffering under man's control and to do so makes use of the conquest of science and of technical skills."

Introduction

Emilio Ambrogio

Direttore Generale dei Servizi di Medicina Sociale (General Director of Social Medicine Services) of the Republic of Italy

Hon. Tina Anselmi, Minister of Health, was supposed to be present. Unfortunately, she was unable to come and I am here to represent her. The Minister sends her regards and wishes to thank the Floriani Foundation for sponsoring this symposium. The presence of the Italian Health Department witnesses the interest that this initiative has for the Health Ministry.

Assistance toward those who suffer from advanced cancer pain is not only a problem that regards treatment to reduce pain but it involves the deepest aspects of the human soul. It is necessary to create for the dying patient an atmosphere not of pitiful solitude but of full life and of dignified acceptance till the end. In this sense, the most recent studies give great importance to the quality of terminal assistance. And, according to the World Health Organization, this assistance should become part of the tasks of the health services of each nation.

Currently, an increasing number of patients prefer to return home to die in their own bed. This is a natural request and it should not be considered as a way to get rid of the patient and to free a bed, but as a solution that permits the patient to enjoy the comfort and companionship of his family and friends. Therefore, it is necessary to give to the medical and paramedical staff an adequate preparation to provide terminal care at the home of the patient. Although this request involves contact with specialized cancer centers and general hospitals, it is essential that in complying with the patient's wishes we must ensure adequate relief of pain.

The Ministry of Health of the Republic of Italy recognizes its moral, social, professional, and economic obligations to patients with cancer pain and will use whatever resources it is able to muster to fulfill these obligations. With the help of the biomedical scientific community and the health professions we can and should develop an overall national plan to support research by scientists and teaching of physicians so that patients with pain of advanced cancer will be effectively relieved of their suffering. The departments of pain therapy should be given greater national, provincial, and municipal governmental support to fulfill their important missions. These include not only the carrying out of various therapeutic modalities for the relief of pain within the hospital but also the instructing of nurses, social workers, and other paramedical personnel in providing effective psychologic support and relief from suffering to the patient and the family in the home environment.

Importance of the Problem

John J. Bonica

Department of Anesthesiology, University of Washington, Seattle, Washington 98195

The proper relief of pain of advanced cancer is one of the most pressing and most important issues of modern society. This importance stems from several facts: (a) Cancer pain afflicts hundreds of thousands and, indeed, millions of people throughout the world annually. In addition to the severe physiologic, emotional, affective, and economic impact of pain in general, cancer pain has special attributes and significance to the patient and family. (b) All too frequently cancer pain is inadequately managed and, consequently, the patient ends his or her last weeks and months or even years of life in great discomfort, suffering, and disability which precludes "a quality of life" that is vital to these patients. (c) The drugs and other therapeutic modalities available at the present time, properly administered, are effective in relieving the pain of most patients.

In this presentation I will attempt to indicate the magnitude of cancer pain, the deficiencies that currently exist which all too often preclude effective relief, and the reasons for these deficiencies. I hope this will serve as a framework or background for the discussion that follows. Following long tradition throughout the world, we will use "cancer pain" generically to include pain caused by any neoplastic disease or occurring as a consequence of therapeutic intervention for neoplastic disease or both.

MAGNITUDE OF THE PROBLEM

For reasons that will be given below, the magnitude of the problem of the pain associated with cancer throughout the world cannot be defined with any accuracy. However, one can gain some insight by citing statistics about the incidence of cancer and deaths consequent to this dreadful disease in Italy and in the United States. I have been informed that in Italy each year about 250,000 patients develop cancer and there are nearly 110,000 deaths from the disease (31). In the United States, the figures are 700,000 new cases of cancer diagnosed and nearly 400,000 deaths from cancer annually (2). This rate of one death per 645 persons makes cancer second only to heart disease as a killer of Americans. Of these deaths, over 23% are due to cancer of the lung, about 13% to lesions of the large intestines, 8.5% to carcinoma of the breast, about 5% to cancer of the prostate or uterus and ovary, 4% to stomach cancer, and 4% to cancer of the bladder and kidney. Realizing that the incidence of oncologic disease and each specific type varies in different countries, these figures suggest that, throughout the world, well over 5 million people die each year from cancer.

INCIDENCE OF CANCER PAIN

Cancer is not usually painful at its onset or during the early phases of the disease, and a significant percentage of patients are cured through surgical, radiation, or anticancer modalities. However, many of the patients with recurrent or metastatic cancer eventually develop pain which becomes progressively more severe and finally develops into a relentless suffering that greatly aggravates the physiologic and psychologic deterioration of the patient caused by the disease itself. Although there are no data from large-scale national epidemiologic studies on the incidence and severity of cancer pain, the data from several surveys of small groups of patients in specific hospitals suggest that moderate to severe pain is experienced by about a third of the patients with the intermediate stages of the disease and by 60 to 80% of the patients with advanced cancer.

Wilkes (33) reported that among nearly 300 patients admitted to a 25-bed unit in an English provincial city which is especially interested in caring for the dying patient, pain was the major symptom in 58%; it occurred in 82% of the patients with cervical cancer, 75% of patients with gastric cancer, and 45 to 60% of patients with cancer of the lungs, rectum, and breast. Twycross (30) reviewed the records of the patients admitted consecutively to St. Christopher's Hospice, the well-known facility for the care of advanced malignant disease in London. About 500 patients are admitted each year and, through an outpatient and domiciliary service, an equal number are supported at home. He reported that more than 80% of the inpatients received diamorphine for severe pain at some time of their hospital stay.

Another very important series of surveys has been carried out by Foley, Houde, and their co-workers (15) at the Memorial Sloan-Kettering Cancer Center. In one survey of 540 inpatients, pain was experienced by 85% of patients with primary bone tumors, 80% with cancer of the oral cavity, 75% of males and 70% of females with cancer of the genital urinary system, 52% of patients with breast cancer, 45% of patients with cancer of the lung, 20% of patients with lymphoma, and only 5% of patients with leukemia. In a subsequent survey of 397 patients, about 38% had pain related to cancer, but the figure rose to 60% among the terminally ill patients in the hospital.

In another survey carried out in Britain, Parkes (26) found that among patients managed in the hospital, 37% had moderate pain and 22% had severe pain, whereas of the group cared for in the home, 21% had moderate pain, and 50% had severe pain. In still another British study, Cartwright and associates (12) found that 87% of patients who died from cancer had pain prior to death.

Pannuti and associates (25) report that of 290 patients with advanced specific tumors admitted to their service, 64% had moderate to severe pain. The incidence of pain in patients with specific tumors was as follows: 68% with breast cancer, 59% with cancer of the prostate, 58% with intestinal tumors, 57% with lung tumors, 55% with kidney tumors, and 47% with head and neck tumors. Molinari (22) reports that more than 50% of patients with head and neck tumors at the National Cancer Institute in Milan have severe pain especially in the advanced stages.

PHYSIOLOGIC AND PSYCHOLOGIC EFFECTS OF CANCER PAIN

Usually the physiologic and psychologic impact of cancer pain on the patient is greater than that of nonmalignant chronic pain which is now generally considered a major health problem (9). The physical deterioration is much more severe because these patients have greater problems through lack of sleep, lack of appetite, nausea, and vomiting. Moreover, their pain threshold and pain tolerance decreases, possibly in part because of depletion of endorphins. As a result of persistent noxious stimulation, patients with persistent cancer pain develop anxiety and reactive depression, and many have hypochondriasis, somatic preoccupation with disease conviction, somatic focusing, and a tendency to deny life problems unrelated to their physical problem. This cluster of psychologic factors, which Pilowsky, Chapman, and Bonica (27) have labeled "abnormal illness behaviors" is characteristic of chronic pain regardless of etiology.

Many patients with cancer pain, knowing that the causative factors are unremovable, cannot give meaningful purpose to the pain and develop feelings of hopelessness and despair. These, like the sleeplessness, spiral to greater proportion as the patient is subjected to surgical operations, chemotherapy, or radiation therapy, and other anticancer modalities. Each time the patient may experience hopefulness but, if the therapy fails, this is followed by disappointment, gradually increased bitterness, and resentment. Many of these patients become more and more preoccupied with the pain and gradually lose interest in social activities: The pain becomes their central focus and dominates their lives.

The social effects of the uncontrolled cancer pain are equally devastating. Many patients develop interpersonal problems with members of their family, friends, and the community. The fact that most patients with advanced cancer have to stop working poses not only an economic but also an emotional stress and a feeling of dependency and uselessness. The physical appearance and behavior produced by the patient's pain and suffering stress the family emotionally; this, in turn, is perceived by the patient and consequently aggravates the pain and suffering. Some patients with severe intractable pain become so discouraged and desperate as to contemplate suicide. (7) The psychologic and psychosocial aspects of cancer pain are discussed in more detail in later chapters.

CURRENT STATUS OF CANCER PAIN CONTROL

Various sources of information suggest that, like chronic pain in general, cancer pain is improperly managed. A study carried out by Marks and Sachar (20) of Montefiore Hospital in New York revealed that many physicians prescribed inadequate amounts of analgesics for patients with cancer pain (and other medical disorders) and that of the amount prescribed, most patients actually received only about 20 to 25% of the (inadequate) amount prescribed. Consequently, in most patients, moderate to severe pain persisted after narcotic therapy. The reason for the inadequate therapy will be discussed in a later section.

Parkes (26) surveyed 276 patients with cancer pain and found among the hospital patients who had severe to very severe pain during the pre-terminal stage it remained unrelieved during the terminal stage of the disease. Moreover, in 65 cancer patients managed in their homes, 30% had severe to very severe pain which was unrelieved during the terminal phase of the disease.

Additional evidence that many patients with cancer pain are improperly managed is provided by the hundreds of letters received by the National Committee on the Treatment of Intractable Pain, a non-profit organization in the United States with the primary goal of effecting better pain control in patients with advanced cancer (28). Virtually every letter describes one or more relatives who spent the last few months with severe, excruciating cancer pain which remained unrelieved until their death. Although admittedly these are anecdotal reports, the fact that the committee has hundreds of such letters on file suggests that a not-insignificant number of patients who die from cancer spend the terminal part of their lives with unrelieved severe pain. Finally, I have observed hundreds of cancer patients in many medical centers throughout the world who had moderate to severe pain which was unrelieved by the therapy being used.

In view of the great advances in biomedical scientific knowledge and technology, and especially the great amount of interest in cancer research and therapy, why is cancer pain so poorly managed? Serious consideration of this important question during the course of the past quarter-century suggests that it is because of neglect of the problem of pain (in contrast to the cancer) by investigators, teachers in colleges, research institutions, and national and international cancer agencies (5,6,11). Consequently, there are great voids in our knowledge, and whatever knowledge is currently available is improperly applied. Let us consider these two issues.

REASONS FOR INADEQUATE PAIN RELIEF

Lack of Knowledge

There still exist great voids in our knowledge of the basic mechanisms and physiopathology of cancer pain. It is true, of course, that in the century and a half since the reports of Majendie (19), Bell (4), and Mueller (23) stimulated the first truly scientific study of pain, a vast amount of information has become available about pain, especially during the last decade (9,32). Unfortunately, most of this information has not been so beneficial to patients with cancer pain as one might anticipate or as many people believe. This less-than-optimal payoff from the many research efforts, in turn, has been due to the fact that until recent years no attention was paid to the application of new knowledge and technology to the study of chronic pain syndromes in general and cancer pain in particular (6).

In the past, many basic scientists working in the isolation of the animal laboratory were not concerned with clinical pain. As a result of the fragmented, independent research efforts on artificially induced acute pain, hypotheses and concepts were developed which, though reasonable for the times and the scientific data available, were not relevant to chronic pain. Moreover, as pointed out by Melzack (21), pain research and theory remained conceptually stagnant for over a century. Thus, we have little or no scientific information on the exact mechanisms by which cancer and other disease states produce chronic pain. To be sure, many speculations have been proposed, but hard scientific supporting data are lacking.

The relatively small number of clinicians interested in the study of cancer pain and other pain syndromes have consistently faced the frustrating problem of the inability to quantify the pain, let alone study its mechanisms. The fact that pain is a subjective and very personal experience which cannot be seen, touched, or measured by persons other than the individual who has it, has presented almost insurmountable problems to the study of its phenomena in patients. This is especially relevant to patients with cancer where the pain and suffering have special emotional and psychologic substrates. Consequently, clinicians have borrowed the hypotheses of basic scientists developed from acute pain experiments in animals to explain cancer pain and other pain syndromes. On the basis of these hypotheses, therapeutic modalities were developed and applied, some of which are not only ineffective but, not infrequently, produce serious complications of their own.

Another reason for the voids in our knowledge of cancer pain has been the lack of sufficient scientifically trained persons working on this problem. Related to this has been the meager amount or total lack of funds for research or research training in this field. Consequently, there has existed a vicious circle of inadequate scientific manpower → inadequate number of grant applications submitted to the research agencies → inadequate amount of funds budgeted for pain research and research training → discouragement of scientists to pursue cancer pain research and causing them to investigate other areas → inadequate scientific manpower.

Again, I want to emphasize that these problems related to inadequate research on chronic pain in general and cancer pain in particular have existed not only in undeveloped and developing countries, but even in the highly developed, scientifically advanced, and affluent countries. I will mention the situation in the United States where about $1 billion will be spent this year for cancer research by the National Cancer Institute (NCI) and other federal, state, and municipal agencies and by voluntary agencies, private institutions, and the pharmaceutical industry. These funds support the research of hundreds of thousands of scientists, technicians, physicians, and other health professionals who are investigating the cause, prevention, and treatment modalities of every form of cancer. However, until recently, research on *cancer pain* per se, which from the viewpoint of the patient and his family is one of the most important aspects of this dreadful disease, was virtually nonexistent. Analysis of a computer printout for the period 1971 to 1975 revealed that NCI spent a total of nearly $2.5 billion to support its program and of these *only* $560,000 was spent for cancer pain research. This averages about $112,000 annually, which represents 0.022% of the annual budget for those years of the major federal agency which supports cancer research. Fortunately, through the interest and efforts of Dr. Diane J. Fink, Director of the Division of Cancer Control and Rehabilitation, and some of her associates, a pain-control program was mounted some three years ago. As a member of the committee that reviewed applications for cancer pain research and therapy, I have been greatly disappointed by the totally inadequate number of meritorious proposals submitted to the Institute. This reemphasizes the point made that there is an obvious lack of scientific manpower interested in carrying out pain research.

Another impressive and distressing aspect of this whole problem is the fact that there are no accurate data on the incidence and magnitude of cancer pain. Again using NCI as an example, we note that it has a biometry branch and an epidemiologic branch, which carry out very detailed epidemiologic studies on the incidence of every kind of cancer, and have the most sophisticated computer system for data which is stored and easily retrieved. The efforts of these two branches have produced accurate information on every aspect of cancer, including detailed information on the most infrequent types of cancer. However, at the time of this writing, the Institute has no data on the incidence, magnitude, and cost of the *pain* associated with malignant disease. This neglect of epidemiologic studies pervades the entire network of cancer hospitals, cancer centers, and agencies.

Fortunately, things are beginning to improve in the United States in regard to funding for cancer pain research and therapy. In 1976 the NCI spent

$330,000 (more than double the amount spent in 1975), and it spent $661,000 in 1977. In addition, the Institute supported hospice projects and rehabilitation programs which included pain therapy (14).[1] Moreover, the office of the President of the United States has manifested significant interest in cancer pain.

Inadequate Application of Current Knowledge

The second major group of reasons for deficiencies in managing patients with cancer pain has been the improper or inadequate application of knowledge currently available for the care of these patients. The reasons for this include: (a) lack of organized teaching of medical students and physicians and other health professionals in the management of cancer pain, (b) the progressive trend toward specialization, (c) the inability or unwillingness of some practitioners to devote the necessary time and effort to provide optimal pain relief, and (d) the meager amount of published information on the proper treatment of cancer pain.

Review of curricula of the medical schools in the United States reveals that few, if any, teach students the basic principles of the use of narcotics and other therapeutic modalities that effectively relieve cancer pain. Indeed, I have been impressed that many physicians in residency training for specialization in surgical, medical, and radiation oncology receive little or no teaching about the proper management of cancer pain. Usually, the senior house officer, who has vague and scanty information about cancer pain and its proper control, teaches the junior house officer how to deal with the problem in a rather empirical way and passes on some of the misconceptions that will be mentioned below.

Lack of interest in the problem of pain by oncologists is further attested by the fact that very little, if any, information about the proper management of pain is found in the oncology literature, voluminous as it is. Of the many textbooks on various aspects of cancer, only a few deal with the problem of pain-management and then do so in a totally inadequate manner. For example, review of seven of the most important textbooks and monographs on the management of cancer published in English reveals the following facts: Of the two recently published books on surgical oncology, one does not mention pain at all (24), whereas the other devotes one sentence to the problem (29). In a 408-page manual for practitioners published by one of the state chapters of the American Cancer Society (ACS), there is no mention of pain (3), and in another published by the Committee on Professional Education of the International Union Contre Le Cancer (UICC) pain-management is disposed of in 1½ pages (13). In one of the best-known and most widely read books on cancer diagnosis and treatment, pain is mentioned in

---

[1] Subsequent to, and probably partly as a result of, this Symposium, NCI has initiated major programs in the evaluation of pain management teams and epidemiology studies.

connection with each tumor, but its treatment is not considered at all (1). In another 819-page book on clinical oncology, 2½ pages are devoted to pain (18). Finally, in the most comprehensive 2,000-page volume on cancer medicine, only 13 pages are devoted to the problem of pain and its control (17). A recent survey of the same types of books published in Italy and other European countries reveals that the same problems exist in those countries.

As a result of this lack of education of students and graduate physicians and other health professionals, the pain of cancer is treated in an empirical manner. Insufficient knowledge or lack of consideration of the various mechanisms and types of cancer pain and the associated physiologic, emotional, and behavioral responses is partly responsible for mismanagement of the pain. A related reason is the lack of personnel with the interest and expertise in the proper application of these modalities. Consequently, most practitioners rely on narcotic analgesics which, while very useful and having a definite role in the control of pain in cancer, for a variety of reasons are often misused.

In a small percentage of patients, potent narcotics are used initially for mild pain which could be relieved by non-narcotic analgesics alone or combined with sedatives or psychotropic drugs. The practice of some physicians to "snow the patient under" because the patient has recurrent or metastatic cancer denotes a lack of understanding of the problem (10). Because it is difficult to estimate the length of life in individual cases, such false humanitarianism may potentiate the depressant effects of the disease, and the patient will have narcotic-induced anorexia, nausea, and vomiting, which will aggravate the physiologic effects of the cancer. Even patients with terminal cancer should *not* be subjected to excessive narcotic analgesics and the consequent respiratory depression and stupefaction which preclude the "quality of life" that these patients deserve.

At the other end of the spectrum, many, if not most, patients with moderate to severe pain of advanced cancer are given inadequate amounts of narcotics. The very high incidence of undertreatment of cancer pain is due to inadequate knowledge of the pharmacology of these drugs and, particularly, to serious misconceptions among physicians, nurses, and other health professionals about the "risk of addiction." As part of the study previously mentioned, Marks and Sachar (20) surveyed 102 physicians in training in two major hospitals and found that because of inadequate knowledge most physicians underestimated the effective dose range of narcotics, overestimated duration of their action, and had an exaggerated opinion of the dangers of addiction. Apparently, this problem of inadequate knowledge and misconception about addiction is widespread because many others have reported similar findings. The findings of Parkes (26) and Cartwright and associates (12) have been cited.

This misconception about the problem of "addiction" is further aggravated by the fact that narcotic drugs are carefully monitored by federal and state governments, and physicians in prescribing such medication and pharmacists in filling such prescriptions follow strict regulations in handling these drugs. Thus, tight government control, clinicians' lack of understanding of the pharmacology of narcotics and other drugs that may be used as adjuncts, and the physicians' and nurses' concern about addiction have provided a milieu which has prevented adequate management of pain in patients with cancer.

In some patients, systemic drugs are not sufficiently effective and other modalities need to be used alone or in combination with drugs. These include nerve blocks and neurosurgical interruption of pain pathways and some of the old and newer psychologic techniques which have been shown to be effective in helping or totally relieving cancer pain. Unfortunately, for the aforementioned reasons, the efficacy, indications, and advantages, as well as the limitations, disadvantages, and complications of these other therapeutic modalities, are not known or applied by most practitioners and even by many oncologists. Consequently, in most patients who could be more effectively relieved by one of these procedures or a combination of two or more of these, these other therapeutic modalities are not considered or, if they are considered, this is done too late. Related to this is the lack of personnel with interest and expertise in the proper application of these other therapeutic modalities.

RECOMMENDATIONS FOR IMPROVEMENT

I believe that more effective management of patients with cancer pain requires a multipronged attack consisting of:

1. *Much greater research efforts* which should include: (a) comprehensive epidemiologic studies on the incidence and magnitude of cancer pain with each type of tumor; (b) study of the neurophysiologic and biochemical and physiopathologic mechanisms of cancer pain; (c) evaluation of the efficacy of the methods currently used to relieve cancer pain; and (d) the development of new therapeutic modalities;
2. *Intensive educational programs* for medical students and other health professionals, as well as physicians in practice, including: (a) knowledge about the causes and mechanisms of pain; (b) the efficacy, indications, limitations, and complications of current methods of pain relief; and (c) specific guidelines about proper management of these patients;
3. *Intensive educational campaigns* for the public, patients, and families, as well as federal agencies;
4. *Provision of better sources of information* through the oncologic literature, books and special articles, and brochures on cancer pain.

Future research should provide much new information on the exact biochemical, neurophysiologic, and psychologic substrates of chronic pain in general and cancer pain in particular. Once such information is available, we can use the vast amount of knowledge and technology now available in chemistry, pharmacology, and biochemistry to develop agents that can act in an exquisitely specific way to prevent or promptly terminate the various biochemical and neurologic factors that act at molecular and cellular levels to produce pain. Such new agents would produce complete relief without any side effects. Moreover, future studies should permit more specific definition of the impact of various emotional, psychologic, sociologic, and environmental factors on cancer pain and how this information could be applied more effectively in its relief.

Until we acquire new information, we should be able to effectively use the knowledge currently available to do a much better job in relieving the suffering and pain of cancer. To achieve this goal, it is necessary for the health professionals responsible for the care of cancer patients to consider the neurophysiologic, biochemical, and psychologic substrates of nociception and pain in general and then consider how these are affected by various types of cancer and cancer therapy in causing pain. In other words, we need to consider the possible causes and mechanisms of cancer pain. Moreover, it is necessary to consider within the framework of current knowledge what role psychologic, emotional, environmental, and sociologic factors play in causing suffering and pain in cancer patients. All of these aspects will be considered in this volume.

Once these are defined, it is essential to evaluate the efficacy, indications, and advantages as well as the limitations, disadvantages, and complications of the various therapeutic modalities available at the present time. These considerations will be the subjects of the following chapters. In addition to considering the mechanism, we will evaluate in detail the various therapeutic modalities that are being used in the relief of certain specific cancer pain syndromes. Finally, one of the most important aspects of the problem of cancer pain is continuing and terminal care. We are fortunate in having three outstanding authorities who have pioneered or have important roles in the development of these programs in Britain.

All these discussions and considerations will make it obvious that optimal care of the patients with pain of advanced cancer requires the efforts of health professionals from various disciplines working as members of cancer-pain therapy teams (6,8). A team of this type should be part of every comprehensive cancer center. Such a team should be composed of basic scientists and clinicians with special interest and expertise in chronic pain in general and cancer pain in particular who would devote the time and effort to evaluate carefully each patient with severe cancer pain and determine what is the best method or methods of relieving the pain. I will discuss this issue in more detail later.

I close this introductory section by again expressing the hope that this volume will help to improve the care of patients with pain of advanced cancer. I exhort everyone to exert maximum effort in pursuing vigorously each of the specific objectives I mentioned earlier. Hopefully, this will help us to achieve our ultimate goal—optimal pain-relief for all patients with cancer pain.

REFERENCES

1. Ackerman, L. V., and Del Regato, J. A. W., editors (1970): *Cancer Diagnosis, Treatment and Prognosis,* 4th ed., p. 783. Mosby, St. Louis.
2. American Cancer Society (1978): *Cancer Facts and Figures.* American Cancer Society, New York.
3. American Cancer Society—Massachusetts Division (1968): *Cancer: A Manual for Practitioners,* p. 408. American Cancer Society, Boston.
4. Bell, C. (1811): *Idea of a New Anatomy of the Brain Submitted for the Observations of His Friends.* Strahan & Preston, London.
5. Bonica, J. J. (1959): Management of Cancer Pain. *GP,* 10:35–43.
6. Bonica, J. J. (1978): Cancer pain: A major national health problem. *Cancer Nurs. J.,* 4:313–316.
7. Bonica, J. J. (1976): Cancer pain: A national health problem. Presentation to C.C.G.R. Committee, National Cancer Institute, June 28, 1976.
8. Bonica, J. J. (1974): Organization and function of a pain clinic. In: *Advances in Neurology, Vol. 4,* edited by J. J. Bonica, pp. 433–443. Raven Press, New York.
9. Bonica, J. J., and Albe-Fessard, D., editors (1976): *Advances in Pain Research and Therapy, Vol. 1.* Raven Press, New York.
10. Bonica, J. J. (1953): *The Management of Pain.* Lea & Febiger, Philadelphia.
11. Bonica, J. J. (1954): The management of pain of malignant disease with nerve blocks. *Anesthesiology,* 15:134 (March) and 280–301 (May).
12. Cartwright, A., Hockey, L., and Anderson, A. B. M. (1973): *Life Before Death.* Routledge & Kegan Paul, London.
13. Committee on Professional Education of U.I.C.C. (1973): *Clinical Oncology (A Manual for Students and Doctors),* p. 322. International Union Against Cancer. Springer-Verlag, Berlin.
14. Fink, D. J. (1978): Personal communication to J. J. Bonica, August 1.
15. Foley, K. M. (1979): Pain syndromes in patients with cancer. In: *Advances in Pain Research and Therapy, Vol. 2,* edited by J. J. Bonica and V. Ventafridda. Raven Press, New York.
16. Ford, G. (1979): Terminal care from the viewpoint of the National Health Service. In: *Advances in Pain Research and Therapy, Vol. 2,* edited by J. J. Bonica and V. Ventafridda. Raven Press, New York.
17. Holland, J. F., and Frei, E., III, editors (1973): *Cancer Medicine,* p. 2018. Lea & Febiger, Philadelphia.
18. Horton, J., and Hill, G. J., II, editors (1977): *Clinical Oncology,* p. 819. W. B. Saunders, Philadelphia.
19. Majendie, F. (1822): Experiences sur les fonctions tes racines des nerfs rachidiens. *J. Physiol. Exp. Pathol.,* 2:276–279.
20. Marks, R. M., and Sachar, E. J. (1973): Undertreatment of medical inpatients with narcotic analgesics. *Ann. Intern. Med.,* 78:173–181.
21. Melzack, R. (1973): *The Puzzle of Pain.* Basic Books, New York.
22. Molinari, R. (1979): Therapy of cancer pain in the head and neck. In: *Advances in Pain Research and Therapy, Vol. 2,* edited by J. J. Bonica and V. Ventafridda. Raven Press, New York.
23. Mueller, J. (1826): *Zur Vergleichenden Physiologie des Gesichtssinnes des Menschen und der Thiere nebst einem Versuch über die Bewegungen der Augen und über den Menschlichen Blick.* Cnobloch, Leipzig 32:462.
24. Najerian, J. S., and Delaney, P., editors (1976): *Advances in Cancer Surgery,* p. 608. Stratton Intercontinental Medical Book Corp., New York.

25. Pannuti, F., Martoni, A., Rossi, A. P., and Piana, E. (1979): The role of endocrine therapy for relief of pain due to advanced cancer. In: *Advances in Pain Research and Therapy, Vol. 2*, edited by J. J. Bonica and V. Ventafridda. Raven Press, New York.
26. Parkes, C. M. (1978): Home or hospital? Terminal care as seen by surviving spouse. *J. R. Coll. Gen. Pract.*, 28:19–30.
27. Pilowsky, I., Chapman, C. R., and Bonica, J. J. (1977): Pain, depression and illness behavior in a pain clinic population. *Pain*, 4(2):183–192.
28. Quattlebaum, J. (1978): President of the National Committee for the Treatment of Intractable Pain. Personal communication.
29. Raven, R. W., editor (1977): *Principles of Surgical Oncology*, p. 510. Plenum Medical Book Co., New York.
30. Twycross, R. G. (1974): Clinical management with diamorphine in advanced malignant disease. *Int. J. Clin. Pharmacol.*, 93:184–198.
31. Ventafridda, V. (1978): Incidence of cancer in Italy. Personal comment.
32. Wall, P. D., and Gutnick, M. (1974): Ongoing activity in peripheral nerves: The physiology and pharmacology of impulses originating from a neuroma. *Exp. Neurol.*, 43:550–593.
33. Wilkes, E. (1974): Some problems in cancer management. *Proc. R. Soc. Med.*, 67:23–27.

Neurophysiology of Nociception, Pain, and Pain Therapy

Manfred Zimmermann

II. Physiologisches Institut, Abteilung Zentralnervensystem der Universität, Im Neuenheimer Feld 326, 6900 Heidelberg, GFR

What is commonly labeled by the word *pain* covers a wide range of subjective phenomena from the perception of an experimental noxious stimulus (e.g., heating the skin), to the most severe and excruciating chronic or recurrent pain in patients with, e.g., terminal cancer, thalamic syndrome, or trigeminal neuralgia, all of which may profoundly alter the personality traits of the patient. Most of what we know on nervous mechanisms refers to experimentally induced pain, whereas knowledge of the physiologic basis of chronic pain remains to be elucidated.

Many new results have come from animal experiments. We conclude from the observation of motor, vegetative, and behavioral expressions (such as flexor-reflexes, blood pressure increases, tachypnea, vocalization) that some sort of behavioral state occurs in higher mammals which corresponds to pain in man, since all these nocifensive reactions of animals also are concomitants of human pain-perception and behavior. This suggests that the basic nervous system mechanisms involved are similar in all higher mammals, including man.

This chapter is aimed at giving a short outline only of the neurophysiologic basis for pain. A number of recently published comprehensive review articles and monographs are available (4,5,6,12,16,20,21,25,27,31,33,42,44,47).

PERIPHERAL ENCODING AND CONDUCTION OF PAIN INFORMATION: NOCICEPTORS AND NOCICEPTIVE AFFERENTS

Afferent Fibers

In most cases pain is produced by the excitation of specialized receptors, the nociceptors, or of their afferent fibers. The existence of such nervous elements was deduced, about 50 years ago, from experiments using electrical stimulation of skin nerves (Fig. 1): nocifensive reactions (in animals) and pain sensations (in man) occurred when the stimulus strength was above

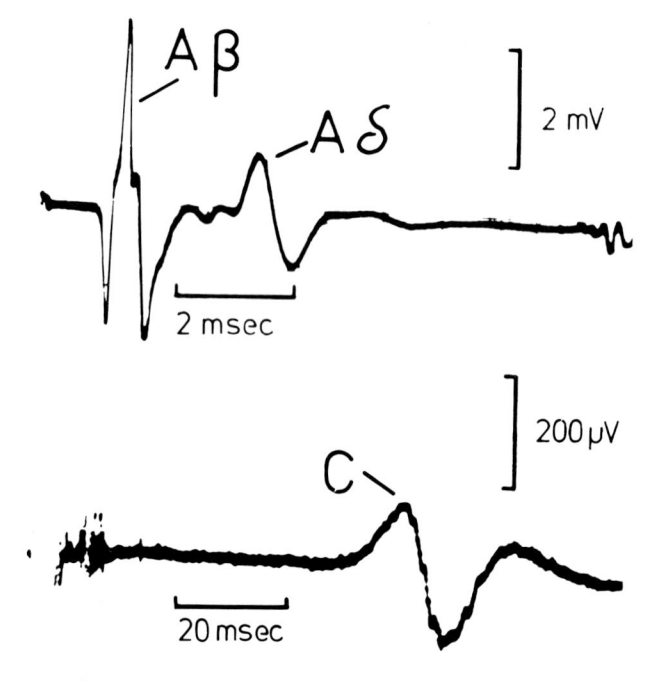

FIG. 1. Compound action potential after electrical stimulation of a cutaneous nerve (sural of the cat) displayed at two vertical gains and sweep speeds to show the three main fiber components. Conduction distance was 70 mm. The table indicates the functional types of afferents in each fiber class. Aβ. sensitive mechanoreceptors; Aδ. sensitive mechanoreceptors (hairs), cold receptors, mechanosensitive nociceptors; C. sensitive mechanoreceptors (hairs), warm receptors, mechanosensitive nociceptors, heat nociceptors, polymodal nociceptors.

threshold for the thin myelinated (Aδ, or Group III) fibers; when stimulus strength was sufficient to recruit nonmyelinated C-fibers (or Group IV afferents) the pain was increased and was of a burning quality.

Through research initiated by the pioneer work of Zotterman in 1939 (46), the existence of specialized nociceptors has been well established, especially during the last decade. However, not all of the Aδ- and C-afferents have nociceptive functions; there are also low-threshold mechanoreceptors and thermoreceptors in these fiber classes (see table in Fig. 1); in addition a large proportion of C-fibers in all nerves are sympathetic efferent fibers. Nociceptors are ubiquitous in practically all organs. I have estimated that about half of the afferent fibers entering the spinal cord via the dorsal roots are nociceptive.

Nociceptors

Best known are the nociceptors of the skin, based on single-fiber studies in animals. Recently nociceptors have been investigated in man by recording

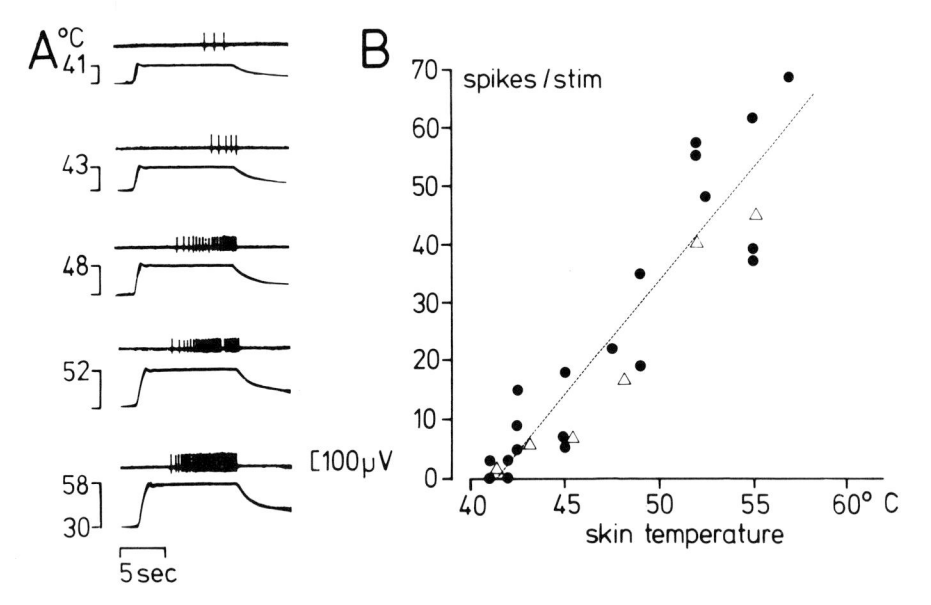

FIG. 2. Discharges of a single cutaneous C-fiber to noxious heating of the skin. **A:** Oscilloscope displays of nerve impulses (*upper trace*), recorded synchronously with skin temperature (*lower trace*); a controlled radiant-heat source was directed to the receptive field of the fiber on the hind foot of the cat. **B:** Relationship between skin temperature and no. of impulses per 10 sec of heat stimulation (●) or during the last 4 sec of heat (△). Conduction velocity of fiber was 0.6 m/sec. (From Beck et al., ref. 3, with permission.)

from single C-fibers with percutaneous microelectrodes (47). Fig. 2 shows an example of, a nociceptor of the cat's foot responding to noxious heat, i.e., when the skin temperature reached a level near 45°C. The response, i.e., the number of impulses per 10-sec heating, was linearly related to the temperature beyond threshold. This suggests that the nociceptor not only signals the mere presence of a noxious stimulus, but that it transmits information on stimulus intensity which is encoded in the impulse frequency.

These electrophysiologic findings on single nociceptors are in accordance with psychophysical measurements in human subjects: the threshold for heat pain is around 45°C skin temperature; various levels of skin temperature above this threshold can be well discriminated by the subject [cf. the psychometric Dol-scale according to Hardy et al. (15)].

The most common excitants of nociceptors in skin, muscles, tendons, ligaments, and visceral organs are strong mechanical deformation, chemical substances released by pathological processes (see below), and ischemia. The majority of nociceptors respond to various excitants, e.g., mechanical, thermal, chemical; these are called polymodal nociceptors.

Knowledge of visceral and muscle nociceptors is less advanced than that of cutaneous nociceptors. Some visceral mechanoreceptors respond to distention combined with contractions of the smooth-muscle wall of hollow organs (32); this mechanism most probably is involved in spasmodic colic pain. Since muscle nociceptors, including cardiac nociceptors, can be excited by chemical substances, it is thought that muscle and cardiac pain are mediated by chemical mediators such as bradykinin (see below).

MECHANISMS FOR CHRONIC PAIN

Noxious stimuli impinging on the skin, such as those used in the laboratory for the investigation of pain (Fig. 2), can be terminated quickly in daily life by an appropriate behavioral response (escape, avoidance). Therefore they usually do not result in a chronic pain state. However it is the persistence which makes pain a most urgent problem in medicine. Some basic physiologic mechanisms of chronic pain will be considered here.

Compression of Nerves

Excitation of nerves takes place not only at the sensory end-organ; nerve impulses can also be elicited anywhere along the sensory fiber in the nerve trunk by electrical stimulation or by local mechanical distortion. Persistent compression (e.g., by dislocation of vertebral discs, by the carpal ligaments) often produces ongoing discharges in afferent fibers which are perceived as paresthesias or pain and are localized by the patient in the innervation territory of that nerve. Some neuralgias which are characterized by irradiation of pain to the territory of a peripheral nerve or dorsal root may have such an origin.

A long-lasting compression, which also might produce some local ischemia of the nerve, eventually can result in a conduction block, which is preferential for $A\beta$-fibers (i.e., tactile afferents). This has been shown in experiments on man and animals. The persistence in these cases of ongoing activity in nociceptive afferents, and the absence of concomitant discharges in tactile afferents, might be the reason why the resulting pain is particularly disagreeable.

Chemical Excitation and Sensitization of Nociceptors

Pathologic alterations of the skin and viscera, e.g., trauma or inflammations, are accompanied by release or enhanced production of chemical substances such as KCl, serotonin, bradykinin, prostaglandin E. Each of these endogenous chemicals can either excite or sensitize nociceptors depending on their local concentrations. They are called algogenic substances (22). Such chemical influences on nociceptors have been reported to occur in the skin (2), in muscle (24,29,30), and in the viscera (18,26). Their increased production during muscle ischemia, particularly in cardiac ischemia (38), has been suggested to be a causal link in ischemic pain, e.g., angina pectoris.

Most probably several of the algogenic substances liberated upon tissue injury combine to excite nociceptors. The time-course of endogenous production and decomposition of the algogenic substances usually is slow, resulting in a long-term excitation of nociceptors.

In moderate tissue injury the concentrations of algogenic chemicals often are not sufficient to excite the nociceptors. However, they can produce sensitization in these cases, i.e., enhancement of responses and/or decrease of threshold of a nociceptor to another adequate stimulus. It is tempting to assume that sensitization of nociceptors by various endogenous chemicals is the physiologic basis for states of increased pain sensitivity which accompany pathologic conditions such as inflammation or sunburn: hyperalgesia and hyperpathia.

The involvement of prostaglandin E in sensitization and excitation of nociceptors during inflammation provides a plausible explanation for the peripheral analgesic effect of acetylsalicylic acid (aspirin): this drug is an inhibitor of prostaglandin synthesis (8). In the presence of acetylsalicylic acid the concentration of this local hormone is greatly reduced and likewise its facilitatory effect upon nociceptors. Thus, in pain involving prostaglandin E, acetylsalicylic acid and similarly acting drugs (e.g., indomethacin) can produce analgesia.

Regenerating Nerves

Nerve transections (e.g., by traumatic lesions, amputations, or neurosurgical transections) induce a powerful stimulus for the fibers of the proximal stump to regenerate. Such sites often are sources of severe pain, particularly when a neuroma has developed. Can this pain arise at the sprouts of the regenerating fibers? Experiments have been conducted recently in rats in which a neuroma was induced by placing the proximal stump of the cut sciatic nerve into a plastic cap (9,40). In such preparations ongoing impulse activity was found in $A\delta$- and C-fibers (Fig. 3); this was initiated at the fiber sprouts in the neuroma. No such ongoing activity occurred in $A\beta$-fibers. It is tempting to assume that many of the spontaneously active $A\delta$- and C-fibers previously had nociceptive endings, so that the impulse flow in these fibers would be interpreted by the central nervous system (CNS) as coming from a noxious stimulus.

Two additional results emerged from these investigations on experimental neuroma (Fig. 3): the ongoing impulse discharge was enhanced by perfusion of the neuroma with noradrenaline (norepinephrine), and suppressed by electrical stimulation of the nerve fibers. The effect of norepinephrine is circumstantial evidence that sympathetic efferents might exert some stimulatory action on nociceptive fibers in the neuroma, a mechanism which had been claimed to operate in causalgia, a pain syndrome that often occurs in patients with a neuroma (see also p. 19).

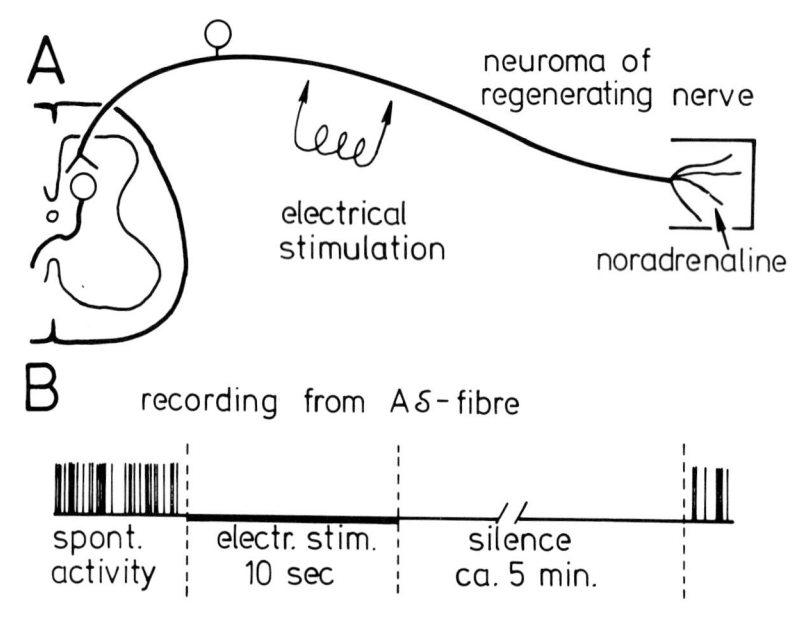

FIG. 3. Properties of nerve sprouts in a neuroma (schematic). **A:** A neuroma had been induced in transected rat nerves by putting a plastic cap over the proximal stump. Afterwards the nerve was prepared for stimulation, recording, and perfusion of the neuroma. **B:** Spontaneous activity in Aδ-fibers arising in the neuroma could be silenced for a long time by a short period of repetitive electrical nerve stimulation. Schematic drawings according to results by Wall and Gutnick (40).

A short period (e.g., 10 sec) of repetitive electrical stimulation of the nerve at a strength above threshold for the single fiber under study completely stopped the ongoing discharge for several min (Fig. 3B). This is a possible foundation for analgesia produced by transcutaneous nerve stimulation in amputees. Apart from this peripheral analgesic action the stimulation will elicit inhibitory processes in the CNS (see below, Inhibition of Spinal Neurons by Afferent Nerve Stimulation).

When a regenerating nerve reaches its peripheral innervation territory (e.g., in the skin), hyperpathia can be observed in patients (37). This situation has been simulated in animal experiments (11). When the sprouting fibers had reached the skin, nociceptors having similar functional characteristics to those in normal skin immediately developed. However, the threshold to noxious heating was significantly reduced by 4°C in the regenerated C-nociceptors, which might account for hyperpathia to thermal stimuli in patients with regenerated nerves.

Implications of Motor and Sympathetic Reflexes in Chronic Pain

Usually motor and sympathetic reflexes to noxious stimuli are aimed to counteract the noxious effect; they can be considered as negative feedback mechanisms to protect the organism from injury (e.g., flexor reflex, hyperemia of an injured organ). However, such reflexes might sometimes function as a positive feedback; i.e., they increase rather than decrease the effect of a noxious stimulus (Fig. 4).

A motor reflex, for example, initiated by a cutaneous or visceral pain stimulus might set up activity in muscle or tendon nociceptors by the muscle contraction (Fig. 4A). This in turn can increase the motor reflex, which eventually will lead to a self-sustained reflex muscle spasm and, concomitantly, to ongoing pain.

Such a vicious circle is also possible in the case of sympathetic reflexes (Fig. 4B). Positive feedback might be considered as causative in the clinically well-known syndrome of sympathetic reflex dystrophy. The sympathetic effector then enhances rather than decreases the excitation of the nociceptors. Several mechanisms can account for such a deleterious effect: vasoconstriction and ischemia; vasodilatation and increase in vascular permeability, thus changing the extracellular fluid environment; contracture of smooth muscle surrounding the nociceptor; direct action of locally released neurotransmitters, neuromodulators; and algogenic chemicals (e.g., norepinephrine, substance P, serotonin, bradykinin, prostaglandin). These adverse effects of sympathetic efferent influences, although apparent from many clinical observations, still lack a physiologic foundation. A systematic investigation of these problems is highly desirable.

Therapeutic actions should be aimed to interrupt the positive feedback or self-excitation loop, either by a regional analgesic block in the afferent or efferent branch of the reflex, or by activating inhibitory systems in the CNS. Local anesthesia of the afferent nerve yields pain-relief which often outlasts, by days or even weeks, the duration of pharmacologic action of the anes-

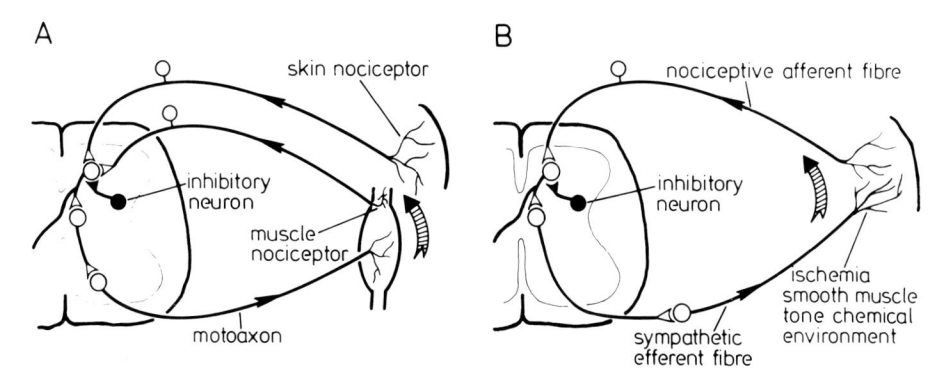

FIG. 4. Hypothetical mechanisms of self-excitation of nociceptors by spinal reflexes (schematic). **A:** Motor reflex induced by skin or/and muscle nociceptors, the contraction acting as a stimulus on muscle nociceptors. **B:** Sympathetic reflex evoked by nociceptors; various sympathetic effector mechanisms are indicated, which can enhance the excitability of the nociceptors.

thetic. This enduring pain-relief lends support to the assumption that the pain really was of the self-sustaining type. Another method of interrupting the positive feedback loop is to activate neuronal inhibition in the spinal cord, as indicated in Fig. 4 (see below).

CENTRAL NERVOUS SYSTEM MECHANISMS OF PAIN AND ANALGESIA

The physiology of nociception and pain is much more complex in the CNS than it is in the peripheral nervous system. A center for pain, comparable to the mapped projections of tactile, visual, and auditory senses onto the cortex, does not exist. Afferent input from nociceptors sets up activity in many subsystems of the CNS. Some of the subsystems and a typical example of related functions are listed below.

Spinal cord:	Motor and sympathetic reflexes
Brain stem:	Control of circulation and respiration, reticular activating system
Hypothalamus:	Homeostasis; release of hormones from the pituitary
Limbic system:	Affective-motivational components of behavior
Neocortex:	Cognitive components of behavior

These CNS subsystems are involved in all of the various behavioral states of a subject; therefore, we argue that pain behavior may be based upon a characteristic pattern of activity in, and interaction among, these brain parts.

This general concept implies that it might be inappropriate to search for central neurons which are specifically related to nociceptive afferents, but not to others. Presumably any central neuron will share in many different functions. In principle, information about noxious stimuli can be extracted from a population of neurons, none of which is specifically excited by such stimuli (45). So, the investigation of the physiology of pain should emphasize these questions: (a) In which neurons can information be found on noxious peripheral events, irrespective of whether or not a particular neuron has additional non-noxious inputs; and (b) are there neuronal mechanisms by which this pain-related information in the central neurons can be modified?

The best-studied examples of neurons yielding answers to these questions are the dorsal horn neurons in the spinal cord (Fig. 5). Here are the central terminals of the $A\delta$- and C-fibers from nociceptors in the skin, viscera, and muscles. Noxious information received by the dorsal horn neurons is dispensed to contribute to spinal motor and sympathetic outflow, some pathophysiologic implications of which have been emphasized above (Fig. 4). Long axons of some dorsal horn neurons ascend to the brain, e.g., in the anterolateral tract (41), transection of which (cordotomy) may give pain-relief. However, there are additional spinal ascending pathways to

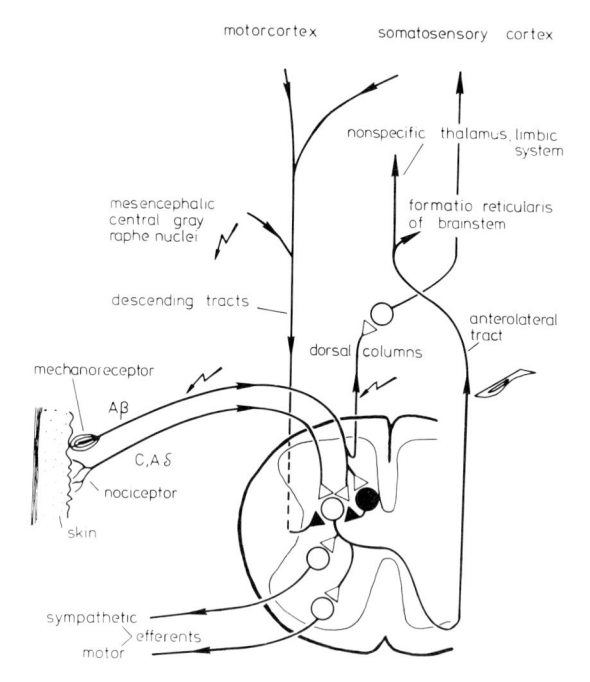

FIG. 5. Functional diagram of the dorsal horn neuron (highly schematic). Afferent fibers synapse onto dorsal horn neurons, which in turn conduct their impulses to segmental motor and sympathetic efferents and to ascending tracts. The dorsal horn neuron can be inhibited; inhibitory synapses and neuron drawn in black. Voltage arrows indicate sites where stimulation can produce inhibition of the dorsal horn neuron; the scalpel indicates cordotomy for pain-relief.

carry pain information, which explains why pain can persist or recur after a cordotomy. Many brain areas, e.g., those mentioned above, may be reached by the pain information transmitted through the ascending pathways, mainly via the brainstem reticular formation and the nonspecific thalamic nuclei (Fig. 5). Tactile skin stimuli, on the other hand, activate mechanoreceptors which project, via the dorsal columns, to the specific somatosensory system in the thalamus and cortex.

However, sensory systems generally are not organized as one-way streets for excitatory impulse traffic. As is indicated in Fig. 5, some segmental and suprasegmental descending inhibitory influences can affect information flow through the dorsal horn neuronal system. Some details of these modulatory mechanisms, which might be regarded as representative for neuronal interactions in pain neurophysiology, will be considered below.

Dorsal Horn Neuronal Responses to Noxious Skin Stimuli

Radiant heat applied to our skin is very painful when the skin temperature is above 45°C. We know that such controlled heating is a practically selective stimulus for nociceptive Aδ- and C-afferents in the cat's hind foot (3). We used radiant heat as a purely noxious stimulus to study the functional characteristics of the neuronal circuitry in the dorsal horn.

About 50% of lumbar dorsal horn neurons respond vigorously to skin-heating (Fig. 6). Varying the intensity of the heat stimulus resulted in a linear relationship between skin temperature and mean discharge frequency, which is quite similar to that found in the C-nociceptors (Fig. 2B). However, there were differences between the discharges of C-nociceptors and spinal neurons: (a) The discharge frequencies were higher by a factor of 10, indicating considerable convergence of many C-fibers to each neuron. (b) The dorsal horn neuronal discharges displayed a build up of responsiveness during repetitive electrical C-fiber stimulation, which indicates temporal facilitation to occur in the synaptic transmission. (c) The discharge frequency slowly decayed within 10 to 100 sec after cessation of the heat stimulus (Fig. 6). These temporal features can be explained by assuming that a synaptic transmitter is involved which has slow kinetics of release, post-

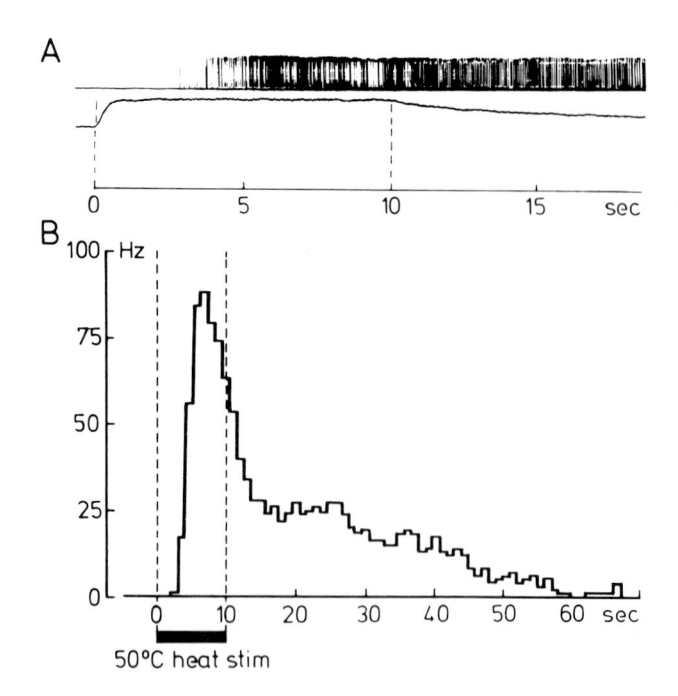

FIG. 6. Impulse discharge of a single dorsal horn neuron in the cat's spinal cord to noxious heat stimulation of the skin. **A:** Oscillographic record of nerve impulses (*upper trace*) and of the skin temperature (*lower trace*), when heating to 50°C, 10 sec in duration, was performed on a 1-cm^2 skin area of the footpad. **B:** Same discharge plotted as histogram, i.e., impulse frequency vs. time, during and after heat stimulation. The period of heating is indicated by the vertical broken lines. (From Dickhaus et al., ref. 10, with permission.)

synaptic action, and inactivation. These and other results hint at substance P, a polypeptide contained in small-diameter primary afferents, to be the synaptic transmitter (17).

These neuronal characteristics correlate with psychophysiologic phenomena of pain sensation. First, the intensity of a painful stimulus can be judged by the subject, based on the frequency modulation in nociceptors (Fig. 2B), whose coding principle obviously is preserved at the synaptic relay to the dorsal horn neurons. The temporal facilitation of neuronal responsiveness corresponds to enhancement of pain when stimulation is repeated at certain rates. The long afterdischarge of the neurons to noxious heat is reminiscent of aftersensations that often are felt subsequent to a painful stimulus.

Descending Control of Spinal Pain Transmission

It is well established now that in all sensory systems the ascending information is modulated by centrifugal influences from the brain. In the somatosensory system such backward modification is exerted via pathways descending in the white matter of the spinal cord. Such descending controls originate in the cortex, the diencephalon, and the brainstem (Fig. 5). In the context of pain, brainstem systems are of great importance. Inhibition of nociceptive messages in dorsal horn neurons has been reported to originate in the mesencephalic periaqueductal gray (PAG), in some of the raphe nuclei which contain serotonergic descending neurons, in the locus coeruleus (noradrenergic neurons), and in parts of the reticular formation.

An example is given in Fig. 7. Spinal neuronal responses to standardized noxious stimulation are shown as histograms in B and C. Repetitive electrical stimulation of the PAG was performed before and during the heat-response in C: This discharge clearly was inhibited to less than ⅓ of the control (B). The particular site of stimulation in the PAG is shown in Fig. 7A, along with effective electrode placements from other experiments.

When this procedure was repeated to a series of heat stimuli at varying heat intensities, the relationship between discharge frequency and skin temperature, i.e., the characteristic line of intensity coding, was affected as shown in Fig. 7D: A decrease in slope to typically less than 50% of control occurred, whereas the threshold remained the same. The inhibitory system arising in the PAG thus may be interpreted as controlling the gain of pain transmission in the spinal dorsal horn (7). There are other descending inhibitory systems which do not change the slope, but produce a shift, of the intensity-coding line to higher thresholds and lower discharge frequencies. Thus, the interactive network of spinal and brainstem neurons might provide a functional system of great dynamic capabilities.

The descending brainstem systems have been characterized also in terms of

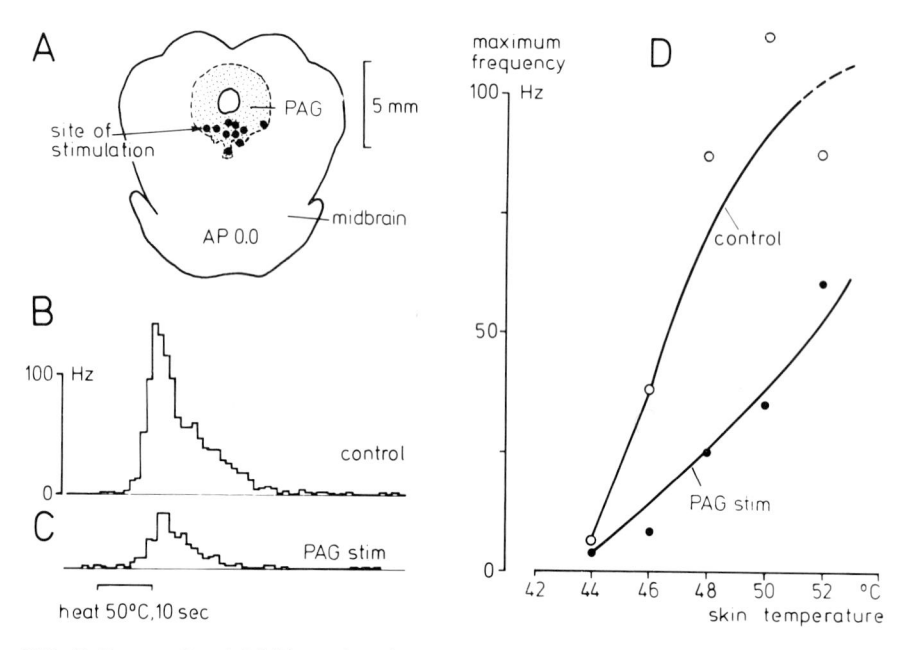

FIG. 7. Descending inhibition of cat's spinal neuron by stimulation in the midbrain. **A:** Histological confirmation of sites in the periaqueductal gray (PAG) of the midbrain (at stereotaxic coordinates AP 0) where stimulation produced inhibition in the spinal cord. **B:** Discharge of a dorsal horn neuron in the lumbar spinal cord to noxious heat (50°C, 10 sec) applied to the receptive field on the pad. **C:** Same heat stimulus; however, repetitive electrical stimulation was given before and during recording of the heat-evoked discharge to the site labeled by arrow in A. Parameters of PAG stimulation were: square impulses 300 μA, 0.1 msec in duration, 100-Hz trains during 0.1 sec, trains repeated at 3 Hz. **D:** Peak frequency of heat-evoked discharges is plotted against the temperature of the skin-heating, under control conditions (○) or during PAG stimulation (●). Data from Carstens et al. (7).

neurochemistry. Thus, serotonin and various neuropeptides have been identified to play a role as neurotransmitters or neuromodulators in these systems (12,27,31). A dramatic advance in this field was the discovery of endogenous opiate-like peptides, the enkephalins and endorphins (13,23,35). The endogenous opiates and morphine both are suggested to activate the descending inhibitory system via the same neuronal receptors (42). Details of neurochemical knowledge will be presented in the following chapter by Benedetti.

In the behaving animal, analgesia or hypalgesia can be produced by electrical stimulation (25), and by microinjection of morphine (42) in the brainstem. Also, in human patients brainstem stimulation has been used for treatment of severe pain (1,34).

The antinociceptive effects are suggested to be due to descending inhibition in the spinal cord and, possibly, also to inhibitory influences ascending to more rostral brain areas (Benedetti, *this volume*).

Inhibition of Spinal Neurons by Afferent Nerve Stimulation

It is a general principle of nervous system function that any sensory inflow not only excites nerve cells, but also produces inhibition. Inhibition is a stabilizing factor in nervous system function. Nociceptive afferents too are subject to, and produce, inhibition.

The inhibition normally operating in the spinal dorsal horn (Fig. 5) can be enhanced by intentional afferent stimulation, as has been shown in animal experiments: Neuronal responses to noxious skin-heating were partially or totally suppressed during repetitive electrical stimulation of afferent cutaneous nerves (Aβ strength) or of the dorsal columns (14). The inhibition ceased immediately at the end of the stimulation period, which lasted a few seconds.

A longer time-course of inhibition was observed when the periods of electrical nerve stimulation were prolonged to several minutes (Fig. 8). The discharges to noxious skin-heating (50°C, 10 sec), plotted as histograms

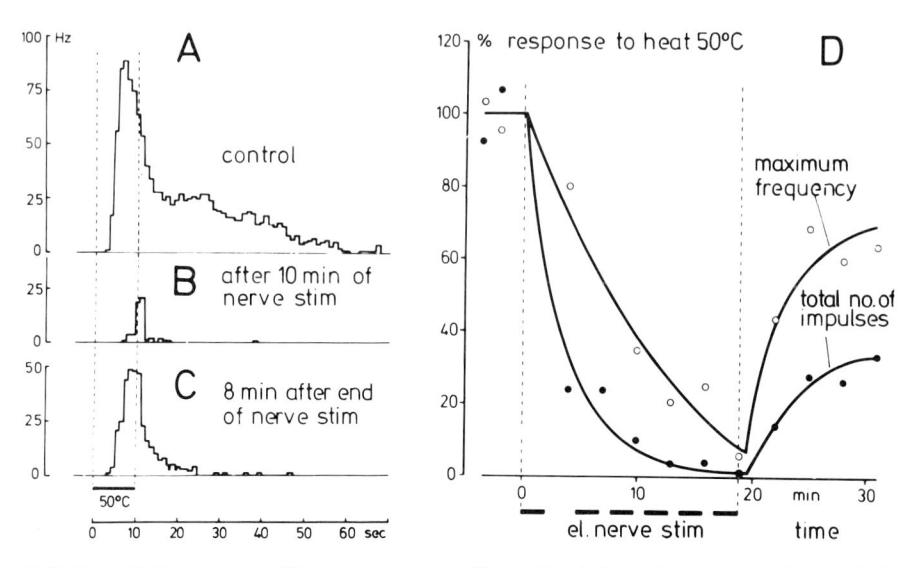

FIG. 8. Inhibition by repetitive, cutaneous A-fiber stimulation of responses in a spinal neuron of the cat evoked by noxious heat stimulation of the skin. **A:** Histogram of the discharge of a lumbar dorsal horn neuron evoked by heating (50°C, 10 sec) the cutaneous receptive field on the hind footpad. **B:** Same heat stimulus as in A was applied, being however preceded by a total of 10 min of repetitive (50 Hz) electrical stimulation of the A-fibers of the posterior tibial and superficial peroneal nerves. **C:** Response to the heat stimulus (as in A) 8 min after cessation of electrical A-fiber stimulation amounting to 12 min totally. **D:** Time-course of peak discharge (○) and total no. of impulses (●) per heat-evoked response of the dorsal horn neuron, during and after the electrical A-fiber stimulation; repeated 2-min periods of electrical nerve stimulation indicated below abscissa. Discharge measures were relative to control values recorded before the period of electrical nerve stimulation. (From Dickhaus et al., ref. 10, with permission.)

(A to C), revealed a considerable suppression even when the repetitive electrical nerve stimulation (50 Hz, $A\beta$ strength) was restricted to the period between the noxious heat stimuli produced at a 3-min rate (as indicated by bars under the time scale in Fig. 8D). Thus, after nerve stimulation amounting to a total of 10 min, the discharge to heat stimulus was reduced to a few percent of control (Fig. 8B). It should be pointed out that the inhibition affected predominantly the afterdischarge to the noxious stimulus, which is suggested to contribute to the aftersensation and therefore will make pain of this type so disagreeable.

After the end of the electrical stimulation, the responsiveness of the neuron to noxious heat slowly recovered (Fig. 8C, D). In a systematic study of this type, time-courses of between 10 sec and more than 10 min were found for the build-up and decay of inhibition. In practically all cases, however, inhibition considerably outlasted the period of electrical stimulation, which has so far not been previously reported (10).

Concerning the neuronal mechanisms involved in these slow alterations, several possibilities might be proposed: (a) The observed time-courses (Fig. 8D) might reflect the turning on and off of inhibitory system(s), being of spinal or/and of supraspinal origin, or (b) alterations in the extra- and intra-cellular ionic compositions (e.g., of K^+), which in turn affect membrane transport mechanisms and, hence, membrane excitability (10,43).

The inhibition in Fig. 8 is reminiscent of hypalgesia produced by transcutaneous nerve stimulation and by stimulation through acupuncture needles in man, where stimulation periods of 10 to 30 min have often been required for the hypalgesia to develop fully. Both these methods of hyperstimulation in human patients presumably have common mechanisms, one of these being the suppression of dorsal horn neurons reported here.

SUMMARY AND CONCLUSIONS

Pain sensations usually are based upon activity in nociceptive afferents. Although there is considerable knowledge on nociceptors, both from man and animals, the key mechanisms of chronic pain are only poorly understood. In this regard, systematic investigations in man and animals are required in these fields:

1. Effects on nociceptors of a variety of endogenous chemicals produced in diseased organs; of particular interest are the basic properties and chemical modifications of nociceptors in the deep organs, e.g., viscera, muscles, tendons, and bones.

2. Excitability conditions of nociceptive fibers in regenerated nerves and freshly reinnervated organs; how can the formation of a neuroma be prevented after nerve lesions?

3. Motor and sympathetic reflexes that act upon nociceptors, thus establishing a positive-feedback, self-excitatory loop to maintain chronic pain.

Although there is impressive evidence in patients for such phenomena, we do not know why such reflexes develop.

In the CNS no pain center exists. The cognitive, affective, motivational, and vegetative dimensions of pain-perception and behavior presumably are based on a complex pattern of activity in, and interactions of, many central nervous functional subsystems. Some basic neuronal mechanisms that might be related to pain and analgesia have been studied in the spinal dorsal horn neurons of animals. However, we are far from having a coherent picture of central pain physiology. The following problems need to be investigated intensively:

4. The neurophysiology of supraspinal CNS. Since nociceptive responses presumably are affected by anesthesia, waking, unrestrained animals should be used, enabling correlations of the electrophysiologic and behavioral responses to noxious stimuli.

5. The dorsal horn physiology, including the afferent and descending inhibitory effects, should be studied in animal models for chronic pain, e.g., induced inflammations of skin or joints. The results of such studies, even when conducted under anesthesia, would be more relevant for the understanding of pain and analgesia in man than the present work using acute noxious stimuli, such as pinching or heat.

6. The gap between the neurophysiologic and neurochemical (pharmacological) approaches should be narrowed, e.g., by relating microelectrophysiologic and microelectrophoretic studies with the histochemical identity of the neuron under study.

7. Studies in man, healthy subjects and patients, should be intensified. A great repertoire of methods is available, such as psychophysiologic measurements, EEG, evoked potentials, EMG, microneurography, diagnostic microelectrode recordings during stereotaxic operations and cordotomies.

The future study of pain physiology will require the use of chronic pain in animals. There are, however, enormous ethical objections, since it is difficult to design appropriate experiments and prevent inducing suffering in animals (36,39). A competent multidisciplinary committee should elaborate guiding principles for such work.

ACKNOWLEDGMENTS

The author wishes to thank Frau Ursula Nothoff for typing and bibliographical assistance, Frau Almuth Manisali for graphics, and Dr. E. Carstens for improving the English.

REFERENCES

1. Adams, J. E. (1976): Naloxone reversal of analgesia produced by brain stimulation in the human. *Pain,* 2:161–166.
2. Beck, P. W., and Handwerker, H. O. (1974): Bradykinin and serotonin effects on various types of cutaneous nerve fibres. *Pflügers Arch.,* 347:209–222.

3. Beck, P. W., Handwerker, H. O. and Zimmermann, M. (1974): Nervous outflow from the cat's foot during noxious radiant heat stimulation. *Brain Res.,* 67:373–386.
4. Bonica, J. J. (editor) (1974): *Advances in Neurology, Vol. 4.* Raven Press, New York.
5. Bonica, J. J., and Albe-Fessard, D. (editors) (1976): *Advances in Pain Research and Therapy, Vol. 1.* Raven Press, New York.
6. Boivie, J., and Perl, E. R. (1975): Neural substrates of somatic sensation. In: *International Review of Physiology, Vol. 3: Neurophysiology I,* pp. 303–411; edited by C. C. Hunt. Butterworths, London.
7. Carstens, E., Yokota, T., and Zimmermann, M. (1979): Inhibition of spinal neuronal responses to noxious skin heating by stimulation of the mesencephalic periaqueductal gray in the cat. *J. Neurophysiol. (in press).*
8. Collier, H. O. J. (1971): Prostaglandins and aspirin. *Nature,* 232:17–19.
9. Devor, M., and Wall, P. D. (1976): Type of sensory nerve fibre sprouting to form a neuroma. *Nature,* 262:705–708.
10. Dickhaus, H., Pauser, G., and Zimmermann, M. (1978): Hemmung im Rückenmark, ein neurophysiologischer Wirkungsmechanismus bei der Hypalgesie durch Stimulationsakupunktur. *Wien. Klin. Wochenschrift,* 90:59–64.
11. Dickhaus, H., Zimmermann, M., and Zotterman, Y. (1976): The development in regenerating cutaneous nerves of C-fibre receptors responding to noxious heating of the skin. In: *Sensory Functions of the Skin in Primates,* edited by Y. Zotterman, S. 415–425. Pergamon Press, Oxford, New York, Toronto, Sydney, Paris, Frankfurt.
12. Fields, H. L., and Basbaum, A. I. (1978): Brainstem control of spinal pain-transmission neurons. *Ann. Rev. Physiol.,* 40:217–248.
13. Goldstein, A. (1976): Opioid peptides (endorphins) in pituitary and brain. *Science,* 193:1081–1086.
14. Handwerker, H. O., Iggo, A., and Zimmermann, M. (1975): Segmental and supraspinal actions on dorsal horn neurons responding to noxious and non-noxious stimuli. *Pain,* 1:147–165.
15. Hardy, I. D., Wolff, H. D., and Goodell, H. (1952): *Pain Sensations and Reactions.* Williams & Wilkins, Baltimore.
16. Hassler, R. (1960): Die zentralen Systeme des Schmerzes. *Acta Neurochir. (Wien),* 8:353–423.
17. Henry, J. L. (1976): Effects of substance P on functionally identified units in cat spinal cord. *Brain Res.,* 114:439–451.
18. Hick, V. E., Koley, J., and Morrison, J. F. B. (1977): The effects of bradykinin on afferent units in intra-abdominal sympathetic nerve trunks. *Quart. J. Exp. Physiol.,* 62:19–25.
19. Horeyseck, G., and Jänig, W. (1974): Reflexes in postganglionic fibres within skin and muscle nerves after noxious stimulation of skin. *Exp. Brain Res.,* 20:125–134.
20. Iggo, A. (editor) (1973): *Somatosensory System. Handbook of Sensory Physiology, Vol. II.* Springer Verlag, Berlin, Heidelberg, New York.
21. Janzen, R., Keidel, W. D., Herz, A., and Steichele, C. (editors) (1972): *Pain: Basic Principles—Pharmacology—Therapy.* Georg Thieme Verlag, Stuttgart.
22. Keele, C. A., and Armstrong, D. (1964): *Substances Producing Pain and Itch.* Edward Arnold Ltd., London.
23. Kosterlitz, H. W. (editor) (1976): *Opiates and Endogenous Opioid Peptides.* North-Holland, Amsterdam.
24. Kumazawa, T., and Mizumura, K. (1977): Thin-fibre receptors responding to mechanical, chemical and thermal stimulation in the skeletal muscle of the dog. *J. Physiol. (Lond.),* 273:179–194.
25. Liebeskind, J. C., and Paul, L. A. (1977): Psychological and physiological mechanisms of pain. *Annu. Rev. Psychol.,* 28:41–60.
26. Lim, R. K. S. (1970): Pain. *Annu. Rev. Physiol.,* 32:269–288.
27. Mayer, D. J., and Price, D. D. (1976): Central nervous system mechanisms of analgesia. *Pain,* 2:379–404.

28. Mayer, D. J., Price, D. D., and Rafii, A. (1977): Antagonism of acupuncture analgesia in man by the narcotic antagonist naloxone. *Brain Res.,* 121:368–372.
29. Mense, S. (1977): Nervous outflow from skeletal muscle following chemical noxious stimulation. *J. Physiol. (Lond.)* 267:75–88.
30. Mense, S., and Schmidt, R. F. (1977): Muscle pain: Which receptors are responsible for the transmission of noxious stimuli? In: *Physiological Aspects of Clinical Neurology,* edited by F. Clifford Rose, pp. 265–278. Blackwell Scientific Publications, Oxford, London, Edinburgh, Melbourne.
31. Messing, R. B., and Lytle, L. D. (1977): Serotonin-containing neurons: Their possible role in pain and analgesia. *Pain,* 4:1–22.
32. Neil, E. (editor) (1972): *Enteroreceptors. Handbook of Sensory Physiology, Vol. III/1.* Springer Verlag, Berlin, Heidelberg, New York.
33. Price, D. D., and Dubner, R. (1977): Neurons that subserve the sensory-discriminative aspects of pain. *Pain,* 3:307–338.
34. Richardson, D. E., and Akil, H. (1977): Pain reduction by electrical brain stimulation in man. *J. Neurosurg.,* 47:178–194.
35. Snyder, S. H. (1977): Opiate receptors and internal opiates. *Sci. Am.,* 236:44–56.
36. Sternbach, R. A. (1976): The need for an animal model of chronic pain. *Pain,* 2:2–4.
37. Sunderland, S. (1968): *Nerves and Nerve Injuries.* Livingstone, Edinburgh and London.
38. Uchida, Y., and Murao, S. (1974): Excitation of afferent cardiac sympathetic nerve fibers during coronary occlusion. *Am. J. Physiol.,* 226:1094–1099.
39. Wall, P. D. (1975, 1976): Editorials in *Pain,* 1:1–2 (1975) and *Pain,* 2:1 (1976).
40. Wall, P. D., and Gutnick, M. (1974): Ongoing activity in peripheral nerves: The physiology and pharmacology of impulses originating from a neuroma. *Exp. Neurol.,* 43:580–593.
41. Willis, W. D., Trevino, D. L., Coulter, J. D., and Maunz, R. A. (1974): Responses of primate spinothalamic tract neurons to natural stimulation of hind limb. *J. Neurophysiol.,* 37:358–372.
42. Yaksh, T. L., and Rudy, T. A. (1978): Narcotic analgetics: CNS sites and mechanisms of action as revealed by intracerebral injection techniques. *Pain,* 4:299–359.
43. Zimmermann, M. (1975): Neurophysiological models for nociception, pain and pain therapy. In: *Brain Hypoxia—Pain: Advances in Neurosurgery, Vol. 3,* edited by H. Penzholz, M. Brock, J. Hamer, M. Klinger, and O. Spoerri, pp. 199–209. Springer-Verlag, Berlin, Heidelberg, New York.
44. Zimmermann, M. (1976): Neurophysiology of nociception. In: *International Review of Physiology, Vol. 10, Neurophysiology II,* edited by R. Porter, pp. 179–221. University Park Press, Baltimore.
45. Zimmermann, M. (1977): Encoding in dorsal horn interneurons receiving noxious and non noxious afferents. *J. Physiol. (Paris),* 73:221–232.
46. Zotterman, Y. (1939): Touch, pain and tickling: An electrophysiological investigation on cutaneous sensory nerves. *J. Physiol. (Lond.),* 95:1–28.
47. Zotterman, Y. (editor) (1976): *Sensory Functions of the Skin in Primates.* Pergamon Press, Oxford.

Neuroanatomy and Biochemistry of Antinociception

Costantino Benedetti

Department of Anesthesiology, University of Washington School of Medicine, Seattle, Washington 98195

Professor Zimmermann has, in the preceding chapter, effectively and extensively reviewed the peripheral and central nociceptive system and has alluded to antinociceptive mechanisms. Now I would like to give an overview of the presently known systems which are involved in the modulation of pain and, in particular, a system which is located in the central nervous system (CNS) and is activated either by endogenous morphine-like substances (enkephalins or endorphins), or by exogenous opioids.

In 1965, after many years during which pain research received very little scientific attention, Melzack and Wall (30) published the Gate Control Theory. Even if the original hypothesis of the Gate Control Theory has to be modified, it nonetheless had a great impact, because in the following years many researchers turned their attention to a neglected area of research—pain (64).

ELECTRICAL STIMULATION ANALGESIA

In 1968, Reynolds reported his experience with electrical stimulation of specific areas of the rat brain (39). By implanting electrodes in the periaqueductal gray (PAG) of rats and electrically stimulating them after the animals had recuperated from the original neurosurgery, he was able to induce, in some animals, sufficient analgesia to allow the performance of laparotomies. Following surgery, when the electrical stimulation was discontinued, Reynolds noted that residual skin analgesia remained for a few minutes, but within 5 min, vigorous, aversive responses to painful stimulation had returned.

In 1971, Mayer et al. (29) repeated this experiment in more detail and under more-controlled experimental conditions. They found that electrical stimulation of subcortical loci could indeed cause profound analgesia without apparent accompanying motor or motivational deficits, and the majority of animals appeared to have no impaired response to visual, auditory, or tactile stimuli. In fact, some were hyperreactive to light touch. The animals were analgesic not only to mechanical noxious stimuli, but also to other noxious events, and the analgesia outlasted brain stimulation by 30 sec to 5 min. In light of these observations, the investigators postulated that the electrical brain stimulation activated an endogenous neurophysiologic system that blocked or at least decreased noxious input.

In a similar experiment, Samanin and Valzelli (43), showed that stimulation for 1 hr of the dorsal raphe nuclei before the subcutaneous injection of morphine markedly enhanced the analgesic effect of this drug, while lesions of the nucleus raphe medianus antagonized morphine analgesia. These authors further observed that the analgesic effect paralleled the increase of 5-hydroxyindoleacetic acid (a metabolic by-product of serotonin) in the forebrain. This finding was in agreement with the results of Aghajanian et al. (2), who had previously demonstrated that electrical stimulation of raphe nuclei, in the vicinity of the central gray, released serotonin in brain synapses.

ROLE OF NEUROTRANSMITTERS

In an attempt to elucidate the interrelationship of pain modulation and serotonin, Tenen (50) lowered the serotonin concentration in rats and reported that these experimental animals developed hyperalgesic behavior, which could be reversed by injecting replacement doses of the serotonin precursor, 5-hydroxytryptophan. Sicuteri et al. (45) inadvertently induced similar hyperalgesia in humans suffering from migraine or other headaches by administering, for headache therapy, parachlorophenylalanine, an inhibitor of tryptophan hydroxylase which causes decrease of serotonin synthesis. They found that 20% of the patients developed hyperalgesia which lasted for 5 to 10 days after the discontinuation of the drug, a period consistent with the usual duration of action of the drug. However, normal subjects did not show this response (44).

The further demonstration that the decrease of serotonin concentration caused a reduction of the analgesia elicited by morphine or other opioids (49) led Akil and Liebeskind (3) to study the roles which the three cerebral monoamines (norepinephrine, dopamine, and serotonin) might play in analgesia. They found that the simultaneous depletion of all three neurotransmitters severely inhibited not only the analgesic effect of morphine, but also the effect of electrical stimulation at specific brain sites. The original level of analgesia could be restored by injection of the precursor of either serotonin (5-hydroxytryptophan) or dopamine (L-dopa). Selective depletion of serotonin reduced the analgesia, whereas elevation of its concentration at the synaptic cleft enhanced it. Pimozide (which blocks dopamine receptors) decreased the analgesia, while apomorphine (a dopamine-receptor stimulator) or L-dopa increased it. On the other hand, depletion of only norepinephrine enhanced the analgesic action of these substances, whereas its increase caused reduction of the analgesic state. If the norepinephrine level was depressed and the dopamine elevated, the analgesic effect was particularly potentiated. Therefore, it appears that dopamine and serotonin are necessary neurotransmitters to facilitate the analgesia whereas norepinephrine depresses it. In accordance with this result is the recent report by Wang (59), who found that 100 to 200 µg of serotonin administered in the lumbar subarachnoid space of rats produced profound analgesia lasting up to 40 min. Behavioral and morphological observation fail to show any adverse reaction.

Bonica (8), in 1953, had already reported that patients suffering from chronic pain sometimes improved after treatment with amphetamines; and since this drug probably acts on the serotonin receptors of the brain, this observation is also in accordance with the above findings. Recently, it has been clinically demonstrated that 10 mg of dextroamphetamine almost doubles the analgesic effect of 12 mg of morphine, while at the same time it decreases the respiratory depression and the lethargy caused by the opioid (14).

SIMILARITIES BETWEEN OPIOID ANALGESIA AND STIMULATION-INDUCED ANALGESIA

The observations that (a) morphine action is dependent on the availability of serotonin and on the integrity of certain raphe nuclei, and (b) electrical stimulation of the dorsal raphe nuclei enhances morphine's action and increases serotonin by-product in the forebrain, suggested that both periventricular electrical stimulation and morphine activated a similar inhibitory mechanism. Akil, Mayer, and Liebeskind (6) reported that analgesia induced by electrical stimulation of PAG was reduced, like morphine analgesia, when the raphe nuclei were lesioned or when the brain level of serotonin was lowered (4). They further observed that a pure opioid antagonist like naloxone reversed the analgesic effect of electrical stimulation (5). All these data strongly indicate that morphine and brain electrical stimulation are very similar in action and that both activate the same nociception-suppressing descending system. The system appears to be tonically active at least in some animal species, since lesioning of the raphe nuclei leads to hyperalgesia in the animals.

OPIATE RECEPTORS

In the early 'seventies other laboratories were actively investigating the mode of action of morphine with particular attention to the mechanism of addiction. In 1973, Pert and Snyder (36) isolated opiate receptors from the synaptosomal fraction of brain homogenate and more specifically from the synaptic membrane. These structures are proteolipid and have a characteristic chemical and physical configuration which makes them stereospecific and bind only the active opioid isomers in a manner similar to the action of a proper lock and key (15). Opiate receptors are present only in the vertebrates (35), and they are distributed in different areas of the body including the brain, spinal cord, and gastrointestinal tract. In both human and lower primates the brain contains the highest concentration of receptors (25). The amygdala, hypothalamus (parts of the limbic system which largely mediate emotional behavior), corpus striatum, caudate nucleus, periaqueductal gray, and thalamus are the areas most heavily endowed. The grey matter of the spinal cord also contains opiate receptors and most of them are located in the substantia gelatinosa. The cerebellum is devoid of opiate receptors whereas the cerebral cortex has a low concentration of them (36). It has been hypothesized that the combination of the opioid agonist with the receptor causes membrane changes that initiate the pharmacologic response, an event which does not occur when an antagonist binds to the receptor.

DISCOVERY OF ENDOGENOUS OPIOIDS

The existence of receptors in the brain which would bind with a substance found in the opium poppy, is certainly a peculiar occurrence. Researchers began to believe that the exogenous opiate must activate a neuromodulation system that is normally mobilized when an endogenous substance, similar in action to morphine, binds to the receptors specific to that substance. In 1975, both Terenius (56) and Hughes (20) independently succeeded in isolating a substance from the brain which had actions similar to opioids and these actions were reversible by naloxone. These findings indicated that endogenous substances with opiate-like actions do indeed exist.

These reports were soon confirmed by other investigators. Cox et al. (11) reported the isolation of a morphine-like substance from the pituitary gland, and Pasternak et al. (34) were able to isolate a similar substance from rat brain. Hughes et al. (21), shortly afterward, reported that the substance was a peptide of molecular weight of about 900 daltons and he termed it *enkephalin*. A few months later, Hughes and colleagues (22) again reported the identification of two related pentapeptides with potent opioid agonistic activity from pig-brain homogenate. The two peptides were identical except for the fifth amino acid, which was either methionine or leucine. These authors also reported that the amino acid sequence of met-enkephalin is identical to the 61–65 amino acid fraction of β-lipotropin, a polypeptide hormone of 91 amino acids from pituitary glands of sheep, pig, and man as represented in Fig. 1. Other fractions of this same molecule contain the amino acid sequence of other brain peptides such as β Melanocyte Stimulating Hormone (β-MSH) and part of ACTH. Subsequently, numerous other investigators have reported the isolation, structure, synthesis, and mode of action of various morphine-like substances.

Bradbury et al. (9) studied the effects of other fragments of β-lipotropin hormone. They found the 61–91 sequence of amino acids had opioid agonist

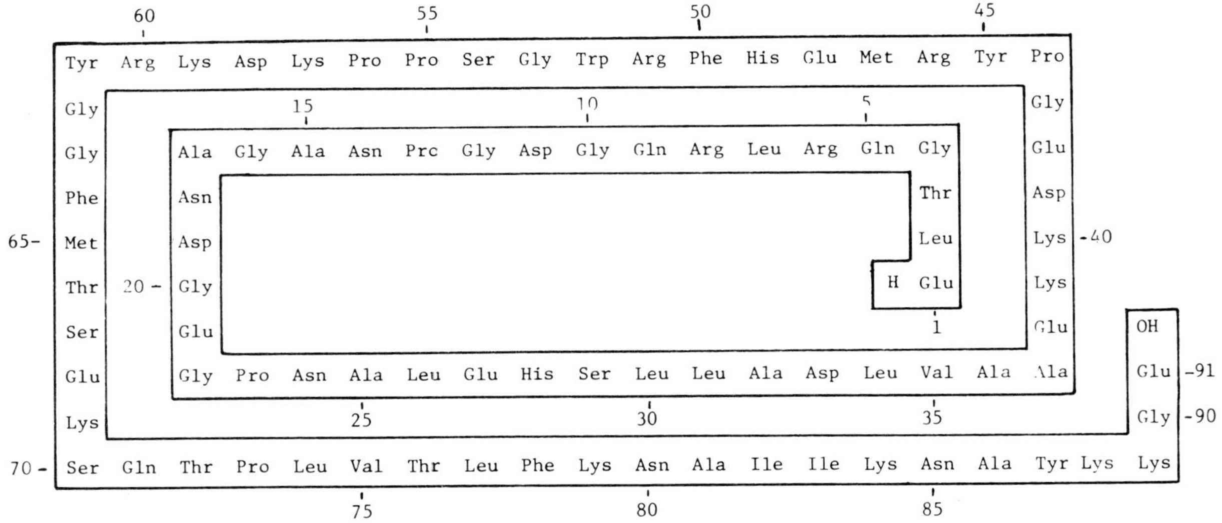

                                                                    45
                                                        50
Tyr Arg Lys Asp Lys Pro Pro Ser Gly Trp Arg Phe His Glu Met Arg Tyr Pro
Gly | Gly
                                     10
Gly   Ala Gly Ala Asn Pro Gly Asp Gly Gln Arg Leu Arg Gln Gly   Glu
Phe   Asn   Thr   Asp
Met   Asp   Leu   Lys –40
Thr 20– Gly   H Glu   Lys
Ser   Glu | Glu
Glu   Gly Pro Asn Ala Leu Glu His Ser Leu Leu Ala Asp Leu Val Ala Ala
Lys | |
                                     25   35
                                                                  OH
                                                                  |
70– Ser Gln Thr Pro Leu Val Thr Leu Phe Lys Asn Ala Ile Ile Lys Asn Ala Tyr Lys Glu –91
                         | | Gly –90
                         75   80   85

65–

60

55

50

Trp : Tryptophan
Tyr : Tyrosine
Val : Valine

Ala : Alanine   His : Histidine
Arg : Arginine   Leu : Leucine
Asn : Asparagine   Lys : Lysine
Asp : Aspartic acid   Met : Methionine
Gln : Glutamine   Phe : Phenylalanine
Glu : Glutamic Acid   Pro : Proline
Gly : Glycine   Ser : Serine
Ile : Isoleucine   Thr : Threonine

FIG. 1. Amino acid sequence of pituitary human β-lipotropin hormone (β LTH). Sequence 1–55 represents α-lipotropin hormone, 41–58 β Melanocyte Stimulating Hormone (β-MSH), 61–65 met-enkephalin, 61–76 α-endorphin, 61–77 γ-endorphin and 61–91 β-endorphin. The amino acid sequence 47–53 is common to ACTH, β MSH and α-lipotropin hormone. This sequence has been shown to have opioid analgesia antagonistic activity.

activity. Cox, Goldstein, and Li (10) tested the entire β-lipotropin hormone molecule and found it devoid of opioid activity, whereas they confirmed that the 61–91 fragment had about the same potency as met-enkephalin. They elected to call this compound *β-endorphin* (endogenous-morphine) in contrast to another fragment 61–76 described by Guillemin et al. (17) and named *α-endorphin*.

Soon thereafter met-enkephalin and other endorphins were produced synthetically and tested on experimental animals. It became apparent that met-enkephalin is more potent than leu-enkephalin and that both are soon inactivated, probably by amino peptidase, since their half life is less than 1 min. β-endorphin is more resistant to plasma inactivation, and it can be injected intravenously to cause analgesia up to 2 to 3 hr (57). Lately, a synthetic enkephalin analog has been produced which shows effects even after oral intake (41). The cross-tolerance between these various endogenous ligands with morphine has been noted. Abstinence symptoms caused by discontinued administration of morphine soon disappear after injection of endorphin. Also, chronic administration of the endorphins causes tolerance and withdrawal symptoms after removal of the drug or reversal by naloxone (58).

From *in vitro* studies using both endogenous and exogenous opioids, multiple receptors have been demonstrated. In addition to the receptors which bind the classic morphine-like substances, others have been identified which show preferred selectivity for opiate peptides and naloxone has less affinity for these receptors. Different tissues have different populations of these receptors, but their distribution in the body and in particular in the CNS is not yet known (27,46,53).

Of similar importance to the discovery of endogenous opioids was the realization that endogenic antagonistic substances exist. Initially, Winter and Flataker (62) had demonstrated that ACTH reduced the analgesic effect of morphine. This work was confirmed and extended by Paroli (33), who found that the antagonistic effect of ACTH was dose-related. Zimmermann and Krivoy (63) have reported that not only ACTH, but also β-MSH has an antagonistic effect on morphine analgesia.

Terenius et al. (51,54) tested these earlier observations in an *in vitro* preparation of opioid receptors. They found that antagonistic activity of ACTH, β-MSH and other smaller peptides was dependent on the presence of the amino acid sequence Met-Glu-His-Phe-Arg-Trp-Gly (47–53 of β-lipotropin hormone) which is common to the above-mentioned hormones and lipotropin hormone (Fig. 1). This sequence is essential for the antagonistic effect and these peptides show affinity to the opiate receptors, which, however, is not so marked as the affinity of the endorphins. Wiegant et al. (61) have recently confirmed the antagonistic effect of this peptide on opioid analgesia in an animal model. This peptide does not possess any intrinsic analgesic properties; however, it can elicit non-analgesic effects in rats, such as excessive grooming, which is also seen with low doses of morphine. This could indicate that this peptide has both agonistic and antagonistic properties.

NEUROANATOMY AND NEUROPHYSIOLOGY OF ANTINOCICEPTION

By means of immunohistochemical analysis, attempts have been made to study the distribution of these polypeptides. It is interesting to note that β-endorphin is located mostly in the pituitary gland and hypothalamus (19) and, in particular, in the same cells which contain ACTH and it is released concomitantly with this hormone (18). In contrast, the enkephalins and in particular met-enkephalin, have a much wider distribution. Met-enkephalin, in fact, is located not only in the brain, but also in the spinal cord, in the nerve plexi of the gastrointestinal tract, and more recently has been found also in the exocrene cells of the stomach and intestine (37).

In the spinal cord it appears that met-enkephalin is located in interneurons of the substantia gelatinosa and/or in the proprioceptive afferents (19), since its level does not change after cordotomy. Immunohistochemical analysis also shows that there is a strict relationship between met-enkephalin and substance P, an excitatory peptide that is necessary for transmission of noxious impulses from the periphery to the higher centers of the brain (24). The demonstration of opiate receptors on the superficial laminae of the dorsal horn and their marked decrease after dorsal rhizotomy suggest their presynaptic localization on primary nociceptive afferents (26). The binding of enkephalin or morphine to these receptors apparently inhibits the release of substance P, preventing the synaptic transmission of noxious impulses (23).

While enkephalin acts on the segmental level of the spinal cord, other antinociceptive descending systems have now been established. Descending substance P pathways have been identified (19), and they may also be involved in the analgesia created by electrical stimulation of mesencephalic brain areas. Substance P, being a stimulating neurotransmitter, may activate the enkephalin neurons in the dorsal horn causing the release of this peptide (19). This is substantiated by the fact that small quantities of substance P given intraventricularly or systemically causes a naloxone-reversible analgesia (28,48).

Another descending antinociceptive system has been known for the last few years. This system is either activated by the electrical stimulation of the periaqueductal gray, or by the action of morphine-like substances (Fig. 2). Neurons in the ventrocaudal area of the gray matter surrounding the aqueductus cerebri make synaptic contact with a cluster of nerve cells which are located ventrally to the fourth ventricle and form the nucleus raphe magnus (42). All these neurons have high concentration of met-enkephalin, substance P, and opiate receptors (19). These neurons send their axons centrif-

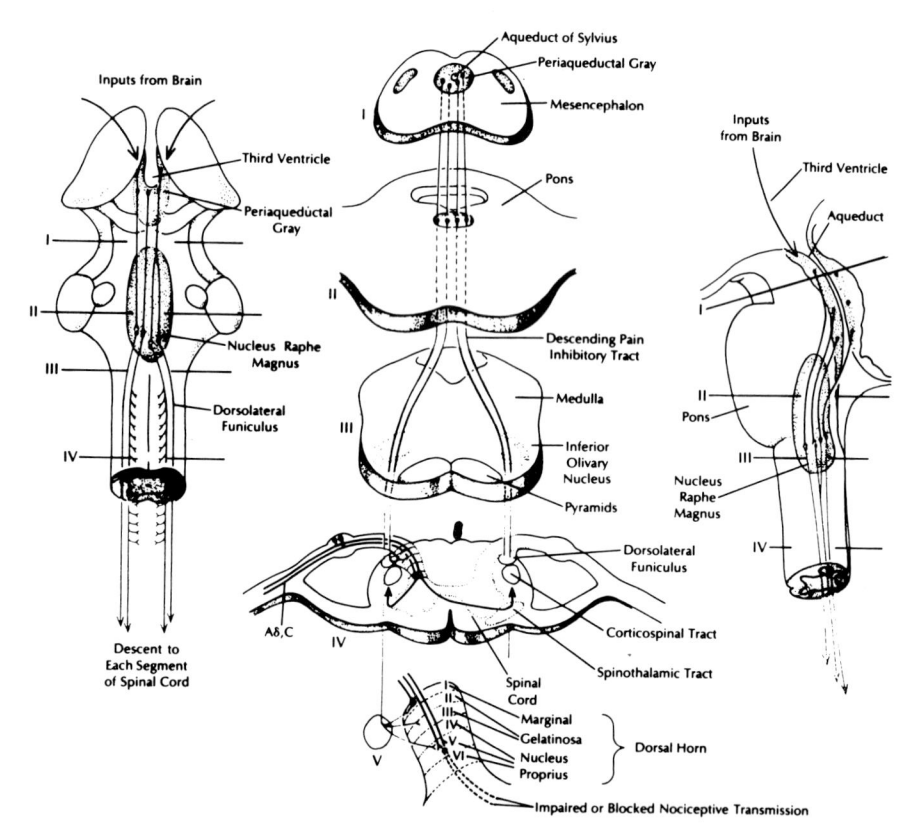

FIG. 2. Schematic drawing of the neuroanatomy of the descending inhibitory system activated by opioids and electrical stimulation of periaqueductal gray. [Courtesy of Dr. John J. Bonica: Pathophysiology of pain. *Hosp. Pract.* (Special Report), January 1978, p. 9.]

ugally in the dorsolateral funiculus just lateral and posterior to the motor axons which form the pyramidal tract and enter the dorsal horn at various levels of the spinal cord (7). These axons, which release serotonin at their synaptic terminals (4,12,16), make contact with nerve fibers located in laminae I, II, and V. This serotonergic system probably inhibits transmission of noxious impulses by axo-axonic influence on the primary nociceptive neurons in the dorsal horn (13,38). It should be noted at this point that some neurons in other raphe nuclei (raphe medianus and dorsalis) send their axons rostrally to innervate many regions such as the hypothalamus, hippocampus, corpus striatum, septum, and cortex (31). Their involvement in pain-modulation is not yet defined, but they appear to contain dopamine and norepinephrine as neurotransmitters, which have been shown to be involved in the modulation of pain (3).

SUMMARY

The data now available indicate that morphine analgesia mimics the action of endogenous morphine-like substances, termed *enkephalins* and *endorphins* and that electrical stimulation of specific areas of the brain causes their release. Strong evidence suggests that a peptide included in ACTH and β-MSH molecules acts as an endogenic opioid antagonist, at least for analgesia.

Since β-endorphin is located mainly in the pituitary-hypothalamic area and the enkephalins are located in other parts of the central nervous system, it appears that at least two major endorphin-releasing systems exist (52). One which is located in the pituitary gland may exert a prolonged hormonal activity owing to the long half-life of β-endorphin (57). The other, where met-enkephalin is the major modulator, acts both in a direct and indirect manner. Direct inhibition occurs when the enkephalin, released by the interneurons of the substantia gelatinosa cells (probably the same cells of the Gate Control Theory), binds to the opiate receptors located at the synapse of the nociceptive afferents and prevents the release of substance P and therefore, nociceptive transmission. Strong experimental evidence indicates that these enkephalin neurons are activated whenever axons descending from the upper centers of the central nervous system or primary proprioceptive afferents secrete substance P at the synaptic junction. Indirect modulation occurs when the neurons of the periaqueductal gray release endorphin. This substance activates a descending inhibitory system which includes neurons located in the nucleus raphe magnus. Their axons run in the dorsolateral funiculus and make axo-axonic synapses with the peripheral nociceptive afferents as they enter the dorsal horn. The release of serotonin at this junction causes nociceptive inhibition.

The observation that dopamine is directly involved in the modulation of pain and that this neurotransmitter is not present in the spinal cord suggests that the analgesic mechanism of endorphins and morphine may involve other inhibitory systems located in the brain. Further research will be needed to elucidate both this mechanism and the pathways of the norepinephrine system which appear to counteract morphine analgesia. Since changes of psychologic state alter the concentration of certain hormones and of neurotransmitters implicated in the endorphin system, it seems plausible that different psychologic states may activate or deactivate this mechanism of pain-modulation.

IMPLICATIONS FOR CANCER PAIN

Having briefly reviewed the endorphin antinociceptive system, let us consider what implications it may have in relation to cancer patients suffering severe pain.

In addition to the fact that the tumors produce noxious stimuli by causing inflammation of the surrounding areas, destruction of tissue, compression of nerve roots, obstruction of a hollow viscus and pressure, the above information suggests that these patients may possibly be hyperalgesic. This can be explained by multiple biochemical mechanisms. In fact, Terenius and Wahlström (55) and Sjölund et al. (47) have found that endorphins in the cerebrospinal fluid (CSF) are decreased in patients suffering from both chronic and cancer pain. Other substances are also implicated. As Dr. Chapman will emphasize in the paper that follows, the majority of patients suffering from a chronic illness, or knowing or suspecting affliction by a neoplastic disease, develop varying degrees of depression and are continuously under abnormal psychologic and physical stress. Distress is known to produce an increase in secretion of ACTH and norepinephrine, substances which act as antagonists at different levels of this antinociceptive system, as previously described. In addition, there are strong indications that depression is accompanied by diminished levels of serotonin, and recent preliminary observations in our institution seem to indicate that depressed patients are usually affected with chronic pain and experience a decrease in pain threshold. Both the decreased amount of serotonin and the increased amount of ACTH and norepinephrine will contribute to hyperreactivity of cancer patients to noxious input.

The ability to change or improve this psychologic state either by pharmacologic means or by psychotherapy will possibly help relieve the pain sensations of the patient. This is possibly the mode of action of amphetamines as observed and reported by Bonica (8) for treatment of some chronic pain states. Drugs used to block pituitary activities, as reported in this volume by Pannuti, and chemical hypophysectomy, developed by Moricca (32) to relieve diffuse cancer pain in terminal patients, may very well affect this endogenous antinociceptive system by altering the interdependent concentrations of the agonist and antagonist substances in favor of the agonist.

Direct application in the clinical setting of pure experimental techniques has also been reported. Richardson and Akil (40) and Adams (1) inserted electrodes in the periventricular gray matter of patients suffering from intractable chronic pain, and they were able to induce a pain-free state by electrical stimulation of this area. The analgesia ensued after 1 to 2 hr of stimulation and outlasted it for about 20 hr. Levels of morphine-like substances increase after the electrical stimulation and naloxone reverses this type of analgesia (personal communication with Akil).

CONCLUSION

To conclude, I would like to emphasize that this new area of biologic research will help us to understand how pain is modulated and possibly help us to explain the individual variation of pain-sensitivity in health and disease. It will also help to explain different psychologic disorders, since preliminary indirect observations seem to indicate that the endorphins are implicated in certain psychiatric conditions (60).

However, an enormous research effort is still needed to elucidate fully how the nervous system modulates noxious input under different situations, and to find therapeutic modalities which will activate these or other yet-unidentified autoanalgesia systems. The discovery of endorphin-selective receptors may yet enable us to develop pure analgesics without the undesirable side effects caused by the presently known narcotics (52).

REFERENCES

1. Adams, J. E. (1976): Naloxone reversal of analgesia produced by brain stimulation in the human. *Pain,* 2:161–166.
2. Aghajanian, G. K., Rosecrans, J. A., and Sheard, M. H. (1966): Serotonin release in forebrain by stimulation of midbrain raphe. *Science,* 156:420–423.
3. Akil, H., and Liebeskind, J. C. (1975): Monoaminergic mechanisms of stimulation-produced analgesia. *Brain Res.,* 94:279–296.
4. Akil, H., Mayer, D. J. (1972): Antagonism of stimulation-produced analgesia by p-CPA, a serotonin synthesis inhibitor. *Brain Res.,* 44:692–697.
5. Akil, H., Mayer, D. J., and Liebeskind, J. C. (1976): Antagonism of stimulation-produced analgesia by naloxone, a narcotic antagonist. *Science,* 191:961–962.
6. Akil, H., Mayer, D. J., and Liebeskind, J. C. (1972): Comparaison chez le rat entre l'analgésie induite par stimulation de la substance grise periaqueducale et l'analgésie morphinique. *C. R. Acad. Sci. [D] (Paris),* 274:3603–3605.
7. Basbaum, A. I., Clanton, C. H., Fields, H. L. (1976): Opiate and stimulus-produced analgesia: Functional anatomy at a medullospinal pathway. *Proc. Natl. Acad. Sci. USA,* 73:4685–4688.
8. Bonica, J. J. (1953): *The Management of Pain.* Lea & Febiger, Philadelphia, p. 532.
9. Bradbury, A. F., Smyth, D. G., Snell, C. R., Birdsall, N. J. M., and Hulme, E. C. (1976): C fragment of lipotropin has a high affinity for brain opiate receptors. *Nature,* 260:793–795.
10. Cox, B. M., Goldstein, A., and Li, C. H. (1976): Opioid activity of a peptide [β LTH (61–91)], derived from β lipotropin. *Proc. Natl. Acad. Sci. USA,* 73:1821–1823.
11. Cox, B. M., Opheim, K. E., Teschemacher, H., and Goldstein, A. (1975): A peptide-like substance from pituitary that acts like morphine. *Life Sci.,* 16(12):1777–1782.
12. Dahlström, A., and Fuxe, K. (1965): Experimentally induced changes in the intraneuronal amine levels of bulbospinal neuron systems. *Acta Physiol. Scand. (Suppl. 64),* 247:5–36.
13. Fields, H. L., Basbaum, A. I., Clanton, C. H., and Anderson, S. D. (1977): Nucleus raphe magnus inhibition of spinal cord dorsal horn neurons. *Brain Res.,* 126(3):441–53.
14. Forrest, W. H., Brown, B. W., Brown, C. R., Defalque, R., Gold, M., Gordon, H. E., James, K. E., Katz, J., Mahler, D. L., Schroff, P., and Teutsch, G. (1977): Dextroamphetamine with morphine for the treatment of postoperative pain. *N. Engl. J. Med.,* 296(13):712–715.
15. Goldstein, A., Lowney, L. I., and Pal, P. K. (1971): Stereospecific and nonspecific interactions of the morphine congener levorphanol in subcellular fractions of mouse brain. *Proc. Natl. Acad. Sci. USA,* 68(8):1742–1747.
16. Guilbaud, G., Besson, J. M., Oliveras, J. L., and Liebeskind, J. C. (1973): Suppression by LSD of the inhibitory effect exerted by dorsal raphe stimulation on certain spinal cord interneurons in the cat. *Brain Res.,* 61:417–422.
17. Guillemin, R., Ling, N., and Burgus, R. (1976): Endorphines, peptides, d'origine

hypothalamique et neurohypophysaire á activité morphinomimétique. Isolement et structure moléculaire de l'α-endorphin. *C. R. Acad. Sci. [D] (Paris),* 282:783–785.
18. Guillemin, R., Vargo, T., Rossier, J., Minick, S., Ling, N., Rivier, C., Vale, W., and Bloom, F. (1977): β-endorphin and adrenocorticotropin are secreted concomitantly by the pituitary gland. *Science,* 197:1367–1369.
19. Hökfelt, T., Ljundahl, A., Terenius, L., Elde, R., Nilsson, G. (1977): Immunohistochemical analysis of peptide pathways possibly related to pain and analgesia: Enkephalin and substance P. *Proc. Natl. Acad. Sci.,* 74:3081–85.
20. Hughes, J. (1975): Isolation of an endogenous compound from the brain with pharmacological properties similar to morphine. *Brain Res.,* 88:295–308.
21. Hughes, J., Smith, J., Morgan, B., and Fothergill, L. (1975): Purification and properties of enkephalin-the possible endogenous ligand for the morphine receptor. *Life Sci.,* 16(12):1753–1758.
22. Hughes J., Smith, T. W., Kosterlitz, H. W., Fothergill, L. A., Morgan, B. A., and Morris, H. R. (1975): Identification of two related pentapeptides from the brain with potent opiate agonist activity. *Nature,* 258:577–579.
23. Jessell, T. M., and Iversen, L. L. (1977): Opiate analgesics inhibit substance P release from rat trigeminal nucleus. *Nature,* 268:549–551.
24. Konishi, S., and Otsuka, M. (1974): The effects of substance P and other peptides on spinal neurons of the frog. *Brain Res.,* 65:397–410.
25. Kuhar, M. H., Pert, C. B., and Snyder, S. H. (1973): Regional distribution of opiate receptor binding in monkey and human brain. *Nature,* 245:447–450.
26. Lamotte, C., Pert, C. B., and Snyder, S. H. (1976): Opiate receptor binding in primate spinal: Distribution and changes after dorsal root section. *Brain Res.,* 112: 407–412.
27. Lord, J. A. H., Waterfield, A. A., Hughes, J., and Kosterlitz, H. W. (1977): Endogenous opioid peptides: Multiple agonists and receptors. *Nature,* 267:495–499.
28. Malick, J. B., and Goldstein, J. M. (1977): Substance P: Analgesia following intercerebral administration in rats. *Fed. Proc.,* 36:994.
29. Mayer, D. J., Wolfle, T. L., Akil, H., Carder, B., and Liebeskind, J. C. (1971): Analgesia from electrical stimulation in the brainstem of the rat. *Science,* 174: 1351–1354.
30. Melzack, R., and Wall, P. D. (1965): Pain mechanisms: A new theory. *Science,* 150:971–978.
31. Messing, R. B., and Lytle, L. D. (1978): Serotonin-containing neurons: Their possible role in pain and analgesia. *Pain,* 4:1–21.
32. Moricca, G. (1976): Neuradenolysis for diffuse unbearable cancer pain. In: *Advances in Pain Research and Therapy, Vol. 1,* edited by J. J. Bonica and D. Albe-Fessard, pp. 863–869. Raven Press, New York.
33. Paroli, E. (1967): Indagini sull effetto antimorfinico dell' ACTH, Relazioni con il corticosurrene ed i livelli ematici degli 11-OH steroidi. *Arch. Ital. Sci. Farmacol.,* 13:236–237.
34. Pasternak, G. W., and Snyder, S. H. (1975): Identification of novel high affinity opiate receptor binding in rat brain. *Nature,* 253:563–565.
35. Pert, C. B., Aposhian, D., and Snyder, S. H. (1974): Phylogenetic distribution of opiate receptor binding. *Brain Res.,* 75:356–361.
36. Pert, C., and Snyder, S. (1973): Opiate receptor: Demonstration in nervous tissue. *Science,* 179:1011–1014.
37. Polak, J. M., Sullivan, S. N., Bloom, S. R., Facer, P., Pearse, A. G. E. (1977): Enkephalin-like immunoreactivity in the human gastrointestinal tract. *Lancet,* 1:972–74.
38. Proudfit, H. K., and Anderson, E. G. (1974): New long latency bulbo-spinal evoked potentials blocked by serotonin antagonists. *Brain Res.,* 65:542–546.
39. Reynolds, D. V. (1968): Surgery in the rat during electrical analgesia induced by focal brain stimulation. *Science,* 164:444–445.
40. Richardson, D. E., and Akil, H. (1977): Pain reduction by electrical brain stimulation in man. *J. Neurosurg.,* 47:178–83.

41. Roemer, D., Buescher, H. H., Hill, R. C., Pless, J., Bauer, W., Cardinaux, F., Closse, A., Hauser, D., and Huguenin, R. (1977): A synthetic enkephalin analogue with prolonged parenteral and oral analgesic activity. *Nature*, 268:547–549.
42. Ruda, M. A. (1976): Autoradiographic examination of the efferent projections of the midbrain central grey in the cat. Ph.D. Thesis, University of Pennsylvania.
43. Samanin, R., and Valzelli, L. (1971): Increase of morphine-induced analgesia by stimulation of the nucleus raphe dorsalis. *Eur. J. Pharmacol.*, 16:298–302.
44. Sicuteri, F. (1976): Headache: Disruption of pain modulation. In: *Advances in Pain Research and Therapy*, Vol. 1, edited by J. J. Bonica and D. Albe-Fessard, pp. 871–880. Raven Press, New York.
45. Sicuteri, F., Anselmi, B., and Del Bianco, P. L. (1973): 5-hydroxytryptamine supersensitivity as a new theory of headache and central pain: A clinical pharmacological approach with p-chlorophenylalanine. *Psychopharmacologia*, 29:347–356.
46. Simantov, R., and Snyder, S. H. (1976): Morphine-like peptides, leucine enkephalin and methionine enkephalin: Interactions with the opiate receptor. *Mol. Pharmacol.*, 12:987–998.
47. Sjölund, B., Terenius, L., and Eriksson, M. (1977): Increased cerebrospinal fluid levels of endorphins after electroacupuncture. *Acta Physiol. Scand.*, 100:382–384.
48. Stewart, J. M., Getto, C. J., Neldner, K., Reeve, E. B., Krivoy, W. A. and Zimmermann, E. (1976): Substance P and analgesia. *Nature*, 262:784–785.
49. Tenen, S. S. (1968): Antagonism of the analgesic effect of morphine and other drugs by p-chlorophenylalanine, a serotonin depletor. *Psychopharmacologia*, 12:278–285.
50. Tenen, S. S. (1967): The effects of p-chlorophenylalanine, a serotonin depletor, on avoidance acquisition, pain sensitivity and related behavior in the rat. *Psychopharmacologia*, 10:204–19.
51. Terenius, L. (1975): Effect of peptides and amino acids on dihydro-morphine binding to the opiate receptor. *J. Pharm. Pharmacol.*, 27:450–451.
52. Terenius, L. (1978): Endogenous peptides and analgesia. *Annu. Rev. Pharmacol. Toxicol.*, 18:189–204.
53. Terenius, L. (1977): Opioid peptides and opiates differ in receptor selectivity. *Psychoneuroendocrinology*, 2:53–58.
54. Terenius, L., Gispen, W. H., and DeWied, D. (1975): ACTH-like peptides and opiate receptors in rat brain: Structure-activity studies. *Europ. J. Pharmacol.*, 33:395–399.
55. Terenius, L., and Wahlström, A. (1975): Morphine-like ligand for opiate receptors in human CSF. *Life Sci.*, 16(12):1759–1764.
56. Terenius, L., and Wahlström A. (1975): Search for an endogenous ligand for the opiate receptor. *Acta Physiol. Scand.*, 94:74–81.
57. Tseng, L. F., Loh, H. H., and Li, C. H. (1976): β-endorphin as a potent analgesic by intravenous injection. *Nature*, 263:239–240.
58. Tseng, L. F., Loh, H. H., and Li, C. H. (1976): β-endorphin: Cross tolerance to and cross physical dependence on morphine. *Proc. Natl. Acad. Sci. USA*, 73(11):4187–9.
59. Wang, J. K. (1977): Antinociceptive effect of intrathecally administered serotonin. *Anesthesiology*, 47:269–271.
60. Watson, S. J., Berger, P. A., Akil, H., Mills, M. J., Barchas, J. D. (1978): Effects of naloxone on schizophrenia: Reduction in hallucinations in a subpopulation of subjects. *Science*, 201:73–75.
61. Wiegant, V. M., and Gispen, W. H. (1977): ACTH-induced excessive grooming in the rat: Latent activity of $ACTH_{4-10}$. *Behav. Biol.*, 19(4):554.
62. Winter, C. A., and Flataker, L. (1951): The effect of corticosterone, desoxycorticosterone and adenocorticotrophic hormone upon the responses of animals to analgesic drugs. *J. Pharmacol. Exp. Ther.*, 103:93–105.
63. Zimmermann, E., and Krivoy, W. (1973): Antagonism between morphine and

the polypeptides ACTH, ACTH$_{1-24}$ and β MSH in the nervous system. *Prog. Brain Res.*, 39:383–394.
64. Zimmermann, M. (1976): Neurophysiology of nociception. In: *International Review of Physiology. Neurophysiology II., Vol. 10,* edited by R. Porter, pp. 179–221. University Park Press, Baltimore.

Psychologic and Behavioral Aspects of Cancer Pain

C. Richard Chapman

Departments of Anesthesiology, Psychiatry and Behavioral Sciences and Psychology, University of Washington School of Medicine, Seattle, Washington 98195

Pain often emerges as a severe problem for patients with advanced cancer. Viewed from the biologic perspective, it is an aversive sensory experience that signals progression of disease, and it is best controlled by destroying pain pathways or by administering analgesic medications. From the viewpoint of behavioral science, however, pain is part of the total human response to the sickness. In part, pain reflects the way in which the patient experiences the pathologic process, what the disease means to him, and how this meaning affects his interaction with others. Both perspectives offer valuable approaches to the management of the suffering patient, but it is the biologic that dominates current medical practice. The purpose of this chapter is to offer a conceptual framework for the management of cancer patients in pain that encourages the integration of biomedical with biosocial therapies.

THE BIOMEDICAL MODEL

Engel (4) has recently described the biomedical model of sickness that determines current medical practice. This model, which has the status of a dogma in contemporary Western medicine, holds that disease is deviation from the norm of measurable biologic variables. Within the model, psychologic and social aspects of illness are irrelevant. As applied to pain-management, the model requires that pain be viewed as a by-product of disordered biochemical or neurophysiologic processes that exist independently of behavioral and social factors. Recent acknowledgment of the epidemic occurrence of chronic pain disorders (1) suggests that the biomedical framework, despite its many brilliant achievements, has failed to solve the problem of persistent pain.

A fundamental limitation of the biomedical model is that it must construe pain problems as arising consequent to disease and that such troubles will subside when the disease is cured or controlled. This perspective is not incorrect but rather incomplete. Contemporary theories of pain emphasize that sensation, emotion, and meaning are intrinsic parts of the experience (2,11). In developing the McGill Pain Questionnaire, Melzack and Torgerson distinguished among the sensory, affective, and evaluative dimensions of pain. The biomedical model lags behind contemporary concepts of pain and current directions in pain research. Furthermore, as Fordyce (5) and others have emphasized, learning processes can occur when illness behavior is reinforced, and social factors such as financial compensation can sometimes force patients into situations where illness behavior supports the vested interests of the patient better than well behavior. In such cases, pain complaints may persist when the noxious sensory barrage disappears. When this occurs, as it sometimes does in patients who have chronic pain without malignancy, the biomedical model becomes entirely inappropriate in patient care.

PSYCHOLOGIC FACTORS IN CANCER PAIN

The literature indicates that psychologic disturbances are important in almost all kinds of medical disorders, as well as in cancer-related pain problems. Stoeckle, Zola, and Davidson (16), studied psychologic distress in medical patients. In reviewing the literature in this area they noted that in most accounts of office medical practice between 5 and 40% of patients

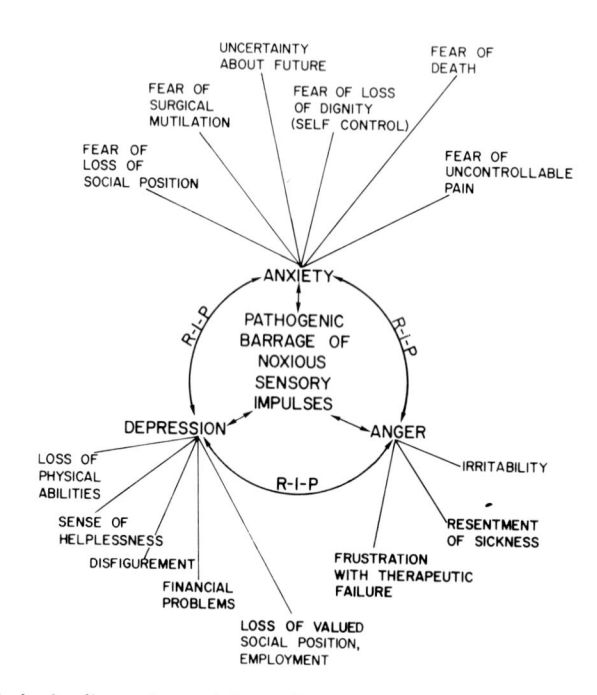

FIG. 1. Psychologic dimensions of the pain experience in the patient with advanced cancer. Anxiety, depression, and anger are presented for visualization purposes as three independent components of the patient's experience, but it should be recognized that these three problems mutually support and feed one another. The relationship among the three dimensions is defined as the rational-imaginative process (R-I-P).

showed a notable amount of basic psychiatric illness. When the concept of psychologic distress was expanded to include stress disorders, psychiatric complaints, and psychosomatic problems, the figure rose to as high as 70% or more. Indeed, in all forms of significant sickness, psychologic problems can arise which reflect the physical distress occasioned by the disease and the impact of disease on the life-style of the patient. When the diagnosis of cancer is made known to the patient, the situation becomes even more complicated. The patient is confronted with the realization that he has a dreaded and possibly terminal disease. Responses of fear, resentment, anger, and frustration are likely to occur. All of these factors enter into the experience of pain and contribute to the patient's pain behavior.

Figure 1 presents a model for the pain associated with advanced cancer. The basic building-block of this pain experience is the barrage of noxious sensory impulses that arises in diseased or damaged tissues. While the nociceptive barrage may be a by-product of neoplastic disease, for the patient with advanced cancer it may be generated by other sources as well. Iatrogenic disease, for example, is not uncommon in individuals who have been operated on multiple times, subjected to radiation or chemotherapy, and given other powerful drugs. In addition, painful neurologic disorders may occur consequent to cancer therapy. Herpes zoster, for example, commonly afflicts patients subjected to immunosuppressant therapies. This disease is exquisitely painful in its onset and throughout its course. In addition, post-herpetic neuralgia may remain as a severe and debilitating problem for an indefinite length of time. The problem is further complicated since the patient's invalid status may lead to severe changes in activity levels, postural changes, and other stresses that may generate pain of muscular origin.

Anxiety

The barrage of noxious sensory impulses gives rise to the conscious experience of pain only after it has been filtered by attentional mechanisms at higher central levels and amplified by various other psychologic factors. One of the principal contributors to the pain experience for the cancer patient is anxiety. Once the patient knows that he has cancer, there is a fear or a sense of dread of the death experience. In addition, patients fear the loss of social position that is a consequence of increasing invalidism, possible loss of control with the progression of the metastatic process and increased medication, and possible surgical mutilation.

Much of the fear experience that characterizes the cancer patient is a function of uncertainty, a factor that has been linked to anxiety and its associated physiologic arousal patterns in the psychologic literature (10). Chronic anxiety is known to result in disturbed autonomic and endocrine function, and it may lead to a variety of well-known psychosomatic symptom complexes such as tension headache, peptic ulcer, or spastic colon. Psychiatric patients with anxiety problems tend to have a large number of pain complaints (3). The presence of nociceptive impulses feeds the cancer patient's anxiety state because it may signal the spread of a disease to a new area. In turn, anxiety has an impact on attentional mechanisms so that the patient becomes hyperreceptive to noxious signals that may indicate changes in the disease process. Anxiety and nociception coexist reciprocally, as though in a vicious circle, as indicated by the bi-directional arrow in Fig. 1. Indeed, many patients experience intense fear with any ache or pain associated with normal living, because such sensations could possibly be symptoms of spreading disease.

Depression

As the patient becomes more and more disengaged from his normal social functioning and increasingly dependent on care-providers and the medical establishment, a sense of helplessness develops. As the disease progresses and reaches advanced stages, the patient typically evolves from repeated bouts of feeling helpless to a general theme of hopelessness and despair. Such depression can be increased by financial problems that face his family because of his inability to work and his mounting medical costs. A sense of self-grief is often evident in these patients, as well, since they undergo a severe loss of valued social position and employment status, and they lose certain physical abilities associated with good health. Many, especially women, suffer grief consequent to surgical disfigurement associated with breast amputation, limb amputation, or facial surgery. Biologic changes associated with depression are well documented in the psychiatric literature. Current theories hold that environmentally precipitated depression may be associated with the depletion of critical neurotransmitter substances such as serotonin. Such biochemical disturbances alter the body's ability to modulate pain states, as Dr. Benedetti described in the previous chapter. Von Knorring (17), Singh (15), and others have shown that pain may emerge as a major complaint in depressed psychiatric patients, even if there is no other specifiable organic disease.

Anger

Because patients perceive and interpret their own suffering and the losses associated with the progress of the disease, many tend to respond with anger, which takes different forms. It is not uncommon for patients to ask, "Why me?" Resentment and bitterness may develop over time as patients develop a sense of hopelessness. Such anger is consequent, in part, to frustration with therapeutic failure. Repeatedly, the patient finds that he is given hope by his physicians only to learn that yet another failure has occurred and the disease has again eluded treatment. When anger is turned inward, it feeds depression. This is represented by the bi-directional arrows connecting the depression and anger parts of Fig. 1. In addition, physiologic changes during anger, similar to those associated with anxiety, may help contribute to information-processing of noxious sensory input. Anger may feed anxiety when the patient begins to fear further frustrations that may provoke him to anger or irritability.

It must be emphasized that the anxiety, depression, and anger described in Fig. 1 are not necessarily abnormal or neurotic responses. Such reactions to the incredible stress of terminal disease are best considered normal and reasonably appropriate when considered from the patient's perspective. Of course, many patients have neurotic tendencies, and these will lead to heightened problems with certain aspects of the psychologic response pattern. Such problems need to be dealt with psychotherapeutically.

Thought Processes

Figure 1 includes a factor that represents the dynamic interrelationship among anxiety, depression, and anger, which is labeled the rational-imaginative process (R-I-P). This process involves the patient's rational interpretation of his problem within his own framework of understanding and the interaction of this interpretation with his imagination about therapeutic outcome and progress of the disease. In brief, the concept represents ongoing thought processes, and it is through such thinking mechanisms that anxiety states help to feed mood disturbances, and vice versa.

While most contemporary therapy is aimed at the pharmacologic control of anxiety and mood disturbance, manipulation of the rational-imaginative processes may provide a viable alternative. The patient's thinking processes are sensitive to information provided by health-care professionals, and, indeed, anger, anxiety, and depression may respond to counseling or proper psychotherapeutic intervention. More importantly, in the cancer patient, prophylactic psychotherapeutic control of such problems can be achieved.

ILLNESS, DISEASE, AND PAIN

Basic Concepts

One of the most useful conceptual schemes for dealing with the problem of cancer-pain management can be derived not from a psychologic framework, but from anthropology. This framework has been most clearly articulated for medical practice by Kleinman and his associates (9). These investigators have offered a conceptual distinction between disease and illness which may be usefully applied to the cancer patient. A *disease* is defined within this context as an abnormality in the function or structure of body organs and systems. It involves the malfunction or maladaptation of certain biologic processes in the patient. In contrast, *illness* is construed as the patient's personal reaction to the disease and associated discomfort. Illness may take a variety of forms depending on the cultural factors that govern the perception of, the classification of, and the explanation of the sickness experience. From the viewpoint of the behavioral scientist, illness refers to the way sick persons perceive, experience, and explain their diseases. Such reactions reflect not only the evaluation of the individual, but also the reactions of the family, the patient's immediate social network, and the culture.

Illness, as defined by Kleinman et al. (6,7,8,9), incorporates the beliefs and attitudes about the sickness held by the patient as well as by his family and his peers. Patients behave, during sickness, in ways that are consistent with the conceptualizations they hold about their problems. They present their symptoms, including their pain complaints, in a way that is rationally related to their illness concerns, interpretations of symptoms, and personal beliefs. To the extent that the patient depends on his doctor for an explanation of what is wrong, the doctor assigns a set of illness-behavior expectations to the patient, and by so doing, determines that patient's social role behavior. But as Kleinman et al. (9) have noted, there is often a discrepancy between the perspective of the health-care professional and that of the patient, his family, and his friends. Indeed, there may be a significant conflict or divergence in beliefs, attitudes, and interpretation among these people for an important health problem. Such conflicts result in poor patient-compliance, searches for quack and folk remedies, and general frustration for both doctor and patient.

The Physician's Perspective

From the viewpoint of the anthropologist, the physician behaves as he does because he has been socialized according to the biomedical model. Trained to maintain the biomedical perspective, physicians and other health-care professionals share a unique "medical" subculture that differs from attitudes toward disease shared by the rest of society. Furthermore, they share a language of technical terms that can be unintelligible to others outside of the medical subculture. Even when the patient strives to understand the physician's perspective on a disease problem, he may be stymied by a language barrier. It is not surprising, therefore, that the patient and the doctor often construe the sickness experience in very different ways.

In general, the physician focuses intensely on disordered biologic processes and looks for ways of applying modern technology so that these destructive trends can be stopped or reversed. In contrast, the patient is concerned with the ways in which the disease and its treatments alter his normal life and social identity. Illness problems involve disturbances in normal daily routine, limitation of activities, psychologic stress experiences such as anxiety, frustration, or a sense of hopelessness, and possible loss of position in the society due to disease-inflicted limitations.

Patient's Perspective

For the cancer patient there are often illness concerns related to fear of death, disturbance of family life, and fear of the unknown course of the disease and uncontrollable pain. Patients need help with these and other illness problems. Further difficulties include changes in premorbid social status and social role, sanctioning of a certain kind of sickness role, financial troubles related to the onset of disease, problems related to family stresses that have grown out of the sickness episode, and problems related to the patient's and the family beliefs about the cause and significance of the sickness.

Most patients expect help from the medical community in dealing with these difficulties. Indeed, such issues may elicit more concern from the patient than the physical symptoms that are so critical to the doctor. In other cases, the patient and his family do not even realize that these problems need attention. Identifying illness problems is an important step in helping such patients and their families, and the long-term consequences for the family of dealing with such problems before death occurs are particularly beneficial. Family crises often emerge after the prolonged illness, suffering, and death of a family member with cancer, but this can be averted in most cases if illness problems are faced and solved while the patient is still living.

Rationale for a Behavioral Perspective

The implication of the medical anthropologic framework for the management of the cancer patient is that both disease and illness problems need to be recognized and managed. The importance of applying all the advantages of medical technology to the problems faced by the cancer patient cannot be denied, but the perspective of medicine has been limited by the biomedical model so that the illness problems surrounding cancer have not been properly appreciated and dealt with in the majority of cases.

In addition, the biomedical model is unable to account for the perceptual complexity of pain. Just as the physiology of vision cannot explain the perceiver's appreciation of a masterful painting, the physiology of pain is inadequate to account for the nature of the pain associated with terminal cancer. Perception is a psychologic experience that involves more than information transmission in the nervous system.

PATIENT BELIEFS AND CANCER PAIN

The Explanatory Model

The rational-imaginative process in Fig. 1 emphasizes the importance of patient beliefs and attitudes in determining the nature of the pain experience.

Kleinman (7) has emphasized that both patients and their families hold explanatory models (EMs) for the occurrence of sickness. These models are systems of beliefs and attitudes that express the lay understanding of the cause, the course, and the nature of the sickness problem. It also incorporates the way that these individuals assign meaning or significance to the problem, as well as the treatment goals that they maintain. Patient EMs are conceptual schemes that derive partly from the patient's culture, his educational experiences, and his family history. In general, American and western-European folk models for disease are rough approximations of the biomedical model held by the physician, but sometimes these approximations are rather poor. It is common to observe in the United States, for example, that patients suffering with a herniated disk will explain that "My back went out" or "I slipped a disk."

In the clinical encounter, the doctor generally explains his model for the disease process to the patient and his family, but it is sometimes presented in a technical idiom which cannot be understood by patients. This is particularly problematic if there is a socioeconomic or cultural difference between the physician and the patient. Often, little or nothing of value is communicated in such an interchange. The author recalls once meeting a poorly educated American black lady from the rural south, who explained that her mother had come down with "Smilin' Mighty Jesus," which was all she could derive from the term *spinal meningitis*.

In the management of cancer pain, the patient's EM is an extremely important factor because it determines his understanding of the situation, his hopes for the future, and his fears for what is yet to come. Some of the suffering observed in patients with advanced cancer is due to the confusion and uncertainty in the patient's thinking and his inability to understand the doctor's EM. In some instances there is a marked discrepancy between the patient and family EMs, which further stresses the patient. Sometimes, and particularly in ethnic subcultures, family members will interpret the disease in terms of a folk medicine or a religious explanation, criticizing the patient for his dependence on physicians and the health-care establishment.

A Cultural Comparison

A fundamental EM cultural contrast in the management of the cancer patient centers around the issue whether or not the victim should be told that he has cancer. Broadly speaking, there are substantial culturally based differences in practice among the various countries of the world. For convenience, it is interesting to compare the United States with Italy. In the United States, most patients are told when cancer is diagnosed. Although there are exceptions to this rule, it is generally considered to be the patient's "right" to know his diagnosis. This news comes as a blow to most patients, and the effects on the patient's psychologic well-being are profound. Most American physicians make strong efforts to explain the patient's situation as best they can; that is, there is an effort to fit the patient's EM to the physician's EM. All too often, unfortunately, this is a failure. The popularity of diet therapies and folk remedies of all sorts bears a silent testimonial to this problem. Recently, for example, the infatuation of American patients with the drug Laetrile led to a public demand that became a major issue in American medical ranks (12,13).

A contrast in cancer-patient management can be observed in Italy where in most instances the patient is not told that he has cancer when it is diagnosed. Usually the family is informed, and doctors elicit their help in actively seeking to mislead the patient into believing that he does not have a malignant disease. The physician and the family both go to great lengths to help the patient develop an EM for his problem that excludes any possibility of cancer, even if the patient is admitted to a cancer hospital. On a covert level the patient may or may not believe what he is told, but on a more overt level he is forced to cooperate in acknowledging that his disease problem is not that of cancer. Whether or not the patient's true beliefs follow the dictates of the family and physician is of little consequence socially, because the patient will not engage in behaviors inconsistent with the beliefs given him by family and authorities.

It would be meaningless to cite the relative advantages of these two patient-management practices, for they are cultural behavior patterns rather than therapeutic strategies. The contrast, however, serves to illustrate the central importance of the patient's EM in the cancer experience.

CONSIDERATIONS FOR PAIN DIAGNOSIS AND THERAPY

Kleinman (8) has suggested that medical-care delivery could be improved by: (a) including a parallel evaluation of illness and disease problems in diagnosis; and (b) undertaking both illness and disease interventions. Table 1 provides parallel lists of cancer-pain–related illness and disease problems. While the listing is incomplete and only suggestive, it illustrates how such an approach might be developed. This approach could be employed in a problem-oriented medical record.

Saunders (14) has provided an example of how important the first item on the illness-problem list can be. She described a 54-year-old woman with advanced carcinoma of the cervix and metastasis to the vulva. Pain was a major complaint. A few days after admission the patient confided a preoccupation with guilt and her beliefs that her disease was related to past sins which had cut her off from God. The chaplain was called, and he was able to successfully allay her fears. As a result she spent her last days in a "tranquility and acceptance that never failed to the end and compelled admiration from us all." Such illness interventions clearly have a place in the care of the dying patient.

TABLE 1. Considerations in cancer pain diagnosis

Illness problems	Disease problems
Conflicting beliefs about the cause, nature, significance of the sickness	Metastatic progression
Family distress	Iatrogenic surgery
Loss of social position, status	Therapy-related disease (such as herpes zoster)
Financial difficulties	Side effects of radiation, chemotherapy
Unsatisfactory communication with care-givers	
Fear of death	

Illness and disease interventions should be planned jointly and listed for formulation and recommendation as suggested in Table 1. Some illness interventions may be carried out by the primary care physician but others may require other health-care specialists or expert services from the community such as legal assistance. The best approach is that of a multidisciplinary team that diagnoses and plans comprehensive treatment for pain problems.

The following concerns are basic illness interventions that would benefit most cancer patients with pain (based on Kleinman) (8):

1. presentation in simple language of the physician's EM for the disease and the pain
2. comparison of patient and physician EMs with negotiation between the two viewpoints
3. family therapy
4. financial counseling and planning assistance
5. ongoing monitoring of noncompliance or dissatisfaction with medical care
6. counseling aimed at resolving fears of death and dying.

By allaying the psychologic distresses of anxiety, depression, and anger, these interventions can substantially contribute to the control of suffering and the complaint of pain in the patient with advanced cancer.

FINAL CONSIDERATIONS

Pain is a complex perceptual experience that cannot be reduced to a problem of disturbed physiology in the cancer patient. The impact of prolonged major disease on the psychologic well-being of the patient is enormous, and the stresses imposed on his family by his invalidity add to his burden. The beliefs that the patient holds about the disease, its course, the cause of pain, and his future contribute intimately to the moment-to-moment perception of painful disorders.

The dichotomy between illness and disease discussed previously is in some ways an artificial one. It is important to acknowledge that most therapeutic interventions have an impact on both disease and illness. Placebo treatment, for example, is an illness intervention presented in the disguise of a disease intervention. But to the extent that the placebo rallies the patient's resources or resistance to disease, it becomes a disease therapy. Conversely, nerve blocks, surgical procedures, and other straight-forward disease interventions often have an incidental impact on patient attitudes and beliefs, thus affecting illness. Nonetheless, the dichotomy may serve a useful purpose in the management of cancer pain, since its use helps ensure that illness needs are not unnoticed, untreated, or inappropriately treated by disease interventions. Furthermore, the dichotomy, if employed in diagnosis, can help guarantee that the patient's illness problems will be directly and aggressively dealt with rather than incompletely and incidentally treated, as they are at present in many settings. Pain is often the focus of the patient's enormous suffering, and management of the dying cancer patient in pain must require treatment of both organic disease processes and illness behavior problems.

REFERENCES

1. Bonica, J. J., and Albe-Fessard, D. (1976): Preface. In: *Advances in Pain Research and Therapy, Vol. 1*, pp. v–vi. Raven Press, New York.
2. Chapman, C. R. (1977): Sensory decision theory methods in pain research: A reply to Rollman. *Pain*, 3:295–305.
3. Delaplaine, R., Ifabumuyi, O. I., Merskey, H., and Zarfas, J. (1978): Significance of pain in psychiatric hospital patients. *Pain*, 4:361–366.
4. Engel, G. L. (1977): The need for a new medical model: A challenge for biomedicine. *Science*, 196(4286):129–136.
5. Fordyce, W. E. (1976): *Behavioral Methods for Chronic Pain and Illness*. C. V. Mosby Company, St. Louis.
6. Kleinman, A. (1978): Clinical relevance of anthropological and cross-cultural research: Concepts and strategies. *Am. J. Psychiatry*, 135(4):427–431.
7. Kleinman, A. M. (1975): Explanatory models in health care relationships, In: *Health of the Family* (National Council for International Health Symposium), pp. 159–172. NCIH, Washington, D.C.
8. Kleinman, A. M. Recognition and management of *illness* problems: Therapeutic recommendations from clinical social science. *Massachusetts General Hospital Series on Psychiatric Medicine*, (in press).
9. Kleinman, A., Eisenberg, L., and Good, B. (1978): Culture, illness and care: Clinical lessons from anthropological and cross-cultural research. *Ann. Intern. Med.*, 88:251–258.
10. Mandler, G. (1975): *Mind and Emotion*. John Wiley & Sons, Inc., New York.
11. Melzack, R., and Casey, K. L. (1968): Sensory, motivational and central control determinants of pain. A new conceptual model. In: *The Skin Senses*, edited by D. Kenshalo, pp. 423–443. Charles C. Thomas, Springfield, Ill.
12. Moertel, C. G. (1978): A trial of Laetrile now. *N. Engl. J. Med.*, 298(4):218–219.
13. New York Academy of Medicine (1977): Statement on Amygdalin (Laetrile). *Bull. N.Y. Acad. Med.*, 53(9):843–846.

14. Saunders, C. (1976): Control of pain in terminal cancer. *Nurs. Times,* 72(29): 1133–1135.
15. Singh, G. (1968): The diagnosis of depression. *Punjab Med. J.,* 18:53–59.
16. Stoeckle, J., Zola, I. K., and Davidson, G. (1964): The quantity and significance of psychological distress in medical patients. *J. Chron. Dis.,* 17:959–970.
17. Von Knorring, L. (1975): The experience of pain in depressed patients. *Neuropsychobiology,* 1:155–165.

# Discussion

Part I. Basic Considerations

J. Bonica and C. Morpurgo (Moderators)

Vignali (Massa): Dr. Benedetti, why don't endorphins produce addiction?
Benedetti (Seattle): As I mentioned in my paper, endorphins do produce addiction exactly as morphine does. So far we cannot see this substance as the "all-healer" for easing pain.
Meglio (Rome): Is it possible to measure beta endorphin in body fluids? How? If it has been done in humans, what are the relative concentrations of the drugs?
Benedetti: We can measure endorphins in the cerebrospinal fluid. A solution is made with receptors together with a solution of radioactive morphine. Then we let this solution react with organic liquids, and we measure how much of the isotopic morphine is taken away from the receptors. These tests have been carried out also on humans, and it is interesting that patients affected by cancer and suffering chronic pain have a reduced concentration of these endorphins or similar substances in the spinal fluid.
Questioner: Man can acclimatize to hot climates in 6 to 8 weeks. Is there any evidence that man can acclimatize to chronic pain?
Bonica (Seattle): I would like to answer that question both as one who has observed patients with chronic pain over the past 30 years and one who has himself suffered pain for the past 12 years or so. I think, if anything, the individual becomes more sensitive and probably there is a gradual decrease of the endorphins which help the individual to cope with the pain. So, the earlier the therapy, the better for the patient and the less chance of complications.
Zimmermann (Heidelberg): Not only is there a lack of adaptation to chronic pain, often there is recurrence of chronic pain after a treatment which is successful initially. So, pain seems to be a sensory system which is very difficult to interfere with because it is basically important for life.
Procacci (Florence): Do endogenous substances always produce a sensitization or a modulation sometimes positive, sometimes negative?
Zimmermann: Concerning your first question, there are experimental findings in man and animals that with manipulations which normally produce a sensitization of receptors, the sensitization is sometimes preceded by a period of desensitization, a period of reduced sensitivity, and it might be that this is also due to the early stage of action of some endogenous substances which are released in response to noxious stimulus, such as bradykinin or serotonin.
Bricolo (Verona): As one of your slides has shown us, there would appear not to be a specific central point for the pain reception. Such a hypothesis is in contrast with that recently reported by Kitahata and his group when testing bulbar cells which respond to pain stimulation. If there is no pain center in the CNS, treating pain is a critically difficult problem for neurosurgeons.
Zimmermann: Thank you for this very basic and important question: Are there neurons in the central nervous system that are specific and specifically related to a noxious stimulus? In animal experiments, there have been found some neurons,

for example, in the spinal cord, that respond specifically to a noxious stimulus, but the majority of neurons that respond to noxious stimulation also respond to other forms of afferent input. And this is quite expected in the nervous system. The motor output that can be activated by a command for movement or by a command for speech can also be activated by a nociceptive input, and so there must be in the nervous system a mixing up of several modalities which determine behavior. So from this standpoint, it must be expected that the most relevant information concerned with pain is contained in the activity of nerve cells that are not only related to a noxious stimulus. Of course, there are some bypasses, for example, the spinothalamic tract where the information on noxious stimulus or on a pain state in the periphery is transmitted high up to the brain; and at this strategic site, one can produce pain-relief by a cordotomy. But, the spinothalamic or anterolateral tract is not only concerned with pain; that is also well established. And the assumption that in the central nervous system there is no pain tract and no nucleus specifically involved in pain does not exclude that a neurosurgical procedure is successful in removing pain because there is a strategic site through which all the pain related information must go.

Bonica: When one considers that cordotomy will relieve pain for many months; and then, despite the fact that analgesia still persists, the pain recurs, one has to consider that perhaps some of the other systems are also involved.

Pain Syndromes in Patients with Cancer

Kathleen M. Foley

Department of Neurology, Memorial Sloan-Kettering Cancer Center, New York, New York 10021

INTRODUCTION

Pain complicating cancer is often a difficult and frustrating clinical problem. A wide variety of complex pain problems in patients with cancer is encountered in a cancer hospital where, since the treatment available is often palliative and noncurative, the assessment and treatment of pain assumes the utmost importance. Pain in the patient with cancer may be caused by any of the pathophysiologic alterations which affect the general population and does not necessarily imply recurrent or persistent cancer. To facilitate appropriate diagnostic and therapeutic approaches for such patients, some knowledge of the common and uncommon causes of pain in patients with cancer and their clinical presentation is essential.

Existing data assessing the prevalence of pain in patients with cancer come predominantly from terminal-care facilities, where 50 to 60% of terminal patients are reported to have pain (8). These data do not report the incidence of pain in patients undergoing active therapy for cancer and do not attend to the causes of the pain. Therefore, we undertook to (a) assess the prevalence of pain in cancer patients and (b) define the common pain syndromes in patients with cancer.

Prevalence

Between January 1974 and December 1977, 3,424 (9%) of the 36,800 admissions to Memorial Sloan-Kettering Cancer Center (MSKCC), a 561-bed active cancer center, had pain of sufficient magnitude and complexity to require consultation from the Pain Service. This 9% figure represents patients with difficult diagnostic or therapeutic pain problems which the oncologists had had trouble in either assessing or treating.

Such a figure obviously underestimates the overall incidence of pain. To estimate the true incidence of pain in hospitalized patients with cancer, we surveyed the entire inpatient cancer population during a 1-week period (4). Postoperative pain was not included in this study. Of 540 patients evaluated,

TABLE 1. *Types of cancer associated with pain: adult group (143)*

Type	No. pts.	% Total pts.[a]
Breast	46	52
Lung	30	45
Bone	6	85
Oral cavity	12	80
GI	20	40
GU—Male	10	75
Female	14	70
Lymphoma	4	20
Leukemia	1	5

[a] % total pts. admitted with tumor type.

156 (29%) had pain which required the use of analgesic drugs. Primary cancers associated with pain in adults are presented in Table 1. When the number of patients with pain for each tumor type were compared with the number of patients in-hospital at that time with the same tumor type, the percentage of patients with specific types of cancer and pain could be demonstrated. Eighty-five percent of patients with primary bone tumors and 52% of patients with carcinoma of the breast had pain, whereas only 5% of the patients with leukemia had pain. In children, 13 of 39 (33%) had pain. The types of cancer associated with pain in the pediatric group revealed a high incidence of primary bone tumors, with 8 of the 13 pediatric patients having this cancer diagnosis.

A second study was undertaken in 1977. Pediatric postoperative and non-cancer patients were excluded from the study; 420 patients were personally questioned, and 397 agreed to a full interview. Data about the severity of their pain, onset, nature, specific pain syndrome, primary tumor, and previous and concurrent therapy were recorded. Of the 397 patients interviewed, 152 (or 38%) complained of pain; 39 of these 397 were terminal, and 23 of the 39 (or 60%) had significant pain.

Based on these two surveys and other clinical experience we have attempted to classify according to etiology specific pain syndromes occurring in patients with cancer in order to facilitate diagnosis (Table 2). The pain syndromes fit into three major groups, according to etiology: (a) 77% of patients in this series had pain caused by tumor invasion or compression of pain-sensitive structures (bone, nerve, and hollow viscus); (b) 19% had pain caused by or associated with cancer therapy; and (c) 3% had pain unrelated to their cancer or their cancer therapy. Before considering these syndromes, certain general principles should be adhered to closely in the evaluation and treatment of patients with pain and cancer.

TABLE 2. *Pain syndromes in patients with cancer*

I. Pain associated with direct tumor involvement
   A. Tumor infiltration of bone
      1. Base-of-skull metastases
         a. jugular foramen
         b. clivus
         c. sphenoid sinus
      2. Vertebral-body metastases
         a. subluxation of the atlas
         b. C_7-T_1 metastases
         c. L_1 metastases
         d. sacral metastases
   B. Tumor infiltration of nerve
      1. peripheral neuropathy
      2. brachial, lumbar, sacral plexopathy
      3. meningeal carcinomatosis
      4. epidural spinal-cord compression
   C. Tumor infiltration of hollow viscus
II. Pain associated with cancer therapy
   A. Pain occurring post-surgery
      1. post-thoracotomy pain
      2. post-mastectomy pain
      3. post-radical neck pain
      4. phantom-limb pain
   B. Pain occurring post-chemotherapy
      1. peripheral neuropathy
      2. post-herpetic neuralgia
      3. steroid pseudo-rheumatism
      4. aseptic necrosis of bone
   C. Pain occurring post-radiation therapy
      1. radiation fibrosis of the brachial plexus and lumbar plexus
      2. radiation myelopathy
      3. radiation-induced peripheral-nerve tumors
III. Pain unrelated to cancer or cancer therapy
   A. Diabetic neuropathy
   B. Cervical- and lumbar-disc disease
   C. Rheumatoid arthritis

Evaluation of Pain in Patients with Cancer

Clarification of the Pain Complaint

A careful history of the pain complaint can often provide the diagnosis. One must attempt to elicit a clear description of the onset of pain, its characteristics, the referral pattern, and exacerbating and relieving factors. Further information about the associated signs and symptoms can often clarify the diagnosis: e.g., in a patient complaining of severe back pain exacerbated by lying down, the associated complaint of difficulty in urinating would suggest the diagnosis of epidural spinal-cord compression.

Examination of the Site of the Pain

There is no substitute for a careful physical and neurologic examination to provide objective data and to substantiate the clinical history. The neurologic examination is particularly useful in differentiating local pain from referred pain and peripheral-nerve involvement from plexus or cord involvement. For example, in a patient with low-back pain and radicular symptoms, reflex changes may suggest root rather than plexus disease.

Use of the Appropriate Diagnostic Tools

Since the diagnosis of metastatic disease may be elusive, the limitations of the available diagnostic procedures should be recognized by the physician ordering such studies. Plain X-rays are a useful screening procedure, but a normal study should not overrule a strong clinical impression of bony metastases. There must be a 40 to 60% change in bone density to detect changes on X-ray, and pain can occur with lesser changes. The bone scan provides a more sensitive method for demonstrating abnormalities often 3 to 4 months before changes appear on plain films. Plain X-rays are inadequate to assess certain areas of the body where bone shadows overlap, such as the base of the skull, C_7-T_1 area, and sacrum. Tomography is necessary to discern bony changes in such areas. Computerized transaxial tomography (CT scan) allows for even further detailed visualization of soft tissue and bone and is rapidly becoming the procedure of choice to evaluate the retroperitoneal, paravertebral, pelvic, and skull-base areas. Cisternal and lumbar myelography and cerebrospinal fluid (CSF) cytologic evaluation are other diagnostic procedures which can further help to delineate the pain diagnosis. These diagnostic procedures should be personally reviewed with the specialist interpreting them to ensure adequate visualization of the area under study.

Evaluation of the Extent of Disease

A clear evaluation of the extent of metastatic disease may help to confirm the diagnosis of a specific pain syndrome. For example, in a patient with carcinoma of the colon, perineal pain and negative X-rays and the presence of a rising CEA antigen can suggest local nerve infiltration as the etiology of pain. It is important to remember that the incidence of second primary tumors is increased in patients with a past history of cancer, and in patients in whom the presentation is atypical or the response to therapy different from predicted, needle biopsy or surgical exploration should be performed to establish a tissue diagnosis.

Early Treatment of Cancer Pain

Establishing an accurate diagnosis is the key to providing appropriate therapy, and a cooperative patient is necessary to facilitate this workup. Generally analgesics are the mainstay of therapy, and adequate pain-control will allow the patient to undergo the necessary diagnostic procedures. In patients with epidural spinal-cord compression or diffuse, painful bony metastases, high-dose steroids dramatically relieve their pain, with a concomitant reduction in their analgesic-drug requirements.

SPECIFIC PAIN SYNDROMES IN PATIENTS WITH CANCER: PAIN ASSOCIATED WITH DIRECT TUMOR INVOLVEMENT

Tumor Infiltration of Bone

Pain from invasion of bone by either primary or metastatic tumor is the most common cause of pain in patients with cancer. The pain may be the presenting complaint, as for example in patients with multiple myeloma, or it may represent the first sign of metastatic disease, as occurs in patients with carcinoma of the breast. The patient may have his pain at the site of the lesion, e.g., rib pain, or the pain may be absent locally but referred to a distant area of the body, e.g., knee pain associated with metastatic hip disease. The characteristics of the pain vary with the site involved, but in general the pain is constant and usually grows progressively more severe. A detailed description of pain in metastatic bone disease is beyond the scope of this chapter. However, several important pain syndromes are often misdiagnosed because physicians are unfamiliar with the characteristic signs and symptoms. Some of these syndromes are considered below:

Metastases to the Base of Skull

The syndromes reported here all share two common features. Pain is the earliest complaint, often preceding neurologic signs and symptoms by several weeks to months, and documentation with plain X-rays is often difficult.

Syndromes

Jugular-foramen syndrome. Occipital pain, often referred to the vertex of the head and ipsilateral shoulder and arm, is an early presenting symptom. The pain is often exacerbated by head movement and associated with local tenderness over the occipital condyle. The patient's signs and symptoms vary with the cranial nerve involved, but can include hoarseness, dysarthria, dysphagia, neck and shoulder weakness, and ptosis. The neurologic examination can help to localize the lesion by determining the function of the IXth, Xth, XIth, and XIIth cranial nerves since involvement of all four of these nerves suggests jugular foramen and hypoglossal-canal involvement with secondary nerve dysfunction. The presence of a Horner's syndrome suggests sympathetic involvement extracranially but in close proximity to the jugular foramen.

Clivus metastases. Pain characterized by a vertex headache exacerbated by neck flexion is a common mode of presentation of this entity. Lower-cranial-nerve dysfunction (VIth–XIIth) usually begins unilaterally, but often progresses to bilateral lower-cranial-nerve dysfunction.

Sphenoid-sinus metastases. Severe bifrontal headache radiating to both temples, with intermittent retro-orbital pain, suggests this entity. The patient often complains of nasal stuffiness or a sense of fullness in the head, with a concomitant diplopia. The neurologic sign of unilateral or bilateral VIth nerve palsy helps further to suggest the diagnosis.

Diagnostic Workup

Base-of-skull metastases occur more commonly in patients with nasopharyngeal tumors, but can occur with any tumor type which metastasizes to bone. A lateral X-ray of the neck to assess the retropharyngeal space is an important aspect of the initial workup. Tomography of the skull and CT scan are the procedures of choice to delineate body changes and associated soft-tissue masses. At times, biopsy of the nasopharynx or sphenoid sinus may be necessary to establish the tumor diagnosis.

Differential Diagnosis

Primary nerve and bone tumors (e.g., meningioma, neurofibroma, or chordoma) are commonly associated with these syndromes and should be differentiated from metastatic disease. Meningeal carcinomatosis should be similarly ruled out by CSF cytologic evaluation.

Metastases to Vertebral Bodies

These syndromes share the common feature of pain as an early symptom which, if not accurately diagnosed, may lead to irreversible neurologic deficits, e.g., paraplegia.

Cervical Vertebrae

Subluxation of the atlas. Metastatic disease involving the odontoid process of the axis (C_1 vertebral body) can result in a pathologic fracture with secondary subluxation of it and resulting spinal-cord or brainstem compression. The early symptoms include severe neck pain radiating over the posterior aspect of the skull to the vertex, exacerbated by movement, particularly flexion of the neck. Neurologic signs include progressive sensory and motor signs beginning in the upper extremities with associated autonomic dysfunction. Neck-manipulation in these patients is dangerous, and tomography is generally necessary to confirm the diagnosis.

C_7-T_1 *metastasis*. Pain originating from metastatic disease to the C_7-T_1 vertebral bodies is usually localized to the adjacent paraspinal area and characterized by a constant, dull, aching pain radiating bilaterally to both shoulders. There may be tenderness to percussion over the spinous process at this level. With nerve-root compression, radicular pain in the C_7-C_8-T_1 distribution occurs most commonly unilaterally in the posterior arm, elbow, and ulnar aspect of the hand. The neurologic symptoms include paresthesias and numbness in the 4th and 5th fingers, with progressive hand weakness and triceps weakness. The presence of a Horner's syndrome suggests paravertebral sympathetic involvement. Metastatic bone disease at this level results from either hematogenous spread to bone or, more commonly, from tumor originating in the brachial plexus or paravertebral space and spreading along the nerves to the contiguous vertebral body and epidural space.

Diagnostic workup. Plain X-rays of the cervical and thoracic spine do not provide adequate visualization of the C_7-T_1 area because of overlapping cardiac and bony structures. Coned-down views, tomography, or CT scan, in that order, may be necessary to define the presence of metastatic disease. In patients with bilateral radicular symptoms or signs of spinal-cord dysfunction, myelography should be performed to rule out an associated epidural spinal-cord compression.

Lumbar

L_1 *metastases*. Dull, aching mid-back pain exacerbated by lying or sitting and relieved by standing is the usual presenting complaint. Radicular pain in a girdle-like manner anteriorly or to both paraspinal lumbosacral areas may also be present. Occasionally patients will have only pain referred to the sacroiliac joint and/or the superior iliac crest. Lack of knowledge of these referred points for L_1 disease leads to inappropriate X-rays of the sacroiliac joint and iliac crest, without visualization of the L_1 area.

Diagnostic workup. AP, lateral, and oblique views of the lumbar spine, bone scan, and tomography, in order, should be the diagnostic approach. Myelography may be necessary to define the presence of epidural disease.

Sacral metastases. Aching pain, beginning insidiously, in the low back or coccygeal region, exacerbated by lying or sitting and relieved by walking is the common clinical complaint. Increasing pain, with the neurologic signs and symptoms of perianal sensory loss, bowel and bladder dysfunction, and impotence help to localize the site of disease.

Diagnostic workup. Plain X-rays of the sacrum are usually inadequate. AP and lateral tomography of the sacrum and the CT scan are the most useful diagnostic procedures in evaluating metastatic disease in this region. A barium enema and IVP can also be helpful to define the presence of presacral tumors.

Differential Diagnosis

Degenerative disc disease, osteoporosis, and epidural spinal-cord compression are the common differential diagnoses to consider in patients with cancer and complaints of neck or back pain from metastatic bony disease.

Degenerative disc disease rarely occurs at the C_7, T_1 or L_1 areas, and this fact should suggest a need for further workup of pain complaints involving these areas. Osteoporosis can often mimic the signs and symptoms of metastatic bone disease. Radiographic differentiation of these two entities can also be difficult, particularly in the case of vertebral-body collapse. Bone scans are positive in both metastatic and osteoporotic vertebral-body collapse. Tomography and CT scanning have been more useful in delineating the nature of the collapse. Tomography in osteoporotic vertebral-body disease reveals intact vertebral-body bony plates and symmetrical bony collapse, in contrast to metastatic disease where the vertebral plates are eroded with associated pedicle destruction and asymmetric collapse of the vertebral body.

Epidural spinal-cord compression is associated with vertebral-body metastases in 85% of patients (5), and a careful neurologic history and examination can help to establish evidence of spinal-cord dysfunction. If there are signs of neurologic dysfunction, myelography should be performed to delineate the extent of epidural disease and to define the appropriate radiation portals.

Tumor Infiltration of Peripheral Nerve, Plexus, Root or Cord

Peripheral Nerve

Constant, burning pain with hypesthesia and dysesthesia in the area of sensory loss is the usual clinical presentation. Tumor compression of peripheral nerve proximally occurs most commonly in association with paravertebral or retroperitoneal tumor. The pain is radicular and unilateral, and a careful sensory examination can often delineate the site of nerve compression. Metastatic tumor in rib often produces intercostal nerve involvement. In this entity, pain is the earliest symptom, with progressive sensory loss distal to the site of nerve compression.

Brachial Plexus

Radicular pain in the shoulder and arm is the earliest presenting symptom. This syndrome, often referred to as the superior pulmonary sulcus or pancoast syndrome, results from tumor infiltration of the lower brachial plexus. It is characterized by pain radiating to the ipsilateral shoulder, posterior aspect of the arm and elbow, in a C_8-T_1 distribution. The neurologic symptoms of pain and paresthesias in the fourth and fifth fingers may precede objective clinical signs for several weeks to months. These paresthesias progress to numbness and weakness in a C_7, C_8, T_1 distribution. The supraclavicular and axillary regions may be normal. The presence of a Horner's syndrome suggests involvement of the sympathetic chain in the paravertebral space.

Diagnostic Workup

This should include a chest X-ray with apical lordotic views, coned-down views of the C_7-T_1 area, and a bone scan. In certain instances, tomography and CT scan are more sensitive to delineate a mass in this region. It is not uncommon for tumor to spread along the nerve root into the epidural space and, if epidural extension is suspected, myelography may be necessary to define the extent of tumor infiltration. This information is particularly useful in defining the ports for radiation therapy. Needle biopsy or surgical exploration may be necessary to ascertain a tissue diagnosis.

The differential diagnoses include brachial neuritis, rotator-cuff tear at the shoulder joint, cervical-disc disease, and radiation fibrosis. They are the common pain syndromes which are often misdiagnosed in patients who have brachial plexus tumor infiltration. Each of these syndromes has characteristic neurologic signs and symptoms and has been previously well described (1,13–15).

Lumbar Plexus Tumor Infiltration

This entity occurs most commonly in patients with genitourinary, gynecologic, and colonic cancers from local tumor extension into adjacent lymph nodes and bone. The pain varies with the site of plexus involvement and is generally of two types: radicular pain in an $L_{1,2,3}$ distribution to the anterior thigh and groin, or down the posterior aspect of the leg to the heel in an L_5-S_1 distribution. Referred pain without local pain may also occur and presents a more difficult diagnostic problem. L_1 pain has been discussed previously. Pain in the anterior thigh, lateral aspect of the calf or heel, and associated palpable local tenderness are often misinterpreted as suggesting local pathology. X-rays and bone scan of these tender areas are often taken without clear awareness that these pains represent referred pain from lumbar plexus tumor infiltration. The neurologic symptoms include paresthesias followed by numbness and dysesthesias, with progressive motor and sensory loss in a plexus distribution. The presence of asymmetric or absent reflexes on neurologic examination often suggests root involvement. The absence of palpable tumor in the pelvis or groin does not preclude the diagnosis.

Diagnostic Workup

Since nerves are not radio-dense, X-rays in general are often unhelpful in discerning tumor infiltration in nerve plexuses, and one must rely on changes in contiguous bony or soft-tissue structures to suggest tumor infiltration. Tomography and CT scanning are more appropriate to define soft-tissue masses or bony abnormalities in the lumbosacral and pelvic regions. Specific studies like lymphangiography and certain radionuclide scans (gallium scan in patients with Hodgkin's disease) may give the necessary added information to suggest the presence of tumor in adjacent lymph tissue. At times, all of these radiographic studies may be negative, and to ascertain the diagnosis, surgical exploration and biopsy may be necessary. As previously noted, tumor infiltration of the epidural space may occur from infiltration along contiguous nerve roots. Myelography may be required to rule out the extension of tumor from lumbar plexus into the epidural lumbar space, to allow for appropriate radiation ports to be established, and for adequate treatment to be given.

The differential diagnosis includes most commonly lumbar neuritis, postsurgical lumbar plexopathy, radiation fibrosis, and lumbar-disc disease. Each of these entities has a characteristic neurologic presentation and should be differentiated from tumor infiltration of the lumbar plexus.

Sacral Plexus Tumor Infiltration

Dull, aching midline pain with sensory loss beginning in the perianal area is the usual clinical presentation. This entity occurs more commonly in patients with colonic, genitourinary or gynecologic cancers. The sensory findings are initially unilateral, with progression to bilateral sacral sensory loss and autonomic dysfunction including impotence and bowel and bladder dysfunction.

Diagnostic Workup

Sacral tomography in the anterior-posterior plane and CT scan are the procedures of choice in evaluating this area. Neither procedure can delineate sacral nerves except to define pre- or postsacral masses and bony destruction in proximity to the sacral nerves. Surgical exploration or needle biopsy may be necessary to establish a tissue diagnosis.

The differential diagnosis includes posttraumatic neuromas in patients with previous local surgery, localized infection, radiation fibrosis, and a series of syndromes characterized as the tension myalgias of the pelvic floor.

Meningeal Carcinomatosis

This is a clinical entity in which there is tumor infiltration of the cerebrospinal leptomeninges with or without concomitant invasion of the parenchyma of the nervous system (10). Pain occurs in 40% of patients and is generally of two types: (a) headache with or without neck stiffness characterized by a constant pain; and (b) back pain most commonly localized to the low back and buttock regions. Pain results from traction on tumor infiltrated nerves and meninges.

Diagnostic Workup

Lumbar puncture is the procedure of choice to detect malignant cells in the cerebrospinal fluid (CSF) of such patients. An elevated CSF protein and low glucose concentration are often associated findings. In patients with low-back and buttock pain, myelography can be helpful to delineate tumor nodules along the nerves in the cauda equina.

The differential diagnosis varies with the site of neurologic involvement. However, in patients with known cancer, signs and symptoms of neurologic dysfunction at several levels of the neuraxis should suggest this possible diagnosis. Alternate considerations may include fungal meningitis, cauda-equina epidural tumor, and arachnoiditis.

Epidural Spinal-Cord Compression

Severe neck and back pain is the hallmark of this entity. Gilbert et al. (5) reviewed 130 patients with epidural spinal-cord compression and found that pain was the initial symptom in 96% of patients, and in 10% was the only symptom of this entity. The pain occurs from local bone or root compression and is generally of two types: (a) local pain occurring over the involved vertebral body; or (b) radicular pain occurring unilaterally in patients with cervical or lumbosacral compression, and bilaterally in patients with thoracic cord compression. The neurologic symptoms vary with the site of epidural disease and commonly include motor weakness progressing to paraplegia, a sensory level, and loss of bowel and bladder function. Eighty-five percent of patients in Gilbert's series had associated vertebral-body tumor.

Diagnostic Workup

Plain X-rays of the spine do not delineate the integrity of the epidural space, and lumbar and cisternal myelography are necessary diagnostic procedures to delineate the extent of the epidural block. It is imperative to define the full extent of epidural tumor to provide the appropriate treatment. Epidural tumor often extends beyond the level of associated vertebral-body metastasis and may be independent of bone disease, and these observations have supported the need for myelographic definition of the problem.

PAIN SYNDROMES ASSOCIATED WITH CANCER THERAPY

This category includes those clinical pain syndromes which occur in the course of, or subsequent to, treatment of cancer patients with the common modalities of surgery, chemotherapy, or radiation therapy. The onset of pain to the cancer patient who fears recurrent tumor and to the physician unfamiliar with the clinical presentation of these nonmalignant syndromes portends a serious clinical problem.

Postsurgery Pain

Postthoracotomy Pain

Pain in the distribution of an intercostal nerve following surgical injury or interruption occurs in a small percentage of patients undergoing thoracotomy. The incidence of this entity is unknown. Pain becomes evident 1 to 2 months following the surgical procedure and is characterized by a constant pain in the area of sensory loss with occasional intermittent shock-like pains. Dysesthesias in the scar area, with hypesthesia in the surrounding zone, are often prominent symptoms. Movement exacerbates the pain, and these patients may develop a concomitant frozen shoulder characterized by limitation of movement at the shoulder joint and disuse atrophy of the arm. Early recognition of this syndrome and its sequelae can often prevent the development of further shoulder limitation.

Diagnostic Workup

The diagnostic workup should include a careful history to delineate the onset of the pain as well as the appropriate radiographic views, including plain X-rays, tomography, or CT scan, to rule out recurrent disease. Disuse atrophy of the humerus has a characteristic appearance on plain X-rays which should not be confused with metastatic disease, although the bone scan is positive in this entity as well. We have observed several instances in which, because of the clinical symptoms of pain and limitation at the shoulder joint, the X-ray findings of the humerus were interpreted as metastatic disease and patients were radiated for disuse atrophy of the arm without evidence of metastatic disease.

Differential diagnosis includes tumor infiltration of the peripheral nerve, rib, chest wall or paravertebral space. Awareness of the postthoracotomy pain syndrome and a careful history are essential to early diagnosis.

Postmastectomy Pain

Pain in the posterior arm, axilla, and anterior chest wall in patients following radical mastectomy occurs from interruption of the intercostobrachial nerve, a cutaneous branch of T_1 nerves. The onset of pain is usually 1 to 2 months following the surgical procedure and is more common in patients with a complicated postoperative course of either excessive local swelling or infection. The pain is characterized as a tight, constricting, burning pain in the posterior arm and axilla which radiates across the anterior chest wall. There is usually no associated lymphedema of the arm. The pain is exacerbated by arm movement, and patients often posture the arm in a flexed position close to the chest wall. As occurs in postthoracotomy pain, a frozen shoulder may develop, producing a second problem of increased pain and limitation of movement at the shoulder joint.

Diagnostic Workup

The diagnostic workup should include a careful history to delineate the onset of the pain as well as the appropriate radiographic workup of plain X-rays, tomography, or CT scan to rule out recurrent disease.

The differential diagnosis includes tumor infiltration of the brachial plexus, but the clinical history should make the diagnosis.

Postradical Neck Dissection Pain

Pain following radical neck dissection occurs from surgical injury or interruption of the cervical nerves. The pain is characterized by a constant burning sensation in the area of sensory loss. Dysesthesias and intermittent shock-like pain may also be present.

Diagnostic Workup

This should include a careful history of the onset of pain and appropriate X-rays of the painful area to rule out recurrent disease. Recurrent tumor involving the cervical spine or base of the skull is the major differential diagnosis.

Phantom-limb Pain

Pain following surgical amputation of a limb is generally of two types: stump pain and phantom-limb pain. These painful clinical entities are separate from phantom-limb sensation, which occurs in all patients following limb amputation. The true incidence of phantom-limb pain in patients following amputation for cancer is unknown. The phantom-limb pain is usually characterized by a burning, cramping pain in the phantom limb, often identical in nature and location to preoperative pain. The underlying mechanisms of such pain are controversial (2).

Diagnostic Workup

This should include a careful definition of the phantom-limb pain, and etiological factors such as local stump pathology.

Postchemotherapy Pain

The group includes a series of pain problems which occur in cancer patients receiving chemotherapy. The major features of each of these entities is briefly described below.

Peripheral Neuropathy

Painful dysesthesias following treatment with the *Vinca* alkaloid drugs occur as part of a symmetrical polyneuropathy (11). Both vincristine and vinblastine are neurotoxic drugs in the doses required to achieve an antineoplastic effect. The dysesthesias are commonly localized to the hands and feet, and are characterized by burning pain exacerbated by superficial stimuli. In children, a more diffuse syndrome occurs from the use of these drugs. It is characterized by generalized myalgias and arthralgias, often beginning with jaw pain and progressing to a symmetrical polyneuropathy including cranial-nerve dysfunction.

Steroid Pseudo-rheumatism

This entity occurs from both rapid and slow withdrawal of steroid medications in patients taking these drugs for either short or long periods of time (12). The syndrome consists of prominent diffuse myalgias and arthralgias, with muscle and joint tenderness on palpation but without objective inflammatory signs. A sense of generalized malaise and fatigue is a common feature of this entity. These signs and symptoms revert with reinstitution of the steroid medication.

Aseptic Necrosis of Bone

Both aseptic necrosis of the humoral and, much more commonly, the femoral head are known complications of cancer therapy, specifically chronic steroid therapy (6). Pain in the shoulder or knee and leg are the common presenting complaints, with X-ray changes occurring several weeks to months after the onset of pain. Limitation of joint movements, with progressive inability to use the arm or hip functionally, is the natural history of this illness. It occurs most commonly in patients with Hodgkin's disease, although it can occur in any patient on chronic steroid therapy. The bone scan is the most useful diagnostic procedure and is usually positive before changes in the plain films appear.

Post-herpetic Neuralgia

This is a well-described clinical entity (9) characterized by pain which persists after the cutaneous eruptions from herpes zoster infection have cleared. In patients with cancer, herpes zoster infection commonly occurs in the area of tumor pathology or in the port of previous radiation therapy. The true incidence of post-herpetic neuralgia in patients with cancer is unknown, but it appears to be more common in patients who develop the infection after the age of 50. There are generally three types of pain: (a) a continuous, burning pain in the area of sensory loss, (b) painful dysesthesias, and (c) intermittent, shock-like pain.

Postradiation Therapy Pain

Radiation Fibrosis of the Brachial Plexus

Pain occurring in the distribution of the brachial plexus following radiation therapy (RT) occurs from fibrosis of the surrounding connective tissue and secondary injury to nerve (13,14). It may appear as early as 6 months or as late as 20 years following radiation treatments. It represents a difficult diagnostic problem in that it must be differentiated from recurrent tumor. The clinical symptoms include complaints of numbness or paresthesias in the hand, usually in a C_{5-6} distribution. Pain occurs later in the course of this clinical entity and is often characterized as diffuse arm pain. Lymphedema in the arm and radiation skin changes and induration of the supraclavicular and axillary areas are often present. The neurologic signs include sensory changes in a $C_{5,6,7}$ distribution, with motor weakness most prominent in the deltoid and biceps muscles. These signs progress to the development of a painful, useless, swollen extremity. In contrast, tumor infiltration of the brachial plexus presents with pain as its earliest symptom, with sensory changes in a C_8-T_1 distribution and motor weakness beginning distally rather than proximally. The associated signs with radiation injury include evidence on X-ray of radiation injury to the lung, rib, or humerus. These findings may help to confirm a history of radiation injury in the absence of appropriate radiation data.

Radiation Fibrosis of Lumbar Plexus

Pain occurring in the leg from radiation fibrosis of the lumbar plexus represents a similar diagnostic problem of radiation injury versus recurrent tumor. Pain occurring late in the course of progressive motor and sensory changes in the leg is more common with radiation fibrosis but is not the most reliable clinical symptom. A previous history of radiation treatment and local skin changes or lymphedema of the leg with X-ray changes demonstrating radiation necrosis of bone may help to establish this diagnosis.

The diagnostic workup to differentiate nerve fibrosis from nerve infiltration by tumor should include plain X-rays of the area to delineate radiation changes in bone or evidence of recurrent metastatic disease. The CT scan has not been helpful in this differential diagnosis except to define an enlarging soft-tissue mass, representing tumor in the area in question or recurrent bony erosion. In certain instances, surgical exploration may be necessary, particularly in patients free of known metastatic disease, to determine further cancer management.

Radiation Myelopathy

Pain is an early symptom in 15% of patients with this entity (7). The pain may be localized to the area of spinal-cord damage or may be referred pain, with dysesthesias below the level of injury. Clinically, the neurologic symptoms and signs are that of a Brown-Sequard syndrome (ipsilateral motor paresis with contralateral sensory loss with a cervical or thoracic level) which progresses to a complete transverse myelopathy. The diagnostic workup should include careful plain X-rays of the spine and myelography, both of which are usually normal. Occasionally widening of the cord at the injured area may be noted. The differential diagnoses include intramedullary tumor, epidural spinal-cord compression, arteriovenous malformation, or a transverse myelitis.

Radiation-induced Peripheral-nerve Tumors

A painful, enlarging mass in an area of pervious irradiation suggests this entity. We have reported a series of 9 radiation-induced nerve tumors (7 malignant and 2 atypical schwannomas) occurring 4 to 20 years following RT (3). Seven of the 9 patients presented with pain and a progressive neurologic deficit, with a palpable mass involving the brachial or lumbar plexus. Surgical exploration and biopsy is necessary to establish this diagnosis. The important differential diagnoses include radiation fibrosis and recurrent tumor.

PAIN UNRELATED TO CANCER OR CANCER THERAPY

Approximately 3% of the pain syndromes which occur in cancer patients have no relationship to the underlying cancer or cancer therapy. Degenerative disc disease, thoracic and abdominal aneurysms, and diffuse osteoporosis are the most common noncancer pain syndromes observed. This category serves to emphasize the point that pain in a cancer patient does not necessarily imply recurrent or persistent disease, and it supports the thesis that a careful diagnostic evaluation in the cancer patient is necessary to define the specific pain syndrome before embarking on a therapeutic course.

REFERENCES

1. Cailliet, R. (1966): *Shoulder Pain.* F. A. Davis, Philadelphia.
2. Carlen, P. L., Wall, P. D., Nadvorna, H., and Steinbach, T. (1978): Phantom limbs and related phenomena in recent traumatic amputations. *Neurology,* 28:211–217.
3. Foley, K. M., Woodruff, J. M., Ellis, F., and Posner, J. B. (1975): Radiation-induced malignant and atypical schwannomas. *Neurology,* 25:354.
4. Foley, K. M., Roger, A., and Houde, R. W. (1978): Pain in patients with cancer: A quantitative reappraisal. *Proc. Am. Soc. Cancer Res.,* 19:357.
5. Gilbert, R. W., Kim, J-H., and Posner, J. B. (1978): Epidural spinal cord compression from metastatic tumor: diagnosis and treatment. *Ann. Neurol.,* 3:40–51.
6. Ihde, D. C., and DeVita, V. T. (1975): Osteonecrosis of the femoral head in patients with lymphoma treated with intermittent combination chemotherapy (including corticosteroids). *Cancer,* 36:1585–1588.
7. Jellinger, K., and Sturm, K. W. (1971); Delayed radiation myelopathy in man. *J. Neurol. Sci.,* 14:389–408.
8. Lipman, A. (1975): Drug therapy in terminally ill patients. *Am. J. Hosp. Pharm.,* 32:270–276.
9. Noordenbos, W. (1959): *Pain,* pp. 68–89. Elsevier, Amsterdam.
10. Olson, M. E., Chernik, N. L., and Posner, J. B. (1974): Infiltration of the leptomeninges by systemic cancer: A clinical and pathological study. *Arch. Neurol.,* 30:122–137.
11. Rosenthal, S., and Kaufman, S. (1974): Vincristine neurotoxicity. *Ann. Int. Med.,* 80:733–737.
12. Rotstein, J., and Good, R. A. (1957): Steroid pseudorheumatism. *Arch. Int. Med.,* 99:545–555.
13. Stoll, B. A., and Andrews, J. T. (1966): Radiation-induced peripheral neuropathy. *Br. Med. J.,* 1:834–837.
14. Thomas, T. E., and Colby, M. Y. (1972): Radiation-induced or metastatic brachial plexopathy: A diagnostic dilemma. *JAMA,* 222:1392–1395.
15. Tsairis, P., Dyck, P. J., and Mulder, D. M. (1972): The natural history of brachial neuropathy. *Arch. Neurol.,* 27:109–117.

The Role of Cerebral Cortex in the Pain of Advanced Cancer

C. V. Morpurgo

Istituto Ortopedico G. Pini, Piazza Card. Ferrari 1, 20122 Milan, Italy

Pain has an important biologic function in the organism's defense against external and internal noxious events. However, when cancer is the noxious agent, pain often fails to signal the onset of the disease in time for successful therapy. On the contrary, it usually becomes intense and extremely difficult to treat in the advanced stages of cancer.

What role does the cerebral cortex play in such a situation? Our experimental and clinical observations suggest the following hypotheses: a) body areas with a small cortical representation have late onset of pain when cancer occurs; b) constant pain can induce an increase in the cortical representation of the affected area.

Moreover we have noticed that if the patient has had previous significant pain experiences in proximity of the body area affected by cancer, there is a high incidence of "incorrect" referred pain. In these particular cases the perception of the correct site of the noxious stimuli produced by the cancer will occur very late.

Recent neurophysiologic and psychophysiologic data have called attention to the structural changes taking place in the central nervous system (CNS) when the subject must cope with unusual situations (2,4,9). When repetitive unusual experiences occur during the period of growth, irreversible changes in the cortex can take place (10). The relative permanence of changes due to early experiences during initial developmental periods is well known to behavioral scientists. Recent findings indicate that this phenomenon also influences perceptual functions, including pain (7,11).

At birth only small parts of the cortex are committed to specific tasks. The rest will be shaped by experience. If part of this experience is repetitive and is related to the endeavours of the subject to adjust to the environment or to fight it, an increasing number of neurons become specified for that particular task so that the organism is able to accomplish it skillfully (5).

Some groups of neurons maintain functional flexibility; others are so highly specific that they can perform only a single task. After months or years these neurons, excited by nonspecific stimuli, will produce the perception of the specific stimulus that caused the changes in the brain.

The term *plasticity* is used by neurophysiologists to define the permanent modifications occurring in the functional units of the brain when excited by repetitive experiences relevant for the subject. Plasticity probably implies the strengthening of some synapses and the weakening of others in order to develop mechanisms that permit skillful performance of complex functions of the cortex (memory, recognition, decision, learning). We consider perception related to these high functions.

The plastic changes, when well consolidated, will become "unerasable" or irreversible.

Plasticity means flexibility to become specific. This can occur in relationship to unusual experiences: In this case plasticity will involve uncommitted units as well as neurons which in the normal individual are specified for a different task.

When specified by a long-lasting experience in the early stages of life (6,13) at which time plasticity is marked, the functions of a unit cannot be easily changed. However, in the adult, different experiences, even though stronger, will be ineffective because the flexibility of the system is markedly reduced.

Kittens exposed to repetitive noxious stimuli in a body part with small cortical representation have shown a dramatic change of the contralateral cortical representation as compared with the unaffected, opposite side (8). As pain experience continued, larger and larger areas of the cortex became involved and a higher number of neurons became specific to pain.

A second evaluation, after several months without any pain stimuli, revealed persistent alterations in the cortical map, as recorded at the end of the training. These data suggest that at the brain level the pain experiences produce complex mechanisms of perception, involving a large number of neurons and causing an abnormal sensitivity to noxious stimuli.

These changes in cortical projection seem to be supported by concomitant changes of the anatomic aspect of the posterior sigmoidal gyrus observed in the experimental animals.

A corresponding increase in the firing of pain neurons has been recorded by Albe-Fessard (1) in the thalamus in rats experiencing chronic pain due to unilateral deafferentation of the spinal cord from C5 to T2. Moreover, it has been demonstrated very recently that pain itself enhances the plasticity of the CNS. Unpublished findings by Spinelli (12) demonstrate that the training time necessary to alter the function of neurons in visual cortex in kittens can be dramatically reduced to $\frac{1}{30}$ by associating pain with visual stimulation. These observations suggest that the cortical representation of different parts of the body can be modified by the experience of the subject. In the same way the cortical projection of a region chronically affected by pain would be predicted to increase according to the intensity and duration of the noxious stimuli.

This means that a strong, long-lasting pain can produce dramatic, irreversible changes in the perceptual processes and induce an increase in the cortical representation of the affected areas. This will lead the patient to perceive pain differently than a naive patient who has not suffered persistent pain.

Meanwhile the affective and perceptual state of hypersensitivity produced by pain will render unbearable every sensation. So the patient will tend to isolate in a state of sensory deprivation in which pain alone influences the activity of the cerebral cortex. The start of a vicious circle (pain increases the perceptual mechanism → increased perception enhances the sensibility to pain, and so on) must be suspected when a patient tends to isolate himself and focuses all of his attention on pain. At this point, pain is no longer a useful warning signal, but becomes aggressive, unbearable, and difficult to handle. If the circle is not interrupted, pain will become intractable and predominant over all the other symptoms, aggravating the physical and psychic condition of the patient.

This is the end result when the problem of pain is not properly considered and treated promptly.

In order to compare the experimental data with clinical observations, we have reviewed all the patients admitted to the Centro Oncologico of the Instituto Ortopedico G. Pini of Milano. The total number is small because the activity of the section started only two years ago, but it is evident that cancer affecting parts of the body having a larger cortical representation will cause intense pain more frequently than cancer of the viscera with little or no cortical representation.

In agreement with the data presented at this meeting by Dr. Foley (3), 9 (60%) out of our 15 patients with cancer of the femur were resistant to simple treatment with analgesic and required combined therapy for pain relief. It was also noted that cancer and metastases affecting parts of the body well represented on the somatosensory cortex caused severe pain, whereas tumors of the viscera were often painless or produced very little pain. In 3 patients with a long history of pain, the visceral cancer gave rise to "incorrect" referred pain.

Of our group of patients, 50% were hospitalized with major pain problems and only 2 patients had no pain. Pain was severe in 22 of 40 patients who had somatic localizations of the cancer and in only 1 of 15 who had visceral lesions.

It will be important to study a larger number of patients to ascertain: (a) whether more intense pain occurs with lesions in parts with large cortical representation compared with lesions involving parts with small somatosensory cortical representation; (b) whether an earlier experience of pain plays any role in determining the characteristics of a subsequent cancer pain. (In one of our patients a long history of lumbar pain made it very difficult to discover a pancreatic cancer because of an incorrect referred pain, until the outset of the signs of metastatic compression of the right ileo-inguinal nerve).

In future investigations of the role of the cortex in cancer pain we should consider that: (a) Chronic pain can produce changes in the cerebral cortex affecting the mechanism of pain perception; (b) perception of chronic pain arising in the various parts of the body will vary depending on the extent of their cortical projection as predetermined by the genome and determined by repetitive pain experiences; (c) in a cancer patient without any interest in life, chronic pain should be promptly controlled to avoid its natural tendency to become intractable.

CONCLUSIONS

Clinical observations in agreement with experimental neurophysiologic and psychophysiologic data suggest that the cerebral cortex plays an important role in determining the modality of pain perception in patients with advanced cancer.

REFERENCES

1. Albe-Fessard, D. (1978): Personal communication.
2. Dunn, A. J. (1976): Biochemical correlates of training experiences: A discussion of the evidence. In: *Neural Mechanisms of Learning and Memory*, edited by M. R. Rosenzweig, and E. L. Bennett, pp. 311–320. The MIT Press, Cambridge, Mass., and London.
3. Foley, K. (1979): Pain syndromes in patients with cancer. In: *Advances in Pain Research and Therapy, Vol. 2*, edited by J. J. Bonica and V. Ventafridda. Raven Press, New York.
4. Hirsch, H. V. B., and Spinelli, D. N. (1970): Visual experience modifies distribution of horizontally and vertically oriented receptive fields in cats. *Science*, 168:869–871.
5. Hirsch, H. V. B., and Spinelli, D. N. (1971): Modification of the distribution of receptive fields orientation during development. *Exp. Brain Res.*, 13:509–527.
6. Hubel, D. H., and Wiesel, T. N. (1970): The period of susceptibility to the physiological effects of unilateral eye closure in kittens. *J. Physiol. (Lond.)*, 206:419–436.
7. Morpurgo, C. V., and Spinelli, D. N. (1976): Plasticity of pain perception. *Brain Theory Newsletter*, 2:14–15.
8. Morpurgo, C. V., and Spinelli, D. N. (1978): Unpublished data.
9. Pettigrew, J. D., Olsen, C., and Barlow, H. B. (1973): Visual experience without lines: Effect on developing cortical neurons. *Science*, 182:599–601.
10. Spinelli, D. N., Hirsh, H. V. B., Phelps, R. W., and Metzler, J. (1972): Visual experience as a determinant of the response characteristics of cortical receptive fields in cats. *Exp. Brain Res.*, 15:289–304.
11. Spinelli, D. N., Metzler, J., and Phelps, R. W. (1975): Neural correlates of visual experience in single units of cat's visual and somatosensory cortex. *Neurosci. Abstracts, Soc. for Neurosci., 5th Annual Meeting.*
12. Spinelli, D. N. (1978): Personal communication.
13. Wiesel, T. N., and Hubel, D. H. (1965): Extent of recovery from the effects of visual deprivation in kittens. *J. Neurophysiol.*, 28:1060–1072.

Psychologic and Emotional Aspects of Cancer Pain

M. R. Bond

Department of Psychological Medicine, Southern General Hospital, Glasgow. G51 4TF

"Cancers are diseases and pain is a symptom." It is important to keep this statement in mind when discussing emotional aspects of painful malignant disease, because the development of a particular form of it, knowledge of its presence, and its significance to the sufferer produce changes in feelings and behaviour which are altered further by the presence of pain. Moreover, the state of emotion produced by the disease influences the severity of the pain and any changes in the former are reflected in the latter. The way in which an individual responds to illness, and in particular to one of the chronic and possibly painful and potentially fatal cancer group, is determined by his or her premorbid emotional characteristics, experiences of previous illness, and attitudes towards illness amongst members of the family and the cultural group to which he or she belongs.

It has been estimated that cancer is responsible for 20% of all deaths in the United States and other Western countries (22), including Britain. Approximately half the 30,000 who die from cancer each year in Britain have pain, of whom about a quarter experience severe pain at times. The pain is usually chronic but fluctuates in severity, being influenced by many factors, some physical and some psychologic, and it is the latter that are of particular interest and importance and yet so often neglected by those who care for the patient. This is surprising, for as Hanay (9) has pointed out, cancer is one of the most researched disease entities, and moreover it is one viewed with the greatest fear by the general public, one that affects many lives and families and one that is very expensive to Society.

EMOTIONS AND CANCER

The Role of Personality in the Development of Cancer

A considerable amount of time and energy has been devoted to examining the possibility that certain personality attributes predispose towards the development of cancer, a concept which, if it were correct and sufficiently specific, would have important implications for the prevention and treatment of this group of diseases.

Rassidakis and others (22) are of the opinion that certain premorbid personality characteristics are associated with the development of cancer and that these include early childhood conflicts and a sense of isolation through life, inability to express hostile feelings and difficulties in interpersonal relationships, and loss of a close relationship which produces depression and despair. In support of their view they quote Engel (7) who earlier reported that where circumstances in life lead to feelings of hopelessness, an organic illness may ensue. It is certainly true to say that in a situation of this kind, as after a bereavement, the incidence of all forms of ill-health amongst widows during the first year after their husband's death is significantly greater than in nonwidowed women of similar age.

The illness may be mental rather than physical for it has been shown by Brown et al. (5) that a depressive illness may occur where an individual develops feelings of helplessness and lowered self-esteem secondary to the loss of loved ones or important sources of value in life. Perris and Pierce (19) were critical in their analysis of the literature and stated that early attempts to find a "cancer type" rarely made it possible to distinguish among psychologic characteristics which might be causative factors, those which might be typical reactions to any serious disease, and those which showed purely accidental variations.

In a review dealing with possible psychologic precipitants of cancer, Surawicz (26) noted that early searchings for a "specific causogenic personality" were not fruitful insofar as many of the claims initially made have not been substantiated. However, it is accepted that individuals who adapt poorly to psychologic and physical stresses may develop one of several physical diseases, including cancer, and that prior to their onset, anxiety or the state of hopelessness and helplessness predominates.

Hanay (9) commented on another aspect of this issue and pointed out that life events of a stressful kind also determine the extent to which each person attends to his or her body and the nature of an individual's behavior when ill, that is, the way he or she perceives, evaluates, and acts upon messages and sensations of the body. In other words he noted that "illness behavior," the term first used by Mechanic (16), differs from person to person once an illness has been established.

Thus it seems that perhaps the individual who develops the cancer may well do so after a period of emotional stress which produces feelings of helplessness and hopelessness. The same emotional combination also produces depression—a state of mind which reflects capitulation and resignation and which is associated with increased levels of pain when present and a reduced ability to cope with it.

The General Emotional Effects of Cancer

Studies of the emotional characteristics of patients who have cancer reveal several interesting facts. First, those general to all patients with malignant disease; second, those specific to patients who also have pain. Chronic illness, whatever its form, is viewed with foreboding by most individuals, and cancer in particular is associated in the minds of many with pain, destruction, loss and often with death. Individuals are concerned not only about the eventual outcome of their illness but also with the possibility of further suffering, especially severe pain, before their lives end. Thus the disease brings with it a sense of helplessness, a feeling of total inability to control events, and a futility too, making life seem meaningless and bringing difficulties in tolerating pain which itself seems to have no biologic purpose and which is often referred to as "useless pain."

Specific anxieties arise and include fear of separation from the family and friends, loss of work, loss of life's goals, and the consequences of illness for others. Patients fear increasing dependency, loss of their faculties, and mutilation by surgery. In the case of carcinoma of the breast, a form of malignant disease of which members of the public are very aware and afraid and which is associated with severe pain at times in its later stages, Maguire (15) has shown that psychiatric morbidity begins as soon as the afflicted woman notices a breast lump. Amongst patients he studied 52% were moderately to severely anxious at this stage, and only 8% claimed they were free from all anxiety. A quotation from one of his patients crystallizes the reaction of women to the discovery that they have a breast tumour:

I don't know whether it's me or not, but the feeling is just indescribable. Unless you've experienced it you just don't know. . . . I was so frightened. All I could think of was the children. If anything is going to happen to me they're so young, that's what I latched on to. . . . My feelings were indescribable. I think I touched absolute hell, I didn't want to die and I didn't know if I'd got cancer. It's the thing everyone dreads. At first you think it can't be happening to you. Then, by God— it is.

He also commented that patients have to live with the knowledge that they have a disease which is potentially fatal and deal with fears that it may recur after treatment and invade other areas of the body causing pain and other very unpleasant symptoms. They must also deal with the side effects or consequences of treatments themselves, which include mutilation, the production of anesthesia, baldness, failure of bladder function, and major disturbances of other kinds.

EMOTIONS AND CANCER PAIN

The General Emotional Effects of Chronic Pain

The presence of chronic pain whether arising from benign or malignant diseases causes individuals to become withdrawn, introspective, and neurotically depressed. Many exhibit hostility and anger, which is an important emotion, for as Pilowsky and Spence (21) have shown, those who suppress anger tend to have more affective disturbance than those who experience and express it. Pain also causes increased preoccupation with other physical symptoms; in other words it leads to hypochondriasis. Examination of the effects of chronic pain on personality as measured by the Eysenck Personality Inventory or the Minnesota Multiphasic Personality Inventory reveals that it causes an increase in levels of neuroticism (2,11,14,23) and that the level of neuroticism falls when pain is relieved (11,24).

As a consequence of debility and lessened mobility there is less contact with friends and a reduction in social activities. The pattern of coping behavior adopted by any given person varies depending upon his or her premorbid personality characteristics; for example, some become dependent upon their family and friends to an unnecessary extent, whereas others attempt to do more than is compatible with their physical and emotional state.

Emotional Changes in Patients with Cancer Pain

The difficulties imposed by the exhausting and stressful nature of painful malignant disease deter many from working with patients with this form of ill-health, and as a result there are relatively few papers dealing with the psychologic characteristics of cancer patients with pain. However available studies show that, as in the case of patients with chronic pain due to benign disorders, most sufferers from painful cancer have raised levels of neuroticism. However, Kissen and Eysenck (12) and Bond and Pearson (4) have reported that men with lung cancer and women with cancer of the cervix, respectively, who were pain-free, had extremely low levels of emotionality. Both groups argued this is due to operation of the mental mechanism of denial brought about by exposure of the patient to the intolerable stresses imposed by the illness they suffer. Further, Bond (3) notes that this is not a permanent change, for he has observed that low levels of neuroticism in some cancer patients with intractable pain rise after the pain is relieved by percutaneous cervical cordotomy. The scores of patients with high levels of neuroticism fell after operation, leaving an overall impression that personality factors are distorted by the presence of severe illness and pain and that in the case of the latter, some restoration in the direction of normality of personality is achieved if it is relieved.

Woodforde and Fielding (28) examined cancer patients with and without pain using the Cornell Medical Index and demonstrated that the former group were significantly more emotionally disturbed than the latter and that they responded least well to treatment of their cancer and died sooner. The main cause of emotional morbidity was found to be depression, although hypochondriasis and psychosomatic symptoms were also recorded. They were uncertain whether the depression was a primary or secondary event but commented that the combination of intractable pain and depression represents symptoms that indicate a state of helplessness, of inability to cope with the disease, damage to the body, and the threat to life, and that, as was stated earlier, this is a response to having a progressive and potentially fatal illness. The implication of these observations is that if each individual's confidence and self-esteem can be restored by the provision of appropriate and alternative goals, the level of suffering may be reduced. This has been reported by Goldfarb et al. (8) and Blumberg et al. (1), although their findings were not conclusive.

Regarding hypochondriasis, it is a state of mind in which there is absorption with physical and mental symptoms. Kenyon (10) suggests that the word *hypochondriasis* implies that "hypochondriacal traits, symptoms, ideas and fears should carry with them the implication that there is morbid preoccupation with mental and bodily functions or state of health." Pilowsky (20) takes the view that, in broad terms, hypochondriasis is a specific set of attitudes towards health and showed that cancer patients have higher levels of hypochondriasis than healthy people and nonhypochondriacal psychiatric patients. Raised levels of hypochondriasis in cancer patients with pain were recorded by Bond (2) in patients who also had high levels of neuroticism as measured by the Eysenck Personality Inventory. He also showed that the lowest levels of hypochondriasis were found in pain-free cancer patients who exhibited low levels of emotionality. Looked at in another way, the degree of pain and neuroticism irrespective of its form correlate highly—the more neurotic the patient, the greater is his or her pain. This relationship is well known and is fundamental to the psychologic and pharmacologic methods of pain-relief based upon reduction of emotional tension.

The Consequences of Physical Treatment upon Emotion in Cancer Patients

Physical treatments available for patients with painful malignant diseases include drugs of various kinds and in particular analgesics, surgery, radiation therapy, and the use of cytotoxic drugs. Each form of treatment has its hazards, and these are increased where multiple therapies are in use. It is not possible to comment in detail on all forms of therapy, and indeed there are relatively few papers in the literature dealing with the emotional consequences of the treatment of cancer and even fewer dealing with the specific emotional and social needs of patients receiving treatment and those who have had treatment (15).

Considering surgery, it is undoubtedly true that if successful in relieving pain and other symptoms this form of treatment lessens patients' emotional tensions and reactions to their disease. However it is often not appreciated that a considerable number of patients have persistent emotional symptoms, and unfortunately these may go unheeded. For example, Lee and Maguire (13) reported that after surgery for breast cancer as many as one-third of the patients had significant levels of anxiety and that marital problems and sexual difficulties actually increased in the year after operation. They also showed that the husbands of the women they studied exhibited an increased level of emotional disturbance matching that of their partner. Devlin et al. (6) made similar comments about patients undergoing surgery for anorectal cancer, noting the adverse emotional and social effects of colostomy. Thus it has been estimated that at least 1 in 4 patients who have had a mastectomy or surgery for rectal cancer develop depressive illness, anxiety neurosis, sexual problems, or marital difficulties.

In the case of radiation treatment, Peck and Boland (18) found that among 50 patients, 60% of whom had been told they had cancer, all arrived unprepared for their treatment and as a consequence they believed that radiation treatment was "bad news," that it was potentially dangerous and damaging and could actually cause cancer, and seldom believed that it would produce a cure. After treatment only a third felt it had improved their health; and whereas 60% had evidence of depression and anxiety beforehand, this increased to 80% immediately after treatment.

The Consequences of Staff-Patient Interactions upon Emotion and Pain

These observations lead naturally to a consideration of what individual patients feel about those who are responsible for treating them in terms of dealing with their anxieties and fantasies about the illness and treatment to be given. Mitchell and Glicksman (17) interviewed 50 patients and found that 52% of them were inadequately prepared for radiation therapy and that the patients did not believe that the referring doctor or technician who gave the treatment were people with whom they could discuss their worries and fears. Maguire (15) reports similar attitudes amongst women with breast cancer and comments from two of his patients summarize the feelings of many. One said, "I felt I had no right to burden them (the medical and nursing staff) with my worries. . . . I just put a face on it," and the other, "They didn't seem interested in what I really felt." It appears that only 5% of patients in this series were asked about their emotions after surgery, and it seemed that surgeons were unwilling to explore their patients' emotions and often failed to appreciate their depth if they were aware of any distress.

Careful studies of interactions between staff and patients on wards for cancer patients reveals that treatment transactions involving analgesics for pain are subject to the influence of culturally determined attitudes of both patients and staff to illness behavior. Indeed, the classic studies of Zborowski (29) supported by the work of Sternbach and Turskey (25) and Turskey and Sternbach (27) lead to the conclusion that the factor governing the behavior of individuals in pain seems to be the level of approval given by society for the public expression of emotions. British attitudes are reflected in recent work by Bond (3) on two groups of patients in Scottish hospitals. He found that irrespective of the source of their pain, all patients believed they should bear it as long as possible. Moreover, in another study it was found that patients' complaints of pain and requests for analgesics were not necessarily taken at their face value by nurses who, despite the evidence that potent drugs were required, tended to give ones of low potency without any attempt to provide emotional support either. On the other hand, independent decisions by nursing staff to give drugs often seemed to lead to the administration of powerful analgesics, indicating that they felt their judgment of patients' needs were more appropriate to the level of pain. It is not surprising therefore that they failed on many occasions to realize that the patients' complaints of pain have a more general purpose in that they signaled distress not only about physical discomfort, but emotional and social problems too.

To conclude, the emotions aroused by the presence of cancer are many and varied, and all are exacerbated by the presence of pain. This is well recognised, although not on the whole handled well by doctors and nurses other than those in special centers where specific training programs exist. Even less recognition and attention is paid to the persisting emotional difficulties of cancer patients, with and without pain, who have had treatment and who have emerged from hospital to live in the outside world. This is a matter which deserves close attention in the future.

REFERENCES

1. Blumberg, E. T., West, P. M., and Ellis, F. W. (1954): A possible relationship between psychological factors and human cancer. *Psychosom. Med.,* 16:277–290.
2. Bond, M. R. (1971): The relation of pain to the Eysenck Personality Inventory, Cornell Medical Index and Whiteley Index of Hypochondriasis. *Br. J. Psychiatry,* 119:671,678.
3. Bond, M. R. (1978): Unpublished data.
4. Bond, M. R., and Pearson, I. B. (1969): Psychological aspects of pain in women with advanced carcinoma of the cervix. *J. Psychosom. Res.,* 13:13–19.
5. Brown, G. W., Harris, T., and Copeland, J. R. (1977): Depression and loss. *Br. J. Psychiatry,* 130:118.
6. Devlin, H. B., Plant, J. A., and Griffin, M. (1971): Aftermath of surgery for rectal cancer. *Br. Med. J.,* 3:413–418.
7. Engel, G. L. (1962): *Psychological Development in Health and Disease.* Saunders, Philadelphia.
8. Goldfarb, C., Driesen, J., and Cole, D. (1967): Psychophysiologic aspects of malignancy. *Am. J. Psychiatry,* 123:1545–1552.
9. Hanay, C. H. (1971): Illness behaviour and psychosocial correlates of cancer. *Soc. Sci. Med.,* 11:223–228.
10. Kenyon, F. E. (1976): Hypochondriacal states. *Br. J. Psychiatry,* 129:55–60.
11. Kissen, D. M. (1964): The influence of some environmental factors on personality inventory scores in psychosomatic research. *J. Psychosom. Res.,* 8:145–149.
12. Kissen, D. M., and Eysenck, H. J. (1962): Personality in male lung cancer patients. *J. Psychosom. Res.,* 6:123.
13. Lee, E. G., and Maguire, P. (1975): Proceedings: Emotional distress in patients attending a breast clinic. *Br. J. Surg.,* 62:162.
14. Lovell, R. R. H., and Verghese, A. (1967): Personality traits associated with different chest pains after myocardial infarction. *Br. Med. J.,* 2:327–330.
15. Maguire, P. (1976): The psychological and social sequelae of mastectomy. In: *Modern Perspectives in the Psychiatric Aspects of Surgery,* edited by J. G. Howells, pp. 390–422. Brunner/Mazel, New York.

16. Mechanic, D. (1977): Illness behaviour, social adaptation, and the management of illness. *J. Nerv. Ment. Dis.,* 165:79–87.
17. Mitchell, G. W., and Glicksman, H. S. (1977): Cancer patients: Knowledge and attitudes. *Cancer,* 40:61–66.
18. Peck, A., and Boland, J. (1977): Emotional reactions to radiation treatment. *Cancer,* 40:180–184.
19. Perris, G. M., and Pierre, I. R. (1959): Psychosomatic aspects of cancer. *Psychosom. Med.,* 21:397–401.
20. Pilowsky, I. (1967): Dimensions of hypochondriasis. *Br. J. Psychiat.,* 113:89–93.
21. Pilowsky, I., and Spence, N. D. (1976): Pain, anger and illness behaviour. *J. Psychosom. Res.,* 20:411–416.
22. Rassidakis, N. C., Evotocritou, A., and Volidou, M. (1976): The psychopathology of cancer. In: *Modern Perspectives in the Psychiatric Aspects of Surgery,* edited by J. G. Howells, pp. 48–60. Brunner/Mazel, New York.
23. Sternbach, R. H. (1974): *Pain Patients, Traits and Treatments,* p. 17. Academic Press, New York.
24. Sternbach, R. H., and Timmermans, G. (1975): Personality changes associated with reduction of pain. *Pain,* 1:177–181.
25. Sternbach, R. H., and Turskey, B. (1965): Ethnic differences among housewives in psychophysical and skin potential responses to electric shock. *Psychophysiol.,* 1:241–246.
26. Surawicz, F. G., Brightwell, D. R., Weitzel, W. D., and Othner, E. (1976): Cancer, emotions and mental illness: The present state of understanding. *Am. J. Psychiatry,* 133:1306–1309.
27. Turskey, B., and Sternbach, R. H. (1967): Further physiological correlates of ethnic differences in responses to shock. *Psychophysiol.,* 4:67–74.
28. Woodforde, J. M., and Fielding, J. R. (1975): Pain and cancer. In: *Pain: Clinical and Experimental Perspectives,* edited by M. Weisenburg, pp. 332–336. The C. V. Mosby Co., St. Louis.
29. Zaborowski, M. (1952): Cultural components in responses to pain. *J. Soc. Issues,* 8:16–30.

Pain in Children with Cancer

J. Gerald Beales

Department of Rheumatology, University of Manchester, Manchester, England

INTRODUCTION

The increasing attention which has, in recent years, been paid to cancer pain and its treatment has focused almost exclusively upon adult patients. Pain in children with cancer has attracted comparatively little interest. In the pediatric oncology literature, references to pain are surprisingly infrequent, and when pain is mentioned it is usually in terms of its implications for diagnosis rather than as a symptom demanding treatment in its own right. Pain on presentation is generally better described in the literature than pain in the later stages of childhood malignant disease.

To some extent, this relative neglect of the subject of pain in child cancer patients simply reflects the lack of study devoted to pain in children as a whole. In part, it may also be a result of a general belief that pain is less of a problem among children with cancer than it is among adults. For many children, cancer is, indeed, substantially painless. But, for many others, pain is an important and distressing feature of their disease. The excruciating intractable pain which afflicts a significant proportion of adult cancer patients does seem to be rare in children, but the pain of children with cancer is nonetheless often quite severe. Furthermore, it could be argued that, if a child has cancer, even relatively mild pain is serious and demands relief.

A child who must die has the right to do so with the absolute minimum of suffering. But even where the prognosis is less gloomy, the relief of pain is equally necessary. Improvements in cancer therapy are now creating a growing pool of children who will survive into adult life, and it is therefore important to ensure that the normal psychologic development of these children is disrupted as little as possible by the disease or the treatment. Continual pain can have emotional consequences which seriously interfere with such development, as well as reduce the child's willingness to cooperate with therapy. The minimization of pain is therefore an important requirement in any chronic childhood disease.

Pain is a complex phenomenon. It is the final product of several processes and is consequently capable of being acted upon at a number of levels and by numerous means. Anticancer radiotherapy or chemotherapy may remove pain by acting directly on the pathology from which pain-producing signals originate. Analgesics, or neurosurgery, can be used to interfere with the transmission of those signals to the brain. But the experience of pain is also influenced by processes which operate within the brain—by psychologic mechanisms—and the manipulation of these mechanisms is a potentially valuable means of reducing or avoiding pain. This is true not only of that pain which is considered to have psychologic origins, and is labeled "psychogenic," but also of pain which arises from a detectable physical insult produced by disease itself or the treatment of disease. There are reasons, which will be discussed later, for suggesting that some psychologic mechanisms involved in the perception of pain may be manipulated much more easily in children than in adults. Yet, this particular approach to the treatment of pain in children with cancer has seen very little systematic use. The aim here will therefore be to consider some of the precise psychologic factors likely to be involved in the pain experienced by children with malignant disease, and to suggest means by which these factors might be acted upon in order to avoid or relieve pain.

THE ROLE OF PSYCHOLOGIC INTERVENTION

The manipulation of psychologic mechanisms has a place in the treatment of all three basic types of pain encountered in child cancer patients. These are: pain which is directly attributable to malignant disease; pain produced by anticancer therapy; and pain which appears to have its immediate origin in the emotional rather than the physical state of the child.

Pain produced by tumor may be relieved for a time at least by direct action upon the malignancy. Bone pain, associated with skeletal destruction occurring in the primary bone tumors and histiocytosis X, and commonly in leukemia and neuroblastoma, often responds well to local radiotherapy. Headache caused by the raised intracranial pressure of brain tumor may disappear with the reduction of that pressure by surgical or chemotherapeutic means. In cases of intraspinal malignancy, pain resulting from compression of a nerve root may be relieved by surgical decompression.

Analgesics are required in order to relieve pain until specific anticancer therapy is able to exert its effect, where no such therapy is available, or where advancing disease no longer responds to therapy. In the later stages of childhood cancer, pain may become increasingly severe, and it may be necessary to resort to the more potent drugs (8). The value of psychologic intervention is likely to be in complementing the role of the analgesics.

Where a clear organic cause of pain is discernible, it is easy to assume that the pain is entirely and directly determined by the physical pathology. Yet the extent of physical pathology by no means always correlates with the severity of pain experienced. This appears to be particularly true of bone pain associated with skeletal destruction. Some children with extensive bone lesions deny pain altogether. Others, with several lesions, report pain from only one site. Toddlers with lower-limb involvement often present with a limp which is apparently unaccompanied by pain. But, in other cases, pain is reported before any lesion becomes radiologically detectable (7,9).

These variations may be the result of cerebrocortical mechanisms inhibiting pain-producing signals in some cases and augmenting them in others. There is convincing evidence that psychologic processes are capable of alleviating or blocking pain despite extensive injury (3). Such processes would also seem capable of producing pain from weak signals emanating from minimal tissue damage. Where pain is directly attributable to malignancy, the contribution of psychologic intervention may therefore be to reduce cerebrocortical augmentation of pain-producing signals and to encourage inhibition.

When a child who has previously suffered well-defined and well-localized pain begins to complain of vague, generalized pain in the absence of demonstrable organic pathology, the new pain is likely to be labeled "psychogenic." A common assumption is that pain of this kind is entirely a product of psychologic factors and has no organic origin. But it is possible that so-called "psychogenic" pain is the result of cerebrocortical augmentation of signals arising from damage so slight as to be undetectable by radiologic or other clinical means. It has been suggested (8) that if a new pain is abolished by tranquilizers alone, it is unlikely to indicate a metastatic lesion. But if tranquilizers exert their effect on pain by reducing psychologic augmentation of weak signals, this cannot be assumed. The origin of the signals may be innocent—the result of normal bodily wear and tear—but it may not. In the case of a child with cancer, the distinction between "organic" and "psychogenic" pain may be an inappropriate and a misleading one.

Psychologic augmentation of pain-producing signals, from whatever source, may be influenced by the use of drugs. But it may be acted upon more precisely through normal sensory channels: by talking to the child, in particular. Words can have a powerful effect, but they are capable of exerting their effect in either direction. They may reduce cerebrocortical augmentation of signals, or they may increase it. In fact, much of what is said to the child with cancer, by doctors, nurses, parents, or fellow patients, may unintentionally make his pain worse. What is said to the child often makes it likely that he will experience signals produced by minimal tissue damage as painful, or that he will suffer unnecessary pain as a result of therapeutic procedures.

Much of anticancer therapy is potentially painful. Vincristine frequently produces pain in the abdomen, jaw, or limbs (6,14). Bone-marrow aspiration, lumbar puncture, and venipuncture are regularly inflicted upon many children. In some centers, those procedures which are potentially most painful are conducted only under a general anesthetic, but this practice is by no means universal. Mennie (12) has complained that the measures taken to relieve pain during episodes of therapy are frequently inadequate or nonexistent. But the withholding of drugs is not the only means by which pain may be caused unnecessarily. As will be explained later, if one follows recommendations in the literature about what the child should be told prior to potentially painful therapy, the likelihood of his experiencing significant pain will probably be increased.

Because of the manner in which psychologic mechanisms involved in pain may be influenced, it is hardly possible for those concerned with the child to avoid acting upon them. It is not only the words which are said that may exert an effect: What is not said can also have an impact upon psychologic modulation of pain-producing signals. It has to be ensured, therefore, that the influence which is exerted is in the direction of avoiding or reducing pain, rather than increasing it.

PSYCHOLOGIC MECHANISMS THAT MAY MODULATE PAIN

Pain comprises a combination of sensation and negative affect (11). It occurs when physical insult gives rise to sensation and that sensation is experienced as unpleasant. If sensation is not unpleasant, there is no pain. Sensation and negative affect involve different areas of the brain and can be modulated independently. Pain may be relieved or avoided by inhibiting sensation or by reducing the extent to which sensation is experienced as unpleasant.

Removing or reducing the unpleasantness of a sensation may be accomplished to some degree by surgery or drugs, but it may be achieved with a greater degree of success and precision by purely psychologic means.

Studies of visual perception in man have indicated that the direction and degree of affect which become linked to particular sensation depend on the meaning which the object giving rise to that sensation has for the individual. If the object has pleasant associations for the individual, then simply seeing the object comes to be experienced as pleasant. Although different sensory modalities have their own specialized receptors and nerve pathways, it seems likely that they are influenced by similar psychologic processes. There is evidence to suggest that the pain experienced by patients with physical pathology depends to some extent on the meaning which that pathology has for them (10). If a certain injury becomes associated with actual attainment of some important goal, the sensation resulting from the injury may itself evoke no feeling of unpleasantness (3). Where, as is more usual, the pathology has unpleasant associations for the individual, the degree of negative affect linked with the sensation—and therefore the degree of pain—may be related to the extent of those unpleasant associations.

For example, in a study of children with juvenile chronic arthritis, it was found that older children associated their disease with considerably more frustration of their goals than did younger children (1). They also indicated more severe joint pain than did younger children. When the sensation and negative-affect components of pain were measured separately, the older children reported only slightly more sensation from their joints, but considerably more negative affect. Some of the younger children denied pain altogether: They claimed that the sensation which they experienced from their diseased joints was not at all unpleasant (2).

The unpleasantness of a sensation may therefore be partly dependent upon the extent to which the pathology it indicates has undesirable consequences for the child. But it may also depend upon whether or not the sensation is recognized as indicating pathology in the first place. A child has to learn that sensations of a particular kind indicate that there is something wrong with his body. Clearly, it is easier for him to link a sensation with physical damage if that damage is immediately visible—if it occurs at the body surface. Because it is much more obvious to them, younger children are primarily concerned with, and most disturbed by, insult to their body surface. They have little or no concept of their internal makeup, and little idea of what the implications may be if it goes wrong. Consequently, in younger children, cerebrocortical augmentation of the negative-affect component of pain is more likely to occur if the responsible injury is cutaneous than if it is internal. The older the child, and the greater the awareness of the possible sinister meaning of an internally originating sensation, the less this difference in the effect of psychological mechanisms upon negative affect might be expected to be.

The sensation component of pain is particularly influenced by the mechanisms of attention and distraction (10). If the individual's attention is focused upon certain signals, he will detect them more quickly, and at lower strengths than he would otherwise do. He might experience sensation from signals so weak that under normal circumstances they would not have impinged upon consciousness. Conversely, distraction of attention has the effect of raising the signal strength necessary to produce conscious sensation. Although many factors may influence the individual's state of attention or distraction at any particular time, there is likely to be an age difference here too. Younger children will be on the look-out for pain-producing signals if placed in a situation in which they anticipate damage to their body surface. Older children who have, or fear, internal pathology, may focus their attention on signals having an internal origin.

PSYCHOLOGIC INTERVENTION IN CHILD CANCER PAIN

In respect of *pain directly attributable to malignancy*, the principal aim of psychologic intervention should be to act on the meaning which the disease has for the child. It may be possible to reduce the negative-affect component of pain by reducing the unpleasant consequences associated with the disease. The younger the child, the easier such modification of meaning is likely to be.

There is a tendency to assume that cancer has only one real meaning for the child: death. And therefore it may be difficult to appreciate how the disease can be made less of a disaster for the patient. But studies have shown that young children either have little awareness of death or do not recognize its full implications (4,13). They may deplore their disease simply because it interferes with play and cuts them off from their friends. If they fear death at all, they may do so because they fear separation from the love and protection of parents.

It is important not to assume that children must inevitably share the reactions of adults to a potentially fatal disease. It should not be taken for granted that, if a child is dying, nothing else is of importance to him. All who are concerned with the treatment of the child with cancer should be fully aware of the child's own point of view and of the things which matter to him personally. Ensuring that there is minimal disruption of the child's play activities, that he is not separated prematurely from parents and friends, and that he is allowed to lead as normal a life as possible for as long as possible may go a considerable way to reducing the negative meaning which the disease has for him.

The older the child, the closer the concept of death approaches to that held by the adult, and the greater its importance may seem. But even where the implications of death are recognized, apparently trivial things may still be of importance to the patient, and interference with them may be a source of additional distress. With the older child, therefore, it is equally necessary to know how the patient himself views his cancer and to be aware of all the unpleasant associations which it has for him. It may well be possible to remove some of those associations quite easily: for example, by making it possible for the child to continue some favorite activity, or by paying particular attention to the protection of his self-esteem.

Death, however, is no longer the inevitable prognosis for all child cancer patients. Therefore, even in the case of the older child, it will not necessarily figure prominently in the patient's appraisal of his condition. Children who are not primarily concerned with death will react to their cancer in the same way as children with any chronic disease. Modifying the meaning of chronic disease to the patient is generally easier with children than with adults. The adult's interests, ambitions, and way of life are well established. Those of children are undergoing change, and because of their flexibility, they may be adapted to compensate for the restrictions on activities imposed by the disease. Younger children can be encouraged to develop alternative play interests; older children can be guided toward a career which is not incompatible with their physical condition.

Making it possible for a child with cancer to lead as normal a life as possible for as long as possible might also have specific impact on the sensory component of pain through the mechanism of distraction. If the child's attention is directed toward play or schooling, for example, he is less likely to become preoccupied with his disease and to focus upon his symptoms. Because of their greater appreciation of what is happening inside them, older children are particularly likely to be on the look-out for any signals indicating the spread of their cancer, and comparatively weak signals resulting from minimal tissue damage may therefore give rise to pain. If *pain unrelated to malignancy* or any other significant organic pathology does develop, it might perhaps be relieved by amending the child's interpretation of it. He may cease to concentrate his attention upon the pain if he is reassured that it has no sinister significance. Some pain of this kind might be avoided by reminding older children with cancer that their bodies are subject to the same normal wear and tear as those of other children, and that every internally originating signal does not indicate malignancy.

It was suggested earlier that much of the *pain caused by anticancer therapy* is avoidable: Painful treatment is often performed without adequate analgesia. Perhaps the reason for this is that medical personnel concerned with therapy are not always aware of the amount of pain which they are inflicting on their young patients. It is by no means easy to assess pain accurately in young children, whose ability to express their pain verbally may be limited or nonexistent. Crying may be attributed to fear rather than pain. Furthermore, it may be assumed that prolonged exposure to pain leads to a greater tolerance of it, so that a child who has had, for example, extensive skeletal lesions for some time may be thought to be inured to pain and unlikely to be distressed by anything inflicted on him in the course of treatment. This assumption, in fact, seems to be quite widespread, although, as Green (5) has pointed out, there is no evidence to support it.

It is particularly easy to underestimate pain caused by therapeutic procedures in children who fail to complain of pain despite extensive malignancy. It might understandably be concluded that if a child does not have pain despite considerable skeletal destruction or a large abdominal mass, he must have an exceedingly high "pain threshold," and therefore will be safe from pain as a result of venipuncture, or lumbar puncture, or having his dressings changed. But it is wrong to assume that a child has a single pain threshold which applies in all situations, for all types of physical insult. Because young children are more concerned about the body surface than what lies beneath it, they may be far more distressed by even a mild insult to the skin than by considerable subcutaneous pathology which is out of sight and consequently out of mind. Therefore, they may experience more pain from it. Because of the meaning which surface damage has for them—because they find it so unpleasant—the unpleasantness of the resultant sensation may be augmented.

Unnecessary pain may also be caused by focusing the child's attention on pain-producing signals during treatment episodes. It is now widely recommended in the pediatric oncology literature that, prior to painful therapy, the child should be informed that pain will be inflicted, in order to ensure that he continues to trust those responsible for his care. But the expectation of pain has the effect of allowing weaker signals to be experienced as conscious sensation, and pain may thereby be actually increased. However, the best of both worlds may perhaps be obtained by warning the child reasonably well in advance of possible pain, but attempting distraction during the treatment episode.

Pain resulting from therapy can often be reduced or even avoided altogether by the use of distraction. But when distraction is attempted during a potentially painful procedure, it is usually in an impromptu and unorganized way, with a junior nurse frequently taking the initiative. If it were used more systematically, with adequate preparation being made to ensure that the child's attention could be engaged in some pleasant activity at the time when pain might be caused, the child might be spared a great deal of suffering. Distraction is undoubtedly easier to achieve in children than in adult patients. Young children in particular will probably accept a game or story as perfectly valid in this situation and allow themselves to become absorbed in it. Adults tend to regard therapy as being so serious a matter that they may consider any attempt to draw their attention away from it as improper.

Of course, it is not always necessary to inform a child that pain might be caused by therapy for him to anticipate pain. The mere suspicion that something unpleasant is about to happen to him may encourage him to create a fantasy in which the level of damage inflicted on him far exceeds reality. The best way of avoiding such fantasies is to give the child as much accurate information about his treatment as he is capable of assimilating, given his age and level of intelligence. It should not be assumed that if a young patient does not ask for information, he does not want to know what will be done to him. It may be his fear which prevents him from asking.

The presence of a parent during treatment episodes may help to reduce the child's fear. But parents are not always encouraged to stay. Some clinicians claim that if a parent is present the child is inclined to exaggerate pain and is generally more difficult to handle. It is undoubtedly true that some parents can lead their child to feel pain, simply by demonstrating, with gasps and appropriate facial expressions, that they are already suffering on his behalf. But if parents are told of what will happen during therapy and warned not to communicate their own anxieties to the child, they can do much to ease his suffering.

The treatment of pain in children with cancer by the manipulation of psychologic mechanisms is not just a job for the doctor. *Everyone concerned with the care of the child has a contribution to make.* Parents are of importance, not simply for the reassurance they can provide during episodes of treatment, but also because they can play a considerable part in minimizing the unpleasant associations which the disease has for their child. During periods of remission, when the child is at home, they can do a great deal to distract the child's attention away from his disease and symptoms. However, parents cannot be expected to undertake this task successfully without guidance and support. Many will be naturally inclined to overprotect a seriously ill child, restricting his activities beyond those precluded by the cancer. Therefore, unless they are given proper help and advice, they may unintentionally increase the negative meaning which the disease has for the young patient, and so perhaps increase his pain through the augmentation of the negative-affect component. Unless warned of the specific dangers, they may pass on their own anxieties about the disease to their child and so make it more likely that his attention will be focused on signals which might indicate a worsening of his physical condition.

Ensuring that augmentation of pain by psychologic mechanisms is minimized, and that cerebrocortical inhibition of pain-producing signals is encouraged, is a full-time activity and a team responsibility. All social contact with the patient may have an influence, for good or ill, on the pain he experiences directly or indirectly as a result of his cancer. It is not enough simply to administer an analgesic to a child if, in the process of so doing, one says something to him which is likely to cause psychologic processes to exert their effect in the direction of increasing pain. Indeed, saying the right words in such a situation may sometimes be of greater value from the point of view of relieving pain than the actual drug administered.

Although it has been possible to suggest the likely identity of some of the psychologic mechanisms involved in the modulation of pain, and to indicate means by which those mechanisms could be manipulated, there is clearly a need for considerably more research in this area. The cerebral cortex has undoubted ability to increase, reduce, and abolish pain, but comparatively little effort has been made to understand, and thereby learn how to make use of, the means by which it can exert this control. Greater study here may produce results of real benefit to those who suffer pain— including children with cancer.

ACKNOWLEDGMENTS

I should like to express my gratitude to Drs. P. J. L. Holt, D. Pearson, and C. Bailey for their help during the preparation of this paper.

REFERENCES

1. Beales, J. G., Holt, P. J. L., Keen, J., and Mellor, V. (1979): Juvenile chronic arthritis: The child's perception of the disease. (*in preparation*)
2. Beales, J. G., Keen, J., and Holt, P. J. L. (1979): Juvenile chronic arthritis: Age and the experience of pain. (*in preparation*)
3. Beecher, H. K. (1959): *Measurement of Subjective Responses*. Oxford University Press, New York.
4. Burton, L. (1974): Tolerating the intolerable. In: *Care of the Child Facing Death*, edited by L. Burton. Routledge & Kegan Paul, London.
5. Green, M. (1967): Care of the dying child. *Pediatrics*, 40(3):492–498.
6. Heyn, R. M., Beatty, E. C., Jr., Hammond, D., Louis, J., Pierce, M., Mur-

phy, M. L., and Severo, N. (1966): Vincristine in the treatment of acute leukemia in children. *Pediatrics,* 38(5):82–91.
7. Jones, P. G., and Campbell, R. E., editors (1976): *Tumors of Infancy and Childhood.* Blackwell Scientific Publications, Ltd., Oxford.
8. Lane, D. M. (1973): Principles of total care—psychologic support. In: *Clinical Pediatric Oncology,* edited by W. W. Sutow, T. J. Vietti, and D. J. Fernback. The C. V. Mosby Co., St. Louis.
9. Marsden, H. B., and Steward, J. K., editors (1976): *Tumors in Children.* Springer Verlag, Berlin.
10. Melzack, R. (1973): *The Puzzle of Pain.* Penguin, New York.
11. Melzack, R., and Casey, K. L. (1968): Sensory, motivational, and central control determinants of pain: A new conceptual model. In: *The Skin Senses,* edited by D. Kenshalo. Charles C Thomas, Springfield, Ill.
12. Mennie, A. T. (1974): The child in pain. In: *Care of the Child Facing Death,* edited by L. Burton. Routledge & Kegan Paul, London.
13. Nagy, M. H. (1959): The child's view of death. In: *The Meaning of Death,* edited by H. Feifel. McGraw-Hill, New York.
14. Sutow, W. W., Berry, D. H., Haddy, T. B., Sullivan, M. P., Watkins, W. L., and Windmiller, J. (1966): Vincristine sulfate therapy in children with metastatic soft tissue sarcoma. *Pediatrics,* 38(1):465–472.

Sociologic Effects of Cancer Pain

Margo McCaffery

Consultant in the Nursing Care of Patients with Pain, Santa Monica, California 90404

The sociologic perspective encompasses how the inner states of the individual affect his relationships and interactions with his social environment. People interact with many social environments, ranging from the family or significant others to the large, impersonal agencies and bureaucracies.

The problems the patient has with the community and large institutions are not my focus nor my area of knowledge. But problems exist in these areas and some are easily observed. As an example, the patient with cancer faces possible loss of his job and associated fringe benefits if the employer learns of the patient's diagnosis. This is illustrated by a woman with pain and suspected pancreatic or intestinal cancer who had been a top designer in the clothing industry for more than 30 years. She remained amazingly energetic and made every effort to hide her pain, but suspicions were aroused by her weight-loss. One afternoon she was fired without warning. Five people had to be hired to take the place of this one woman. Although her productivity would have decreased gradually, she could have been an asset to the company up until about 3 months prior to her death almost 2 years later.

Just as industry is learning that it is often less expensive to rehabilitate an alcoholic than to replace him, industry might also find some ways of benefiting from the skills of employees with cancer pain who may die and/or gradually reduce their working time. Certainly there is the need for education and exploration in this area.

My focus, however, is concerned with factors that may hamper the patient's relationships with significant others, especially his family and close friends. I have selected a few somewhat overlapping but seemingly significant factors:

1. differences between the patient's pain-related attitudes and behaviors and those expected of him by others,
2. role-change adjustments,
3. expressions of affects such as anger and depression, and
4. the fight between dependence and independence.

Anthropologic and sociologic studies have shown clearly that early in life people begin learning very specific and detailed cultural expectations regarding pain and that these expectations may differ greatly from one sociocultural group to another. These findings are clinically relevant, but not because they tell us how a person from a particular sociocultural group will respond to pain. Rather these studies reveal the myriad of attitudes and responses regarding pain that may be present to some extent in any person regardless of his cultural background. For example, Zborowski found that the Irishman was proud of being able to handle pain by himself and tended to go through a long period of struggling with his pain before he sought assistance from a physician (4). However, this response may be exhibited by a patient who does not possess an ounce of Irish blood. Further, his family and close friends, while seemingly members of the same sociocultural group, may have opposing views.

When significant others in the patient's environment do not share the patient's attitudes and beliefs about pain-related behavior, their interpersonal interactions may be severely damaged. People tend to view their learned responses to pain as correct and normal. Responses that are different from their own are often regarded as improper, abnormal, or wrong. Therefore, the family member or friend who differs from the patient regarding how to handle pain usually finds it quite difficult to be understanding, compassionate, or even tolerant of the patient's behaviors.

Arguments and social isolation are among the possible outcomes of differing pain-related beliefs. A previously described characteristic associated with the Irishman serves as an example. The spouse may believe that it is senseless to endure pain, especially when a disease such as cancer has been diagnosed, and that pain-relief should be sought immediately. The husband and wife may argue about these differences daily.

Consider the woman who cries easily about her pain and feels that this is a natural response that need not be suppressed. Friends who value minimal expression of pain may begin to avoid her for several reasons. For instance, they may want to spare her the embarrassment they believe she feels when she cries in their presence. On the other hand, if she feels that crying is childish and her efforts to control it are unsuccessful, she may fear that others will be disgusted or uncomfortable with her. Consequently she may impose her own social isolation.

The degree to which a person is expected to discuss and share his problems is also partially determined by cultural expectations. This is particularly significant for the patient with cancer pain, since discussion of death-related topics tends to be especially taboo.

One study showed that many patients with pain say they do not like to discuss their pain with others or are ambivalent about it. But usually the reason they give for this reticence is that they feel others are not interested in their pain. For example, one patient with metastatic cancer commented, "I don't feel anybody's really interested. . . . Oh, they're interested, but I mean, well not really. . . . They've got their problems too, probably, so I just feel, why burden them with mine." Patients with cancer pain seemed especially aware of the social stigma attached to complaining about pain. This study found that when patients do talk about their pain, the person they most frequently talk with is the spouse (1). When pain is of long duration and associated with cancer and death, the spouse obviously will have personal needs and at least occasionally will find it difficult to talk with the patient.

Role-change represents another area of disruption in interpersonal relationships. Illness and pain lasting only a few days will interfere with role-function. This problem is enormously increased when pain and illness are prolonged and lead to death.

Roles vary of course from person to person, but more importantly the patient's roles have varying significance to him and to those around him. Some roles are heavily invested emotionally, whereas other roles are of a more practical nature. For example, a man may find that cancer and pain prevent him from fulfilling his role as financial provider for himself and his family. This poses practical and serious economic problems for the entire family. But in addition to this, work may have been a very gratifying activity for the patient and a major contributor to a positive self-concept.

One study of patients with bone metastasis from breast cancer found that the necessary limitations on movement were extremely hard on women with young children. Mothering was a much more difficult role to relinquish than that of housekeeping (3).

When the patient is no longer able to function in a particular role, the activities associated with this role may have to be assumed by others. This may be depressing for the patient to witness, and it may impose a great hardship on those who must assume the patient's previous responsibilities. The husband who must now wash dishes and feed the children may become genuinely, although irrationally, resentful toward his ill wife.

Another factor that may hamper the patient's relationships with others is the effect of certain emotions associated with having cancer pain. A sociologist who was also in pain shared with me his experiences in this area. He felt that the anxiety, fear, depression, and other feelings elicited by pain tend to heighten the patient's interpretations of various situations. As a result the patient exacerbates and discolors minor events in social interactions. The patient is often angry and irritable and makes exaggerated responses to his environment. The other person involved in the interaction usually is not sophisticated enough to identify the part that pain plays in what the patient says or does. Hence, the response of the person with whom the patient interacts will tend to increase in intensity to match that of the patient. This often leads to a highly emotional climate. As the interaction continues, each person is responding with greater intensity and the process spirals upward.

He pointed out that in addition to the emotions associated with the illness and the pain, side effects from medications may further complicate interpersonal interactions. Among these side effects may be irritability, fatigue, drowsiness, confusion, weakness, and increased or decreased libido.

The previously discussed factors along with other factors contribute to the conflict between dependence and independence. Some patients struggle against depending upon others in meeting emotional and physical needs. Such patients may resent the assistance offered by others. Those who wish to help the patient may be hurt or baffled by the patient's response to their well-intentioned actions.

On the other hand, some patients are not threatened by certain degrees of dependence upon others. In this case the problem may be that the people upon whom the patient depends may find the situation too demanding. They may lack the time, interest, or energy to respond to the patient's dependency needs. The egocentricity that so often accompanies prolonged pain and illness may render the patient insensitive to these feelings (2). The balancing of the patient's needs for dependence and independence against the needs of others is clearly problematic regardless of which way the pendulum swings.

In summary, there are many factors related to cancer pain that may hamper the patient's relationships with others. There is no single solution to this. However, a simple but significant beginning might be to provide the patient and others close to him with counseling, perhaps by a nurse or social worker, for the purpose of identifying and discussing the basic dynamics of their interpersonal problems.

REFERENCES

1. Jacox, A., and Stewart, M. (1973): *Psychosocial Contingencies of the Pain Experience.* University of Iowa Press, Iowa City.
2. McCaffery, M.: *Nursing Management of the Patient with Pain,* 2nd ed. J. B. Lippincott, Philadelphia.
3. McCorkle, M. R. (1973): Coping with physical symptoms in metastatic breast cancer. *Am. J. Nurs.,* 73:1034–1038.
4. Zborowski, M. (1969): *People in Pain.* Jossey-Bass, Inc., San Francisco.

Sociological and Nursing Aspects of Cancer Pain

Ada G. Rogers

Analgesic Studies Section, Sloan-Kettering Institute for Cancer Research, New York, New York 10021

Recorded history and anthropological discoveries have revealed that cancer has been prevalent in man and animals since the dawn of civilization. Until the 20th century, it was classified by many as an incurable disease. Even today, despite all the advances that have been made in its treatment, there are those including some health-care professionals who feel that cancer is an incurable disease, accompanied by intractable pain, ending only in death. We recognize that this is not true; not all cancer is incurable and in some cases, even when the disease is far advanced, pain may not be a problem. However, when one considers the history of cancer and its slow evolution, one can understand these attitudes.

Prehistoric man used rituals and superstitions as a weapon against cancer, and in some cultures this has prevailed up to the present time. Hippocrates the "Father of Medicine" recognized the disease, defined its grave prognosis, and named it *karkinos,* meaning "a crab." The name described the appearance of advanced breast cancer. The Latin word *carcinoma* is derived from the Greek *karkinos* (9). Although the Greeks had temple-hospitals where care was given primarily by priests, patients with cancer were removed to the seclusion of nearby woods, abandoned, and left to die. Conversely, the Romans did everything they could to effect a cure and the sick, even their slaves, were treated at home, nursed by the women of the household (10).

During the next 1,500 years, essentially the only advances made were in recognizing the different forms of cancer. Galen listed 61 types but included among them inflammation, swelling, and ulceration. In the 16th century, Giovanni Fillippo Ingrassia, Professor of Medicine and Anatomy at Naples and called the "Sicilian Hippocrates," extended the list to 287 varieties (9). The treatment and understanding of this "horrible" disease was still based on astrological charts, handwriting analysis, the use of strong odors, e.g., garlic and onions, "trapping the evil spirits," and "the evil eye." During this time, the care of the sick was under the auspice of religious groups, both Jews and Christians. This seemed appropriate, since disease and pain were thought of as punishment or atonement for sins. The monasteries had absolute control over their members, and their great purpose was the moral and spiritual discipline of the young and old, of the sick and well, of those who minister and those who were ministered to. Nursing was learned through practice and had special virtues. Because of the hard work and distasteful duties, it was considered to be an effective way for mortifying the flesh and developing humility, patience, and other Christian virtues. Some of these monasteries had a place for the shelter of travelers and these were called *hospices*. Religion continued its influence in the care of the sick.

The world's first cancer hospital was established at Rheims in France by Bishop Jean Godinet in the middle of the 18th century, but it was closed in 1778 because the public thought that cancer might be contagious. It was not until 1840 that French hospitals admitted cancer patients, but in separate blocks. In England at the end of the 18th century, a cancer ward was established at the Middlesex Hospital. However, little was done in the treatment of the cancer patient until 1851, when the first cancer hospital was founded. It was later called the Royal Cancer Hospital (4). In America, progress in the field of cancer was even slower.

Our first American institutions for care of the sick were a combination of municipal hospital, poorhouse, insane asylum, house of correction, and orphanage. Cancer patients were included among these. Bellevue Hospital in New York City was a classic example of this type of institution. The care-givers were prostitutes, drunks, and petty criminals. It took almost a hundred years to recognize that the care-giver should be trained and its trainees come from a better class. In 1873, one of the first nursing schools to use the Nightingale system was established at Bellevue. Since cancer had the stigma of venereal disease or some hereditary deficiency, the wealthy class were treated at home. They feared that if the presence of cancer were divulged, their families would be disgraced as well as their descendents.

The well-to-do class was responsible for establishing better hospitals, but unfortunately, they imposed their own ignorance and prejudices on the admission of cancer patients. In 1847, The New York Hospital admitted 1,022 patients with typhus fever, 177 with fractures, 280 with syphilis, but only 4 with cancer. If by accident, cancer patients were admitted, they were promptly discharged as "improper objects" or "disorderly" (4). A man who fought against the injustices to patients with cancer was Dr. James Marion Sims. Sims specialized in feminine ills, and he was responsible for the founding of the Women's Hospital in New York City. Sims and his colleagues, seeking a cure for uterine cancer, admitted women who were suffering from this disease into the hospital. The Lady Managers opposed this practice and for years there was constant opposition. Eventually, Sims gave up the fight and resigned his position; however, his dedication to this cause continued.

In a letter to his friend, John Parsons, who was John J. Astor's lawyer, he wrote: "A cancer hospital should be built on its own foundation wholly independent of all other hospitals. Its medical board ought to be men who go into it with zeal, determined not only to give temporary relief to human suffering, but to do something towards discovering better methods of treatment. It is time we turn a listening ear to the cries of humanity." The letter received widespread publicity in the New York newspapers and led to a meeting of a group who were a minority of the Board of Governors of the Women's Hospital who had sided with Sims. Out of this meeting came the basic plans and proposals for a cancer hospital. In 1884, the New York Cancer Hospital, the first hospital specializing in the treatment of cancer patients, was established in America. This should have ended public opposition, but it did not. The New York Cancer Hospital at West 105th Street and Central Park, was called by many "The Bastille."

In an attempt to lessen the stigma still attached to cancer, the name of the hospital was changed in 1888 to the General Memorial Hospital for the Treatment of Cancer and Allied Diseases. Owing to financial problems caused by insufficient public funds and the cost of cancer care, private surgical patients with benign disease had to be admitted. By 1913, only 10% of the cases handled involved cancer, and those patients were walled off from the others by a partition in two least-desirable wards away from the park, but a rebirth of Memorial was soon to come through the deep interest of Dr. James Douglas, who had lost a daughter to cancer, and the timeless devotion of Dr. James Ewing, who became President of the Medical Board. There were many changes over the next few years. In 1915, the word "General" was dropped from the name of the hospital. In 1917, with funds provided by Douglas, a new research laboratory was opened. In 1922, the X-ray extension was added; in 1923, a dental clinic was established; and in 1924, the outpatient extension was opened. In 1927, John D. Rockefeller, Jr. started making contributions of $60,000 a year for research and clinical development, and six clinical fellowships were established. Rockefeller's generosity did not stop there. He donated the site of the present Memorial Sloan-Kettering Cancer Center in 1936 (6).

The battle toward the conquest of cancer was on its way through treatment, research, and education. Nevertheless, the emotional impact on and reaction of every patient to this disease, and the effects on his family, friends, and even health-care professionals is still a problem that is not fully appreciated. In the last few decades, some efforts have been made to understand and cope with these problems. In 1969, Dr. Elizabeth Kübler-Ross (8) published a book entitled *On Death and Dying* in which she states that the patient goes through five emotional stages in the course of terminal disease: denial and isolation, anger, bargaining, depression, and acceptance. However, it is not uncommon to find that the patient may continue in one stage until the end, and this may also be true for his family, friends, and professional care-givers.

When pain is present it can emphasize the hopelessness of terminal disease, and inadequately controlled pain contributes to greater anxiety, fear, desperation, guilt, hostility, depression, and even attempted suicide. Old taboos still play a role: The religious beliefs that disease and pain are punishment for sins committed in this life or in another life, that we must suffer to attain a greater glory after death, and that cancer is contagious or hereditary and that we may be passing it on to our loved ones.

In addition to knowing one has cancer, the treatments may cause suffering. How often does the patient who has lost a part of his body have the opportunity to mourn openly for that loss and how well is he adjusting to disfigurement and/or changes in bodily functions? Some patients never verbalize their feeling of embarrassment, of being dirty and foul-smelling, uncomfortable, fearful, and socially unacceptable—they just go and hide and become anti-social and lonely.

To many Americans, the added financial burden of this illness is of considerable concern. The head of the household will worry about if and when he will be able to go back to work, and, indeed, whether or not his job will still be there when he is able to return. Financial problems are increased with multiple hospitalization, as his medical insurance may not cover the hospital and doctor bills. The housewife will be concerned about being able to care for her family and the home. One lovely lady was upset because she would not be able to cook for her husband; no one else had cooked for him for 30 years. She was afraid he would be angry with her and she would lose his love. Cooking for him is what she talked about, but there were many other things she could not do for him that she did not discuss. Sexual problems are seldom discussed, and yet, sexual activity is an important function that may be changed permanently. By and large, female patients will not discuss this aspect with male physicians and even many male patients may not. Wise (11) has stated that: "It has been observed that cancer patients with poor prognoses wish to have various forms of physical closeness with their spouses, if not direct genital intercourse." Consideration of these needs has been sadly neglected by the medical and nursing professions.

Nausea and vomiting, major changes in eating and sleeping habits, constipation, diarrhea, dehydration, weakness, metabolic, motor, or sensory changes may contribute to discomfort, fear, and anxiety. There are many other situations that the staff may be unaware of that may be causing distress: A patient with a language barrier who cannot communicate with the staff may feel that the staff is not concerned about him; changes in awareness of world and local events; changes in degrees of independent behavior and personal privacy; presence of unfamiliar machines and mechanical devices; inadequate explanations of treatments; unfamiliar or new staff members; presence of a severely ill or noisy roommate; and perhaps most important, hospital routines that are designed for the benefit of the staff and not the patient.

Patients need a feeling of friendliness around them and this is too often forgotten by the hospital staff. Staff-patient relations can be improved when patients feel free to call the staff by their first names. Some staff members object to this, believing that over-friendliness may result in a loss of objectivity. However, as one patient stated: "Good nursing and good doctoring is not destroyed because of first names. I like the intimacy—it makes me feel that the doctors and nurses care. After all, the hospital is another family and another life for me. I like to think that I am leaving a legacy of intimacy, that I am worth something here." Perhaps there would be better understanding of how the patient feels if we think of the patient as a member of our own family—mother, father, sister, brother, son, or daughter—and how we would want them to be treated. Most patients want to be known as "good patients," and many patients will not complain because they fear reprisal, particularly if a staff member has been abusive, hostile, and mean. Even patients who feel they are coping with the disease and treatment have confided that this is the one fear they have.

It was not too many years ago that the rehabilitation of cancer patients with or without advanced disease was thought of as foolish, ridiculous, and a waste of money. After all, these patients were going to die eventually, so why bother? Rehabilitation service in the United States before 1967 was only given if the patient was 18 months post-surgery, without evidence of metastases, and had full-time employment. This 18-month waiting period was exempt for part-time workers or housewives. Some funds were available from the Vocational Rehabilitation Administration of the Department of Health, Education and Welfare. In 1972, accelerated federally supported programs were instituted for rehabilitation and counseling as part of an all-out attack against human cancer (7). Similar efforts were made in other countries.

Emphasis was placed on the team approach and the effort and supportive role of each member of the team. Change in attitude was directed toward the quality of life, hope, and the will to live. The services of psychiatrists, psychologists, social workers, dieticians, clergymen, physical therapists, occupational therapists, self-help groups, volunteers, and nurses all play an important role in these changes.

In the last two decades, nursing has had to take a new look at the care of patients with cancer to keep in step with the advances being made in the treatment of cancer. Today, schools and colleges of nursing have Cancer Nursing as part of their curricula. Cancer hospitals and cancer units have had to update their inservice education programs in order to ensure better patient care. The American Cancer Society has held two national conferences on cancer nursing (2) in the last 5 years, and each year the local divisions of the American Cancer Society as well as State Nurses Associations have workshops and/or symposiums to keep their nurses informed of the latest advances in cancer.

Cancer nursing is now a recognized specialty (2). The University of Pittsburgh, School of Nursing awards a Master's Degree in Cancer Nursing and the Oncology Nursing Society held its Third Annual Convention in Washington, D.C., April 5–7, 1978. *Cancer Nursing,* an international journal for cancer care, had its premier issue this past February. The Editor-in-Chief Rachel Ayers and Senior Editor Carol Reed-Ash (3) in a Message from the Editors wrote:

Cancer is a part of the work of every nurse, and practitioner, teacher, administrator, researcher, and student alike face an exposure of knowledge associated with caring for people living with cancer. Every nurse from the experienced specialist who cares exclusively for cancer patients to the general practitioner who must coordinate cancer care with other equally important assignments, has a common need and cause—to learn, to explore new approaches, and to share their experiences, awareness and understanding of cancer nursing, advances in treatment, and the implications of research findings.

This is indicative of the importance being placed on cancer nursing and the advancement being made.

However, this is not the case when we speak of the role of the nurse in the management of pain due to cancer. There is lack of knowledge and understanding, and this is quite evident when, too often, you see and hear the nurses' negative responses to the patient who has pain. This aspect of the care of the patient with cancer has not been fully developed. There are nurses who have had the opportunity to become involved with patients with pain due to advanced cancer and they have responded with sensitivity and compassion to these patients but, unfortunately, their numbers are too few. Pain due to cancer presents special problems with which most nurses are unprepared to cope. The patient with cancer may be facing a life-threatening situation. If the cancer causes persistent pain or the pain reappears after definitive treatment, the patient may feel that the original treatment has failed and that he is doomed.

Although most patients will accept the temporary use of narcotics, many will reject their continuous use. Most patients are extremely concerned about taking too much medication. Many of them will suffer needlessly by refusing to take medications because of misunderstandings about the nature of addiction. This may be reinforced by the nurses, and this produces more anxiety and guilt. The nurse may withhold an analgesic in order to prevent addiction and may even tell the patient he is taking too much narcotic and that he will become a drug addict. When the nurse administers an analgesic, she sometimes acts as though she is doing the patient a favor. Some patients may feel that nobody believes he has pain.

Unfortunately, many nurses do not know the basic pharmacology of analgesics, and this is also true of some physicians. For example, some physicians will write orders for parenteral and oral narcotics in the same milligram dose, typically meperidine 50 mg i.m. or PO q. 4 to 6 hr prn. If the nurse is busy, she will probably give the oral form—it is easier. But, if at one time or another, the patient should receive the parenteral dose and reports good relief, the nurse and doctor will conclude that he just "likes" the injection. However, oral meperidine is only ¼ as potent as the parenteral dose and is about equivalent to 650 mg of aspirin. Also, meperidine is a relatively short-acting narcotic and may be effective for only 2 to 3 hr. In addition, the patient whose pain comes on suddenly, will prefer the injection since peak effect of most parenteral narcotics occurs within 1 hr, whereas peak of oral effect may occur as late as 2 hr after administration. The ratio of oral versus parenteral potency of narcotics will vary with the drug. Methadone is twice as potent by parenteral route; morphine 6 times as potent.

The continuous use of narcotics will inevitably produce tolerance. This is often confused with addiction.

The first sign of tolerance is that the duration of effect has lessened. Patients will request their medication before it is scheduled. These patients are labeled first "clock-watchers" and then "addicts" who have lost control of themselves. The tendency for the doctor is to order another narcotic, usually in an inappropriately low dose, or to order a less-potent drug. The patient then continues to complain of inadequate relief. After several changes of narcotics with the same results, both the nurse and doctor become frustrated. This leads to hostility toward the patient who is called "a chronic complainer," "a neurotic," and again, "an addict." Nobody believes that he has that much pain, and they are convinced that the patient's pain must be supratentorial or that he is overreacting. The next step often taken is to try to modify the patient's behavior rather than treat his pain. Very often, it is the nurse who will suggest to the doctor that the patient needs a tranquilizer or even a placebo.

In our experience, we have found that the addition of a tranquilizer or a sedative does not potentiate the analgesic effects of narcotics but instead will not only sedate the patient, but cause confusion and disorientation, and in some instances, may cause the patient to act in an irrational manner, especially if his pain is not being controlled.

By now, we all should understand the effects of a placebo. The patient who has confidence in his doctor and nurses, will almost always have a positive response to the placebo even when his pain correlates with demonstrated organic disease.

Since patients with cancer are often candidates for complications, one cannot assume that the cause of pain will necessarily be the same from day to day. Before giving an analgesic, the nurse should ask the patient if the pain is the same or if there has been some change. If there has been a change, she should obtain more information about it. Any new pain should be reported to the patient's physician as soon as possible. Some complications, if not treated promptly can lead to irreversible effects, such as cord compression.

There are times when the nurse should anticipate when the patient may require an analgesic. These times may be:

1. Before a patient is sent for a procedure that may be painful or uncomfortable and may require several hours (e.g., skeletal survey, scans, I.V.P., etc.). Patient may be unable to lie on a hard table because of pain and may refuse to complete the procedure. These patients are often sent back to the hospital floor with the notation that the patient was uncooperative. The nurse should be aware of the nature of these procedures and explain them to the patient, and she should encourage the patient to take his medication before the pain becomes unbearable so that the medication ordered would be most effective.
2. Before ambulation (if pain increases on movement or on sitting).
3. Before meals (if the patient's pain increases while he is eating or shortly after).
4. At bedtime (if the patient states the pain gets worse at night or he can't fall asleep even with sedation because the pain keeps him awake).

To be effective, a nurse must be aware and sensitive to all the problems that these patients may be facing. It is not enough just to know the disease process and the cause of pain. Her role as a care-giver requires understanding and a willingness to attend to even the little things.

Today, the public is more educated and is demanding better understanding of health-care services and that their rights and expectations, interests, needs, and concerns be recognized. Since 1913, the American Cancer Society has been involved in cancer control, public education, and services. In their 1978 publication, *Cancer Facts and Figures,* they discuss basic data, why early detection is vital, early detection and high-risk groups, the cancer checkup, cancer trends, treatment trends, and the function of the American Cancer Society in public education and information, professional education, service and rehabilitation, research, cost of cancer, and their sources of income and the allocation of ACS Funds.

Although it would be important to discuss all these aspects in more detail, two areas that warrant more emphasis are public education and information and costs of cancer.

The American Cancer Society allocated 30.2% of their 1976–1977 budget to research ($37,987,000) and the next highest figure, 16.7%, to public education ($20,973,000). Special emphasis is placed on projects involving person-to-person contact. A 1977 Gallup study indicated a broad receptiveness to that kind of cancer education. To help advance the person-to-person education concept, the Society now is using specialized volunteers who are individuals already trained professionally in certain skills that can be adapted to fighting cancer. Ex-smokers are leading Quit-smoking Clinics to help smokers "kick the habit." Nurses are teaching the breast self-examination (BSE) and encouraging women at or after menopause to have endometrial-tissue samplings taken.

Other programs include the new "Early Start to Good Health" in an attempt to introduce good health-habits to children in kindergarten through the third grade. During the annual ACS Cancer Crusade, volunteers made personal home visits urging individuals to protect themselves against cancer. Last year, local public education programs involving two-way communication reached more than 22.5 million people throughout the United States, and in conjunction with business and industry, 1.3 million workers.

It is difficult to estimate the impact of public-information programs. Surveys have shown, for example, that only one woman in three practiced breast self-examination (BSE), however, 9 out of 10 said they had heard of it and 36% were interested in learning. Teenage girls are smoking more. In this age group, it has increased by 5% from 1964 to 1975 to a level of 27%. The number who smoke a pack or more a day quadrupled. Teenage boys held steady at 30%. The Society's antismoking campaign through mass media has been accelerated with a new series of TV spots, new pamphlets, such special events as writing contests and no-smoking days. It is unfortunate that scare tactics may not always work; in fact, in many instances, the negative approach may actually defeat the purpose. The person who may have a cancer phobia may be too afraid to seek medical advice for he may think it is too late and nothing can be done anyway. On the other hand, a patient may go from doctor to doctor and be labeled a hypochondriac. In the last several years, many of our motion-picture films or films made for television have been based on those who have died of cancer rather than on those who have been cured of cancer or are living with cancer.

Although the American Cancer Society has issued a new booklet entitled *The Hopeful Side of Cancer*, in which they mention community and patient services that are available, this information and information of the costs of cancer is seldom conveyed to the public via the mass media. The total cost of cancer is now estimated to be, including earning loss, at over $18.9 billion a year in the United States. The Third National Cancer Survey of the United States Department of Health, Education and Welfare placed the average cost of cancer hospitalization in 1969 and 1970 at $2,529—about $90 a day—over a 28-day period. The Health Insurance Institutes' latest statistics show the average community-hospital costs per day for 1975 were $151, which would raise the 28-day cancer stay to $4,228. A 1973 study by Cancer Care, Inc. of New York City reported overall cancer expenses ranging from $5,000 to $50,000 with a median of $19,000 spent over 2 years (1). Because of inflation, the cost of hospitalization, physicians' services, drugs, treatments, nursing services, and equipment is even higher today. The public has no idea of these costs until it happens to them, and the health-care professionals know even less. Although prevention, early detection and public education are vital, the public should be better informed as to what can be done for the patient who has advanced cancer and pain. The patient expects to be treated as a whole human being; therefore, every effort should be made to look at him as a whole person—his social, cultural, and economic environment in and out of the hospital, social-psychological factors in his illness, and patient–professional health-care-team interaction (5). Our aim for the patient who has pain due to advanced cancer is an understanding of his suffering and, through understanding, relief.

ACKNOWLEDGMENTS

Supported in part by grants awarded by the National Institute on Drug Abuse (DA 01707–02).

I wish to thank Miss Julie Franchi and Mr. George Heidrich, R.N., B.S.N., for their assistance in the literature search and Miss Natalie M. Rogers for her assistance in the preparation of the manuscript.

REFERENCES

1. American Cancer Society (1978): *Cancer Facts and Figures.* American Cancer Society, New York.
2. American Cancer Society (1977): *Proceedings of the Second Nursing Conference on Cancer Nursing.* American Cancer Society, New York.
3. Ayers, R., and Reed-Ash, C. (1978): Message from the editors. *Cancer Nurs.,* Vol. I, No. I.
4. Butler, F. (1955): *Cancer Through the Ages: The Evolution of Hope.* Virginia Press, Fairfax, Va.
5. Chasca, N. (1977): Medical Sociology for Whom? *Mayo Clinic Proc.,* 52:813–818.
6. Considine, B. (1959): *That Many May Live.* Memorial Center for Cancer and Allied Diseases, New York.
7. Hardy, R. E., Cull, J. G. (1975): *Counseling and Rehabilitating the Cancer Patient, No. 964: American Lecture Series.* Charles C Thomas, Springfield, Ill.
8. Kübler-Ross, E. (1969): *On Death and Dying.* The Macmillan Company, New York.
9. Shinkin, M. B. (1977): *Contrary to Nature.* United States Department of Health, Education and Welfare, Public Health Service, National Institute of Health, Washington, D.C.
10. Time-Life Books (1966): *Great Ages of Man: A History of the World's Culture.* Time-Life Books, New York.
11. Wise, T. (1978): Sexual functioning in neoplastic disease, *Med. Aspects Hum. Sexuality,* 12(1):16–31.

Discussion

Part I. Basic Considerations (continued)

K. Foley and G. Martino (Moderators)

Chapman (Seattle): Dr. Beales, to what extent are the parents' beliefs and fears about the child's disease likely to become a factor in the developing pain of the child?

Beales (Manchester): The parents' attitudes are of vital importance because how the child interprets what is going on inside his own body is greatly influenced by learning, and he is very much dependent upon other people's telling him what signals might mean. If the parents themselves are very anxious about a particular type of condition, there is a fair chance that the child will present at some time or other symptoms which seem to indicate that kind of condition. It very frequently happens that the parents pick up the slightest indications the child gives that he has this kind of problem and become anxious; the child himself becomes anxious, and it can be extremely difficult for the clinicians to reassure the parents or the child that there is, in fact, nothing wrong.

Bond (Glasgow): In addition to learning about the usually accepted significance of pain, mainly that it indicates organic damage of some kind, children also learn from their parents the other meaning of pain; that pain can be used to manipulate people, that pain can be equated in gaining pleasure and affection and so forth. One should bear this in mind when looking at pain problems in young children.

Mascia (Brooklyn): Dr. Bond, can you comment on the remarkable reactivation or remobilization of patients following psychological interventions?

Bond: I think there is not a simple answer. One can look at the question of the effect of the disease on the individual, the effect of the response of those around him or her to the illness, that is, both the medical personnel and the family; and I think the various factors involved have been mentioned during the course of the day by Chapman, myself, and others. Psychologic intervention usually means reestablishing contact with the patient, it may mean the making of a diagnosis of depressive illness which does occur in such people which, when treated, can produce considerable improvements in mood and motivation. It may mean removing the sense of helplessness, of hopelessness, of loneliness which often afflicts people who feel that doctors have nothing more to offer.

Bistolfi (Genova): Dr. Foley, have you had any experience about the worsening of radiationmyelitis by subsequent BC and U treatment?

Foley (New York): Patients with any neurological illness commonly become much worse when they receive chemotherapy. We do not see it as commonly with BC and U as we see it with vincristine or vinblastine or with high doses of methotrexate, since both drugs are neurotoxic in high doses.

Giugiaro (Torino): Dr. Morpurgo, what is the role of the following components in decoding the pain symptom: physiological cortex representation of the sensitive areas; progressive expansion of the representation of the diseased neoplastic area; drastic reduction of the exogenous stimuli following the patient's isolation? Furthermore, by which means do you define the body image present in cats? How are the registrations made?

Morpurgo (Milano): We had the impression that the progressive expansion of the area is the determining factor, while the reduction of the stimuli is less important because the visual perception associated with the painful stimulus and the large reduction of the training time would show that the pain stimulus itself is capable of occupying areas other than its own, independently of whether other areas are occupied or not. Everybody here knows that when we have a toothache, it is difficult to follow a show. So I would say that the other sensory inputs are considerably reduced by pain. As for the technique, we follow all the other researchers, from Mountcastle to Albe-Fessard and Spinelli. The cortical area which has to be explored is evidenced by means of electrodes that progressively penetrate it. Every time the machine shows a stable activity due to a neuron, then we analyze peripherally the areas from which such activity is generated. This way we can correlate the cortical image to what happens peripherally.

Raineri (Genova): Dr. Bond, do the patients who know of their disease and the ones who do not show any difference as regards pain sensitivity?

Bond: I think the answer lies in levels of anxiety. When people are told unpleasant things and become anxious, their tolerance tends to fall. So any circumstance which reduces the tendency to raise anxiety, and perhaps being treated at home may, in some circumstances, lower anxiety, whereas, in others, for reasons we have heard, may raise anxiety. Any situation which lowers anxiety will tend to keep pain thresholds up.

Martino (Milano): Italian physicians do not give explanations to the patient more than is necessary and are also reluctant in administration of analgesics. We should know that a percentage of patients, larger than we had thought, is capable of knowing the truth and its conditions, and that hiding the truth can give as much anxiety, even more than knowing the truth. As for hospitalization, it does not improve the survival, and it is isolating both in structure and in practice. Such inconvenience is indirectly confirmed by the literature, which shows a higher percentage of pain incidence in hospitalized patients than in those at home. However, also in this regard, there is no rule. Home can also be isolating depending on the social, cultural, and financial conditions of the family. For this reason, to carry out a correct analgesic therapy, we must estimate, in every single case, not only the psychological conditions of the patient, but also the social and cultural conditions of his home environment. In our experience, the pain symptom in the ambulatory patient is often a signal of his social discomfort. In these cases, to carry out a correct analgesic therapy, we should also work with the family, supporting it psychotherapeutically and financially.

Introduction to Management of Pain of Advanced Cancer

John J. Bonica

Department of Anesthesiology, University of Washington, Seattle, Washington 98195

In this chapter we begin consideration of the various modalities currently available for the management of pain of advanced cancer. As is well known this revolves around three main methods of approach: (a) use of anticancer modalities intended to decrease or eliminate the neoplasm and consequently eliminate the etiology and mechanism of the pain; (b) control of the pain without affecting the neoplasm; and (c) a combination of these.

Anticancer modalities include the use of: (a) *chemotherapy,* (b) *endocrine therapy,* (c) *radiation therapy,* (d) *radioisotope therapy,* and (e) *palliative surgery,* including excision of the tumor, bypass operation, and destruction or excision of endocrine organs such as hypophysectomy, adrenalectomy, and castration. It is important to emphasize, however, that regardless of which of the major approaches is to be used that physiologic and psychologic support of the patient and his family is an essential, if not the most essential, part of the management of patients with cancer pain. This will require a well-coordinated, concerted effort by the medical team, sociologists, and religious counselors.

When the aforementioned measures prove totally or partially ineffective or not feasible, it is necessary to control pain symptomatically without affecting a neoplasm (2,3,4). The modalities in current use include: (a) *systemic drugs* consisting of nonaddictive analgesics, sedatives, ataractics, psychotropic drugs, and potent (addictive) narcotics; (b) *therapeutic nerve blocks* which can be achieved either temporarily with a local anesthetic or for a prolonged period by injecting neurolytic agents; (c) *neurosurgical operations,* which may either be ablative, intended to interrupt pain pathways, or use stimulation of pain-modulating mechanisms including transcutaneous stimulation, peripheral-nerve stimulation, dorsal-column stimulation, and stimulation of the brain; (d) *psychologic methods* which include traditional psychotherapy, hypnosis, biofeedback, and operant conditioning. Many patients with cancer pain also need rehabilitation programs, which may include physical therapy, occupational therapy, exercise and support by psychologists, nurses, theologians, etc.

In determining which one or combination of therapies is to be used, it is essential to adhere to certain principles basic to the practice of medicine in general and to oncologic therapy in particular. In introducing the proper management of pain of advanced cancer, I wish to emphasize some of these principles and issues in order to provide a background for the following chapters. Although most of these are well known, all too often many of them are neglected by therapists. They will be discussed in greater detail in the chapters that follow.

One of the cardinal principles for health care is that optimal therapy of any pathologic process, including cancer pain, requires a correct diagnosis. In regard to pain, the therapist must know and appreciate its etiology, mechanism, and physiopathology. It is becoming clear that chronic pain is due to prolonged and persistent dysfunction of peripheral or central neural mechanisms, or psychologic or motivational or cognitive substrates of pain, or, most frequently, a combination of these. In Chapter 2, Zimmermann has already discussed the neurophysiology of nociception and acute pain and some of the peripheral mechanisms of chronic pain. Here I wish to supplement the discussion by presenting some speculations on the mechanisms of chronic pain in general which may serve as background for the discussion of the mechanisms of cancer pain. I emphasize that these are speculations, because scientific data from human studies are meager.

MECHANISM OF CHRONIC PAIN

From a therapeutic viewpoint, it may be useful to classify the suggested mechanisms of chronic pain in a simplistic fashion into "peripheral," "peripheral-central," "central," and "psychologic" mechanisms.

Peripheral Mechanisms

In some patients, including those with cancer, chronic pain is a consequence of a persistent pathologic process that causes persistent biochemical, mechanical, and thermal changes that sustain stimulation of nociceptors or afferent nociceptive pathways in the periphery. Persistent mechanical noxious stimulation probably occurs in various lesions such as tumors which irritate nerve endings or fibers. As Zimmermann has emphasized, sensitization may be caused by some of the pain-producing substances liberated from cellular breakdown or through emotional factors which increase sympathetic hyperactivity. Perl (18) has recently shown that, once the high-threshold A-delta and C-fibers have been damaged or heated and are tested after the evoked discharge has died down, they have become sensitized so that light pressure or mild warming now evokes firing. Moreover, as Zimmermann has mentioned, Wall and Gutnick (21) developed an experimental model for neuroma by cutting rat sciatic nerves and allowing the cut end to regenerate into a sealed polyethylene tube, and thus studied the physiology and pharmacology of the fine sprouts in the neuroma. They showed that the partially damaged nerve membrane and the sprouts within a neuroma become very sensitive to light pressure and to norepinephrine, which is liberated in greater amounts as a result of sympathetic hyperactivity provoked by injury. They also showed that some of the modulation produced by electric stimulation of peripheral nerves resulted from the turnoff of abnormal peripheral nerve generators in the neuroma. The clinical implication of peripheral mechanisms is that pain due to prolonged dysfunction of peripheral parts of the nociceptive system, can be eliminated by interrupting the afferent nociceptive pathways (6).

Peripheral-central Mechanisms

In some patients dysfunction of nociceptor systems initiates in the periphery but subsequently involves parts of the neuraxis. Examples of these are reflex sympathetic dystrophy phantom-limb pain, and the late stages of postthoracotomy and other postoperative-pain syndromes that may develop in cancer patients. Although the exact mechanisms of this persistent dysfunction are not known, the following are among the most important hypotheses proposed.

The "vicious circle" mechanisms. Initial injury produces reflex responses that, in turn, produce abnormal changes in tissues that contribute to the noxious stimulation (13). The reflex skeletal muscle spasm contributes to the afferent barrage; the sympathetic hyperactivity causes vasospasm with a consequent sequence of ischemia, cellular damage, liberation of pain-producing substances, and sensitization of nociceptors to nonnoxious stimuli. The sympathetic hyperactivity also causes increased liberation of norepinephrine in nerve endings that then augment the firing in the small sensory fibers. One or all of these factors cause persistent noxious stimulation that then causes abnormal firing patterns in closed, self-exciting neuron pools in the spinal cord, which in turn produce more intense reflex responses with consequent increased noxious stimulation (13). Thus, a vicious circle of pain, reflex response, and more pain is initiated and sustained. Invariably, psychologic factors contribute to these mechanisms.

Decrease of peripheral inhibition. These mechanisms, based on the Melzack-Wall theory (16), often have been invoked to explain the chronic pain associated with certain peripheral-nerve disorders that reduce the number of active large fibers and cause the loss of their inhibitory influence on synaptic transmission on dorsal horn cells. This mechanism has been suggested for: (a) painful peripheral neuropathies in which there is an actual loss of large fibers, as in diabetes, post-herpetic neuralgia, and certain toxic neuropathies; and (b) painful disorders in which there is mechanical pressure on peripheral nerves. Since large fibers are more vulnerable to pressure than are small fibers, there is consequent loss of large-fiber inhibition. Wall (20) has suggested that this may be the mechanism of pain associated with neoplasm and other diseases that mechanically impinge on axons and peripheral nerves.

Central biasing mechanism. A hypothesis somewhat related to the preceding two is that of Melzack (15), by which he proposed to explain the pain of phantom limb, causalgia, and other peripheral-nerve injuries. It is based on some of the aforementioned recent data pertaining to the neural systems that exert powerful inhibitory influences on various parts of the neuraxis. According to this concept, a portion of the brainstem reticular formation acts as a central biasing mechanism by exerting a tonic inhibitory influence or bias on transmission at all synaptic levels of the somatosensory system, including the "gate" in the dorsal horn and at other levels of the neuraxis. This inhibitory function of the central biasing mechanism is dependent in part on a normal sensory input. Loss of input to the system, as occurs with peripheral-nerve lesions and amputation, weakens the inhibition and thus causes persistent pain. Emotional stress and certain drugs can also impair the efficacy of the biasing mechanism, thus aggravating the spontaneous pain. Contrarily, increased sensory input by mechanical stimulation or by direct electrical stimulation of the skin or nerve would increase the inhibition and decrease the pain.

Melzack has used this concept to explain the therapeutic efficacy of peripheral tactile and electrical stimulation in peripheral-nerve injuries. He has also used the concept to explain the therapeutic efficacy of nerve blocks in the treatment of causalgia and other reflex sympathetic dystrophies. The nerve block permits temporary return to normalcy by breaking up the activity in the self-sustaining neuron pools, and it thus produces relief of pain that may outlast the pharmacologic effect of the block. After the block has worn off, stimulation again triggers sustained activity, but because of the time necessary for it to spread to a sufficiently large number of neurons within the pools, pain-relief outlasts the action of the local anesthetic. Moreover, the relief of pain permits increased use of the limb, which produces patterned, temporarily dispersed inputs, particularly from the muscles that are out of phase with the rhythmically firing neuron pools, and disrupts their activity. This delays resumption of self-sustaining firing.

Denervation hypersensitivity. To explain the pain, dysesthesia, and paresthesia that often accompany peripheral-nerve injuries and complicate surgical interruption of pain pathways such as rhizotomy and cordotomy, Loeser et al. (14), among others, have proposed that loss of normal sensory input produces an abnormal firing pattern in the somatosensory system proximal to the deafferentation (9). In animal models, he found seizure-like abnormal firing patterns in deafferented dorsal-root fibers and lateral caudate nucleus. He also has recorded high-frequency bursts distal to a spinal-cord injury in a patient exhibiting paraplegic pain and flexor spasm. Black et al. (1) have shown similar abnormal firing patterns following trigeminal denervation consequent to tooth-pulp extraction and section of the nerve. Since damage to a peripheral nerve causes chromatolysis of ganglion cells, and since it has been shown that chromatolytic motor neurons become hyperexcitable, Wall (20) has suggested that peripheral-nerve section produces either a partial central deafferentation with consequent hyperexcitability, or a change of the location of central terminals.

Central Pain Mechanisms

Disease of certain parts of the central nervous system (CNS) often produces what is generally referred to as "central pain," characterized by spontaneous burning, aching pain, hyperalgesia, dysesthesia, and other abnormal sensations (8). Central pain often accompanies thalamic lesions (so-called "thalamic pain"), surgical interruption of certain parts of the pain pathway, tabes dorsalis, and other painful diseases of the CNS (2,8). Mechanisms of these disorders are not known, but it has been suggested that there is a loss of descending inhibitory influences, or that interruption of certain parts of the pain pathway disturbs the normal balance between the discriminative and motivational systems.

Psychologic Mechanisms

In addition to the important role psychologic factors play in chronic pain produced by injury or disease, in a significant number of patients, chronic pain primarily due to psychologic factors develops. This group can be arbitrarily subdivided into four categories: (a) psychophysiologic mechanisms; (b) operant mechanisms; (c) psychogenic mechanisms; and (d) psychiatric mechanisms (6).

Psychophysiologic (psychosomatic) mechanisms. In some individuals, severe emotional stress, through psychophysiologic (corticofugal) mechanisms, produces skeletal-muscle spasm, local vasoconstriction, visceral dysfunction, liberation of pain substances, or a combination of these (2,19). One or more of these produces peripheral noxious stimulation, with its consequences of pain, reflex responses, and affective reactions, all of which aggravate the emotional stress. This, in turn, provokes more psychophysiologic impulses, thus sustaining the vicious circle of pain. This is probably the mechanism of tension headache and pain due to spasm of muscles in the shoulder girdle, low back, and chest. Psychophysiologic mechanism has also been invoked to explain migraine headache, in which emotional factors provoke the liberation of substances that produce the characteristic vasoconstriction and vasodilatation. It has long been appreciated that this is the probable mechanism of coronary artery disease, peptic ulcer, and colitis, each of which is often accompanied by chronic pain.

Operant mechanism. This mechanism, first proposed by Fordyce (11,12), is responsible in a significant number of patients in whom chronic pain behavior develops following a disease or injury that often is of a minor nature.

The initial injury provokes operant responses and pain behavior on the part of the patient that are reinforced by favorable consequences or reactions on the part of those important to the patient. Thus, a husband who for years has been inattentive to his wife becomes solicitous and concerned and gives special attention when she sustains an injury—favorable consequences that reinforce her pain behavior. This concept involves well-established principles of operant conditioning that state that behavior is subject to the influence of, or under the control of, learning factors, and to a considerable degree is governed by consequences in the environment.

Chronic pain behavior continues as long as the consequences are favorable, and eventually becomes independent of the underlying pathology and persists even after the original pathogenic factor is gone. Under such conditions, a "pain habit" that is real and is readily accounted for by learning or conditioning has developed. The important therapeutic implications are that, to change the chronic pain behavior, it is necessary to eliminate the favorable consequences that are acting as positive reinforcers to the behavior, rather than to seek out and try to eliminate underlying pathology.

Mechanisms of "psychogenic" pain. A significant number of patients who have chronic pain have what is traditionally referred to as "psychogenic" pain, which really means pain due to psychologic causes. It deserves strong emphasis that these patients are not imagining the pain, but that the pain is as real as and is felt and described in much the same way as "somatogenic" pain. The difference between these two major groups is that psychogenic pain is less adequately explained in physical terms. In view of this, Sternbach (19) suggested the definition that "psychogenic pain" refers to "pain which is better understood in psychologic than in physical language." The psychodynamics of "psychogenic" pain have been detailed by Sternbach. Briefly, in these patients' early lives, pain was associated with anxiety and fear of bodily harm and loss of love. Later, the experience of one evokes the sensation of the other: Pain provokes "unnecessary anxiety," or anxiety can cause "psychogenic pain." Anxiety is the affect associated with the experience of acute pain. When what is feared actually does come to pass, depression replaces anxiety. Psychogenic pain symbolizes conflict among unmet emotional needs, internal prohibition, and external realities.

Psychiatric mechanisms. Chronic pain is occasionally a symptom of depression, hysteria, or other psychiatric disorders. The psychodynamics of these are described by Merskey and Spear (17).

Cancer can cause pain by one or more of the following mechanisms: (a) bone tumor invasion, (b) compression of nerve roots, nerve trunks, or plexuses; (c) infiltration of nerves by tumor cells; (d) obstruction of hollow viscera; (e) occlusion of large blood vessels; (f) infiltration, contraction, and swelling in tissue invested snugly by fascia, periosteum, or other pain-sensitive structures; or (g) necrosis, infection, inflammation, and ulceration of pain-sensitive structures produced by the lesion.

MECHANISM OF CANCER PAIN

As emphasized by Foley (10), the etiology of cancer pain may be classified into one of three major categories: (a) pain caused by the oncologic process; (b) pain that develops as a result of therapy; and (c) pain that develops coincidentally with, but is unrelated to, the cancer. In the average cancer-hospital population, pain is caused by the oncologic process in three-quarters of the patients, posttherapy pain is present in 20% of the patients, and about 5% have coincidental pain (10). Although Foley has described the most important causes of pain in cancer patients, the following brief section is intended to summarize the subject. Those aspects discussed in detail by Foley will only be mentioned here.

Pain Caused by the Oncologic Process

The following classification of cancer-induced pain is a modification of the one first proposed by Bonica (2,3) a quarter-century ago and taking into consideration recently acquired information about basic mechanisms as well as the information provided by Foley.

Bone Tumor Invasion

As Foley has indicated, tumor invasion of bone by either primary or metastatic lesion is the most common cause of pain in patients with cancer. This is discussed in greater detail by Foley (*this volume*).

Compression of Nerve Roots, Nerve Trunks, and Plexuses

Compression of nerve roots, nerve trunks, or plexuses by an enlarging tumor or lymph glands or metastatic fracture of bones adjacent to the nerves results in a radiculopathy or neuropathy which is accompanied by fairly sharp, localized neuralgic pain projected to the distribution of the nerve structure involved. In such instances, it is likely that noxious mechanical stimulation produces dysfunction of the nociceptive system which is limited to the periphery for a time, but then it may activate peripheral-central mechanisms.

Tumor Infiltration of Nervous Structures

Infiltration of a peripheral nerve causes constant, burning pain associated with hyperesthesia and dysesthesia in the area of sensory loss. Tumor infiltration of other plexuses or major nerves will produce burning pain with hyperalgesia, hyperesthesia, and dysesthesia along the distribution of the affected nerve. It is important to note that the quality of the pain is usually burning, resembling that of causalgia and reflex sympathetic dystrophy. In fact, reflex sympathetic dystrophy frequently accompanies perineural infiltration by cancer cells.

Infiltration of Blood Vessels

Infiltration of blood vessels by tumor cells results in vasospasm and a perivascular lymphangitis and consequent irritation of nociceptors or nociceptive afferents. This process produces a diffuse burning or aching pain that does *not* have a peripheral-nerve distribution. In many instances, there develops a reflex sympathetic hyperactivity with a consequent increased liberation of norepinephrine which aggravates the basic physiopathology and sensitizes nociceptors. This type of process probably involves peripheral mechanisms, and the pain can be eliminated effectively by interruption of the affected peripheral nociceptive pathways.

Obstruction of a Hollow Viscus or the Ductal System in a Solid Viscus

It is well known that obstruction of the stomach, intestine, biliary tract, ureters, uterus, or urinary bladder causes intense contraction of the smooth muscles under isometric conditions (i.e., when the exit of the viscus is obstructed) with the production of visceral pain which is characteristically diffuse and poorly localized and referred to dermatomes supplied by the same spinal-cord segments which supply the affected viscus. Recent data show that these structures are supplied by A-delta and C-fibers which are activated by ischemia and chemical agents (7). It is likely that the ischemia causes cellular breakdown with production of "pain-producing substances" and probably lowers the threshold of mechanical nociceptors. A similar mechanism is probably operative in oncologic processes which obstruct the outflow of ductal systems of the pancreas, liver, and other solid viscera. In all of these conditions, persistent obstruction produces progressively greater contractions and finally intense distention with consequent progressively greater pain.

Occlusion of Blood Vessels

Occlusion of blood vessels, either partial or complete, by an adjacent tumor produces venous engorgement or arterial ischemia or both. Venous engorgement will result in a tumor of all the structures that are supplied by the obstructing vessel. The edema, in turn, causes distention of facial compartments and other pain-sensitive structures resulting in progressively more severe, intractable pain. Examples are the progressively more severe headaches consequent to obstruction of the veins draining from the head, and the pain in the upper or lower limb caused by obstruction of the venous outflow from these structures. Ischemia produced by obstruction of a major artery probably causes cellular breakdown with production of "pain-producing substances" which lower the threshold of nociceptors. The pain generated by these mechanisms is usually diffuse and does not follow any particular nerve distribution and usually becomes progressively worse. It is likely that the pain arising from these pathologic processes involves purely peripheral mechanisms and theoretically should be relieved by denervation of the affected part, provided that the interruption is extensive enough.

Tumefaction and Swelling in a Structure Invested Snugly by Fascia, Periosteum, or other Pain-sensitive Structures

This type of process is probably responsible for the pain associated with growing tumors of liver, spleen, and certain types of kidney tumors. Each of these processes produces distention of the investing pain-sensitive structure with consequent stimulation of mechanical nociceptors. If the pain-inducing tumor is a superficial somatic structure, the pain is sharp and relatively well localized; whereas if the tumor is situated in deep somatic structures or the viscera, the pain is dull, poorly localized, and usually referred to dermatomes which receive the same nerve supply as the involved structure.

Necrosis, Infection, Inflammation, and Ulceration of Mucous Membranes and Other Pain-sensitive Structures

These pathologic processes produce pain which is frequently excruciating and most likely to occur with cancer of the lips, mouth, and face, and tumors of the gastrointestinal and genitourinary tracts. It is likely that the inflammatory reaction lowers the threshold of nociceptors so that innocuous stimuli produce excruciating pain usually localized to the region.

Pain Syndromes Associated with Cancer Therapy

Pain that develops as a complication of cancer therapy can be further subdivided into three etiologic subgroups: (a) pain that develops following surgery such as postthoractomy pain, postmastectomy pain, pain after a radical neck dissection and phantom-limb pain; (b) postradiation pain syndromes including radiation fibrosis of the brachial or lumbar plexus, radiation necrosis of bone, and radiation-induced secondary injury; (c) pain that develops following chemotherapy such as the pain associated with peripheral neuropathy from *Vinca* alkaloids, post-herpetic neuralgia that develops as a late effect of immunosuppresive therapy and mucositis in which chemotherapeutic agents produce chemical changes in mucous membranes and other pain-sensitive structures with consequent severe pain particularly in the mouth, throat, and nasal passages.

Postsurgical Pain

Pain following thoracotomy and mastectomy is usually due to damage of the nerves during the surgical operation. The nerves may be partially injured or completely severed. The pain becomes evident 1 to 2 months following the operation and is characterized by constant pain in the area of sensory loss with occasional, intermittent, shock-like pains. Dysesthesia in the scar area and hyperesthesia in the surrounding zone are often prominent symptoms. It is likely that the proximal portion of the severed nerve regenerates and produces small neuromata. Moreover, the surgical trauma usually damages nerve membranes of unsevered nerves. The neuroma and damaged membrane are hypersensitive to pressure and norepinephrine (20,21). Consequently, light touch and movement exacerbate the pain. As a result, some of these patients may develop a concomitant frozen shoulder and consequent limitation of motion and disuse atrophy of the arm, and the patient may develop a true reflex sympathetic dystrophy.

A number of patients who undergo radical neck dissection develop constant burning pain, dysesthesia, and lancinating pain in the region of the neck. The physiopathologic process is similar to that of other postsurgical neuropathies. Following amputation of the limb, the patient may develop two types of pain: pain in the stump and pain in the phantom limb. The stump pain is constant and burning in character, whereas the pain in the phantom limb may be either a burning pain or cramping, proprioceptive pain characterized by abnormal position of the missing distal part of the limb.

In all of these postsurgical pain syndromes, peripheral-central mechanisms are usually operative. Initially, the peripheral nociceptive dysfunction predominates, but eventually the disturbance in the neuraxis plays the most important role. The clinical implication of this is that interruption of pain of peripheral nociceptive pathways is likely to produce little or no pain-relief.

Postchemotherapy Syndromes

Painful dysesthesia and paresthesia following treatment with the *Vinca* alkaloid drugs such as vincristine and vinblastine occurs as part of a symmetrical polyneuropathy which usually develops with the doses of the drug required to achieve an antineoplastic effect (10). Dysesthesias are commonly localized to the hands and feet and are characterized by burning pain exacerbated by noxious stimuli.

Steroid pseudo-rheumatism occurs following withdrawal of steroid medications. Some patients develop diffuse myalgia and arthralgia with muscle and joint tenderness on palpitation but without objective inflammatory signs. These symptoms regress with reinstitution of steroid therapy.

Aseptic necrosis of the head of the femur or the humerus or both with consequent pain in the knee or shoulder joint, respectively, occurs as a complication of cancer therapy, specifically, chronic steroid therapy. This is discussed in detail by Foley.

Post-herpetic neuralgia is a complication of radiation therapy, or it may occur following herpes zoster that develops in the area of tumor pathology. The patient usually experiences continuous, burning pain in the area of sensory loss, painful dysesthesia and intermittent lancinating pain. This condition involves peripheral-central mechanisms and is one of the most difficult pain syndromes to treat.

Mucositis occurs after the administration of certain chemotherapeutic agents which apparently produce biochemical changes in mucous membranes and other pain-sensitive structures with consequent severe pain particularly in the mouth, throat, and nasal passages.

Postradiation Therapy Pain

Following radiation therapy to the region of the brachial plexus or the lumbosacral plexus, *fibrosis* of the surrounding or connective tissue occurs with secondary injury to the nerve structures (2,10). The condition is progressive with consequent increasing pain. The pain is often associated with numbness or paresthesia in the structures supplied by the affected nerves, lymphedema in the arm, and radiation skin changes and induration of the supraclavicular and axillary areas present with brachial plexus fibrosis. Similarly, fibrosis of the lumbosacral plexus produces pain associated with progressive motor and sensory changes and lymphedema in the limb. The fibrosis, which is a slow, progressive process, produces injury to the nerves with consequent abnormal firing that eventually produces abnormal function in the somatosensory system in the neuraxis. Consequently, the peripheral-central mechanism produces the pain, which is not likely to respond to interruption of peripheral pathways.

Radiation myelopathy is an important problem which is discussed in detail by Foley (*this volume*).

SELECTION OF THERAPY

In determining the best therapeutic modality or combination of therapies to effectively relieve the pain, it is essential to consider the characteristics of the pain, the chronology of the disease and of previous therapy, and various other aspects which can only be ascertained by a very detailed history and a comprehensive general physical, neurologic, orthopedic and other appropriate examinations (2,10). Since most patients with cancer pain present a complex array of physical, psychologic, behavioral, and affective manifestations, a total psychologic and social evaluation is mandatory to develop the most appropriate therapeutic strategy. These are essential to define the role that psychologic, social, cultural, motivational, and related factors play in the patient's total pain experience.

History

A careful history of the pain complaint is an essential first step in determining a therapy. It is important to consider the location and distribution of the pain and its possible spread, its quality, severity, and time-characteristics (i.e., whether it is continuous or occurs in bouts), and what factors aggravate and relieve the pain. It is also important to elicit information about associated phenomena including sensory deficits, muscle weakness, and visceral dysfunction. For example, in a patient complaining of severe back pain exacerbated by lying down associated with a complaint of difficulty in urinating suggests a diagnosis of epidural spinal-cord compression.

It is also important to obtain a history of the oncologic process in order to determine which of the major etiologic factors is responsible for the pain. If the pain is directly due to the neoplasm, it is essential to know the type and grade of differentiation and site of spread or metastasis. If the pain is the result of therapy, an attempt should be made to predict its time-course. For example, the pain of postradiation fibrosis of the brachial plexus is progressive in severity and often very difficult to control with drugs. Similarly, post-herpetic neuralgia consequent to immunosuppressive therapy and post-thoracotomy, postmastectomy, and postamputation pain are also progressive and require early application of therapeutic modalities that will eliminate the basic mechanisms which, at this stage, involve only the peripheral nociceptive system. Management of such patients with systemic drugs may relieve the pain temporarily but does not prevent progression of the neural mechanism. These are likely to involve the CNS with a consequent progressive increase in the pain and the associated reflex sympathetic dystrophy which, after a period of months, will not be relieved by anything except very destructive procedures in the higher parts of the neuraxis.

Examination

Careful examination of the painful region and the general physical, neurologic, and orthopedic examinations are also essential to acquire objective data and substantiate the clinical history. A detailed neurologic examination is particularly useful in differentiating local pain from referred pain, and in differentiating pain due to peripheral-nerve involvement from pain due to plexus or cord involvement. For example, in a patient with low-back pain and radicular symptomatology in L5-S1 distribution, together with an absent ankle jerk, nerve root rather than plexus involvement is suggested.

Psychologic and Psychosocial Evaluation

A comprehensive psychologic and social evaluation is essential to develop the most effective therapeutic strategy. This should include a general psychologic and behavioral assessment and the application of appropriate psychometric tests. Psychosocial evaluation should include determination of cultural background, religious beliefs, interaction with spouse and family unit, social activities, and the impact of these on the pain. These will be considered in more detail in later chapters.

Special Diagnostic Tests

Various diagnostic tools may be essential to determine the mechanisms of pain. Since plain X-rays have limitations, it may be necessary to supplement them with bone scan, tomography and, in some special cases, computerized transaxial tomography (CT scan). In addition to the usual laboratory examination, special biochemical procedures may be necessary. Cisternal and lumbar myography and cerebrospinal fluid cytology are sometimes necessary to determine the etiology of the pain. The important role that appropriate nerve blocks can play in ascertaining the mechanisms and pathways of cancer pain will be discussed later. The appropriate use of placebo or hypnosis or both may provide important information about the physiologic and psychologic substrates of pain.

Evaluation of Therapeutic Modalities

Knowledge of therapeutic modalities currently available for the relief of cancer pain is crucial to the selection of the most effective therapy. It is essential to know not only the analgesic efficacy and advantages, but also the limitations and disadvantages of each procedure. Only with such knowledge integrated into the information obtained from the history and physical examination will it be possible to determine which is the best method or methods of relieving cancer pain.

Multidisciplinary Team Management

The importance of a multidisciplinary team effort in managing patients with cancer, especially in the terminal phase, has become well established. For many years, cancer hospitals and cancer units of general hospitals have had oncology groups consisting of oncologic surgeons, radiation therapists, medical oncologists, and pathologists to deal with the pathologic process. More recently, the importance of treating the whole patient (rather than just the lesion) has become appreciated; and consequently oncology teams have added nutritionists, nurses, physical therapists, psychologists, social workers, and various other health professionals and chaplains with special interest and expertise in cancer management. Moreover, much has been written on the physiologic and psychologic needs of cancer patients.

Unfortunately, most of these oncology groups in the United States have ignored or neglected one of the most important aspects of the care of cancer patients—the effective control of pain. This aspect is especially important in patients with advanced and terminal cancer. Except for a few of the comprehensive cancer centers with pain-control teams, the management of pain is relegated to the house staff who, as previously mentioned, have had no formal teaching and consequently treat the pain empirically, usually with narcotics prescribed in totally inadequate doses.

Consideration of the numerous mechanisms of chronic pain in general and cancer pain in particular and of the various modalities currently available for its therapy makes it obvious that no one individual has the knowledge, expertise, and skill to provide optimal relief to each and every patient. I recognized this problem 35 years ago when I was given the responsibility of managing patients with severe intractable pain due to wartime injuries (2). As a result of these experiences, I developed the conviction that the management of complex pain problems is best achieved by well-coordinated, concerted efforts of a team composed of the patient's physician and specialists from different disciplines, each of whom contributes individualized knowledge and skills to the common goal of making a correct diagnosis and developing the most appropriate therapeutic strategy. Following World War II, I proved the usefulness of this concept in a community general hospital, and in 1960, I founded the University of Washington Multidisciplinary Pain Clinic. In the course of 18 years, this group has grown to about 25 health professionals representing some 14 basic science and clinical disciplines (5). Despite the numerous publications and hundreds of lectures given throughout the world, until the early 1970s the concept was ignored by the medical profession. Fortunately, during the past 6 years or so, a number of such multidisciplinary facilities modeled after the University of Washington program have been developed in the United States and several other countries.

A detailed description of the organization and function of the University of Washington facility has been published (5). The unique feature of this facility is that the members of the group have close interaction during the diagnostic workup of the patient. The managing physician and the various consultants continuously communicate during the entire process. Once all of the diagnostic information is collected, it is presented at the conference which is held at frequent intervals. This is followed by vigorous interchange among the members of the group until there is a consensus about the diagnosis and best therapy. Long experience has shown that this type of face-to-face group discussion held during the conferences is much more effective and productive in making a correct diagnosis and formulating the appropriate therapeutic strategy than communication by letter or telephone or through the fragmented, independent efforts inherent in traditional medical practice. In addition to providing highly specialized consultant services to the referring physician and the patient, these conferences serve as an excellent forum for the exchange of ideas and information and thus constitute a highly effective teaching mechanism. Moreover, the frequent interchange among the members of the group enhances the cross-fertilization of new ideas and stimulates independent and collaborative research.

Long experience also suggests that this multidisciplinary team approach is even more effective in managing patients with cancer pain. As far back as 1953, I advocated the team approach to provide a more effective therapy for pain of advanced and terminal cancer (2,4). In the ensuing quarter-century, I have espoused the concept repeatedly in numerous articles and lectures given at regional, national, and international cancer meetings. A multidisciplinary pain diagnostic and therapy team is especially indicated in the larger comprehensive cancer centers. Such a team should be composed of basic scientists and clinicians with special interest and expertise in chronic pain in general and cancer pain in particular who would devote the time and effort to evaluate carefully each patient with severe cancer pain and determine the best method or methods of relieving the pain. Such a team should include medical, surgical, and radiation oncologists, clinical pharmacologists, anesthesiologists, neurosurgeons, psychologists, psychiatrists, social workers, nurses with special knowledge and expertise in pain, theologians and others with special expertise and skills that might be needed in the diagnostic workup and in the development of the most appropriate therapeutic strategy.

REFERENCES

1. Black, R. G., Anderson, L., and Abraham, J. (1971): Neuronal hyperactivity in experimental trigeminal deafferentation. *J. Neurosurg.*, 35:444–452.
2. Bonica, J. J. (1953): *The Management of Pain*. Lea & Febiger, Philadelphia.
3. Bonica, J. J. (1954): The management of pain of malignancies with nerve blocks. *Anesthesiology*, 15:134–142; 280–301.
4. Bonica, J. J. (1954): The management of cancer pain. *GP (American Academy of General Practice)*, 10:34–43.
5. Bonica, J. J. (1974): Organization and function of a pain clinic: In: *Advances in Neurology, Vol. 4: International Symposium on Pain,* edited by J. J. Bonica, pp. 433–443. Raven Press, New York.
6. Bonica, J. J. (1977): Neurophysiologic and pathologic aspects of acute and chronic pain. *Arch. Surg.*, 112:750–761.
7. Bonica, J. J., and Albe-Fessard, D., editors (1976): *Advances in Pain Research and Therapy, Vol. 1: Proceedings of the First World Congress on Pain*. Raven Press, New York.
8. Cassinari, V., and Pagni, C. A. (1969): *Central Pain: A Neurosurgical Survey*. Harvard University Press, Cambridge, Mass.
9. Denny-Brown, D., Kirk, E. J., and Yanagisawa, N. (1973): The tract of Lissauer in relation to sensory transmission in the dorsal horn of the spinal cord in macaque monkey. *J. Comp. Neurol.*, 151:175–200.
10. Foley, K. (1979): Pain syndromes in patients with cancer. In: *Advances in Pain*

Research and Therapy, Vol. 2, edited by J. J. Bonica and V. Ventafridda. Raven Press, New York.
11. Fordyce, W. (1974): Treating chronic pain by contingency management. In: *Advances in Neurology, Vol. 4: International Symposium on Pain,* edited by J. J. Bonica, pp. 585–587. Raven Press, New York.
12. Fordyce, W. E. (1976): *Behavioral Methods for Chronic Pain and Illness.* C. V. Mosby Co., St. Louis.
13. Livingston, W. K. (1943): *Pain Mechanisms.* Macmillan Co., New York.
14. Loeser, J. D., Ward, A. A., Jr., and White, L. E., Jr. (1968): Chronic deafferentation of the human spinal cord neurons. *J. Neurosurg.,* 29:48–50.
15. Melzack, R. (1973): *The Puzzle of Pain.* Basic Books, Inc., New York.
16. Melzack, R., and Wall, P. D. (1965): Pain mechanisms: A new theory. *Science,* 150:971–979.
17. Merskey, H., and Spear, F. G. (1967): *Pain: Psychological and Psychiatric Aspects.* Bailliere Tindall & Cassell, Ltd., London.
18. Perl, E. R. (1976): Sensitization of nociceptors and its relation to sensation. In: *Advances in Pain Research and Therapy, Vol. 1: Proceedings of the First World Congress on Pain:* edited by J. J. Bonica and D. Albe-Fessard, pp. 19–27. Raven Press, New York.
19. Sternbach, R. A. (1968): *Pain: A Psychophysiological Analysis.* Academic Press, New York.
20. Wall, P. D. (1974): Physiological mechanisms involved in the production and relief of pain: In: *Recent Advances on Pain: Pathophysiology and Clinical Aspects,* edited by J. J. Bonica, P. Procacci, and C. A. Pagni, pp. 36–63. Charles C Thomas, Springfield, Ill.
21. Wall, P. D., and Gutnick, M. (1974): Ongoing activity in peripheral nerves: The physiology and pharmacology of impulses originating from a neuroma. *Exp. Neurol.,* 43:580–593.
22. Wall, P. D., Waxman, S., and Basbaum, A. I. (1974): Ongoing activity in peripheral nerve: Injury discharge. *Exp. Neurol.,* 45:576–589.

Role and Limits of Anticancer Drugs in the Treatment of Advanced Cancer Pain

Gianni Bonadonna* and Roberto Molinari**

*Division of Clinical Oncology F, Istituto Nazionale Tumori, Milan, Italy; **Division of Clinical Oncology C, Istituto Nazionale Tumori, Milan, Italy

For nonmedical people, the image of cancer has always been associated with the fear of prolonged, severe, and intractable pain. Today, despite significant progress achieved with specific drug regimens as well as sophisticated supportive measures, a considerable number of cancer patients die with poorly controlled pain due to progressive disease in some "trigger zones."

In recent years, the medical treatment for various forms of neoplastic disease has markedly improved in terms of strategy, number of effective drugs, and incidence of favorable response. The medical approach to advanced cancer can now be regarded as an established method of therapy with either curative or palliative purposes depending on the histology and stage of the neoplasm. Furthermore, in a large number of patients treated in the United States of America and in Europe, specific drug therapy is administered by qualified physicians.

The specific impact of medical treatment on pain produced by advanced cancer has not yet been the subject of a detailed report. The main reason is probably that, by tradition, the response to anticancer drugs has been considered significant only when documented by an objective regression of measurable parameters (Table 1). Because of frequent concomitant supportive measures, subjective improvement alone, including pain-relief, was almost never regarded as a meaningful response to anticancer drugs (3).

The aim of this report is to summarize briefly the current status of medical treatment for advanced cancer and to delineate those clinical situations in which various anticancer drugs, alone or in conjunction with specific local modalities, are indicated to control pain produced by progressive tumors.

ANTICANCER DRUGS AND THEIR ACTIVITY IN ADVANCED TUMORS

A relatively small number of drugs of different classes are now available for the treatment of advanced cancer. Table 2 lists the most important com-

TABLE 1. *Current criteria for objective evaluation of drug response in advanced solid tumors*

1. *Complete Remission (CR)*: Complete disappearance of all known disease including recalcification of all osteolytic metastases for at least 1 month.
2. *Partial Remission (PR)*: A decrease of 50% or greater in the product of the two largest perpendicular diameters of all measurable lesions including partial recalcification of osteolytic metastases for a minimum of 1 month.
3. *Objective Improvement (OI)*: A decrease of 25–50% of the product of the two largest perpendicular diameters of all measurable lesions with no change in osseous metastases.
4. *Progression*: An increase of 25% or greater over original measurements in the product of the two largest perpendicular diameters of measurable lesions, irrespective of concomitant regression in other tumor sites and/or occurrence of new lesions.
5. *Recurrence*: Appearance of new lesions or increase in the product of the two largest perpendicular diameters of measurable lesions by 50% over the size recorded at the initiation of therapy following a period of initial response or a period of no change.

pounds utilized in clinical practice. They are currently being administered in numerous combinations and through a wide range of dose schedules.

The medical literature is overloaded with publications from different institutions reporting the therapeutic results of a variety of drug regimens in different forms of advanced solid tumors. An effort to summarize those results and relate them to specific combinations is beyond the scope of this report, and the readers are referred to specific publications (1,2,4). Table 3 simply outlines the average response rate currently being obtained with anticancer drugs.

The table indicates that, irrespective of the drug combination utilized, many forms of solid tumors are now showing objective response to specific medical therapy. Although a satisfactory control of most forms of cancer is still far

TABLE 2. *Main anticancer drugs utilized in clinical practice*

Class	Drugs
Alkylating agents	mechlorethamine, cyclophosphamide, chlorambucil, melphalan, busulfan
Antimetabolites	methotrexate, fluorouracil, mercaptopurine, thioguanine, cytosine arabinoside
Plant alkaloids	vinblastine, vincristine, VP-16, VM-26
Antibiotics	adriamycin, daunomycin, bleomycin, actinomycin D, mitomycin C
Hormones	androgens, estrogens, antiestrogens, progestogens, corticosteroids
Miscellaneous	procarbazine, dacarbazine, hydroxyurea, cis-platinum, hexamethylmelamine, dibromodulcitol, nitrosoureas (BCNU, CCNU, MeCCNU, streptozotocin), asparaginase

TABLE 3. *Average expected response rate with various drug combinations in advanced solid tumors*

Neoplasia	CR (%)	CR + PR (%)
Hodgkin's disease	70–80	85–95
Non-Hodgkin's lymphomas	50–60	60–80
Wilms's tumor	60–70	70–80
Testicular cancer	60–70	85–95
Ovarian cancer	25–30	70–80
Breast cancer	12–20	50–70
Soft-tissue sarcomas		
children	30–40	70–80
adults	< 10	25–35
Lung cancer		
small-cell cancer	30–40	70–90
non-small-cell cancer	20–30	40–60
Bladder cancer	< 20	50–60
Head and neck cancer[a]	20–30	40–60
Ewing's sarcoma	< 20	50–60
Gastric cancer	< 15	20–35
Colorectal cancer	< 10	20–30
Endometrial cancer	10–20	40–60
Epidermoid ca. (cervix, esophagus)	< 20	30–40
Malignant melanoma	< 10	20–30

[a] squamous

from being obtained, it cannot be denied that available drug treatments are currently able to produce good partial remission (PR) and even complete remission (CR) in some neoplastic diseases for which 10 years ago only supportive therapy was available. As a general rule, the achievement of significant response (CR + PR) is almost always translated into an improved survival compared with nonresponders. Furthermore, in a fraction of patients with specific forms of neoplasia (pediatric tumors, lymphomas, testicular cancer, ovarian cancer) complete remission of the neoplastic disease is followed by a prolonged disease-free survival compatible with cure (1,2,4).

Table 4 summarizes the main reasons for the limited efficacy of available anticancer drugs in advanced neoplastic disease. The words "inherent low susceptibility" oversimplify the fact that many solid tumors (e.g., gastrointestinal, bronchogenic, renal, thyroid, and epidermoid carcinomas, as well as many adult sarcomas) show only a moderate to minimal response to agents which are very effective in other forms of cancer (e.g., lymphomas, Wilms's tumor, embryonal carcinoma of testicle). Our ignorance as to why certain types of neoplastic cells do respond to given drugs whereas others do not remain vast. However, few reasons for the success or failure of medical therapy have been, in part, elucidated through a number of studies carried out in experimental animals.

TABLE 4. *Main reasons for the limited efficacy of anticancer drugs in advanced cancer*

1. Inherent low susceptibility to available drugs
2. High tumor cell burden
    Decreased growth fraction
    Prolonged doubling time
    Increased cell loss
3. Ineffective concentration of drug to the target site for a long enough time (C × T)
4. Development of drug resistance
    Decreased: cellular uptake, activation of drug
    Increased: DNA repair, target enzyme, deactivation of drug
5. Development of drug toxicity
    Acute: e.g., myelosuppression, mucositis
    Cumulative: cardiomyopathy, nephrotoxicity, lung fibrosis

One important reason is represented by the fact that in clinically overt metastatic disease the tumor cell mass ($> 10^{10}$) is too high to be effectively eradicated or reduced by current drug combinations. In large tumor masses many cells are temporarily nondividing (G_0 or prolonged G_1 phase) and are only partially or completely insensitive to drugs, depending on the class of drug and the disease entity. Another reason is related to the pharmacokinetics of drugs in patients. Even if a tumor is susceptible to a drug, it cannot influence the tumor in a favorable way unless the drug reaches the target site and remains there in tumoricidal concentration (C) for a long enough period of time (T) to bring about the desired effect. The effectiveness of an antitumor agent is directly related to its C × T which is markedly affected by dose and schedule. The optimum C × T should kill the maximum tumor cells with minimum lethality in cells of normal tissue.

To be effective, in most cases chemotherapy must be repeated over long intervals. Under these circumstances, repetitive exposure of tumor cells to chemicals can lead to clinical resistance to drugs. The clinician is faced with a two-fold problem: the regrowth of tumor cells between cycles of therapy (which must be separated by intervals sufficient to allow recovery of normal tissue) and reduced amounts of tumor-cell kill with subsequent cycles of treatment owing to the development of resistant cell lines. Largely on the basis of experimental animal systems, various mechanisms have been proposed for the development of resistance.

In susceptible tumors, the eradication of the last neoplastic cell is theoretically possible with chemotherapy, but the toxic effect of drugs on normal cells represents an important limiting factor. Cyclic chemotherapy currently represents the most effective measure to minimize severe bone-marrow suppression as well as oral and intestinal mucositis. Cumulative toxicity can be prevented in the large majority of patients by discontinuing the administration of a given drug before the total risk dose is reached.

ANTICANCER DRUGS AND PAIN-CONTROL OF ADVANCED TUMORS

Several tumor factors are involved in many clinical situations characterized by pain. Table 5 summarizes some of the more obvious mechanisms by which pain is produced in advanced cancer. While a detailed discussion of pain mechanisms is beyond the scope of this chapter, the reader should remember that usually more than one factor can be present at the same time in a given situation (e.g., obstruction plus infection, pressure plus destruction of tissue).

Table 6 outlines the main factors responsible for the limited efficacy of anticancer drugs alone. First of all, solid tumors which often produce pain symptoms usually do not respond well to current drug regimens. In fact, complete remission occurs in less than one-third of patients, and in the large majority of cases is short-lived. Pain is often produced by large tumor masses and, as previously mentioned, a high tumor burden is inversely related to the incidence of a satisfactory drug response. Furthermore, since pain usually develops in late stages of the disease, second- or third-line drug treatments yield a minimal response rate. Finally, in certain target sites (e.g., head and neck area, pelvis) prior radical surgery and especially prior irradiation negatively affect in almost every patient the vascular supply, thus preventing an effective drug $C \times T$.

Despite the aforementioned limitations, effective first-line drug therapy

TABLE 5. *Principal mechanisms by which pain is produced in advanced cancer*

1. Infection	lowered resistance, poor drainage, ulceration of skin or mucous membranes
2. Obstruction	occlusion of a hollow viscus by a tumor mass; occlusion of large vein or artery
3. Destruction of tissue	destruction of bone, skin, soft tissue, and viscera
4. Pressure	growth of tumor in closed areas and/or compression of nervous structures
5. Visceral pain	direct involvement by tumor, rapid enlargement of a viscus due to cancer

TABLE 6. *Main reasons for the limited efficacy of anticancer drugs on pain of advanced malignancies*

1. Many solid tumors associated with pain symptoms are not sufficiently responsive to current drug regimens.
2. Pain usually develops in late stages when the tumor has become resistant to first-line drug therapy.
3. Pain is often produced by large tumor masses.
4. Prior surgery and especially prior radiotherapy applied to the target site almost always prevent effective drug C × T.

does produce pain-relief along with objective tumor regression. Some practical examples are provided in Table 7. For instance, advanced local breast cancer may be painful when inflammatory reaction distends the breast, when local extensive infiltration of the chest wall occurs, and when the tumor ulcerates. In all these situations, medical therapy (chemotherapy and/or endocrine therapy) produces complete plus partial remission in 50 to 70%, and the objective response is almost always associated with marked regression and even disappearance of pain. In contrast, in the presence of skeletal metastases, tumor response to drugs is usually slow, and pain-control is best

TABLE 7. *Activity of current drug regimens on pain characteristics of certain tumors*

Disease	Pain characteristics	Drug activity on pain[a]
Breast cancer	Tumor ulceration, infiltration of chest wall	+++
	Skeletal metastases	++
	Lymphedema of the arm (supraclavicular recurrence)	+
Prostate cancer	Skeletal metastases	+++
Leukemia, myeloma	Periosteal irritation or invasion, medullary pressure	+++
	Headache (meningeal infiltration)	+++
Lymphomas	Back pain (para-aortic adenopathy)	++++
	Spinal-cord compression	++
Testicular cancer	Back pain (para-aortic adenopathy)	++
Lung cancer	Superior sulcus (Pancoast) tumors	+
Colorectal, cervical, or bladder cancer	Low abdominal, perineal, or back pain due to pelvic recurrence	+
Oral, pharyngeal cancer	Tumor ulceration, invasion of nervous structures (e.g., earache)	++
Intracranial tumors	Headache (increased pressure)	+[b]

[a] ++++ complete relief; +++ very good, but incomplete relief; ++ fair relief; + little relief.
[b] Corticosteroids excluded.

achieved by combining drugs with radiotherapy. On the other hand, in prostate cancer, endocrine therapy (orchiectomy, estrogens) produces a high and prompt response rate. Therefore, palliative radiation therapy is utilized only in the late stages of the disease. However, radiation therapy is always the treatment of first choice when supraclavicular adenopathy in breast cancer produces compression of the brachial plexus and lymphedema of the arm.

Diffuse bone pain often occurs at the onset or during the course of multiple myeloma as well as in leukemia with high peripheral blood count. In acute leukemia a frequent cause of pain is meningeal infiltration. In all these situations, initial chemotherapy is successful in producing a prompt remission. This is particularly true in leukemia whereas in myeloma, radiation therapy is often indicated, especially in the presence of bone fractures.

Large retroperitoneal adenopathies can produce back pain. This is promptly and well controlled by anticancer drugs in all types of malignant lymphomas, less well in testicular cancer. The tumors of the thoracic inlet, sometimes called superior sulcus or Pancoast tumors, involve the nerves of the brachial plexus and the sympathetic chain and are characterized by severe shoulder and arm pain. Although combination chemotherapy can produce a fairly prompt objective remission in about 50% of patients, the degree of tumor regression is usually not sufficient to achieve satisfactory pain-control. Therefore, it is always advisable to combine chemotherapy with irradiation. This strategy should also be applied to intracranial tumors (either primary or metastatic) when not resectable. In fact, available drugs such as nitrosoureas do not induce a satisfactory remission rate which could relieve a severe and persistent headache.

Recurrence of various types of tumors in the low abdomen, in the pelvis as well as in the pharyngeal and cervical regions, often produces pain which is difficult to control by means of anticancer drugs. The large majority of tumors with recurrence in these sites have been previously subjected to extensive surgery and irradiation. For this reason, almost always drug C × T is ineffective. To circumvent this situation, intra-arterial drug infusion has been attempted, mainly in head and neck area. In spite of the above-mentioned modifications of blood supply, the immediate results on pain symptoms are often dramatic, irrespective of the degree of objective response. However, intra-arterial chemotherapy can not be continued for more than 15 to 30 days because of frequent local complications. Therefore, remission is commonly for a short period and requires further systemic chemotherapy to be maintained. In spite of some progress recently achieved in head and neck cancer (5), in clinical situations where severe and protracted pain is caused by infiltration of nervous structures, conventional analgesics, nerve blocks, and/or neurosurgical procedures must be considered as the treatments of choice, rather than waiting for the response of a second or third-line chemotherapy.

CONCLUSION

Medical therapy, and especially cyclical combination chemotherapy, can produce a prompt relief of cancer-induced pain only if the tumor is usually well or fairly well responsive to anticancer drugs. To achieve a prompt and satisfactory pain-relief, anticancer drugs should also be administered as first-line chemotherapy, in patients whose target sites were not previously subjected to extensive surgery and/or radiotherapy and in the absence of very large tumor masses. In the large majority of clinical situations, pain-control is the result of a combined team approach which includes medical oncologists, radiation therapists, neurosurgeons, and anesthesiologists. Although several techniques were recently standardized, optimal management is often the result of an individualized approach.

REFERENCES

1. Carter, S. K., Bakowski, M. T., and Hellmann, K. (1977): *Chemotherapy of Cancer.* John Wiley & Sons, New York.
2. Clarysse, A., Kenis, Y., and Mathé, G. (1976): *Cancer Chemotherapy: Its Role in the Treatment Strategy of Hematologic Malignancies and Solid Tumors. Recent Results in Cancer Research, 53.* Springer-Verlag, Berlin.
3. Karnofsky, D. A. (1961): Meaningful clinical classification of therapeutic responses to anticancer drugs. *Clin. Pharmacol. Ther.,* 2:709–712.
4. Holland, J., and Frei, E., III (1978): *Cancer Medicine,* 2nd ed. Lea & Febiger, Philadelphia.
5. Molinari, R., Mattavelli, F., Cantu', G., et al. (1979): Results of a low-dose, double synchronizing sequence of polychemotherapy (VBM) in the palliative treatment of oral and oropharyngeal squamous cell carcinoma. *Eur. J. Cancer (in press).*

Role and Limits of Oncologic Chemotherapy of Advanced Cancer Pain

Georges Brulé

Medical Oncology Unit, Institut Gustave-Roussy, 94800 Villejuif, France

The previous chapter was focused on chemotherapeutics which would delay or inhibit metastatic extension. Unfortunately, despite properly administered medication, a large number of patients do reach the stage of general dissemination, with all the sufferings which accompany this condition. Various mechanisms may be at the origin of oncologic pain including: (a) invasion or compression of the nervous network through the neoplastic process or peritumoral edema; (b) lymphatic or venous stasis; and (c) distant repercussion of a pelvic tumor such as lumbalgia, or renal colic, etc. Therefore, anything which can reduce the size of the tumor will logically lead to relief of pain; chemotherapy manifests its action following this principle but equally by some other processes which still remain obscure.

Antimitotic drugs are far from being harmless and often prove to be highly toxic, particularly in patients in poor general condition either as a result of the disease or previous medication. The whole problem is to find the proper balance between the risk of toxic phenomena and the advantages one may expect from chemotherapy.

It may be recalled that during cancer proliferation, the cells multiply unceasingly and, when the critical mass is reached, their erratic growth leads to the death of the host organism. Moreover, regardless of the mode of cell growth or on the principles of chemotherapy, a given dose of drug will kill a constant proportion and not a constant number of cells, whatever be the number of cells existing during the treatment. Hence, the greater the number of cells existing at the time of medication, the less is the chance of reducing significantly the size of the tumor. It therefore follows that because of this fractional destruction, the proper elimination of the tumor-cell population can only be obtained either by increasing the dose of the drug or drugs within the limit tolerable to the host, or by starting the treatment when the number of cells is still small in the hope of completely destroying the tumor. For patients with advanced cancer, this approach is not possible, because they have already a large number of tumor cells. Therefore, the problem is essentially dosage-oriented. Unlike what very many physicians believe, oncologic chemotherapeutic agents may be more selectively cytotoxic toward cancer cells than normal cells of the host. We will see later that some drugs are more particularly indicated for some anatomic locations or for some types of cancer. Only a fairly small number of cells do proliferate and are chemosensitive, the remainder being quiescent, as they are anoxic or in the process of necrosis.

In order to be effective for most patients, chemotherapy must be repeated at regular intervals so as to allow restoration of normal cell mitosis between each course. Under such conditions, the repeated action of chemical agents or tumor cells may lead to a clinical resistance to the drug. Then, the physician faces a dual problem: (a) the recurrence of tumor growth between courses, which must be sufficiently spaced so as to enable restitution of normal tissues; and (b) reduction of death of tumor cells during later courses because of the occurrence of resistance to drug therapy.

The various mechanisms which may explain the occurrence of this resistance are not known, but it is clear that resistance to anticancer drug makes the problem of advanced cancer treatment even more difficult to solve. The success of any medication depends on the number of resistant lines in the tumor population and the available therapeutic armamentarium as to elaborate effective combination. In addition to the mechanism of cell resistance, other factors inherent in the host may cause an apparent reduction of tumor cells' sensitivity. For example, these factors may interfere with the reduction of the concentration of active ingredient in tumor cells.

The hope of overcoming drug resistance has probably been the most important stimulus for the study of various drug combinations. Similarly, the combination of radiotherapy and chemotherapy has led to target cells in the resting phase which are sensitive to radiotherapy, while they are actually resistant to chemotherapy. Moreover, the toxicity of healthy tissues is different. Normal tissues with a high mitotic index of frequent cell renewal are very sensitive, for example, hematopoietic tissue or digestive epithelium, whereas the conjunctive tissue near the tumor is more sensitive to radiation and allows better penetration of the drug into the tumor. If the combination of radiotherapy and chemotherapy does potentiate the effect of the drug, it also increases the effect of the drug on healthy tissue.

The therapeutic armamentarium of the oncologist has progressed considerably over the last 30 years. Now we have a wide range of drugs having various modes of action, degree of toxicity, and spectrum of effectiveness. Within the framework of this presentation, I cannot describe all of them. Therefore, I shall refer to some drugs used either separately or in combination for some pain syndromes. I will purposefully not discuss dosage because it can vary considerably, depending on the general condition of the patient, the integrity of the core cancer cells, and possible impairment of hepatic and renal functions.

Often patients with advanced cancer have diffuse bone metastases and have in most cases received radiation therapy over a wide target area. Therefore, the initial dosage must be lowered. It must be adapted for each patient. In such circumstances, it is difficult to draw general rules. For most oncologic drugs, administered alone or in combination, it is the destruction of medullar cells which remains the main restriction for the dosage.

A complete hematologic examination just before each chemotherapeutic course is essential. Nevertheless, as these drugs alone or in combination are more effective at full doses, it is preferable to allow more time to elapse between courses than to reduce the doses. In case of severe medullar impairment, adequate precaution may have to be taken, but only a very small number of centers happen to be in a position to cater for such circumstances. Some sensitive tumors may equally, after rapid resorption, cause nephropathy through precipitation of uric acid stones. To prevent this complication, it is therefore essential that the patient takes enough liquid, to keep his urine alkaline and to give him allopurinol during the chemotherapy.

Among 50 drugs currently prescribed by oncologists in specialized hospitals, some are particularly indicated for certain anatomic locations or certain histologic types of tumors which may at times be very specific. The best example is given by hormonodependent carcinomas for which high dose of hormones, often synthetic hormones, will act electively. I will not elaborate on this subject since it will be discussed elsewhere, but it may be recalled that for breast or prostate cancer, it is not a hormonal but a chemical effect which is involved. The best demonstration of this fact is brought by some forms of cancer which apparently have nothing to do with hormones, for example, hypernephroma. In 20% of such cases, the administration of very high doses of progestational agents will give positive results. Such synthetic hormones may equally be indicated not only in endometrial carcinoma but also in some forms of ovarian cancer, even though this mode of action remains debatable.

Streptozotocin, whose mode of action is unknown, is an extremely toxic drug to the kidney, but at the dose of 1 $g/m^2/week$, it manifests specific effectiveness on secretory tumors of the pancreas, that is, tumors of the islets of Langerhans. Similarly, endocrine tumors of the adrenal and their usual pulmonary metastases do not respond to any hormonal treatment, but they are very sensitive to mithotane, a derivative of DTT which manifests a specific necrotic action on normal or pathologic adrenal cortex.

Apart from these two examples of almost specific action on very rarely encountered tumors, many currently administered products show some tropism, either toward some tissues or toward some histologic forms. For example, tumors of the central nervous system, which are protected by the meningeal barrier, are normally resistant to all substances administered by the systemic route because these products do not pool in the nervous tissue. Nitrosourea derivatives offer a striking advantage because they cross the meningeal barrier and enough concentration is obtained in the brain and the spinal cord, so that unlike other products they are effective not only on primarily cerebral tumors, but also in some cases of metastasis. Derivatives of podophyllotoxin, such as VM-26, equally seem to be able to cross the serosa, and that is why the combination VM-26–BCNU may preferably be used in case of cerebrally located secondaries of tumors regardless of the primary location. Finally, it must be mentioned that for meningeal and cerebral localization of acute leukemia, methotrexate may well be injected by the intraspinal route to relieve the terrible headache caused by meningitis during certain forms of leukemia or hematosarcoma, lymphoblastic sarcoma in particular.

5-Fluorouracil is an antipyrimidin extensively used in oncologic chemotherapy. This drug seems to act selectively on the hepatic tissue, particularly on hepatic metastasis of tumors of the colon. Besides this, it also applies to almost all tumors of glandular origin. The more acute the hepatic metastasis with rapid development (whether accompanied by fever or not), the greater are the chances of 5-fluorouracil's being effective. In such cases, the patient is generally very ill, febrile, and suffering dreadfully from the hepatic lesion. Infusions of 15 mg 5-fluorouracil/kg/day during 5 to 6 days will cause dramatic remission in 35% of the patients, and this may extend over several months when courses of 5 days a month are given, even in the absence of corticoids or other products.

When studying the effectiveness of derivatives of doxorubicin, adriamycin, or duborimycin, it occurred to us that duborimycin manifests a particularly specific and unaccountable action on often-unbearable pain of bone metastasis of breast cancer. In a group of 20 patients, pain was relieved in 65% of cases, while radiologically the lesions had remained absolutely unchanged and calcemia had not improved (1). This action of duborimycin is much less marked for adriamycin and seems less obvious for rubidasone, another derivative of this family of drugs.

Mithramycin, which has been abandoned because of its great toxicity at oncologic dose, yields hypocalcemic action at low dose and relieves muscular pain and digestive disorders caused by hypercalcemia, which is so frequent during advanced cancer, particularly in breast cancer.

Very high dose of cyclophosphamide as infusion of 2 g in 30 min often leads to dramatic relief of pain and dyspnea of bronchopulmonary cancer, in particular oat-cell forms which are relatively chemosensitive but grow very rapidly.

Amongst other currently administered drugs, bleomycin seems to show specificity for upper-digestive epidermoid cancer. Described by other authors, this fact has not been confirmed at Gustave-Roussy Institute.

On the other hand, Japanese investigators have reported that mitomycin is particularly effective in large stomach tumors, which do not in general respond to any other chemotherapy. This product is also useful in local or regional spreading which follows such tumors.

It must also be recalled that actinomycin D shows some specificity for embryonary tumors or for some tumors in children, melphalan in ovarian tumors, and decarbazine or DTIC in some melanomas. The effectiveness of the last three products is at times debatable, but it is useful to include them in therapeutic combination which may be used in the treatment of such tumors. For example, in case of melanomas, the combination of decarbazine with vincristine and adriamycin may prove effective.

A wide range of possibilities occurs for the combination of drugs. The same applies for their dosage and schedule of administration. The combination of antimitotic drugs is theoretically based on our knowledge of cell kinetics and biochemical properties of these substances. Actually, clinical results and dogmatic expectations are not always in agreement. Therefore, all these combinations are more essentially based on some empirism and chemotherapeutic experience rather than concrete data. Without going into details, the essential principles are the following:

1. used simultaneously or sequentially, drugs which act at various stages of the cell cycle; for example, an antimetabolite which acts on the synthesis, an alkylating agent which acts on DNA, and a spindle poison which will exert its effect during mitosis. By multiplying the cycles and possibly by changing the substances, one may expect to target a maximum number of cancer cells.
2. all these drugs exert toxic effects on different targets (hematopoietic system, digestive tract, nervous system, kidney, myocardium, etc.) and should therefore be so combined that their respective side effects do not occur concomitantly; hence maximum dosage may be given while avoiding cumulative toxicity.

Table 1 shows a combination which is very often used in the treatment of advanced breast cancer. The first substance used, an alkaloid obtained from the periwinkle, is a poison for the spindle. It acts during mitosis and essentially manifests neurologic toxicity. The second is an alkylating agent and shows mild hematologic toxicity. At times, it causes cystitis. The third one is an antimetabolite. It manifests side effects mainly on the digestive tract and the bone marrow. An interval of 4 weeks between each course causes restoration of normal cells, which occurs more rapidly than for tumor cells.

Examples of such combinations are unlimited in number: For embryonic tumors, actinomycin D is in general combined with cyclophosphamide and methotrexate. In case of resistance to this combination, cis-platinum (CDDP)-bleomycin-vincaleucoblastine sulphate may, in very advanced cases, lead to regression of fairly long duration.

TABLE 1. *Drug combinations used for breast cancer*

Day 1–2	i.v.d. vincristine without exceeding 1 mg
Day 3–4–5–6	i.v.d. Endoxan® without exceeding 400 mg
Day 3–4–5–6	infusion over 1½ hr 5-fluorouracil 500 mg/m²

Moreover, it may be recalled that the adjunction of heparin to all these chemotherapeutics, either alone or in combination, may, according to some authors, potentiate their therapeutic effects without increasing their toxicity.

Hematosarcomas, leukemias, and other such diseases do respond to several drugs. Unfortunately, they have a tendency to relapse, and it is in this type of disease that some products may serve as substitution to classic medications: for example, L-asparaginase or methyl-glyoxal.

L-Asparaginase in blastic transformation of lymphosarcomas may lead to new remission in patients in apparently desperate condition. The same applies with methyl-glyoxal-bis in blastic transformation of chronic myeloid leukemia having become resistant to Misulban® or other classic therapeutics.

Vindesine, the latest alkaloid of the periwinkle, leads to a high proportion of remission in acute lymphoid leukemia. Some resistant cases of lymphosarcoma and Hodgkin's disease respond to this medication. The most effective daily dosage seems to be 2 mg/m^2 administered as i.v. infusion during 2 days.

As already stated, patients suffering from advanced cancer have, in general, new drugs or original drug combinations. In case of success or transitory improvement, this may lead to the elaboration of an optimal chemotherapy for the treatment of disseminated cancer and finally the integration of local or regional neoplasms. Therefore, this approach shows that, in no circumstance, should the oncologist despair even when the patient appears to be in the ultimate stage. He should always attempt to test new combinations and, in so doing, he may be providing a contribution to the care of other patients. The severity of side effects caused by the treatment should be the only limiting factor to the therapeutic regimen. If there is no hope of recovery and if pain remains unbearable, one must not increase the patient's discomfort through therapeutic insistence. On the other hand, in case of intolerable pain, an effort to find new combinations, even including high-dosage corticosteroids, should delay the use of major analgesics with all the side effects which such drugs may have on the patient's personality. [*Editors' Note:* We vehemently disagree with Dr. Brulé's last statement. The patient's pain *must* be relieved by one of the other modalities, including the use of potent narcotics, while chemotherapy is being tried.]

REFERENCES

1. Brulé, G., Chauvergne, J., Clavel, B., Carton, M., Klein, T., Gary Bobo, J., Guerrin, J., and Pommatau, E. (1975): Essai de chimiothérapie anticancéreuse par la Duborimycine. *Bull. Cancer (Paris)*, 63:41–58.

The Role of Endocrine Therapy for Relief of Pain Due to Advanced Cancer

F. Pannuti, A. Martoni, A. P. Rossi, and E. Piana

Division of Oncology, Marcello Malpighi Hospital, 40138 Bologna, Italy

In our experience, pain due to cancer can be basically attributed to: (a) compression and/or infiltration of nerve structures by the neoplastic process; (b) inflammatory process around or within a tumor; and (c) the action of chemical mediators. In the first and second and, more rarely, the third types, pain is located in the region of the tumor or referred to the distribution of the nerves involved and follows the evolution or development of the tumor. In the third type, pain is usually widespread systemically. This report will confine itself to local pain as a direct expression of the presence of neoplastic lesions and in relation to the influence that can be exerted on it by hormonal therapy in the region of so-called "hormone-sensitive tumors."

Of 291 patients with advanced solid tumors treated in our Division of Oncology during the first 4 months of 1977, 186 or 63.9% had moderate to severe pain. The incidence of pain in patients with specific tumors was as follows: 68% with breast cancer (117 of 171 patients); 67% with stomach cancers (14 of 21 patients); 59% with cancer of the prostate (10 of 17 patients); 58% with intestinal tumors (14 of 24 patients); 57% with lung tumors (23 of 40 patients); 55% with kidney tumors (11 of 20 patients); and 47% with head and neck tumors (7 of 15 patients).

Since 1973, we have been carrying out studies on the use of high doses of medroxyprogesterone acetate (MAP) which is capable of having a significant beneficial effect on the pain of these patients (see below). Figure 1 shows the percentage rate of patients who died in pain during the 4-year period 1972 to 1976 (pain evaluation was carried out 15 days before death). Although it is slight, the percentage drop of patients with breast cancer should be noted.

BASIC CONSIDERATIONS

Neoplastic pain is assessed in different ways and with different aims in clinical semiology and pharmacology.

Clinical Considerations

Pain as a symptom can be made use of in diagnosing disease and in the differential diagnosis of several possible disorders. An example is given in

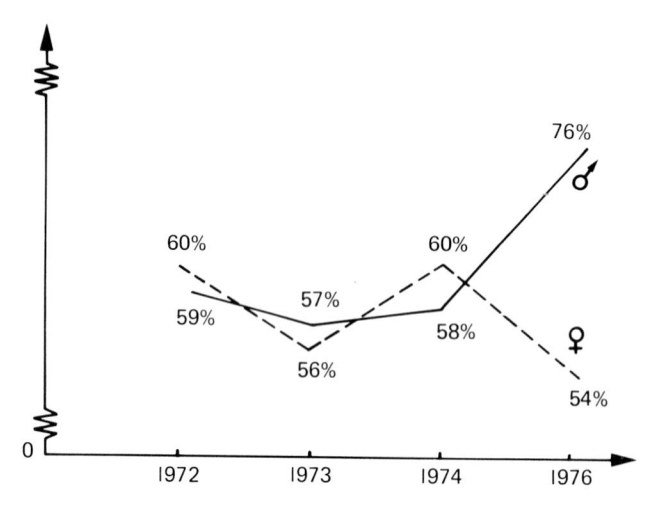

FIG. 1. Percentage rate of patients that die in pain (pain evaluation carried out 15 days before death).

Table 1. The clinical definition of pain is important for a prompt diagnosis of recurrence. The case shown in Fig. 2 refers to a patient who had been subjected to rectal amputation and had intense pain situated in the perineal region. The pain regressed partially only following anticancer therapy. However, clinical evidence for relapse already had existed before the chemotherapy course was effected (location, features, type of pain intensity, lack of sensitivity to anti-inflammatory drugs). Another example is provided by acute colicky pain localized in the liver as an early symptom of hepatic metastases in patients who have had mastectomy for carcinoma of the breast.

Definition of "signal-symptom" includes the clinical, biologic, and hematologic elements capable of characterizing the neoplastic disease in relation

TABLE 1. *Differential diagnosis of painful conditions in the chest*

Characteristics of the pain (location, quality, etc.)	Benign disease of the breast	Cancer of the breast	Angina pectoris	Thoracic neuropathy	Arthrosis
Superficial	+	−	−	+	−
Stable localization	−	+	+	+	+
Diffuse	+	−	−	−	−
Spreading from the breast	−	−	+	+	+
Rapid onset	+	−	+	−	−
Continuous	−	+	−	+	−
Intense	−	−	+	+	+
Upon effort or movement	−	−	+	+	+

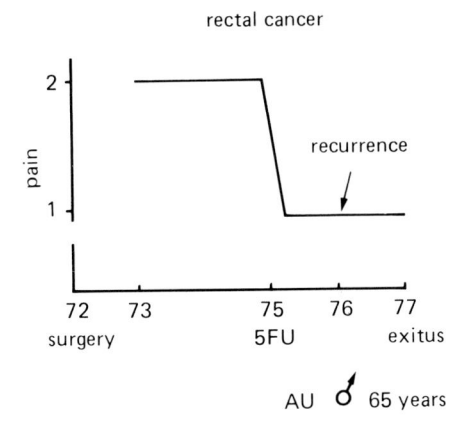

FIG. 2. Patient discussed in text (p. 146) with severe perineal pain partially relieved with 5-fluoro-uracil therapy. Vertical axis pain intensity (2—severe; 1—moderate; 0—none) and horizontal axis time in weeks.

to the treatment adopted. Pain as a signal-symptom in oncology is, by definition, a direct expression of the local presence of the neoplastic lesion and is also capable of indicating with an acceptable degree of clinical approximation the evolution of the disease in relation to the treatment adopted.

Pain as a signal-symptom should be distinguished from non-neoplastic pain and from pain which, even though it is related to the neoplastic process, is not a reliable indication of the evolution of the disease in terms of expansion or regression of the neoplastic mass. An example of the latter is provided by pain due to pathologic fractures of the vertebra. When pain is present as an isolated event during remission of the disease, pain is to be attributed only to fracture rather than to the expansion of the neoplastic process. Even though pain, in this sense, is an index of objective worsening of the patient's conditions (e.g., occurrence of paraplegia in the lower limbs), in itself it is *not* an indication of the failure of the anticancer treatment that may be in progress. It is more probable that the treatment should be integrated into other modalities such as radiotherapy and orthopedic measures.

Pain as a signal-symptom serves to (a) monitor the disease during treatment, and (b) appraise the final results of the treatment. To this end, it should be defined in a qualitative-quantitative fashion. For this purpose, we use the following rating: *grade 0*—absent; *grade 1*—moderate, for which the patient requires not more than one analgesic every 24 hr; *grade 2*—intense, for which the patient requires more than one analgesic every 24 hr. A significant change in pain is referred to only when the change involves the move from one grade to another.

Method of Use of the Pain Rating (43,50)

The patient is told that he can freely avail himself of a certain type of analgesic drug (e.g., acetylsalicylic acid, pentazocine, etc.) in a quantity not exceeding a specified limit in a 24-hr period (e.g., not more than three 0.5-g tablets of acetylsalicylic acid or two 30-mg vials of pentazocine). The physician simply records the quantity of analgesic drug taken during the 24-hr period. These conditions mean that only the *subjective assessment* of the patient is involved.

An advantage of this rating is that only three degrees of intensity of pain are involved. A simple code of this kind is better suited to practical routine clinical evaluations compared with those involving 5 or 6 grades of intensity. Although the latter may be more precise, they are influenced by the fact that both the patient's and the physician's subjective judgments become involved to a greater degree than the simpler rating.

PAIN AND HORMONE THERAPY

From a pharmacologic point of view, pain as a signal-symptom has different meaning and different features in (a) clinical drug tolerance and (b) pharmacodynamics.

Pain and Clinical Drug Tolerance

The administration of hormones for cancer therapy can lead to the production of pain. Obviously, no problems exist in interpreting local pain following intramuscular administration. On the other hand, when the hormone is given intravenously, problems of differential diagnosis can develop. The clinical features that enable a symptom to be categorized as a side effect and not as a symptom of the tumor are the following: (a) continuous pain following administration of the drug; (b) the pain ceases with the end of the metabolic phase responsible for the pain; (c) the site or sites of pain are not subject to change; and (d) the quality of the pain.

An example is provided by pain arising following administration of diethylstilbestrol diphosphate (DES-P). The pain is quite specific, as it arises during intravenous administration and reaches a climax in a few minutes. It then disappears after 5 to 15 min and reappears each time the drug is administered. The pain is usually located in the perineal region (but can also appear at the site of metastases) and is experienced as a burning sensation.

Pain and Pharmacodynamics

Hormone Interference

The concept of hormone dependence is based on Huggins' (24,25) clinical and experimental observation that cancer cells, like the normal cells from which they originate, "depend" on the activity of one hormone or more for their metabolism and proliferation. The term *hormone dependence,* according to Tagnon (23,66), has a tendency to oversimplify the relationship between cancer cells and hormones. The administration of estrogens, for example, can induce breast cancer both in man and in animals, and ovariectomy previous to menopause can induce remission in approximately 40% of patients with advanced breast cancer. However, it is also true that small doses of estrogens stimulate the evolution of the disease, whereas higher doses have an inhibiting effect. This is why Tagnon suggests replacing *"hormone dependence* with the term *hormone sensitivity*. In other words, the breast cancer cells do not necessarily depend on a hormone, but "may" be sensitive to one or more hormones. Some time ago we suggested (51) the use of the term *hormone sensitivity* with the reservation that sensitivity can be "absolute" or "relative" (in relation to one hormone or more, or depending on the different doses of the same hormone).

The tendency to divide clinical hormone therapy into additive and subtractive types may certainly simplify the issue, but also contains the risk of an imprecise and schematic approach to these cancer patients. Ovariectomy, for example, involves on the one hand the removal of hormones synthesized by the ovaries and on the other an excess production of the corresponding pituitary trophic hormones due to the inactivation of the feedback mechanism. It is also known that, in this kind of situation, the adrenal glands are also able to produce greater amounts of sexual hormones in order to effect compensation. It is apparent that, following surgery, we are faced with a situation entailing both addition and subtraction of hormones, which are all capable of interfering with the growth and reproduction of this kind of tumor cell. For example, administration of hormones such as progestins is in itself an "additive hormone therapy" which involves inhibition of the secretion of a series of hormones at different levels (ovaries, pituitary gland, and perhaps adrenal gland) and a "subtractive" effect which occurs concomitant with the "additive" effect brought about by the therapy itself.

The problem is further complicated by the fact that a few hormones are undoubtedly able to carry out pharmacologically autonomous activity in the host organism and also modify the state of the relationship between the tumor and the organism (for example, immunosuppressive activity of MAP), leading finally to important subjective and objective improvements. This situation validates the statement that these hormones are capable of significantly "interfering" with the evolution of the neoplastic disease. The tumor should not simply be considered as a pool of atypical infiltrating and proliferating cells, but a clinical situation which involves a complex relationship between the tumor cells and the organism.

At this point, we believe that the term *hormone interference* as described above can be introduced into oncologic literature alongside the term *hormone sensitivity*. The latter term stresses the possibility of response to hormone treatment, independently of the problems connected with the direction followed by the response, the type of hormone, or the dosage selected. By using *hormone interference* as a term, we are attempting to shift the emphasis from the cancer cells to the hormone employed in pharmacologic terms with the intention of: (a) underlining the complexity of hormone therapy, as it is usually not only "additive" or "subtractive" but both at the same time; (b) underlining the possibility that interference may be effected at the level of tumor-cell kinetics, regardless of the type of effect the hormone will have; and (c) indicating that the hormone also interferes with the evolution of the tumor with the understanding that the neoplastic disease is to be thought of in its widest clinical sense and therefore also in function of the state of the relationship between the tumor and the host organism.

ENDOCRINE THERAPY AND PAIN RELIEF

Most authors reporting results of anticancer treatment in patients with advanced malignant neoplasms have usually been concerned only with measuring the volume-reduction of the tumor masses. Most writers have neglected and often deliberately excluded the assessment of subjective response, including that relative to pain, because this factor was not thought to be a reliable measure of the effectiveness of the treatment. In this chapter we shall indicate the incidence of relief or remission of pain and other general subjective symptoms as assessed and reported by the authors of the papers reviewed. In this regard it is necessary to mention the almost complete lack of rating systems of pain assessment on the part of therapists and this obviously leads to heterogeneous results which cannot be compared precisely.

Advanced Prostate Cancer

Table 2 lists the results (subjective results and pain whenever possible) derived by patients with advanced cancer of the prostate following orchiectomy, adrenalectomy, or hypophysectomy. Table 3 lists results obtained with additive hormone therapy and in particular with diethylstilbestrol diphosphate (DES-P), cyproterone acetate (CP) and high doses of medroxyprogesterone acetate (MAP) in doses of 1,500 mg intramuscularly (i.m.) per day for 30

TABLE 2. Results with hormonal therapy in advanced prostate cancer

Treatment	No. of pts.	Object. rem.	Subject. rem.	Pain rem.	Authors
Hypophysectomy					
surgery	34	n.d.	12(35.2%)	n.d.	Murphy et al. (38)
^{90}Y	13	n.d.	n.d.	11(85%)	Straffon et al. (64)
^{90}Y	74	n.d.	n.d.	51(69%)	Fergusson (19)
Adrenalectomy	4	n.d.	n.d.	1(25%)	Huggins et al. (26)
	10	2(20%)	n.d.	7(70%)	West et al. (74)
	7	n.d.	n.d.	7(100%)	Archimbaud et al. (3)
Orchiectomy	21	n.d.	15(71.4%)	n.d.	Huggins et al. (27)

Legend: Object. rem. = objective remission; Subject. rem. = subjective remission; Pain rem. = pain-remission. Percentages are given in round numbers. n.d. = no data.

TABLE 3. *Results with hormonal therapy for advanced prostate cancer*

Treatment	No. of pts.	Object. rem.	Subject. rem.	Pain rem.	Authors
Estrogens					
(DES-P)	23	n.d.	19/25(76%)	21(91%)	Colapinto et al. (11)
	10	4(40%)	n.d.	5(50%)	Band et al. (5)
	9	4(44%)	n.d.	8(89%)	Susan et al. (65)
Cyproterone	25	n.d.	n.d.	12(48%)	Smith (62)
acetate (CP)	10	8(80%)	n.d.	8(80%)	Scott (59)
Medroxyprogesterone acetate (MAP)					
300 mg/day i.m.	12	n.d.	n.d.	9(75%)	Rafla et al. (54)
500 mg/day i.m.	12	n.d.	n.d.	9(75%)	Bouffioux (8)
1,500 mg/day i.m.	10	n.d.	10/10	10(100%)	Pannuti et al. (53)

Legend: See Table 2.

TABLE 4. *Results of hormonal therapy for advanced prostate cancer pain/subjective remission*

	Additive			Ablative	
	No. of pts.	Pain rem. (%)		No. of pts.	Pain rem. (%)
Oestrogens	42	80	Adrenalectomy	21	71
Cyproterone	35	57	Hypophysectomy	87	71
Medroxy-progesterone acetate (MAP)	22	68			
Total	99	70	Total	108	71

Legend: See Table 2.

days. Table 4 shows that additive and subtractive methods on the average gave the same percentage of pain relief (around 70%). For additive methods, the highest percentage rate was found with MAP and DES-P, while for subtractive methods the percentage rates for adrenalectomy and hypophysectomy were identical. Our experience concerns the use of high doses of MAP. The experience we have is limited and refers to a "pilot study" that preceded the definition of the protocol which is now being followed and which envisages prospective and randomized comparison of MAP versus DES-P in this kind of patient.

Advanced Endometrial Carcinoma

Table 5 shows results obtained with progestins on subjective response in the advanced stage of endometrial carcinoma. The average remission rate

TABLE 5. Results of hormonal therapy (progestins) for advanced endometrial cancer

Treatment	No. of pts.	Object. rem.	Subject. rem.	Pain rem.	Authors
Medroxyprogesterone acetate (MAP)	42	17 (40%)	30 (71%)	n.d.	Smith et al. (61)
(<500 mg/day)	13	2 (15%)	11 (85%)	n.d.	Serment et al. (60)
17-Hydroxyprogesterone	176	58 (33%)	123 (70%)	n.d.	Kistner et al. (29)

Legend: See Table 2.

was 71%. It should be noted that these authors used low doses of MAP (less than 500 mg/day). No data relating to incidence of pain-relief are available in the reports.

Advanced Thyroid Cancer

Although there is a large body of literature on the use of hormones for advanced thyroid cancer, no reliable data relating to subjective response and, in particular, pain, are available.

Advanced Clear-Cell Kidney Cancer

The appearance of kidney tumors in male hamsters following estrogen treatment and inhibition of these tumors employing testosterone or progestins

TABLE 6. Results with hormonal therapy for advanced renal clear-cell cancer

Treatment	No. of pts.	Object. rem.	Subject rem.	Pain rem.	Authors
Progestins					
(other than MAP)	16	2 (12%)	14 (87%)	n.d.	Talley et al. (67)
	33	2 (6%)	12 (36%)	n.d.	Van der Werfmessing et al. (70)
Androgens	11	n.d.	11 (100%)	n.d.	Talley et al. (67)
Corticosteroids	38	n.d.	38 (100%)	n.d.	Talley et al. (67)
Total	98	n.d.	75 (76%)	n.d.	
Medroxyprogesterone acetate (MAP)	8	1 (12%)	7 (87%)	n.d.	Talley et al.[a] (67)
	9	1 (11%)	4 (44%)	n.d.	Van der Werfmessing et al.[a] (70)
	20	2 (10%)	6/14 (43%)	5/12 (42%)	Pannuti et al.[b] (43)
Total	37	4 (11%)	17 (46%)	n.d.	

Legend: See Table 2.
[a] Low doses.
[b] High doses.

(7) suggested the concept of hormone therapy for renal adenocarcinoma. On the basis of these indications, Bloom was the first to use testosterone and subsequently MAP for treating human renal carcinoma, especially the advanced clear-cell variety.

Table 6 lists subjective remission rates obtained by administering androgens, cortisone substances, and progestins with special reference to MAP. Our results refer to the treatment of a group of patients with high doses of MAP (1,500 mg. i.m. per day for 30 days) (46). High doses of MAP are capable of significantly reducing or completely eliminating pain in 42% of the patients with advanced renal cancer. In light of this and considering the low percentage of objective remission, the treatment protocol we are currently using envisages the use of MAP associated with a multiple chemotherapeutic regimen.

Advanced Breast Cancer

Due to the high incidence, the strong tendency to develop skeletal metastases, and the not-infrequent high life-expectancy that advanced cancer patients have, breast cancer is one of the neoplastic situations where pain treatment is most important. There are few details in case statistics assessing pain-remission employing adrenalectomy and castration (see Table 7). The best results reported indicate pain-relief is obtained by a maximum of 44% of the patients.

TABLE 7. Results of hormonal therapy for advanced breast cancer

Treatment	No. of pts.	Object. rem.	Subject. rem.	Pain rem.	Authors
Hypophysectomy					
^{90}Y	100	32 (32%)	42 (42%)	n.d.	Notter et al. (40)
^{90}Y	300	90 (30%)	n.d.	225 (75%)	Denoix (16)
^{90}Y	56	17 (30%)	n.d.	49 (88%)	Abbes et al. (1)
^{90}Y	n.d.	n.d.	n.d.	85%	Juret et al. (28)
Cryohypophysectomy	42	13 (31%)	n.d.	30 (71%)	Abbes et al. (1)
Transsphenoidal-hypophysectomy	146[a]	n.d.	n.d.	140 (96%)	Hardy et al. (22)
Alcohol-injection into pituitary	10	0	0	10 (100%)	Martino et al. (33)
Adrenalectomy	18	8 (44%)	8 (44%)	8 (44%)	Dao[b] (15)
	500	178 (36%)	202 (40%)	n.d.	Fracchia et al.[c] (20)

Legend: See Table 2.
[a] All patients with osseous metastases.
[b] Controlled clinical trial.
[c] In 255 patients + ovariectomy.

TABLE 8. *Results with hormonal therapy (androgens) for advanced breast cancer*[a]

Drug used for therapy	No. of pts.	Object. rem.	Subject. rem.	Pain rem.	Authors
Testosterone propionate	23	3 (13%)	0	n.d.	Brennan et al. (9)
	20	4 (20%)	8–10 (40–50%)	n.d.	Lewison et al. (31)
	27	4 (15%)	9 (33%)	n.d.	Nevinny et al. (39)
	16	2 (13%)	10 (63%)	n.d.	Volk et al. (73)
3β-17β-Androstanedeol	21	2 (10%)	8 (38%)	n.d.	Brennan et al. (9)
11β-OH-17α-Methyl-testosterone	23	2 (9%)	5 (22%)	n.d.	Volk et al. (71)
Fluoxymesterone	25	2 (8%)	8 (32%)	n.d.	Volk et al. (71)
Testost. prop. + 17β-hydroxy-androsten-3-one	25	3 (12%)	? (40–50%)	n.d.	Lewison et al. (31)
2$\alpha\gamma$-Methyldihydro-testost. propionate	23	6 (26%)	14/16 (88%)	n.d.	Volk et al. (72)
6β-Dibromethyl-ene-testost. propionate	23	4 (17%)	9/12 (75%)	n.d.	Volk et al. (72)
6-dehydro-17α-methyl-testosterone	20	0	5 (25%)	n.d.	Nevinny et al. (39)
Norandrolone phenpropionate	26	7 (27%)	9 (35%)	n.d.	Volk et al. (73)
Calusterone	44	4 (9%)	n.d.	16/36 (44%)	Aslam et al. (4)

Legend: See Table 2.
[a] All data from controlled clinical trials.

There are more numerous and consistent indications relating to the effect on pain of operations aiming at removing or destroying the hypophysis (Table 7). This type of treatment provides remission of pain in 82% of the patients on the average (from 71% with cryodestruction to 100% with the Moricca technique of alcohol neuroadenolysis) (36). It should be stressed that the ratio between objective remission and remission of pain was 1:3.

The vast literature relating to the use of androgen refers vaguely to subjective remission obtained in an average of 37% of the patients treated (range: 0 to 87.5%). In almost none of the reports is there specific reference to the anti-pain effect of this hormone (Table 8). The same considerations apply to the use of estrogens. In Table 9 results are shown on the use of anti-estrogens, cortisone substances, L-DOPA and progestins (other than MAP). In the case of tamoxifen, reference is made to the fact that pain may become acute again during the first days of treatment (12,35) but then subsides.

Table 10 shows results obtained using additive hormone therapy excluding

TABLE 9. Results with hormonal therapy for advanced breast cancer

Treatment	No. of pts.	Object. rem.	Subject rem.	Pain rem.	Authors
Antiestrogens					
Tamoxifen	96	17 (18%)	41 (43%)	n.d.	Cole et al. (12)
Nafoxidine	48	18 (37%)	n.d.	8/24 (33%)	Bloom et al. (6)
Cortisone	20	0	4 (25%)	3 (15%)	Dao[a] (15)
Prednisone	23	1 (4%)	3 (13%)	2 (9%)	Colsky et al.[a] (13)
L-DOPA	30	10 (33%)	10 (33%)	10 (33%)	Minton (34)
Progestins (other than MAP)					
9α-Bromo-11β-ketoprogesterone	23	0	8 (35%)	5 (22%)	Colsky et al.[a] (13)
norethisterone acetate	55	21 (38%)	31 (56%)	n.d.	Curwen (14)
	31	14 (45%)	n.d.	19 (61%)	Sonkin et al. (63)

Legend: See Table 2.
[a] Controlled clinical trial.

TABLE 10. Results with hormonal therapy for advanced breast cancer

Drug	No. of pts.	Object. rem.	Subject rem.	Pain rem.	Authors
L-DOPA	30	33%	33%	33%	Abbes et al. (1)
Cortisone	43	2%	16%	12%	Amadori et al. (2)
Androgens	316	12%	37%	44%	Colsky et al. (13)
Antiestrogens	144	24%	43%	33%	Amadori et al. (2)
Progestins (other than MAP)	118	30%	50%	38%	Archimbaud et al. (3)

Legend: See Table 2.

MAP. Compared with an average objective remission rate of 23.5% (range: 2 to 33%), the average subjective remission rate was 35.8% (range: 16 to 50%), and remission of pain took place in 32% of the patients treated (range: 12 to 44%). These give the ratios for objective to subjective results and for objective results to pain relief of 1:1.5.

Medroxyprogesterone Acetate (MAP) and Pain

MAP, a steroid which was synthesized in 1958, has an intense progestative effect on animals, as well as androgen- or estrogen-type effects and a corticoid activity (21). In oncology it has been used, apart from breast cancer, in endometrial carcinoma, renal carcinoma, and prostate carcinoma.

Mechanism of Action of MAP

The anti-tumor effect of MAP would seem to consist of inhibition of the pituitary gland, the ovary, and the adrenal glands, and also a direct effect on the neoplastic cell. In man MAP has a pronounced inhibitory effect on the pituitary-ovary axis (55) and on the adrenal-hypothalamic axis (41) and, in a secondary fashion, blocks the secretion of ovarian hormones and cortisol (57). These effects are brought out in man both with low doses (< 500 mg/day) and high doses.

Our experience can be summarized as follows: High doses of MAP induce a rapid decrease of plasma levels of GH, FSH, and LH—an effect which persists for a few months after treatment is discontinued. On the other hand, prolactin underwent no significant change. MAP also inhibits adrenal function as reflected by the reduction of the excretion of endogenous cortisol and endogenous 17-keto-steroid metabolites (58).

Recently, new information has been acquired concerning hormone receptors. Progesterone and a few synthetic progestins related to MAP are able, *in vitro*, to reduce the bond formed by 17β-estradiol with specific receptors present in breast cancer, and this effect seems to be in proportion to the hormone's concentration (17). MAP also reduces the cell concentration of estradiol receptors (ER) in human endometrium (69) and exhibits competitive effects at hypothalamic level towards estrogens and reduces their capacity to bind to specific receptors (56). Finally, in the uterus of the rabbit, it has been shown that the affinity of MAP for progesterone receptors is approximately 30 times greater than that displayed by natural progesterone (68).

These data lead us to suppose that progestins and particularly MAP are capable of displaying notable interference to hormone-sensitive neoplastic cells at the level of hormone receptor mechanisms.

The response to therapy with a given hormone administered at high doses may be correlated to a direct nonspecific toxic effect of the hormone itself. In fact, with cultured breast cancer cells, identical results are obtained as regards the inhibition of thymidine-tritiate incorporation using both 17α-estradiol and its nonactive isomer 17β-estradiol if the same high concentrations are employed (32).

Results with Low Doses of MAP

The use of MAP in advanced breast cancer goes back to the beginning of the 1960s. The average dose used was 100 mg/day given orally or intramuscularly. Table 11 shows results obtained using "low doses" of MAP with specific reference to remission of pain or subjective remission. The rates of remission are statistically dispersed (range: 18 to 92%). Results relating to remission of pain are also of little significance, and the relative percentage values are lower than 33%.

TABLE 11. *Results with hormonal therapy (low doses of MAP) for advanced breast cancer*

Doses of map	No. of pts.	Object. rem.	Subject. rem.	Pain rem.	Authors
50 mg/os	30	11/30 (37%)	n.d.	9/27 (33%)	Bucalossi et al. (10)
100–125 mg i.m.	27	15/27 (55%)	25/27 (92%)	n.d.	Dogliotti et al. (18)
100 mg i.m. × 3	34	7/34 (20%)	6/34 (20%)	n.d.	Muggia et al. (37)
20–300 mg/day/os	40	4/40 (10%)	n.d.	5/40 (12%)	Klaassen et al. (30)

Legend: See Table 2.

Results with High Doses of MAP

In 1973, we showed it was possible to use daily doses of MAP that were greater than those previously in use (usually less than 500 mg i.m. per day): the maximum tolerable dose (MTD) of MAP given i.m. was found to be 1,500 mg/day for 30 days (52). Subsequently (48), we treated 54 patients suffering from advanced breast cancer with MAP at the MTD, obtaining 44% of objective remission.

Even before objective remission became apparent, treatment with high doses of MAP was shown to be capable of inducing prompt subjective remission and producing an impressive anti-pain effect. During a study aimed at identifying the maximum therapeutic dose (MTD), it was found that MAP was able to induce pain-remission in 90% of the patients treated (52).

Subsequently, in a group of 54 patients treated with doses of 1,500 mg i.m. per day for 30 days the subjective remission rate was 86% (38 of 44) and partial or complete relief of pain occurred in 95% (35 of 37) of the patients (48). Table 12 shows that the remission of pain became apparent as early as 1 week from commencement of treatment and became propor-

TABLE 12. *Pain-remission in relation to time and total doses of MAP in 37 patients with grade 1 and 2 pain*

	Grade 2 (no. of pts.)	Grade 1 (no. of pts.)	Grade 0 (no. of pts.)	MAP total dose (gm)
Before treatment	26	11	8	0
After 1 week	7	25	13	10.5
After 2 weeks	2	24	19	21
After 3 weeks	1	18	26	31.5
After 4 weeks	1	15	29	42
After 5 weeks	0	11	34	50
After 6 weeks	0	11	34	n.d.

Legend: Grade 2 = severe pain; grade 1 = moderate pain; grade 0 = no pain.

tionally greater during the following weeks and while the treatment was still in progress. By 5 weeks of the therapy all of the 26 patients who had severe pain before treatment had been totally or partially relieved of the pain. The anti-pain effect was especially noticeable in patients with very advanced breast cancer with multiple osseous metastases who were forced to keep completely still and were thought to be no longer susceptible to chemotherapy. Together with the anti-pain effect, we also noted an improvement in the ability to walk in 63% (15 of 24) of the patients. For the purpose of assessing the latter, we considered walking-impairment as a signal-symptom and therefore as being correlated to the presence of probable neoplastic foci capable of inducing motor impairments. We used the following rating scale: grade 0—absent or slight; *grade 1*—the patient spends less than 50% of the day in bed; *grade 2*—the patient is forced to spend more than 50% of the day in bed.

In this group of patients, the incidence of objective remission [complete remission (CR) + partial remission (PR)] was 44% (20 of 45) with an average duration of 7 months (48). Prior to therapy 79% of this group of patients had pain and nearly one-half of these had severe pain. After 1 month of treatment only 15% had pain and none had severe pain. However, this remission lasted about 6 months, when pain recurred in 48% of the patients and of these nearly one-third had severe pain. In 23 patients of this group, upon reappearance of pain, we repeated MAP treatment employing higher doses (2,000 mg i.m. per day for 30 days) with a more-concentrated MAP pharmaceutical preparation.[1] As a result of this repeated therapy, we noted remission once again in 21 patients (91%). In this second group of patients the incidence of objective remission (CR + PR) was 18% (49).

Subsequently, we treated another group of 25 patients with the same type of advanced disease with daily doses of 2,000 mg i.m. per day for 30 days. We noted an objective remission rate of 45% and subjective remission rate of 70% (48).

A new group of 92 patients with the same type of disease was studied as part of a prospective, randomized, multi-institute study with the aim of assessing the effectiveness of two different dose-levels of MAP. Forty-six patients received 500 mg/day for 30 days and 46 patients received 1,500 mg/day for 30 days. The drug was administered intramuscularly (47). Statistical analysis of objective results revealed that a larger percent of the patients who received 1,500 mg doses had complete or partial remission but the differences were not significant. However, the remission rates in all the signal-symptoms considered were consistently higher for MAP at the 1,500-mg dose-level (Table 13). Moreover and very importantly, remission of pain which occurred during the treatment was more rapid and greater for the higher dose-level than the lower dose-level (Table 14).

---

[1] Farlutal 500–1,500, F.I. 7401, 200 mg/ml vials.

TABLE 13. *Significant reduction or disappearance of the signal-symptoms present before treatment with high and low doses of MAP*

Symptomatology	Patients tested with MAP 1,500 mg			Patients tested with MAP 500 mg		
	Before therapy	After therapy	Remission rate	Before therapy	After therapy	Remission rate
Pain	26	4	85%	28	7	75%
Dyspnea	9	3	67%	6	3	50%
Asthenia	25	7	72%	24	8	67%
Anorexia	10	0	100%	16	3	81%
Walking-impairment	10	3	70%	12	7	42%

TABLE 14. *Behavior of the pain during the treatment (rate of remission)*

Drug dose (mg)	Patients with pain before therapy	Rate of remission during therapy (weeks) (in % of total patients with pain)			
		1	2	3	4
MAP 1,500	20	40%	60%	70%	80%
MAP 500	21	29%	38%	48%	71%

The results we obtained using high doses of MAP were subsequently confirmed by other authors (2,33). On the whole, MAP induced remission of pain in 83% of the patients (Table 15).

Moreover, review of the literature reveals that with MAP doses of 500 mg or less per day pain-relief was obtained by 21% of the patients compared with the 83% rate achieved with high doses. Although we are well aware of the limitations of retrospective comparisons, the difference in the remission of pain induced by high doses and low doses of MAP appears quite clear.

TABLE 15. *Results with hormonal therapy (large doses of MAP) for advanced breast cancer*

Authors	MAP dose (mg/day i.m.)	No. of pts.	Objective remission		Pain before therapy		Pain remission	
			No.	%	No.	%	No.	%
Pannuti et al. (51)	1,500	44	18	41	40	91	37	92
Amadori et al. (2)	1,000–1,500	44	25	57	37	84	21	57
Martino et al. (33)	1,500	20	6	30	20	100	20	100
Pannuti et al. (44)	500–1,000–2,000	168	76	45	114	70	98	86
Total/Averages		276	125	45	211	76	176	83

TABLE 16. *Effect of MAP orally/2,000 mg on pain of advanced breast cancer*

Effects on pain	Hormone-sensitive tumors (no. of pts. = 9)	Not hormone-sensitive tumors (no. of pts. = 16)	Total of the two groups
Decrease or complete relief	67%	50%	56%
No change	22%	44%	36%
Increase	11%	6%	8%

Administration of 1,500 mg of MAP intramuscularly is associated with a 15% incidence of abscess. Because of this complication, we began a series of studies concerning the oral administration of high doses of MAP (2,000 mg/day for 30 days) aimed at appraising: (a) the effect on the appetite and body-weight of the patient (anabolic effect); (b) the anticancer effect on hormone-sensitive tumors; (c) the effect on pain. At the moment, we have already shown an anabolic effect in 58 patients who experienced a statistically significant increase in body-weight and appetite (45). Studies concerning points b and c are still in progress. Preliminary results regarding pain relief are shown in Table 16.

Table 17 summarizes some of the results obtained with different hormone therapies for advanced breast cancer. It is apparent that of the subtractive measures, those that induced the highest remission of pain involved the destruction of the pituitary gland, whereas among the additive measures were high doses of MAP. In this regard, we should mention an important study made by Martino and Ventafridda (33) who compared the anti-pain effects of pituitary neuroadenolysis (alcohol-injection of the pituitary gland) with those obtained with 1,500 mg/day doses of MAP for 30 days (in the way

TABLE 17. *Results of therapy for advanced breast cancer: hormonotherapy*

	Additive therapy			Ablative therapy	
Drug	Pain rem.	Subject. rem.	Organ	Pain rem.	Subject. rem.
L-DOPA	10/30 (33%)	10/30 (33%)	Hypophysis	454/554 (82%)	42/100 (42%)
Cortisonics	5/43 (12%)	7/43 (16%)	Adrenals	8/18 (44%)	8/18 (44%)
Androgens	16/36 (44%)	77/209 (37%)	Adrenals + ovary	n.d.	202/500 (40%)
Progestins (other than MAP)	24/54 (44%)	39/78 (50%)			
MAP low doses	14/67 (21%)	n.d.			
MAP high doses	176/211 (83%)				

Legend: See Table 2.

TABLE 18. Advanced breast cancer (MAP/500, 1500, 2000 mg/day × 30 days) side effects

Infiltration	12/166	(7%)
Abscess	31/166	(18%)
Facies lunaris	28/166	(16%)
Fine tremors	27/166	(16%)
Sweating	25/166	(15%)
Vaginal bleeding	18/166	(10%)
Thrombophlebitis	2/166	(1%)
Cramps	15/166	(9%)

we first suggested) and with the two therapies combined for patients with very advanced breast cancer. Their patients were no longer responsive to multiple chemotherapy and had very severe, continuous pain which was no longer controllable with narcotic analgesic drugs. They found a more prolonged anti-pain effect in the two groups treated with MAP, compared with the group treated with pituitary alcoholization. Furthermore, in 6 of the 20 patients who had been given MAP there was objective remission of the disease, but none occurred in the 10 patients who had undergone only pituitary alcoholization.

The relative profile for the toxicology of MAP at high doses is reported in Table 18. All side-effects are reversible within 20 days after the end of treatment and do not delay or interrupt further treatment.

CONCLUSIONS

Our experience concerning the effect of MAP on pain in the treatment of advanced hormone-sensitive tumors and especially in breast cancer leads us to conclude that the analgesic effect is at least in part independent of the pure anticancer effect. This conclusion is based upon two considerations: (a) In breast cancer the incidence of remission of pain is considerably greater than the incidence of objective remission of the tumor; and (b) there is a proportion of patients who, although they exhibit progression of the neoplastic disease, also experience reduction of pain-intensity. One comes to the same conclusion when one considers the results of hypophysectomy. These considerations lead one to the attractive hypothesis that there may be an analogy in the mechanisms of action. This is further suggested by the data of Martino and Ventafridda and also by data which show that MAP is capable of inhibiting pituitary-hormone activity in a less destructive fashion and without the immediate and long-term side effects of hypophysectomy.

Although the mechanism of the anticancer activity (direct or mediated by pituitary blocking) may be the prime factor to explain the anti-pain effect of MAP, one cannot rule out that the analgesic effects of this hormone may also be due to its actions on such factors as prostaglandin inhibition, anti-inflammatory effects, etc. These are worthy of study separately and systematically, not only in man but also in suitable pre-clinical experimental animal systems.

Regardless of the possible mechanism of action, it should be stressed that MAP is certainly an anticancer agent which, when given in high doses (as we first suggested), is able to induce remission of pain in hormone-sensitive tumors to an extent that has never been observed previously. The value of this therapeutic intervention certainly takes on greater importance when one considers that it is associated not only with quite considerable objective remission rates, at least in breast cancer, but also with a strong anabolic effect that is no small contribution to the quality of life of cancer patients.

ACKNOWLEDGMENTS

We are grateful to Dr. Antonia Cricca, to Dr. Fiorenza Fruet, and to Ms. Ida Rubino for help in the preparation of this manuscript.

REFERENCES

1. Abbes, M. M., Bourgeon, G., Paillaud, F., Juillard, G., Kermarec, J., Cambon, P., and Namer, M. (1972): À propose de 111 destruction hypophysaires pér yttrium 90 on cryothérapie pour cancer du sein avancé. *Ann. Chir.*, 26:521–531.
2. Amadori, D., Ravaioli, A., and Barbanti, F. (1976): L'impiego del medrossiprogesterone acetato ad alte dosi nella terapia palliativa del carcinoma mammario in fase avanzata. *Min. Med.*, 67:1–14.
3. Archimbaud, J. P., Dex Roseax, M., and Picq, P. (1973): Le traitement des douleurs des métastases osseuses de l'épithélioma prostatique par la surrénalectomie unilatéralle gauche. *J. Urol. Nefrol.*, 79:415–419.
4. Aslam, J., and Maxwell, J. (1977): Calusterone therapy for advanced breast cancer. *Cancer Treat. Rep.*, 61:371–373.
5. Band, P. R., Banergee, T. K., Patwardhan, V. C., and Eid, T. C. (1973): High-dose diethylstilbestrol diphosphate therapy of prostatic cancer after failure of standard doses of estrogens. *CMA J.*, 109:697–699.
6. Bloom, H. J. G., and Boesen, E. (1974): Antioestrogens in treatment of breast cancer: Value of nafoxidine in 52 advanced cases. *Br. Med. J.*, 2:7–10.
7. Bloom, H. J. G., Dukes, C. E., and Mitchley, B. C. V. (1963): Hormone-dependent tumours on the kidney. 1. The oestrogen-induced renal tumour of the Syrian hamster—hormone treatment and possible relationship to carcinoma of the kidney in men. *Br. J. Cancer*, 17:611–645.
8. Bouffioux, C. (1976): Traitement du cancer de la prostate par les agents progestatifs. *Acta Urol. Bel.*, 44:336–353.
9. Brennan, H. J., Beckett, V. L., Kelley, J. E., and Betanzos, G. (1960): Treatment of advanced mammary cancer with 3-β-17-β-androstanediol. *Cancer*, 13:1195–1200.
10. Bucalossi, P., Di Pietro, S., and Gennari, L. (1963); Trattamento ormonico del carcinoma mammario diffuso con un progestativo sintetico: il 6-α-methil-17-α-acetossiprogesterone. *Min. Chir.*, 9:358–366.
11. Colapinto, V., and Aberhart, C. (1961): Clinical trial of massive stilbestrol diphosphate therapy in advanced carcinoma of the prostate. *Br. J. Urol.*, 33:171–177.
12. Cole, M. P., Jones, C. T. A., and Todd, D. H., (1971): A new anti-oestrogenic agent in late breast cancer in early clinical appraisal of ICI 46474. *Br. J. Cancer*, 25:270–275.
13. Colsky, J., Shnider, B., Jones, R., Jr., Nevinny-Stickel, H. B., Hall, T., Regelson, W., Selawry, D. S., Owens, A., Brindley, C. D., Frei, E., III, and Uzer, Y. (1963): A comparative study of 9α-bromo, 11β-ketoprogesterone and prednisolone

in the treatment of advanced carcinoma of the female breast. *Cancer,* 4:502–505.
14. Curwen, S., (1963): The value of norethisterone acetate in the treatment of advanced carcinoma of the breast. *Clin Rad.,* 14:445–446.
15. Dao, T. L. (1961): In: "Progress report: results of studies by the cooperative breast cancer group 1956–1960." *Cancer Chemother. Rep.,* 11:109–141.
16. Denoix, P. (1970): *Breast Cancer: Treatment of Malignant Breast Tumours.* pp. 1–92. Springer Verlag, Berlin.
17. Di Carlo, F., Pacilio, G., and Conti, G. (1975): Sul meccanismo d'azione dei progestinici nella terapia dei tumori mammari ormono-dipendenti. *Tumori,* 61:501–508.
18. Dogliotti, G. C., Gavosto, F., and Molinatti, G. M. (1968): Trattamento del cancro avanzato della mammella con progestatici di sintesi. *Min. Med.,* 81:42–83.
19. Fergusson, J. D. (1971): *Life Sciences Monographs, 1, International Symposium on the Treatment of Cancer of the Prostate.* Pergamon Press, Vieweg.
20. Fracchia, A. A., Randall, H. J., and Farrow, J. H. (1967): The results of adrenalectomy in advanced breast cancer in 500 consecutive patients. *Surg. Gynecol. Obstet.,* 125:747.
21. Glenn, E. N., Richardson, S. L., and Bowman, B. J. (1959): Biologic activity of 6α-methil compounds corresponding to progesterone, 17-α-hydroxyprogesterone acetate and compounds. *Metabolism,* 8:265–285.
22. Hardy, J., Grisoli, F., Leclercq, T. A., and Somma, M. (1975): Hypophysectomie transphenoidale dans les cancers du sein metastatiques (160 cas). *Nuov. Presse Med.,* 4:2387–2390.
23. Heuson, J. C., Kenis, Y., and Tagnon, H. J. (1969): Hormones et cancer mammaire. Base espérimentale et traitment endocrinien. In: *Traitment médicaux des cancers et des léucemies,* Masson et Cie, Paris.
24. Huggins, C. (1956): Control of cancers of man by endocrinologic methods. A review. *Cancer Res.,* 16:825–830.
25. Huggins, C. (1967): Endocrine-induced regression of cancers. *Cancer Res.,* 27:1925–1930.
26. Huggins, C., and Scott, W. W. (1945): Bilateral adrenalectomy in prostatic cancer. *Ann. Surg.,* 122:1031–1045.
27. Huggins, C., Stevens, R., and Hodges, C. V. (1941): Studies on prostatic cancer. II. The effect of castration on advanced carcinoma of the prostate gland. *Arch. Surg.,* 43:209.
28. Juret, P., and Hayem, M. (1974): Pituitary ablation in the treatment of breast cancer. In: *Mammary Cancer and Neuroendocrine Therapy,* edited by B. A. Stoll, pp. 283–311. Butterworths, London.
29. Kistner, R. W., Griffiths, C. T., and Craig, J. M. (1965): Use of progestational agents in the management of endometrial cancer. *Cancer,* 12:1563–1579.
30. Klaassen, D. J., Rapp, E. F., and Hirte, W. E. (1976): Response to medroxyprogesterone acetate (NSC-26386) as secondary hormone therapy for metastatic breast cancer in postmenopausal women. *Cancer Treat. Rep.,* 60:251–253.
31. Lewison, E. F., Trimble, F. H., Grow, G. L., and Masukawa, T. (1963): Results of combined hormone therapy in advanced breast cancer. *Cancer,* 16:1243–1245.
32. Lippman, M., Bolan, G., and Huff, R. (1976): The effect of estrogen and antiestrogen on hormone-responsive human breast cancer in long-term tissue culture. *Cancer Res.,* 36:4595–4601.
33. Martino, G., and Ventafridda, V. (1976): Effetto antalgico dell'alcolizzazione ipofisaria, del medrossiprogesterone acetato ad alte dosi e della loro associazione nel carcinoma mammario in fase avanzata. *Tumori,* 62:93–98.
34. Minton, J. P. (1974): The response of breast cancer patients with bone pain to L-DOPA. *Cancer,* 33:358–363.
35. Morgan, L. R., Schein, P. S., Hoth, D., McDonald, J., Posey, L. E., Beazley, R. W., and Trench, L. (1976): Therapeutic use of tamoxifen in advanced breast cancer: A correlation with biochemical parameters. *Proc. Am. Assoc. Cancer Res.,* 17:126.
36. Moricca, G. (1974): Chemical hypophysectomy for cancer pain. *Adv. Neurol.,* 4:470–714.

37. Muggia, F. M., Cassileth, M. O., Ochoa, M., Jr., Flatow, F. A., Gellhorn, A., and Hyman, G. A. (1968): Treatment of breast cancer with medroxyprogesterone acetate. *Ann. Intern. Med.,* 68:328–337.
38. Murphy, G. P., Reynoso, G., Schoonees, R., Gailani, S., Bourke, R., Kenny, G. M., Mirand, E. A., and Schalck, D. S. (1971): Hypophysectomy and adrenalectomy for disseminated prostatic carcinoma. *J. Urol.,* 105:817–825.
39. Nevinny-Stickel, H. B., Dederick, M. M., Haines, C. R., and Hall, T. (1964): Comparative study of 6-dehydro-17α-methyltestosterone and testosterone propionate in human breast cancer. *Cancer,* 17:95–99.
40. Notter, G., and Melander, O. (1966): Pituitary implantation with ^{90}yttrium in the treatment of advanced breast cancer. *Coll. Int. (Lyons),* pp. 113–121.
41. Novak, E. (1977): Effects of medroxyprogesterone acetate on some endocrine functions of healthy male volunteers. *Curr. Ther. Res.,* 21:320–326.
42. Ortiz, A., Hiroi, M., Stanczyk, F. Z., Goebelsmann, V., and Mishell, D. R., Jr. (1977): Serum medroxyprogesterone acetate (MPA) concentrations and ovarian function following intramuscular injection of Depo-MPA. *J. Clin. Endocrinol. Metab.,* 44:32–38.
43. Pannuti, F., editor (1977): *Il protocollo terapeutico ed i codici di caratterizzazione e di valutazione in clinica oncologica.* Editrice Universitaria Bolognese, Bologna.
44. Pannuti, F., Castellari, S., Camera, P., Di Marco, A. R., Fruet, F., Giusti, H., Lelli, G., Martoni, A., Piana, E., Pollutri, E., Rossi, A. P., and Strocchi, E. (1977): I protocolli oncologici dell'ospedale M. Malpighi. In: *La chemioterapia dei tumori solidi,* edited by F. Pannuti, pp. 517–553. Editrice Universitaria Bolognese, Bologna.
45. Pannuti, F., Fruet, F., Piana, E., Strocchi, E., and Cricca, A. (1978): The anabolic effect induced by high doses of medroxyprogesterone acetate (MAP) orally in cancer patients. *IRCS Med. Sci.,* 6:118.
46. Pannuti, F., Martoni, A., and Cricca, A. (1978): Treatment of renal clear cell carcinoma by high doses of medroxyprogesterone acetate (MAP): Pilot study. *IRCS Med. Sci.,* 6:177.
47. Pannuti, F., Martoni, A., Di Marco, A. R., and Piana, E. (1978): Results of a randomized clinical trial of two different massive dosages of medroxyprogesterone acetate (MAP) in the treatment of metastatic breast cancer *(in press).*
48. Pannuti, F., Martoni, A., Lenaz, G. R., Piana, E., and Nanni, P. (1976): Management of advanced breast cancer with medroxyprogesterone acetate (MAP, F.I. 5837, F.I. 7401, NSC-26386) in high doses. In: *Functional Explorations in Senology,* pp. 253–265. European Press, Ghent, Belgium.
49. Pannuti, F., Martoni, A., Lenaz, G. R., Piana, E., and Nanni, P. (1978): A possible new approach to the treatment of metastatic breast cancer: Massive doses of medroxyprogesterone acetate. *Cancer Treat. Rep.,* 62 *(in press).*
50. Pannuti, F., Martoni, A., Piana, E., and Palenzona, D. (1977): Proposta di un modello di valutazione della tossicità in chemio-ormonoterapia antiblastica. *Min. Med. (in press).*
51. Pannuti, F., Martoni, A., Pollutri, E., Camera, P., and Lenaz, G. R. (1974): Ormonointerferenza da medrossiprogesterone acetato: Risultati relativi a 50 pazienti affetti da carcinoma mammario in fase avanzata. Proposta di una nuova metodologia di caratterizzazione e di valutazione. *Bull. Sci. Med.,* 144:1–43.
52. Pannuti, F., Martoni, A., Pollutri, E., Camera, P., Losinno, F., and Giusti, H. (1976): Massive dose progestational therapy in oncology (medroxyprogesterone). Preliminary results. Acts of the IV symposium on the locoregional treatment of tumours, St. Vincent, 1973. *Pan. Min. Med.,* 18:129–136.
53. Pannuti, F., Rossi, A. P., and Piana, E. (1977): Massive doses of medroxyprogesterone acetate (MAP): Pilot study in the treatment of advanced prostate cancer. *IRCS Med. Sci.,* 5:375.
54. Rafla, S., and Johnson, R. (1974): The treatment of advanced prostate carcinoma with medroxyprogesterone. *Curr. Ther. Res.,* 16:261–267.
55. Rifkind, A. B., Kulin, H. E., Cargille, C. M., Rayford, P. C., and Ross, G. T. (1969): Suppression of urinary excretion of luteinizing hormone (LH) and follicle stimulating hormone (FSH) by MAP. *J. Clin. Endocrinol Metab.,* 29:506.

56. Rosner, J. M., Declercq De Perez Bedes, G., and Gomez, E. (1974): Competition entre l'oestradiol et different progestagens au niveau de l'hypotalamus du rat. *Ann. Endocr.*, 35:173–176.
57. Sadoff, L., and Lusk, W. (1974): The effect of large doses of medroxyprogesterone acetate (MPA) on urinary levels and serum levels of cortisol T4 LH and testosterone in patients with advanced cancer. *Obstet. Gynecol.*, 43:262–266.
58. Sala, G., Castegnaro, E., Lenaz, G. R., Martoni, A., Piana, E., and Pannuti, F. (1978): Hormone interference in metastatic breast cancer patients treated with medroxyprogesterone acetate at massive doses: Preliminary results. *IRCS Med. Sci.*, 6:129.
59. Scott, W. W. (1973): Rationale and results of primary endocrine therapy in patients with prostatic cancer. *Cancer*, 32:1119–1125.
60. Serment, H., Spitalier, J. M., Ayme, E., De Giovanni, E., and Bardin, J. P. (1970): Médroxyprogestérone et adénocarcinomes de l'endométre. *Bull. Fed. Gynecol. Obstet.*, 22:93–97.
61. Smith, J. P., Rutledge, F., and Soffar, S. W. (1966): Progestins in the treatment of patients with endometrial adenocarcinoma. *Ann. J. Obstet. Gynecol.*, 94:977–984.
62. Smith, R. B. (1971): Cyproterone therapy in stage IV. In: *Life Science Monographs, 1, International Symposium on the Treatment of Cancer of the Prostate.* Pergamon Press, Vieweg.
63. Sonkin, R., Coudeyras, M., and Thévenet, M. (1969): L'utilisation de la noréthindrone à doses fortes dans le traitement de certains cancers génitaux hormonodépendants. *Obstet. Gynecol.*, 68:355–372.
64. Straffon, R. A., Kiser, W. S., Robitaille, D. F., and Dohn, D. F. (1968): ^{90}yttrium hypophysectomy in the management of metastatic carcinoma of the prostate gland in 13 patients. *J. Urol.*, 99:102–108.
65. Susan, L. P., Roth, B. R., and Adkins, W. C. (1976): Regression of prostatic cancer metastases by high doses of diethylstilbestrol diphosphate. *Urology*, 7:598–601.
66. Tagnon, H. J., Coune, A., Heuson, J. C., and Van Rymenant, M. (1967): Problems in the treatment of disseminated cancer of the breast: Selection of patients for hormone treatment. In: *New Trends in the Treatment of Cancer*, edited by L. Manuila, S. Moles, and P. Rentchnick, pp. 126–133. Springer-Verlag, Berlin, Heidelberg, New York.
67. Talley, R. W., Moorhead, E. L. Tucker, W. G., San Diego, E. L., and Brennan, M. J. (1969): Treatment of metastatic hypernephroma. *JAMA*, 207:322–328.
68. Terenius, L. (1974) Affinities of progestogen and estrogen receptors in rabbit uterus for synthetic progestogens. *Steroids*, 23:909–919.
69. Tseng, L., and Gurpide, E. (1975): Effects of progestins on estradiol receptor levels in human endometrium. *J. Clin. Endocrinol. Metab.*, 41:402–404.
70. Van der Werfmessing, B., and Van Gilse, H. A. (1971): Hormonal treatment of metastases of renal carcinoma. *Br. J. Cancer*, 25:423–427.
71. Volk, H., Ciprut, S., and Escher, G. (1962): Hormonal therapy in advanced breast cancer. II: Effect of oral 11β-hydroxy-17α-methyl-testosterone compared with fluoxymesterone on clinical course and its effects on metabolism of nitrogen and selected electrolytes. *Cancer*, 15:726–732.
72. Volk, H., Foley, C. J., Sanfilippo, L. J., and Escher, G. C. (1964): Hormonal therapy in advanced breast cancer. III: Effect of 6-β-dibromomethylene-testosterone propionate compared with that of 2α-A-methyl-dihydrotestosterone propionate on clinical course and metabolism of selected serum electrolytes. *Cancer*, 17:1073–1078.
73. Volk, H., Wilde, R. C., Carabasi, R., and Bisel, H. (1965): Anti-tumor efficacy of norandrolone propionate compared with testosterone propionate in advanced breast cancer. *Cancer*, 18:651–655.
74. West, C. D., Hollander, V. P., Whithore, W. F., Jr., Randall, H. T., and Pearson, O. H. (1952): The effect of bilateral adrenalectomy upon neoplastic disease in man. *Cancer*, 5:1009–1018.

Radiation Therapy

S. Basso Ricci

Department of Radiology, Istituto Nazionale per lo Studio e la Cura dei Tumori, 20133 Milan, Italy

Pain and other discomforts of different types and intensity almost always occur with advanced carcinoma. Usually pain is related to the location and extension of tumor and individual reactivity, and it may be localized to the site of the primary tumor or referred elsewhere. The questions relevant to the possibility of getting partial or total regression of pain and other symptomatology are often very important in the therapy of these patients, even though recovery is no longer possible for most of them. The analgesic effect of ionizing radiation employed in the radiotherapy of tumors has long been well known. Although the precise basic mechanism of analgesic action from radiation therapy is not known generally, the most important beneficial effects result from: (a) decrease or removal of pressure on the nervous structures, (b) reduction of heteroplastic infiltration under the action of radiation, (c) disappearance of ulcerations and pressure on hollow organs with consequent elimination of colicky pain, and (d) resolution of inflammatory reaction in the tumor and its periphery.

It cannot actually be predicted to what extent these factors will respond to the radiation treatment or what degree of analgesia will be produced. It is this uncertainty of results which is the main restraint of radiation therapy.

The subject matter I intend to treat is dealt with on the basis of data from reports on this subject by others and from my own personal experience. It is subdivided according to the sites at which tumors manifest themselves, so I shall consider them successively under the following headings: (a) the head and the neck, (b) the chest, (c) the female genital system, (d) the male genital system, (e) the nervous system, and (f) the skeletal system. In the end I'll mention systemic tumors.

TUMORS OF THE HEAD AND THE NECK

If very extended, all these tumors can cause pain and, if there has been no previous radiation treatment, they can all show definite relief of pain and improvement of other symptomatology because of ionizing radiation.

Of the tumors in the rhinopharynx, the cases that I will consider are the ones concerning the sensory branches of the trigeminal nerve. It is known that in cases of recurrence this often involves mechanical or inflammatory processes of these nerves, and a second radiotherapy cycle is likely to produce relief of pain and related symptomatology (3). With tumors in the paranasal cavities and especially in the maxillary sinus, pain often occurs both in the cases that can't be operated and with tumors that recur after previous radiation and surgical treatments. These often produce pain because of the inflammatory process. Moreover, the pain often involves structures with different innervation so that surgical interruption or nerve blocks directed to one branch will not produce adequate relief [*Editors' note:* In such cases the neurosurgical procedure or nerve block must involve all of the branches of the trigeminal nerves that are likely to become involved with future expansion of the lesion. Therefore it is best to destroy the gasserian ganglion or sensory root of the trigeminal nerve. (See p. 537.)]

For large tumors in the oropharynx and the hypopharynx, which often cause local and referred pain, especially lesions in the floor of the mouth and the base of the tongue, the analgesic and curative effect of ionizing radiation is well known. On the other hand, when there is persistence or recurrence of these tumors, there develops ulceration in the infiltration zones which are poorly radiosensitive. Consequently, radiation therapy does not produce pain-relief and is therefore not indicated for analgesic action. In these cases it is better to use chemotherapy.

Radiation therapy of large tumors in the thyroid, which affect the nerves of the neck, produces effective pain-relief in most patients. Metastatic adenopathies of the neck deserve special mention, particularly those which progressively enlarge after previous radiation and surgical therapy. These metastatic lesions affect the nerves of the neck and those of the base of the skull by pressure and infiltration from the extralymphonodal component with consequent severe pain which has different location in different patients. Therefore, radiation therapy to produce analgesia must also include the base of the skull.

TUMORS IN THE CHEST

Advanced cancers in the chest considered here include primary tumors of the lung, primary and secondary tumors in the chest wall, and carcinoma of the breast. It is well known that Pancoast tumor early on infiltrates the brachial plexus and later becomes involved in pathology of the ribs.

Other peripheral pulmonary tumors in an advanced stage spread into the pleura and chest walls, whereas the central ones tend to affect the parabronchial and mediastinal nervous structures. In most cases, thanks to the experience which is now common to all radiotherapists, it is possible to obtain prompt and dramatic relief of pain and other discomforts as Haas and his associates pointed out in 1937 (5,9).

In our Institute, in the presence of pain after radiation treatment or surgical intervention, often we use bleomycin with radioactive indium in order to localize the probable site of recurrence and then start a new schedule of radiotherapy. Pain caused by metastatic lesions in the pleura and chest wall is often relieved by radiation treatment. I have no direct experience nor could I find any information about the response to radiotherapy when pain is caused by primary tumors in the pleura.

Carcinoma in the breast, with big, metastatic lymph nodes or ulcerations of tissues may cause pain which can be promptly relieved by radiation therapy. When pain develops in the distribution of part or whole of the brachial plexus in a woman who has received radiation therapy, we must exclude postradiation fibrosis pain before further therapy is considered.

TUMORS IN THE ABDOMEN

Here we will discuss tumors of the pancreas and the large bowel. For tumors of the pancreas, radical curative therapy is hardly ever feasible, and therefore the main object of radiation therapy is to provide pain-relief. Green and associates (4) state that pain-relief is almost always obtained, even with low doses, and should be considered even when hepatic metastases have already become evident.

Remarkable regression and even elimination of pain and related symptomatology may be obtained in the cases of endopelvic metastases of carcinoma of the large bowel and especially the rectum. These metastases are often in the hypogastrium and sacral regions. In the last 5 years, in our Institute, we have irradiated about 40 patients with this type of lesion with good results in most of them.

Recently, Smoron (13) has reported good results with radiation therapy of carcinoma of the biliary tract, even those which were not amenable to surgical therapy.

TUMORS OF THE FEMALE GENITAL SYSTEM

In these cases pain and related symptomatology is caused by infiltration of the parametrium and by hypogastric, sacral, aortic, and inguinal lymph-node metastases. The hypogastric and sacral metastases affect the sacral and parasacral nervous structures, although sometimes pain is due to a heteroplastic infiltration in the the bony structures.

In a series of 313 patients suffering from endopelvic recurrences of carcinoma of the uterus, Basso Ricci and Bianchi (1) noticed the presence of pain in about a third of the cases, with partial relief following radiation therapy. However, the best results have been obtained with anterolateral cordotomy (10).

TUMORS OF THE MALE GENITAL SYSTEM

These include malignant tumors in the testicle and the prostate. The voluminous metastatic adenopathies of tumors in the testicle, especially in the aortic and inguinal regions, often cause pain because of the pressure and infiltration of the individual nerves and lumbosacral plexus in the paravertebral region. When they are teratocarcinomas, we use radiotherapy to relieve pain only in the cases where chemotherapy proves inadequate. However, because these neoplasms are poorly radiosensitive, we should not expect dramatic or total pain-relief, but only partial analgesia.

Radiation therapy from the outside of tumors in the prostate in D stage with consequent neoplastic infiltration into the endopelvic tissues and organs produces regression of pain and at times total relief (6,12).

TUMORS OF THE URINARY APPARATUS

Renal tumors which have not been radically removed by surgery may cause pain in the hypochondrium or in the lumbar region by producing pressure and irritation of lower thoracic and lumbar nerves in the paravertebral region and also by to the concomitant presence of retroperitoneal lymph-node metastases.

Tumors in the urinary bladder with infiltration of the vesical wall, or lymph-node metastases, or even endopelvic recurrences after total cystectomy, can be successfully treated with radiation therapy to relieve pain and related symptomatology.

TUMORS INVOLVING THE NERVOUS SYSTEM

The neoplastic involvement of the central nervous system (CNS) must be differentiated from the ones involving the peripheral nervous system. As is well known, primary malignant neoplasms of the CNS which cannot be operated or have not been surgically removed produce progressively severe cephalalgia. In such cases radiation therapy can produce regression of the symptomatology, but we must add that the headache in these patients can be cured in most cases with surgical procedures which lessen the increased intracranial pressure and can be remarkably improved with the use of cortisone.

According to Hendrikson (7) the cerebral metastases were associated with severe headache in 30% of the patients, and of these at least 85% derived almost complete regression of the symptom with radiation therapy. The latter is carried out along with the use of cortisone in order to lessen the cerebral edema. It is also known that chemotherapy is not effective in cerebral metastases. In our Institute in the last 5 years we have treated 40 patients with this type of lesion, and our results have been similar to those reported by Hendrikson (7). As Posner (11) has emphasized, extracerebral, epidural, or arachnoid metastases can also be associated with headache if there is pressure or thrombus in the sagittal sinus. For these intracranial lesions which seldom are associated with edema, cortisone is not effective, and the only possible treatment is often radiation therapy. According to Posner (11) even the latter therapy is not effective when the sagittal sinus is thrombosed.

Pain is often experienced when the spinal cord is pressed upon by bony vertebral or epidural metastatic lesions. This pain, which is often of the radicular type, may precede even by months other neurologic symptomatology, especially motor disturbances. Therefore, after thorough study of the case including neurologic examination of the meninges, myelography, and possibly scintigraphy, radiation therapy is used possibly after laminectomy. Metastatic lesions can involve the roots of spinal nerves as well as spinal cord. Moreover, as previously mentioned, metastatic lesions may also involve nerve plexuses and more peripheral nerves.

The cauda equina may also be involved with a radicular pain which may be preceded by the loss of vesical and intestinal functions. I agree with Posner (11) that in such cases radiation therapy is more effective in lessening pain than other symptoms. When radiation therapy proves ineffective, we use neurosurgical procedures or neurolytic blocks (10,15).

TUMORS OF THE BONES

Primary tumors of bones deserve only a brief mention here because they can often be operated upon. Nevertheless in these cases, radiation therapy can produce good pain-relief. Metastatic tumors to bones are more important, because they are often the site of pain whether the tumor is in the bone itself, or in the subperiostal region, or if the metastases causes bony destruction and collapse with consequent pressure on nerve roots. These metastases respond promptly to radiation therapy and pain usually regresses rapidly and disappears after just a few treatments.

The osteolytic metastases react more effectively than the osteoblastic ones. Besides the radiation therapy from the outside, there is also the use of 32 radioactive phosphorus for the metastases of prostatic carcinoma, especially when we take care to increase the use of these isotopes for the metastases with parathormone. Hypophysectomy with radioactive yttrium can also give good results.

SYSTEMIC TUMORS

In the subject we are dealing with, the important cases are the ones where the lymph-node localizations cause pressure on paravertebral nerve structures and when there are meningeal, intracranial, or bony metastases.

SEQUELAE OF RADIOTHERAPY

Among the sequelae that arise in the peripheral nervous system, lesions of the nerve plexus and especially the sacral and brachial plexus are most important. Lesions of the sacral plexus are rather rare (8); on the other hand, those of the brachial plexus are relatively frequent following repeated cycles of irradiation of the supraclavicular region in patients with metastases from breast cancer or head or neck tumors. Irradiation in these cases can improve the symptomatology caused by the metastases but can also cause lesions of the brachial plexus, which produce very intense pain-symptomatology associated with alterations of muscle function in the arms. These are diagnosed by clinical and electrophysiologic examinations (2).

Finally, irradiation of bones, as is done, for example, in the case of bone metastases of mammary cancer with excellent pain-relief, can also cause permanent inhibition of the bone-marrow activity, with anemia, leucopenia, and thrombocytopenia. These alterations can be serious and can reduce survival time.

Early local reactions to radiation therapy, such as skin rash, inflammation of the mucosa, loss of hair, and decrease in salivation, in addition to general reactions such as the so-called "radiation disease" are all transitory and do not merit further comment. More important, however, are the delayed sequelae, most of which are not found at clinical examination because, in general, patients affected by advanced cancer have a brief survival. On the other hand, these sequelae in cases with longer survivals are particularly important, because we are usually dealing with patients subjected to repeated cycles of irradiation. Among the most important of these sequelae are those involving the skin, subcutaneous tissue and mucosa, bones, mediastinum, lungs, nervous tissue, and bone marrow.

The skin, subcutaneous tissue, and mucosa can have necrotic ulcers after repeated radiation treatments, and those which arise on the mucosa can produce intense pain. Necrotic lesions, sometimes of the rhinopharynx, are not infrequently the cause of serious hemorrhage after repeated treatment. The bones can also develop necrosis and consequent bone sequestra of fractures, especially of the mandible, the clavicle, or the upper part of the femur (8).

Among the sequelae in organs in the mediastinum, pericarditis deserves mention although it is very rare (14). Irradiation can cause inflammatory processes in the lung that evolve in fibrosis.

Among the sequelae of the CNS, transverse myelitis is the most important because it is almost always irreversible.

CONCLUSION

The significant radiosensitivity of certain neoplasms, the existence of probable contraindications for chemotherapy or surgery, and the opportunity of delaying the use of drugs represent important indications for radiation therapy for the relief of pain of advanced cancer. The more radiosensitive the neoplasm, the more promptly is its response to radiation therapy. So we must also expect a more obvious beneficial effect from radiation therapy in the cases where pain is caused by simple pressure rather than by infiltration of nerve structures which may also be irreparably damaged. The difficulty of localizing the nervous structures involved by the neoplasm or the involvement of many nerves make surgical intervention difficult. In contrast, radiation therapy, using relatively wide fields of irradiation, can act on more structures at the same time, as often happens for involvement of the base of the skull.

In order to make more complete data available on the extension of neoplasms to be irradiated, we have often resorted not only to the clinical examination and the common radiographic examination, but also to scintigraphy with labeled bleomycin, especially in the presence of recurrence of pulmonary carcinomas.

Contraindications of radiation therapy include previous radiation treatments when the latter have been made recently and with very high doses. Even if we take into account the different radiosensitivity of neoplasms, we do not think it useful to go further than a certain limit of doses to obtain some relief of pain rather than complete relief.

The maximum dose for an analgesic effect is different from patient to patient, but it is always below the one which must be reached for a radical elimination of the neoplasm. Sometimes we notice a worsening of the pain after the first application; but this effect, which is due to an initial congestion caused by radiation, rapidly resolves with the successive therapies. Sometimes we obtain not only regression of pain but also an improvement of the general condition of the patient, because narcotics with side effects can be decreased or eliminated.

REFERENCES

1. Basso Ricci, S., and Bianchi, F. (1966): Terapia delle recidive pelviche del carcinoma del collo dell'utero. *Minerva Ginecol.,* 18:603–609.
2. Basso Ricci, S., Ventafridda, V., Zanolla, R., Cassani, L., and Spreafico, R. (1976): Presentazione di 25 casi di lesioni postirradiatorie del plesso brachiale e loro trattamento. *Tumori,* 62:365–372.
3. Felci, U. (1964): La radioterapia dei tumori della rinofaringe. In: *Corso Superiore sulla terapia dei tumori della testa e del collo,* Milano, 6–11 April, pp. 181–215. CEA, Milano.
4. Green, N., Beron, E., Melbye, R. W., and George, F. W. (1973): Carcinoma of pancreas palliative radiotherapy. *Am. J. Roentgenol. Radium Ther. Nucl. Med.,* 117:620–622.
5. Haas, L. L. (1957): The place of the betatron in radiotherapy. *Arch. Intern. Med.,* 100:190–195.
6. Hazra, T. A. (1974): The role of radiotherapy in management of carcinoma of the prostate. *Maryland Med. J.,* 23:48–49.
7. Hendrikson, F. R. (1975): Radiation therapy of metastatic tumors in the brain. *Semin. Oncol.,* 2:43–46.
8. Kaplan, S. H. (1972): Complications of radiotherapy. In: *Hodgkin's Disease,* pp. 327–339. Harvard University Press, Cambridge, Mass.

9. Milani, F., and Lattuada, A. (1975): La radioterapia nei tumori dell'apice polmonare. In: *I tumori polmonari,* edited by P. Bucalossi, U. Veronesi, H. Emanuelli, and G. Ravasi, pp. 233–237. CEA, Milano.
10. Natale, P., and Miserocchi, E. (1952): La cordotomia anterolaterale nelle sindromi dolorose dell'utero incurabile. *Minerva Ginecol,* 5:1–6.
11. Posner, J. B. (1971): Neurological complications of systemic cancer. *Med. Clin. North Am.,* 55:625–646.
12. Rodriguez, A., Cook, S. A., Jelden, G. L., Hunter, A. T. W., Sraffon, R. A., and Stewart, B. H. (1973): Management of primary and metastatic carcinoma of the prostate. *Am. J. Roentgenol. Radium Ther. Nucl. Med.,* 118:876–880.
13. Smoron, G. L. (1977): Radiation therapy of carcinoma of Gallbladder and biliary tract. *Cancer,* 40:1422–1424.
14. Stewart, J. R., Cohn, K. E., Faiardo, L. F., Hancock, E. W., and Kaplan, H. S.: Radiation-induced heart disease: A study of twenty-five patients. *Radiology,* 89:302–310.
15. Wilson, C. B. (1969): Surgical control of pain in the cancer patients. *Oncology,* 23:44–48.

Palliative Surgery

Leandro Gennari

Istituto Nazionale per lo Studio e la Cura dei Tumori, 20133 Milan, Italy

What is the meaning of palliation? By palliation we mean the effect of all the procedures (such as inhibiting the progression of the disease or minimizing the dramatic events that are often produced by the neoplastic disease) that are used when it is impossible to cure a patient and that improve the quality of his remaining life. Palliative treatment of tumors almost always involves the use of physical means or chemical agents, such as radiotherapy or chemotherapy, whereas surgery is generally considered a means of attempting to solve contingent and grave situations, such as intestinal obstruction or bleeding. Recently, the improved knowledge in the field of oncology has altered this opinion, and surgery as a palliative measure is now being used more extensively. However, the meaning that is given to the term *palliation* is important.

If it is true that an operation is really curative when no residual tumor cells are left in the body, a large number of operations can be considered as palliative. In fact, from the survival data, we can state, for example, that in about 80% of the stomach carcinomas and in 50% of the carcinomas of the large intestine, the surgical operation employed was theoretically curative but in essence only palliative.

Perhaps this is both a philosophic and semantic matter; however, it suggests complex problems, the hypothetical solutions of which are not free from criticism and polemics where everybody is right and nobody is wrong. If the concept of surgical palliation is to be given a more restrictive meaning, all the situations in which surgery is required with a definite palliative purpose must be identified. Four different surgical situations are therefore distinguishable:

1. direct palliative surgery: (a) urgent, (b) reductive, and (c) necessary,
2. indirect palliative surgery,
3. palliative surgery for pain,
4. mediate palliative surgery.

DIRECT PALLIATIVE SURGERY

Urgent Palliative Surgery

Urgent palliative surgery means the surgical practice necessitated by emergency conditions, such as intestinal perforation or serious bleeding. Tumors of the gastrointestinal tract frequently cause heavy bleeding owing to the neoplastic erosion of a blood vessel. In these cases it is almost impossible to employ a raphe because of weak tissue, and it is thus essential to do a resection that may not always be carried out according to oncologic criteria of radicality. The surgeon, in this situation, is more concerned with resolving the emergency than removing all of the clearly metastatic lymph nodes. In the same way, a colostomy is required for a closed stenosis at the rectal-sigmoid junction or if the neoplasm is not resectable, Hartman's or Mukuliecz's operations are necessary when peritoneal or hepatic metastases are present.

Experience has demonstrated that, regardless of association with chemotherapy and/or radiotherapy, the survival of these patients is improved, both in the duration and quality of life, because the pain-symptom, due to local inflammatory events, is decreased by the absence of fecal passage. This kind of surgery is insensitive towards reductive palliative surgery.

Reductive Palliative Surgery

Reductive palliative surgery is so defined because at the end of the surgical treatment a notable reduction in the tumor mass is obtained. The result of such a treatment is that the radiologist and/or the chemotherapist have the opportunity to devise a therapeutic scheme that, even though it has no curative purpose, allows in many cases a recovery of the patient's general conditions, a restoration of some compromised functional capacities, and thus not only an extended survival but, more importantly, an improvement of the quality of life.

We have re-examined a group of patients affected by rectal cancer and treated in a nonradical way with surgery alone or in association with radiotherapy. Palliative surgery or radiotherapy alone resulted in a 1-year survival in 30% of the cases and 0% within 3 years. Association of the two types of treatment gave a 100% survival at 1 year, and 20% of the cases are still alive at 5 years. Such data corroborate the fact that palliative surgery as the only therapeutic treatment is extremely limited, but it has a wider application when used as part of a multidisciplinary approach.

Experimental studies and cell kinetic information have formed the basis for associated surgery-chemotherapy treatments. In such cases, however, the surgeon should not lose sight of the initial indications, limits, and objectives of the treatment, which in any case is palliative.

Palliative surgery is not intended only as a means for prolonging life. Its main purpose has been stated by Pack: "Palliation is not simply the duration of life, but rather the measure of comfortable living the individual enjoys in the remainder of his life." On the other hand, the surgeon must consider some elements objectively before making any decision, even if he does not contest every man's right to live as long as possible, regardless of the kind of life he might have. The surgeon must therefore consider: the operative mortality, the postoperative morbidity, the extent of the mutilation, and the kind of survival.

Each surgical operation, however simple, involves the risk of surgical mortality. However, this is a calculated risk that takes into account the possibility of complete recovery of the patient. On the contrary, knowing that a palliative treatment is useless risks death during or immediately after surgery. In these cases, the surgeon must avoid operating and must not become committed to a useless and dangerous course for reasons of ostentation or technical pride. Finally, the surgeon must not forget that the patient, because of the diffusion of the disease, often has only a weak resistance to the surgery. In fact, a tumor in such an advanced stage that it can not be removed, has already lowered the patient's organic resources so much that a simple laparotomy can cause an irreversible process that could be fatal. The weak resistance to surgical trauma also is largely responsible for postoperative morbidity, and therefore between two possibilities of palliative surgery, it is a good rule to chose the less dangerous one.

For example, in the case of a patient with a stenosis and bleeding carcinoma of the sigmoid colon with distant metastases, the surgeon must decide whether to perform a colostomy, which would solve the mechanical problems of the obstruction but not the oncologic ones, or to perform an intestinal resection, which would solve the immediate and delayed problems but might be followed by a high percentage of complications. In other words, is it better for the patient to undergo an operation that might be dangerous or to begin immediately after colostomy chemotherapeutic or radiologic treatment to relieve pain? Moreover, the surgeon must not forget the implications of the mutilation and the relative quality of the patient's remaining life.

For example, it is technically possible to perform a resection of almost all of the small intestine. In the literature cases are reported of patients who have survived for up to 2 years after a resection that left only from 6 to 18 inches of the small intestine. This fact is surprising if we consider the functions of the small intestine, also because the caloric contribution necessary for survival has been assured by the total parenteral nutrition (TPN). Although the survival of these patients is a fact of clinical relevance, we should ask ourselves if the high surgical mortality and the serious hardships during residual life are not too heavy a price to pay in comparison with the hypothetical advantages.

Finally, the choice of extensive palliative resections is conditioned, more-

178   PALLIATIVE SURGERY

over, by the usual criteria: the duration of the possible remaining life and those factors which influence the outcome of the surgery.

Necessary Palliative Surgery

Necessary palliative surgery means all operations directly performed on primary tumors or metastases and required by their sometimes monstrous growth. Since this kind of surgery is often destructive, is the disarticulation of a limb justified? As long as the above-mentioned rules are taken into account, we feel that such surgery is warranted. In our opinion, such surgery is definitely required in the case of very large, necrotic, ulcerated, infected and malodorous, painful and secreting tumors that result in an early cachexia. In fact, after palliative amputation or disarticulation, patients whose grave general conditions were due to large limb tumors rather than to the presence of pulmonary metastases, have recovered. Moreover, with the improvement of the hematologic picture, these patients can undergo chemotherapy with a greater probability of success. In other words, the two-fold purpose of removing a source of infection and often stabbing pains and of dealing with possible metastases by reducing the tumor mass is realized.

Finally, we should not forget that large superficial tumors, because of the

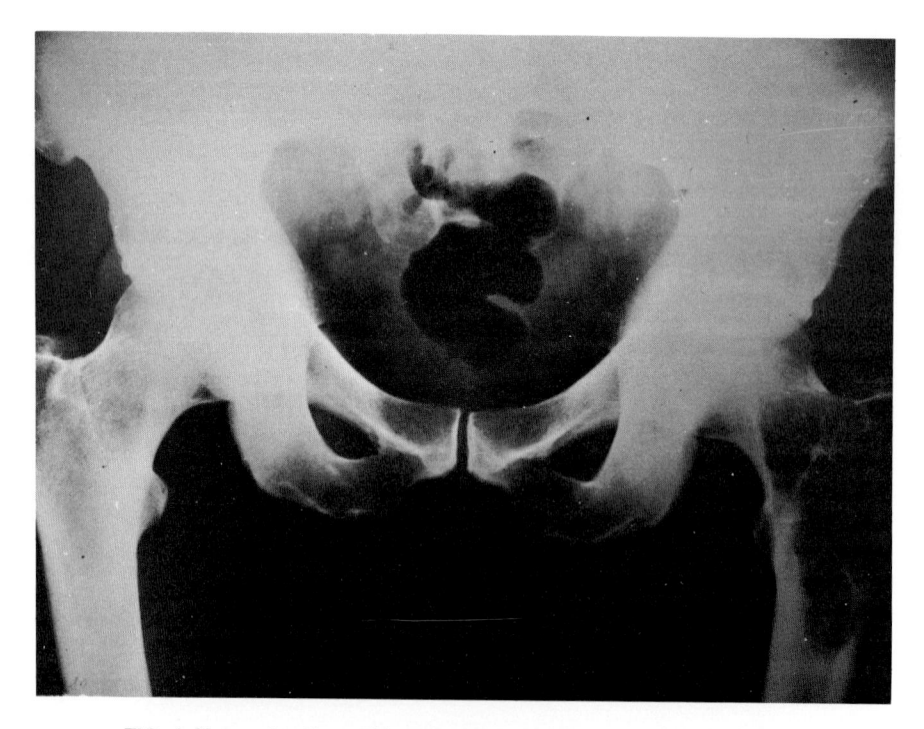

FIG. 1. X-ray of patient with pain in left hip due to metastatic lesion.

obvious discomfort they cause, represent a serious psychologic problem, and their removal gives patients the illusion of a cure that offers, in addition to the physical integrity, a reacquisition of psychologic equilibrium, which is necessary for reinsertion, even if temporary, into society.

Some tumors have a rather restricted activity that is expressed by a late, sometimes single metastasis and by a relatively slow local progression. In these cases, which are represented by bone metastases from thyroid or renal carcinomas, a surgical treatment, aggressive and conservative at the same time, is well justified. We have experimented with such types of surgery and have obtained very good results.

Figure 1 shows the radiogram for a 42-year-old patient who underwent X-ray examination for pain in the hip. The lesion was interpreted as a primary bone tumor, and the tumor was biopsied. The histologic diagnosis

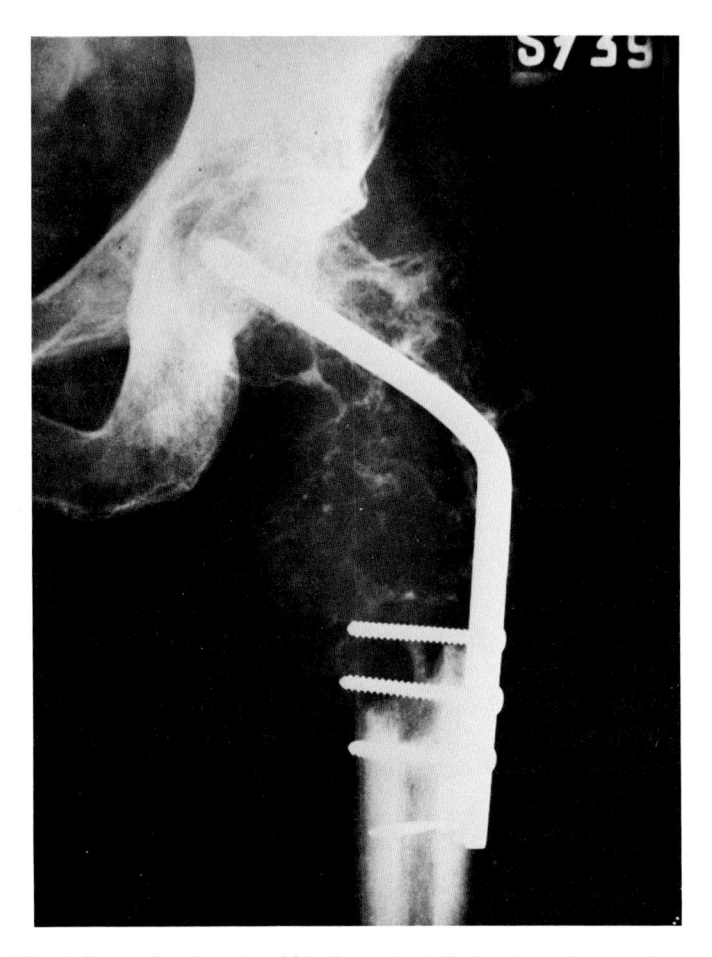

FIG. 2. X-ray showing pin of hip for metastatic fracture of upper femur.

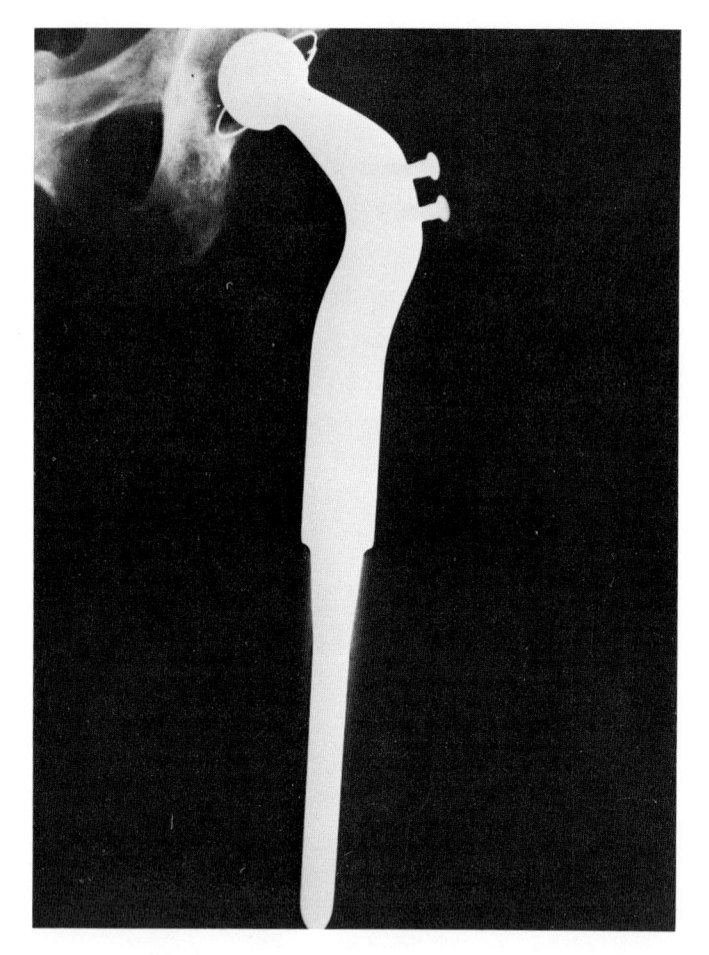

FIG. 3. X-ray showing prosthesis of left hip which resulted in relief of pain.

was "hypernephroma metastasis," and the surgeon performed a nephrectomy. After some time a pathologic fracture was found in the femoral site, and the orthopedist inserted a pin (Fig. 2). The patient remained without additional therapy until December, 1977, when the progressive increase of the femoral metastases caused a complete functional disability. After some time, the metastases were removed, and a prothesis was inserted with good results (Fig. 3).

INDIRECT PALLIATIVE SURGERY

Indirect palliative surgery involves the surgical treatment of organs whose functional activities have an effect on the development of the neoplastic disease. This includes mainly the so-called "ablative surgery" of endocrine organs and is used for patients with metastatic breast or prostatic carcinomas. Of all the forms of palliative surgery, this is the one that has given the best results in terms of response, both subjective (with decrease of pain and recovery of muscle function) and objective (with regression of pathologic parameters). Ablative surgery for ovarian cancer is particularly indicated for younger or premenopausal patients.

The recent finding of the presence of estrogen receptors has been of great assistance in the field of hormone surgery. In other words, on their surfaces, cells of breast cancer may have certain receptors that are able to bind and carry estrogens into the cells. Thus we are able to identify estrogen-receptor–positive (ER^+) and estrogen-receptor–negative (ER^-) tumors. The estrogen-receptor assay could play an important role in the planning of therapy, since it seems that only ER^+ tumors may benefit by an ovariectomy. Castration causes a partial or complete objective remission for an average period of about 6 months in 35% of the cases. Regression of bone and lymph-node lesions is most remarkable and is also accompanied by a complete remission of pain symptomatology.

With the progression of the neoplastic disease, it is possible to perform bilateral adrenalectomy which, however, complicates patient-management because of the necessity of continuous corticosteroid administration. At present, we tend to avoid adrenalectomy, and there is a renewed interest for surgical or radiologic hypophysectomy, not only for the hormonal suppression involved, but also for its analgesic action.

The same theoretical principles are also adopted in the treatment of metastasized prostatic carcinoma. It is generally a neoplasm with a slow evolution, and even after several years important results are obtained with castration or estrogen hormonotherapy. Some important studies, like those of Nesbit and Baum, carried out on 1,818 cases, have led us to conclude that castration is the treatment of choice with respect to estrogen therapy (3). Moreover, surgical treatment, thanks to modern technical devices, is well tolerated by the patient physically and psychologically.

PALLIATIVE SURGERY FOR PAIN

Pain has both a physical and an emotional component; the evaluation of pain-intensity is difficult, chiefly because of the unforeseeable quantification of the subjective component. In this volume, pain has been analyzed in all of its components by renowned specialists. I would like to agree with Pettavel (4) in stating that in a cancer it is the long duration, its increasing severity, and the progressive breakdown of physical and psychologic conditions of the patient that make pain intolerable. Pain is caused by many factors, such as tissue anoxia due to vascular insufficiency, compression, and the deceptive perineural infiltration.

Any palliative surgery, direct or indirect, reductive or mediate, causes a reduction of pain. However, it is sometimes so intense that the analgesic purpose of the surgery can be achieved only by operating on sensitive nerve trunks. It is a good rule to surgically intervene for the alleviation of pain only after all the other therapeutic means, pharmacologic and others, have failed. The main difference between this palliative surgery and the others is represented by the fact that this one tends only to make remaining life more tolerable, whereas the others can also prolong life. There is a wide range of operations for the peripheral nervous system: nerve blocks produced with neurolytic agents such as alcohol or phenol, which have been widely employed, particularly for stabbing pains in the limbs or in the perineal area due to recurrence of rectal carcinoma; and chordotomy, which is the most common operation with the greatest probability of success. Because of complex nervous compromises, blocks for pains in the perineal area must be performed very cautiously, since they can cause unpleasant complications, such as urinary incontinence.

MEDIATE PALLIATIVE SURGERY

Mediate palliative surgery is surgery that acts as an essential tool to carry drugs to the tumor area.

The local administration of antineoplastic drugs is a form of chemotherapy that, if performed on selected cases, gives more advantages than does systemic chemotherapy. Intra-arterial local-regional treatment has been used in various parts of the body and is now considered an important therapeutic tool. Some years ago Dargent (1) obtained good results, of a chiefly analgesic nature, on inoperable or recurrent rectal and uterine carcinomas that were considered beyond the limits of the possibilities of radiotherapy treatment.

For many years hepatic infusion has been performed, according to Watkins and Sullivan (5), via the hepatic artery for patients with metastases from carcinoma of the stomach and, above all, of the large intestine. Results are encouraging, even if not exciting. In a critical review of the treatment of primary and secondary hepatic tumors, Lee (2) reported a mean survival time of 5.6 to 7 months from the moment of diagnosis. Even the best results with chemotherapy, both mono- and polychemotherapy, were only from 17% (with 5-fluorouracil) to 55% (5-fluorouracil + adriamycin + mitomycin), and the duration of remission was also rather brief (about 10 weeks).

Palliative treatment with arterial infusion seems to give more satisfying results. We have treated 44 patients with inoperable primary tumors of the liver or affected by metastases in the gastrointestinal tract, which were responsible in many cases for a pain-symptomatology that was probably due to rupture or involvement of the peritoneal wall because of its proximity. The survival according to the degree of hepatic involvement is very important. For an accurate analysis of the efficacy of infusion treatment, a breakdown by stage is essential. We have adopted the classification of Pettavel (4). The best survival is found for the patients in Stage I and II, with a median survival of more than 1 year. The most impressive fact was the absence of systemic toxicity, even at high doses in a relatively brief time.

The absence of toxicity was apparent mainly when 5-fluorouracil was employed, whereas when adriamycin was used, toxicity was so intense that a patient died following bronchial pneumonia. The lack of systemic toxicity with 5-fluorouracil is probably due to the elimination of the drug partially by the liver and partially by the lungs. Regardless of the extension of survival, infusional treatment has brought about an immediate effect, has diminished severe pain in the hypochondrium, and caused a partial regression of hepatomegaly.

CONCLUSION

In conclusion, even when a radical cure is not feasible, it is possible for the surgeon to carry out an effective therapy, both to improve the quality of the patient's remaining life and to prolong survival. The surgeon must, however, attempt to minimize the physical and psychologic damages that an indiscriminate, aggressive operation can cause in a patient affected by cancer.

REFERENCES

1. Dargent, O. (1977): Lecture given at the National Cancer Institute of Milan, Italy. (Unpublished.)
2. Lee, Y. T. (1977): System and region treatment of primary carcinoma of the liver. *Cancer Treat. Rev.,* 4:195–212.
3. Nesbit, R. M., and Baum, W. C. (1950): Endocrine control of prostatic carcinoma: Clinical and statistical analysis of 1818 cases. *JAMA,* 143:1317–1320.
4. Pettavel, J. (1971): Les limites de la chirurgie palliative du cancer. In: *Oncologie Chirurgical,* edited by F. Saegesser and J. Pettavel. Masson, Paris.
5. Watkins, E., Jr., and Sullivan, R. D. (1964): Cancer chemotherapy by prolonged arterial infusion. *Surg. Gynecol. Obstet.,* 118:2–19.

Hyperthermic Perfusion with Sympathectomy for the Treatment of Advanced Painful Limb Tumors

*R. Cavaliere, **G. Moricca, *G. Stradone, and *F. Di Filippo

*Department of Surgery, **Department of Pain Therapy, Regina Elena Cancer Institute, Rome, Italy

INTRODUCTION

For many years, after the first report by Busch in 1866 (3), investigators have commented on the destructive effect of heat upon cancer cells (8,12,15,22). In previous papers, we have reported on biochemical and clinical studies which demonstrated that hyperthermia is an effective antineoplastic treatment (6,18,19). At the beginning of our clinical attempts, the first problem we were concerned with was the choice of a technique for an effective local heating. Isolation perfusion according to Creech and Krementz (10), but using prewarmed and diluted blood without drugs, seemed to be the right technique for reaching and maintaining a 42.0°C temperature in the perfused area as far as advanced malignant tumors of the limb were concerned.

The first series of hyperthermic perfusions was performed using a sigma-motor heart-lung machine equipped with a digital pump, a disc-oxygenator previously primed with whole, heparinized blood diluted at 50% with an isotonic solution, and a water-circulating heat exchanger unit maintained at about 47 to 48°C. Thermistor needle probes were applied to the arterial line of the circuit, on the skin, in the muscles, and in the tumor. The perfusions were started; no drugs were perfused; pump flows and the perfusion pressure were previously calibrated. Since a long perfusion time has been found to be effective against tumors, the application of a tourniquet was discontinued after the first cases because it caused peripheral nerve dysfunction. Consequently, we have had to standardize flow equilibration and perfusion pressure during the whole time of perfusion in order to control the exchange of blood between the systemic and the perfusing circulations which, when very pronounced, are a considerable handicap to the hyperthermia of the limb and the general condition of the patient.

Many complications occurred in this first series of patients treated with hyperthermic perfusion which was continued until 1967 (6). Nevertheless, the follow-up of this series allowed us to evaluate the long-term results.

These have been encouraging since of all the patients who were alive and well in 1967, only one died of the disease more than 7 years after hyperthermic perfusion; and this patient had a distant metastasis at the time of perfusion.

At that time, we did not have the possibility of dealing with the difficult problem of limb pain, because we were compelled to improve the technique in order to avoid major complications like acute renal failure, amputations, arterial ruptures, and secondary shocks. These trials were successfully accomplished: The heart-lung machine was replaced by a more reliable one; a flowmeter was inserted into the arterial line of the circuit together with a multichannel monitoring system; and, at the heat exchanger, the temperature was supplied by an independent water-circulating thermostat unit. At the beginning of the perfusion, the temperature in the arterial line was about 42.5°C to 43.0°C, and 42.0°C when hyperthermia was achieved. Mannitol was infused slowly but continuously and continued for some days. A beta-blocking agent was injected into the perfusion circuit at the beginning of perfusion with the aim of reducing the reaction to heat at the microcirculatory level, thus limiting arteriovenous shunts and tissue hypoxia due to the exclusion of the capillary bed.

The mortality rate was reduced to about 2% after the modifications were introduced to the technique. The results obtained in 150 patients clinically confirmed that hyperthermic perfusion is able to cause limb tumors to regress, even if the experimental results do not show complete agreement to the clinical experience (5). However, it is noteworthy that a statistical evaluation of our results published in 1977 (19) showed a 5-year survival rate of about 60% of the patients with osteogenic sarcoma and 75% of the patients with melanoma of the limbs. In spite of these excellent results, there remained the problem of the pain which we continually observed.

For a long period of time, we attached no great importance to this problem of "painful limb," allowing ourselves to be convinced that it was a transient problem of the postoperative period, probably due to swelling with venous stasis and blistering, which were frequently observed, sometimes followed by foot drop. The latter was avoided early by routinely performing anterolateral fasciotomy of the leg, but the problem of painful limb remained unchanged and, in the long run, attracted our full attention. These observations or considerations caused us to focus on this problem.

The first observation—truly disappointing—was the answer obtained from a systematic control of the perfused patients, many of whom were found to be suffering from painful limb, although the limb itself was apparently normal. The second observation concerned the discrepancy between the intensity of persistent pain and the gravity of circulatory disturbances following perfusion. The third observation had to do with the definite improvement obtained with sympathetic blocks, whose effectiveness was greater when the blocks were performed as early as possible in the postoperative period. This suggested that the pain was nonmalignant in nature though obscure in its exact mechanisms, and imprecise in its character, which is possibly mediated by the autonomic nervous system. On the basis of descriptions in the literature (1,2,7,25), we think this kind of painful limb may represent a form of reflex sympathetic dystrophy because of the absence of direct nerve damage, the persistent burning pain, the hyperesthesia and, sometimes, the presence of edema or intermittent cyanosis (4). We are in agreement with Gross (13) when he states that the "autonomic irritation syndromes occur either after irritation of the vessel or of the sympathetic trunks." It is a matter of fact that hyperthermic perfusion can reasonably be considered sufficient stimulus to give rise to painful limbs and that it possesses almost all the characteristics of a minor causalgia: the abnormal topography of pain, dyskinesia, dyscrasia, and dystrophy.

On the basis of these considerations, and because we noted complete, but transitory relief of pain following sympathetic blocks, we decided to tackle such a difficult problem at its origin. We therefore tried to find a new surgical approach that could allow us to perform hyperthermic perfusion and sympathectomy at the same time. This report describes the preliminary results obtained with this combined form of therapy.

MATERIAL AND METHODS

Thirteen patients undergoing hyperthermic perfusion for cancer of the limb were included in this clinical trial: 7 had osteosarcoma, 3 had soft-tissue sarcoma, and 3 had recurrent melanoma. Of the 7 patients with osteogenic sarcoma of the lower limbs, 6 had very extensive tumors and had to be amputated some weeks after perfusion in accordance with our protocol regarding the hyperthermic treatment of limb tumors. The 7th patient underwent bone resection followed by endoprosthesis 4 weeks after hyperthermic perfusion.

Of the 3 patients treated for soft-tissue sarcoma, 1 had a rhabdomyosarcoma of the left arm, and the others had large recurrent fibrosarcoma of the thigh and the calf, respectively. The treatment protocol for these tumors is to use hyperthermic perfusion followed by endoarterial antiblastic infusion and, finally, the excision of the tumor.

Of the 3 patients treated for melanoma, 2 underwent hyperthermic perfusion and dissection of involved nodes for recurrent multiple melanomas of the lower limb. The 3rd one underwent perfusion without node dissection for recurrent melanoma with satellitosis of the upper limb.

All the above patients were treated with sympathectomy at the time of hyperthermic perfusion, involving a single surgical approach. The addition of the sympathectomy does not significantly increase the surgical problems: The exposition, insulation, and cannulation of both iliac and axillary vessels are not affected by the modifications to the technique performed in order to remove the sympathetic chain. The surgical procedure is as follows:

For upper limb tumors, the patient is placed in the supine position with the head turned to the opposite side and the arm in abducted position with the palm upward. The incision is made from the midportion of the sternocleidomastoid muscle, 4 cm above the clavicle, laterally and downward along the deltopectoral groove. The clavicle could be divided in its midportion, but this can be avoided and we prefer to do so in order to permit the prompt mobilization of the perfused limb. The clavicular head of the sternocleidomastoid muscle, the omohyoid muscle, and the anterior scalene muscle are divided above the clavicle, obviating retracting the phrenic nerve. The insertion of the major pectoralis muscle over the short head of the biceps muscle is incised, and the tendinous insertion of the pectoralis minor muscle is divided on the coracoid process. At this time, the content of the axilla is bared below the clavicle, while the subclavian artery is exposed in the upper part of the wound. It is easy to divide the thyreocervical arterial trunk, to palpate the stellate ganglion, and to dissect the sympathetic chain in the extrapleural

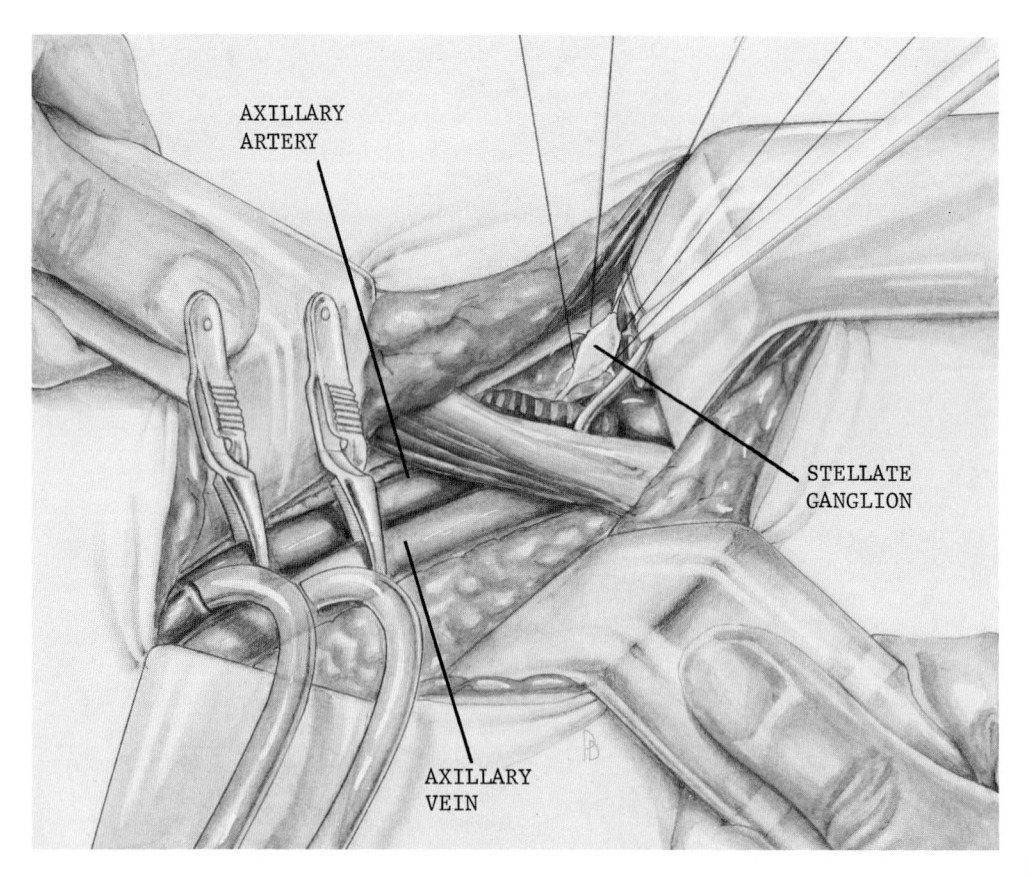

FIG. 1. The stellate ganglion is to be excised above the clavicle (the schematic drawing does not show that the upper part of the ganglion is left *in situ*). Below the clavicle, the axillary artery and vein are cannulated.

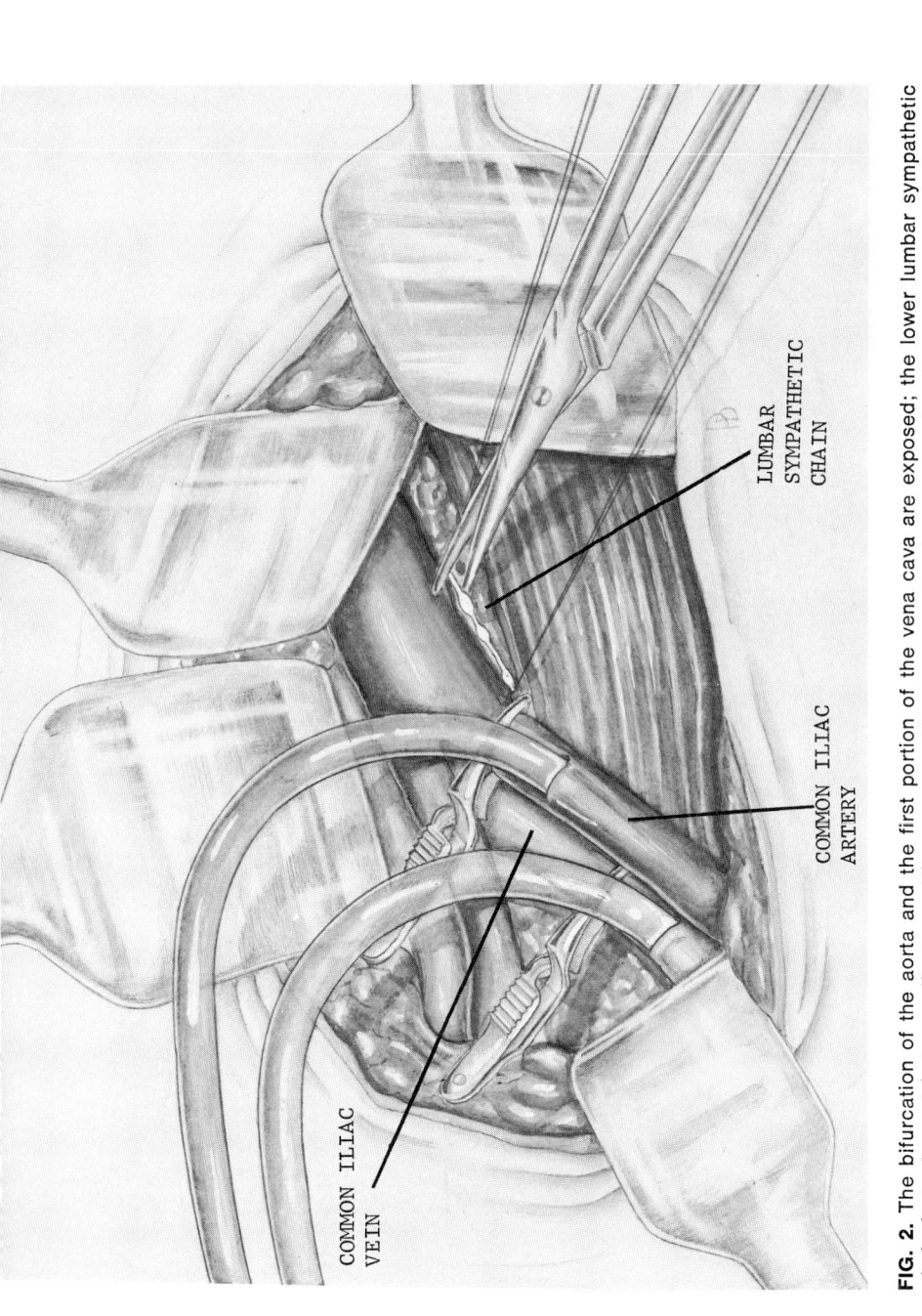

FIG. 2. The bifurcation of the aorta and the first portion of the vena cava are exposed; the lower lumbar sympathetic chain is to be cut between ligatures. The common iliac artery and vein are cannulated.

space. A nerve hook is placed under the sympathetic chain, the various rami are clipped with silver clips, and the chain is divided between the distal part of the stellate ganglion and the 3rd dorsal ganglion (Fig. 1). The cannulation of the axillary vessels and perfusion are performed as described in previous papers (5,19).

For lower limb tumors, the patient is placed in the supine position, and the whole abdomen and the limb to be perfused are included in the operative field. A transverse abdominal incision is made approximately 2 cm below the umbilicus, omolaterally to the limb. The rectus muscle and the external oblique and internal oblique muscles are incised in the direction of the skin incision. The transversus abdominis may usually be incised in the direction of its fibers. The peritoneum is opened; the liver and aortic nodes are exposed. After this maneuver, the peritoneum is sutured, and the peritoneal sac with its contents is bluntly directed medially. The psoas muscle, the distal portion of the abdominal aorta on the left side, or the first portion of the vena cava on the right side, the iliac vessels, and the other structures in the retroperitoneal area come into view. Following Hershey and Calman (14), the sympathetic chain is palpated laterally on the vertebral bodies. By gently lifting the chain with silk threads, the last 3 lumbar ganglions and their rami are identified (Fig. 2). Silver clips are applied between the second lumbar ganglion and the terminal division branches. Other silver clips are applied on the remaining part of the rami, and sympathectomy is performed.

The sympathectomy can be carried out before or after the perfusion; our experience did not show any difference between the two modalities, although it could theoretically be more correct to perform it at the end of the hyperthermic perfusion.

For both upper and lower limbs, a drainage is placed and the incision is closed in layers. No special postoperative care is necessary in relation to adjunctive sympathectomy.

RESULTS

Of the 7 patients treated for osteogenic sarcoma, 6 were suffering from "painful limb," presumably due to the tumor mass's infiltrating the soft tissues around the bone disease. The pain was continuous, markedly increased by palpation and walking, but not well defined in its characters and variable in its intensity. After hyperthermic perfusion and lumbar sympathectomy, the continuous pain was greatly reduced, while the intense and provoked pain disappeared. Neither edema nor venous stasis nor foot drop were observed. These considerations remained until the patient underwent surgery in accordance with the protocol for the treatment of extensive osteogenic sarcoma. The last patient of this group did not present preoperative painful limb; the postoperative period was very comfortable because of the complete absence of pain and of circulatory disturbances. After 4 weeks, he underwent a second operation for bone resection with metallic endoprosthesis; even then, the limb was not painful nor edematous. None of the patients who underwent amputation developed a painful phantom limb.

Of the 3 patients treated for soft-tissue sarcoma, one underwent this combined therapy for a rhabdomyosarcoma of the arm, a very large ulcerated tumor with an important edema of the hand and forearm. The tumor was recurrent and the limb very painful, with a burning, superficial type of discomfort. After the combined treatment, the burning sensation disappeared, although the arm remained heavy; the edema decreased in a few days. These effects cannot, however, be attributed to the therapeutic action of hyperthermic perfusion on the tumor because of their rapidity.

The other 2 patients treated for soft-tissue sarcoma were not suffering from painful limb, although their tumors were large. In these cases, however, the effectiveness of combined therapy was immediately evident in view of the condition of the perfused limb: Swelling, edema, venous stasis, postoperative pain, and foot drop were completely absent, so neither fasciotomy nor debridements were necessary. The patients walked promptly after surgery, and mobility of the limb was also recovered without any trouble.

The same effect of such combined therapy was observed in the 3 patients treated for recurrent melanoma. They did not need fasciotomy or debridements either, and they never complained of painful limb. The only complication encountered was 1 case of Bernard-Horner syndrome, presumably due to a mistake in the identification of the lower portion of the stellate ganglion and first ramus communicans.

DISCUSSION AND CONCLUSION

The first consideration concerns the mechanism of the pain in the limbs. The characteristics of the pain and associated symptomatology suggest that postperfusional circulatory disturbances, such as swelling and edema, can be excluded, because of the persistence of the pain in many patients after their limb had completely recovered. A causative mechanism identified with some direct traumatic action on the vessels appears more likely. A twofold origin can be recognized for such action: at a surgical level, due to the handling of major vessels and/or at a diffuse level, throughout the limb, because of the action of heating on vascular walls. This origin can explain reasonably well why other authors (16,24) who have performed antiblastic hyperthermic perfusion at lower temperatures with shorter durations observed minor incidences of postoperative, long-lasting, painful limb.

The aforementioned preliminary results have convinced us to pursue this clinical trial. The postoperative conditions of the perfused limbs after the association of sympathectomy show such significant differences in comparison with the conditions observed prior to using sympathectomy, that this form of combined therapy should no longer be ignored. Moreover, complications of sympathectomy are few and can be entirely avoided by correct surgical management. At the cervicothoracic level, it is not necessary to accomplish total stellectomy; the goal consists in the excision of the lower part of the stellate ganglion together with the 2nd and 3rd thoracic ganglia. The lower part of the stellate ganglion is identified as the 1st thoracic and may be recognized by its shape and because of the presence of the communicant ramus with the 1st thoracic nerve. The approach we describe permits—without any differences—the perfusion procedure and the excision of the 1st, 2nd, and 3rd thoracic ganglia; and this is sufficient to control the pain even if the innervation of the axilla is avoided (21).

At a lumbar level, surgical implications were emphasized by Simeone (23) and are unchanged in respect to our surgical approach. The only difference concerns the possibility of injuring, on the right side, a large lumbar vein which emerges at approximately the first lumbar vertebra and crosses the sympathetic trunk to enter the vena cava. It can be injured by the retractor because of the reduced direct exposition that our incision permits. On the other hand, such an approach did not present great difficulties if the retractors were correctly applied. Because of the limited extent of sympathetic resection that we have carried out, the first two lumbar ganglia are not affected. This prevents sexual complications (impotence) while allowing us to obtain good physiologic effects, as it prevents the regeneration of preganglionic fibers to the 4th and 5th lumbar ganglia with consequent reactivation of postganglionic neurons whose axons contribute to the femoral and sciatic nerves passing through the lower roots of the lumbosacral plexus. The prevention of regeneration is quite important in our opinion, even in the absence of primary vascular disease, because of the possibility of other kinds of operation such as bone resection or amputation for osteosarcoma, or endoarterial antiblastic infusion for soft-tissue sarcoma, or another perfusion at a different level for melanoma.

The literature indicates it is obvious that postsympathectomy neuralgia is a common complication, occurring to a significant degree in approximately 25% of cases. However, there is great variability between reports, ranging from 2 to 100% (11,17). Fontaine (11) attributes little importance to this complication, observed in 5% of his patients. The nature of the neuralgia is not precisely known, but it is likely due to injury of the somatic lumbar nerves during the operation (1,2). In the opinion of Cooley and Herman (9), the ligature of the sympathetic trunk with nonresorbable thread, as we do, prevents the onset of this kind of postoperative pain. In our limited experience, no complications occurred related to the sympathectomy with the exception of the Bernard-Horner syndrome in 1 patient.

The combined use of sympathectomy with hyperthermic perfusion is to be considered an important achievement, which has encouraged us to continue to use it. As a matter of fact, for the treatment of advanced tumors of the limbs, we are developing a very complex multi-step therapy in which hyperthermic perfusion plays the most important role; but the final goal consists of obtaining limbs definitely free of disease and pain which will be at the same time functional and working. Even if it is too early to draw firmly definite conclusions on this subject, it is our opinion that such a combined approach is an advance toward the solution of the problem and is to be considered a progress because it does not affect the mortality and morbidity in comparison with perfusion alone.

REFERENCES

1. Bonica, J. J. (1959): *Clinical Applications of Diagnostic and Therapeutic Nerve Blocks.* Charles C Thomas, Springfield, Ill.
2. Bonica, J. J. (1953): *The Management of Pain.* Kimpton, London.
3. Busch, W. (1866): Über den Einfluss, welchen heftigere Erypsipeln zuweilen auf organisierte Neubildungen austuben. *Verhandl. Naturh. Preuss. Westphal.,* 23: 28–30.
4. Carron, J., and Weller, H. C. (1974): Treatment of post-traumatic sympathetic dystrophy. In: *Advances in Neurology, Vol. 4: International Symposium on Pain,* edited by J. J. Bonica. Raven Press, New York.
5. Cavaliere, R. (1976): In: *Proceedings of the International Symposium on Cancer Therapy by Hyperthermia and Radiation.* American College Radiology Press, Baltimore, Md.
6. Cavaliere, R., Ciocatto, E. C., Giovanella, B. C., Heidelberger, C., Johnson, R. O., Margattini, M., Modavi, B., Moricca, G., and Rossi-Janelli, A. (1967): Selective heat sensitivity of cancer cells, biochemical and clinical studies. *Cancer,* 20(9): 1351–1381.
7. Challenger, J. H. (1974): Sympathectomy nervous system blocking in pain relief, Monographs in Anaesthesiology. In: *Relief of Intractable Pain,* Vol. 1, edited by M. S. Swerdlow. Excerpta Medica, Amsterdam.
8. Coley, W. B. (1893): The treatment of malignant tumors by repeated inoculations of erypsipelas—With a report of ten original cases. *Am. J. Med. Sci.,* 105:487–511.
9. Cooley, D. A., and Hermann, B. E. (1963): Simple means for prevention of postsympathectomy neuralgias. *Surgery,* 53:587.
10. Creech, O., Jr., and Krementz, E. T. (1961): Cancer chemotherapy by perfusion. *Adv. Cancer Res.,* 6:111–147.
11. Fontaine, R. (1977): Histoire de la sympathectomic lombaire de sa naissuance à ce jour. *Acta Chir. Belg.,* 1:3–16.
12. Fowler, G. A. (*unpublished report*): Effects of acute concurrent infection on cancer in man (Series A)—Pyrogenic infection in inoperable cancer, 152 cases.
13. Gross, D. (1974): Pain and autonomic nervous system. In: *Advances in Neurology, Vol. 4: International Symposium on Pain,* edited by J. J. Bonica. Raven Press, New York.
14. Hershey, F. B., and Calman, C. H. (1967): *Sympathectomy, Atlas of Vascular Surgery,* C. V. Mosby, St. Louis.
15. Johnson, H. J. (1940): The action of short radio waves on tissues—III. A comparison of the thermal sensitivities of transplantable tumors *in vivo* and *in vitro. Am. J. Cancer,* 38:533–550.
16. Krementz, E. T., and Ryan, F. (1972): Chemotherapy of melanoma of the extremities by perfusion: Fourteen years of clinical experience. *Am. Surg.,* 175:900–917.
17. Litwin, M. S. (1962): Postsympathectomy neuralgia. *Arch. Surg.,* 84:121.
18. Mondovi, B., Strom, R., Ratilio, G., Finazzi-Agro, A., Cavaliere, R., and Fossi-Janelli, A. (1969): The biochemical mechanism of selective heat sensitivity of cancer cells. *Eur. J. Cancer,* 5:129.
19. Moricca, G., Cavaliere, R., Caputo, A., Bigatti, A. and Calistro, F. (1977): Hyper-

thermic treatment of tumors: Experimental and clinical applications. *Recent Results Cancer Res.,* 59:112–152.
20. Pettigrew, R. T., Galt, J. M., Ludgate, C. M., and Smith, A. N. (1974): Clinical effects of whole-body hyperthermia in advanced malignancy. *Br. Med. J.,* 4:679.
21. Robb, C. and Smith, R. (1977): *Operative Surgery—Vascular Surgery.* Butterworth, London.
22. Rohdenburg, G. L. (1918): Fluctuations in the growth of malignant tumors in man, with special reference to spontaneous recession. *J. Cancer Res.,* 3:193–225.
23. Simeone, F. A. (1977): The lumbar sympathetic—anatomy and surgical implications. *Acta Chir. Belg.,* 76:17–26.
24. Stehlin, J. S., Giovanella, B. C., et al. (1975): Results of hyperthermic perfusion for melanoma of the extremities. *Surg. Gynecol. Obstet.,* 140:338.
25. White, J. C. (1974): Sympathectomy for relief of pain. In: *Advances in Neurology, Vol. 4: International Symposium on Pain,* edited by J. J. Bonica, pp. 629–638. Raven Press, New York.

Combined Whole-body Hyperthermia and Chemotherapy in the Treatment of Advanced Cancer with Diffuse Pain

*G. Moricca, **R. Cavaliere, †M. Lopez, and ‡A. Caputo

*Department of Pain Therapy, **Department of Surgery, †Department of Medicine, ‡Scientific Department, Regina Elena Cancer Institute, Rome, Italy

INTRODUCTION

The therapeutic effect of high temperatures on neoplastic diseases has been known for several decades. Probably the first clinical report is that of Busch (2), who described a patient who had complete regression of sarcoma of the face after two attacks of erysipelas. Bruns in 1877 (1) reported on a patient with disseminated melanoma who had an attack of erysipelas with a sustained fever of more than 40°C (104°F) for several days. All tumors disappeared, and the patient was alive and free of disease 8 years later. Coley, in 1893 (5) discussed 38 patients with histologically proved advanced cancer who had accidental or deliberate infections of erysipelas with high fever; of these, 12 had complete disappearance of their tumors, and the survival of 2 of the patients with sarcomas was 7 and 27 years, respectively. Subsequently, there were numerous reports on the beneficial effects of high fever or locally applied heat on malignant tumors (17,25,27,28), but much of this information went unnoticed because of the unpredictability of the results related to the methods used to elevate body temperatures.

A renewed interest in the use of heat in the treatment of cancer arose from our demonstration of the selective lethal effect of elevated temperatures on tumor cells, both experimentally and clinically (3). Our successes in tumor control and pain-relief, obtained initially with hyperthermic perfusion and then following Stehlin's experience (23) with hyperthermic-antiblastic perfusion, led us to evaluate the therapeutic possibilities of whole-body hyperthermia alone, and then in combination with antiblastic drugs in the treatment of advanced cancer with diffuse pain.

Table 1 shows the most common methods used to produce total-body hyperthermia. Coley induced hyperpyrexia in cancer patients through the so-called "Coley's toxins" (filtered extracts of *Streptococcus erysipelatis* and *Bacillus prodigious*). Although beneficial effects were recorded for several types of cancer (15), this method fell into disuse because of the great diffi-

TABLE 1. *Methods used to produce whole-body hyperthermia*

Resetting the hypothalamic thermostat using pyrogens:
    live organisms (e.g., malaria, erysipelas)
    vaccines
    bacterial extracts (e.g., Coley's toxins)
    nonspecific proteins (e.g., milk)
Introduction of heat into the body:
    inflation of the lungs with heated gases
    hot-air cabinet
    hot baths
    irrigation of body cavities with heated fluids
    shunt of the blood through a heat exchanger
    diathermy
    electric blanket
    heated wax
    hot-water blanket
Inhibition of the evaporative heat loss
    sealed polyethylene bag

---

culty of standardizing the bacterial toxins biologically, and the correspondingly capricious results.

Apart from this technique, the most commonly employed method of obtaining high body temperature was immersion in hot baths. Schmaberg and Tseng (22), in a review of the literature, found that the water temperatures used varied between 35.5 and 53.3°C (96 to 120°F) with a mean temperature commonly used of 40°C (104°F). The duration of immersion also varied widely, but was generally short, ranging between 4 and 5 min. In their experiments, they concluded that the maximum safe water temperature was 43.3 to 45.5°C (110 to 114°F) and that, at a bath temperature of 40°C (104°F) an immersion of 30 min was necessary to achieve a body temperature of 39.4°C (103°F).

Although von Ardenne (26), from his own Institute in East Germany, with his program of "cancer multi-step therapy" based on extreme hyperthermia induced by hot baths, tumor hyperacidity, and changed glucose concentration, has claimed spectacular successes, the considerable problems of control in the application of extreme hyperthermal procedures led him to stop these experiments. He observed "precollapse or collapse states" also, after about 200 or 300 min of hyperthermia at 40°C in the middle-aged patients, and after 120 min in the advanced-age patients.

In fact, the detailed case reports that we have been able to consult are few. Kirsch and Schmidt (12) reported on 5 out of 48 patients with inoperable cancers who were treated with whole-body hyperthermia in a hot-water bath with additional diathermy: 1 of the 5 patients died shortly after the treatment and the other 4 showed minor clinical improvement. Suryanarayan (24), using combined whole-body hyperthermia at 42°C by immersion in hot baths, and chemotherapeutic drugs, treated 9 patients with advanced cancer. He observed pain-relief and regression in tumor size, but the results were not impressive.

In 1968, we started our experiments with a cabinet in which forced-air ventilation at controlled temperature and humidity was maintained. Under general anesthesia, the patient was put into the cabinet with, above him, a cable from a Siemens 608 Ultratherm diathermy machine. The head of the patient was kept outside of the cabinet and enclosed in a helmet in which cold water circulated continuously. Two patients were treated in this manner, and the preliminary results were reported in a previous paper (14). Because of these not-very-satisfactory results, we modified the technique. After a series of various experimental approaches, among which a two-chamber hyperthermia bath with a cooling head-chamber was also used, a final assessment of the technique was possible.

METHOD

At the present time, we are using the following method: After premedication with atropine and promethazine, the patient is anesthetized with an intravenous barbiturate, curarized, and intubated with an endotracheal canula. Anesthesia is maintained with a 60–40% N_2O and O_2 mixture supplemented as needed with intravenous short-acting barbiturates. Leads for the electrocardiograph are applied on the chest, and an intravenous catheter is inserted to monitor central venous pressure and to replace fluid losses. A nasogastric tube is passed to prevent vomiting due to fluid accumulation, and an indwelling catheter serves to control urine output. Temperature probes are placed in the esophagus, in the rectum, in contact with the tympanic membrane and, whenever possible, in the tumor.

After these procedures, the patient is entirely wrapped in a polyethylene bag to inhibit evaporative heat loss (Fig. 1). (As known, evaporation of 1 liter of sweat from the skin takes 580 kcal from the body.) The major source of heat is a blanket containing water at 50°C that surrounds the polyethylene-enclosed patient (Fig. 2). Endotracheal gases are preheated to 38°C, mainly in order to diminish heat loss in this way.

Core temperature generally rises about 2° to 3°C per hr in relation to body weight, so an average of 2 hr is necessary to obtain the optimal esophageal temperature of 41.8°C. When the esophageal temperature reaches 41°C, the circulation of hot water is stopped. This avoids overshooting of the predetermined temperature, and slows down the rate of heating. By exposing the head and the anterior thorax and adjusting the temperature of the circulating water, it is easy to maintain predetermined esophageal

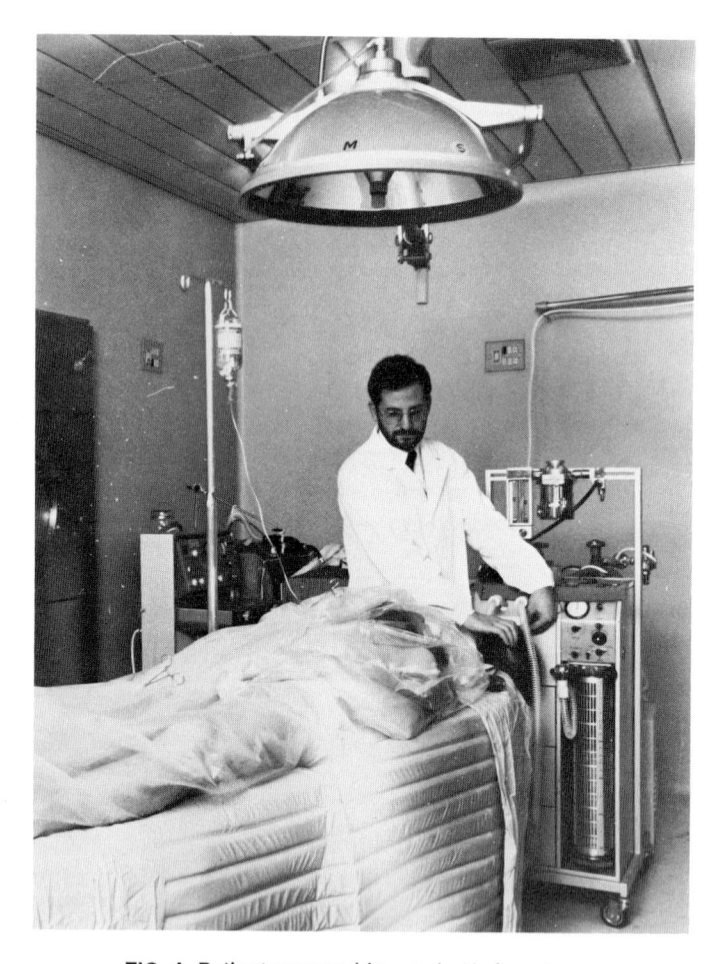

FIG. 1. Patient wrapped in a polyethylene bag.

temperature for the established time (generally 3 hr). If the core temperature rises too rapidly, the procedures designed to diminish the rate of heating are carried out early.

During the treatment, EKG and core temperature are monitored constantly; at intervals, blood pressure, central venous pressure, heart rate, serum electrolytes, urine output, and intratumor temperatures are recorded. Extracellular fluids and serum electrolyte losses are replaced with solutions preheated to 36°C. The monitoring of cerebral function during treatment has proved unnecessary. After treatment, when the water blanket is removed and the patient's body surface is exposed, cooling is rapid, and normal body temperature is reached within 2 hr.

Antiblastic drugs are injected in a single dose when the esophageal temperature of 41°C is achieved. All the drugs used are administered by

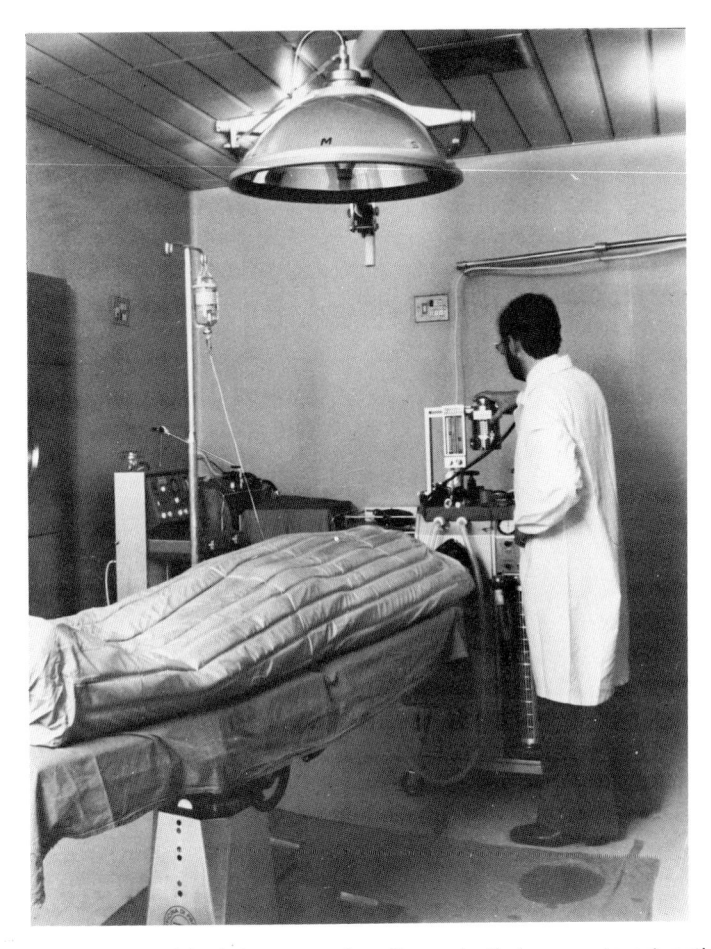

FIG. 2. Hot-water blanket surrounding the polyethylene-enclosed patient.

bolus i.v. injection with the exception of VM-26, a semisynthetic podophyllotoxin derivative, which was given by i.v. infusion over a period of 30 to 40 min in order to obviate the hypotension reported from rapid drug administration (21).

Gastrointestinal and pancreatic carcinomas were treated with 5-flourouracil, 600 mg/m^2, and BCNU, 60 mg/m^2. Breast cancers and soft-tissue sarcomas were treated with vincristine, 1.4 mg/m^2 (maximum dose, 2 mg), and adriamycin (ADR), 60 mg/m^2. The only patient with cerebral neoplasia was treated with VM-26, 100 mg/m^2, and BCNU, 60 mg/m^2, which have a high degree of lipid-solubility and a low molecular weight, i.e., the chemical characteristics required to cross the "blood-brain barrier."

After 4 or 8 weeks depending on the therapeutic schema, bone-marrow toxicity and the patient's clinical response, the thermochemotherapy is repeated. The criteria for response evaluation are both subjective (pain-relief, weight gain, performance status improvement) and objective (tumor regression as seen in serial measurement clinically, or in radiologic changes).

PATHOPHYSIOLOGIC CONSIDERATIONS

The circulatory and biochemical effects of whole-body hyperthermia as seen in our series of patients are the following: The increase in pulse rate was, on the average, 10 beats per min per centigrade degree. In order to avoid undue stress on the heart, we were very careful to avoid overshooting 180 beats per min, both maintaining stable narcosis and administering, if necessary, beta-blocking agents, generally oxprenolol, 2 to 6 mg, intravenously.

Unlike what happened in conscious patients, in whom hypotension and decreased central venous pressure due to peripheral dilatation were observed, there were no significant changes in these parameters in anesthetized subjects. Cardiac dysrhythmias occurred sporadically and generally took the form of ventricular ectopic beats controllable with the usual anti-arrhythmic agents such as lidocaine, initially administered with a bolus i.v. injection of 1 mg/kg body weight, with additional doses every 5 min, either until the arrhythmia was abolished or until 5 mg/kg had been administered.

Out of 6 patients treated with adriamycin, 3 showed ST-T changes returned to normal within 48 hr after treatment. No changes in serum enzymes were observed in adriamycin patients. Fluid losses through sweating were considerable—as much as 500 ml per hour—but serum electrolytes changed remarkably little, and infusions of 700 ml/hour of fluids (we alternated the use of 500 ml of normal saline and 500 ml of 5% dextrose) were generally sufficient to maintain sodium and chloride serum levels within normal limits. Urine output was about 130 ml/hour.

In some cases, a slight fall in the serum calcium and phosphate levels was observed, but normal values were achieved spontaneously within 3 days. Table 2 shows that the average serum activities of lactate dehydrogenase (LDH), alanine aminotransferase (SGPT), aspartate aminotransferase (SGOT), alkaline phosphatase, and gamma-glutamyl-transpeptidase (Gamma-GT) changed little after hyperthermic treatment, and also in patients treated with adriamycin. Significant increases in the serum enzyme activities were observed only when the temperature was held between 42.0°C and 42.3°C for periods of 15 to 20 min. These data agree to a certain extent with those reported by Pettigrew et al. (19).

Renal function tests, serum urea nitrogen and creatinine did not reveal renal dysfunction due to high temperature. Uric acid levels generally rose proportionately to tumor necrosis, so that allopurinol was given (100 mg, 3 times a day, starting 3 days before treatment) to the patients in whom necrosis of large tumor masses was expected.

TABLE 2. Serum enzyme levels before and after hyperthermia

Enzyme	Normal level (U/l)	Before heating	After heating 24 hr	After heating 72 hr
SGOT	< 12	4	6	6
SGPT	< 12	6	9	7
LDH	< 240	163	170	165
Gamma-GT	♂ 6–28	16	22	18
	♀ 4–18	10	15	12
Alk. phosphatase	20–48	31	42	35

Coagulation parameters, prothrombin time (PT), and partial thromboplastin time (PTT) did not change remarkably, whereas platelet counts tended to drop later, mostly in patients treated with BCNU. Nevertheless, neither bleeding diathesis nor disseminated intravascular coagulation (DIC) was observed.

Leukocytosis was observed during hyperthermia, probably related to the letting into the circulation of an amount of white blood cells owing to the hyperthermic stress. Hemoglobin concentration did not change from base-line values, suggesting that hemolysis did not occur at the temperatures involved. This is in accordance with the slight change observed in the serum bilirubin concentration.

RESULTS

Effects on Pain and Neoplasm

As of March 2, 1978, a total number of 15 patients ranging in age from 21 to 77, had been treated with combined whole-body hyperthermia and chemotherapy. The patients were suffering from unbearable diffuse pain due to disseminated cancers and were considered unsuited for further conventional treatments. A total of 39 treatment sessions were carried out and the total number of hours over 40°C was 156. Table 3 shows the data on the malignancies treated, the number of treatment sessions for each patient, the chemotherapeutic agents used, the responses observed, and the survivals as from the start of chemotherapy. The number of treatment sessions to which each patient was subjected was not high, varying from 1 to 4. This reflects our main purpose, which was pain-relief; in the responders, therefore, the interval between courses was prolonged.

The 3 cases of pancreatic carcinoma had a bulky abdominal mass with intractable pain in the epigastrium and in the lower-quadrant areas, radiated to the back. In one patient ascites was present, and another had lung metastases. All 3 patients showed favorable response, with relief of pain and

TABLE 3. *Results of treatment using combined whole-body hyperthermia and chemotherapy*

Type of tumor	No. of patients treated	Previous treatments Surg.	Radio-therapy	Chemo-therapy	No. of treatments	Antiblastic drugs	Objective resp.	Subjective resp.	No resp.	Survival as from start of therapy (wks)
Pancreatic cancer	3	0	1	2	4,2,1	5-FU, BCNU	1	3	0	20,10,5
Gastric cancer	3	3	0	2	4,2,3	5-FU, BCNU	2	3	0	26,8,15
Breast cancer	4	4	4	3	3,4,1,4	VCR, ADR	2	2	2	9,17,2.5, 19+
Soft-tissue sarcomas	2	2	2	2	1,4	VCR, ADR	1	1	1	3, 18+
Colon cancer	2	1	0	1	1,3	5-FU, BCNU	1	1	1	3,12
Cerebral neoplasia	1	1	1	0	2	VM-26, BCNU	1	1	0	9

Legend: 5-FU = 5-fluorouracil; BCNU = 1-3 *bis* (2-chloroethyl)-1-nitrosourea; VCR = vincristine; ADR = adriamycin; VM-26 = 4′-demethyl-epipodophyllotoxin-β-D-thenylidene-glucoside.

discontinuance of opiates, but only one showed objective response with considerable regression of lung metastases (Figs. 3 and 4) and a decrease of more than 50% in the 2 perpendicular diameters of measurable abdominal mass.

Out of 3 patients suffering from gastric carcinoma, 2 had unbearable pain in the epigastrium with anorexia, vomiting, and weight loss. After thermochemotherapy, both subjective and objective response was observed with complete pain-relief, decrease in size of measurable abdominal tumor mass and weight gain. The third patient, with diffuse, severe pain from bone metastases, showed only subjective improvement with pain-relief; he died after 2 months.

Of the 2 patients listed with colon carcinoma, only one demonstrated favorable response with complete pain-relief and decrease of metastatic liver involvement. The other died 3 weeks after treatment with acute hemorrhage, and necropsy showed multiple areas of necrosis in the tumor metastases.

Of the 4 patients with carcinoma of the breast, treated with thermochemotherapy, a 28-year-old woman showed no response. At necropsy, involvement of the liver, pancreas, both kidneys, uterus, both lungs, and skeleton was found. Another patient died 18 days after treatment, without pain-relief, and necropsy showed multiple areas of necrosis in the tumor. Two patients who had diffuse, severe pain had pain-relief and objective regression of measurable lesions and were able to lead a relatively normal life.

Of the 2 patients with sarcomas treated, the nonresponder was a 21-year-old man suffering from recurrent fibrosarcoma in the lateral wall of the left hemithorax, and previously treated with chemotherapy for multiple lung metastases. The second patient was a 65-year-old woman, twice operated on in the past for recurrent retroperitoneal fibrosarcoma. She had unbearable pain due to a very large mass occupying the right hemi-abdomen (Fig. 5). Shortly after the first treatment, pain-relief and decrease in tumor size occurred (Fig. 6). The subjective and objective conditions progressively improved with further treatments.

A favorable response was also obtained in the only patient suffering from recurrent malignant glioma. This patient, obtunded and totally hemiplegic prior to therapy, recovered a normal mental status and had an almost complete return of motor function. Improvement was maintained for 2 months until he died from intratumor hemorrhage.

Complications

Six patients developed herpes labialis, generally following first treatment. In 2 cases, a metabolic acidosis developed, with a base excess of -8 and -10 and a fall in serum potassium to 2.4 mEq/l, respectively. Promptly treated, these situations reversed rapidly.

No problems were encountered in controlling ventricular ectopic beats,

A

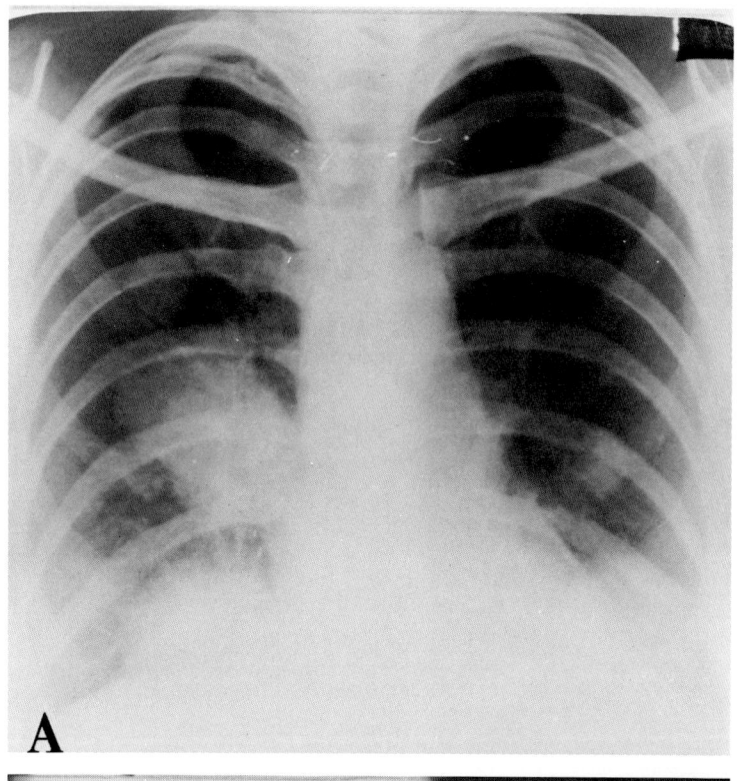

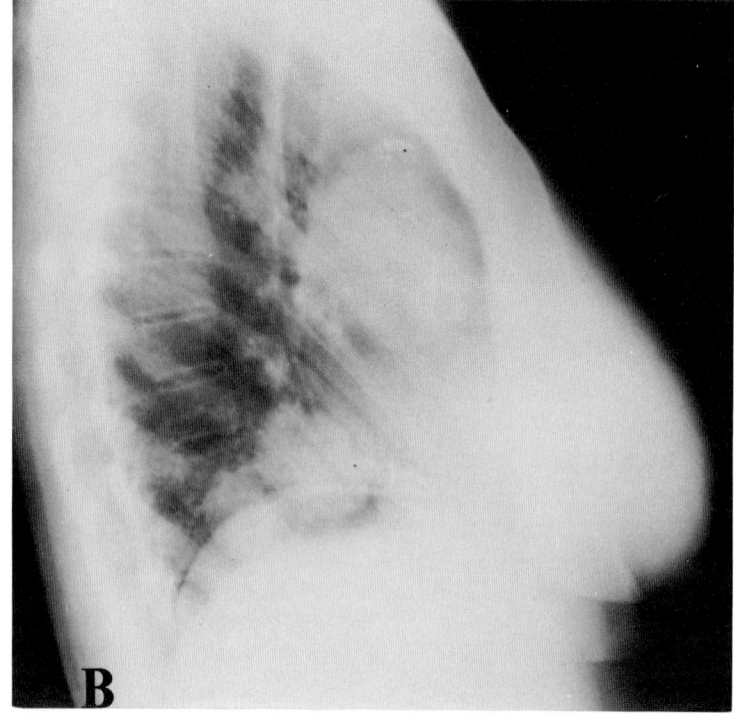

B

generally with lidocaine. Sore throats and superficial burns at recognized pressure points occurred in a few patients. During the recovery period some patients showed restlessness and disorientation, but they returned to normal during the subsequent 2 days.

In our series of patients, no deaths were attributable to the treatment. Adriamycin, a potentially cardiotoxic agent, as mentioned above, caused reversible ST-T changes, but not cardiac dysrhythmias or cardiomyopathy. On the other hand, the 550 mg/m^2 dose limit was not exceeded.

Ventricular fibrillation occurred once in Mackenzie's series (13) and once in Pettigrew's series (20); then it was attributable to the temperature level (43°C) or to biochemical disturbances.

Associated heart disease was not encountered in patients receiving adriamycin. It is our opinion that cardiovascular effects of whole-body hyperthermia do not increase the risk of adriamycin cardiotoxicity in comparison with patients not treated in this way if the patient is carefully controlled in order to prevent other myocardial sensitizer factors.

DISCUSSION

Tumor cures have not been achieved so far with whole-body hyperthermia, and complete clinical remissions have generally been few and short-lasting. Nevertheless, pain-relief with discontinuance of opiates and objective responses obtained in some cases of advanced cancer are sufficient to justify this method for the treatment of advanced cancer unsuited to further therapy by conventional methods. Moreover, the relatively easy method, in experienced hands, permits very short hospitalization times.

With present knowledge and technology, it is not very likely that whole-body hyperthermia can produce total neoplastic cell necrosis. Johnson (11) believes that over 20 hr would be needed at 41.8°C in order to obtain this result. On the contrary, Dietzel et al. (6), in their experiments with high frequency heating, showed that the higher thermosensitivity of the tumor cells is not sufficient to achieve cures in a generalized tumor because of the impossibility of separating nonmalignant cells geometrically, even if they are less thermosensitive.

Therefore, it is likely that the best results can be obtained with short and moderate hyperthermia in combination with chemotherapy. Several workers have observed a synergistic effect between high temperatures and certain antiblastic drugs (7,8,9,10,23), but the explanation of such synergism is not

---

←

FIG. 3A. Chest X-ray image before treatment (lung metastases from pancreatic carcinoma): frontal view. **B.** Chest X-ray image before treatment (lung metastases from pancreatic carcinoma): lateral view.

A

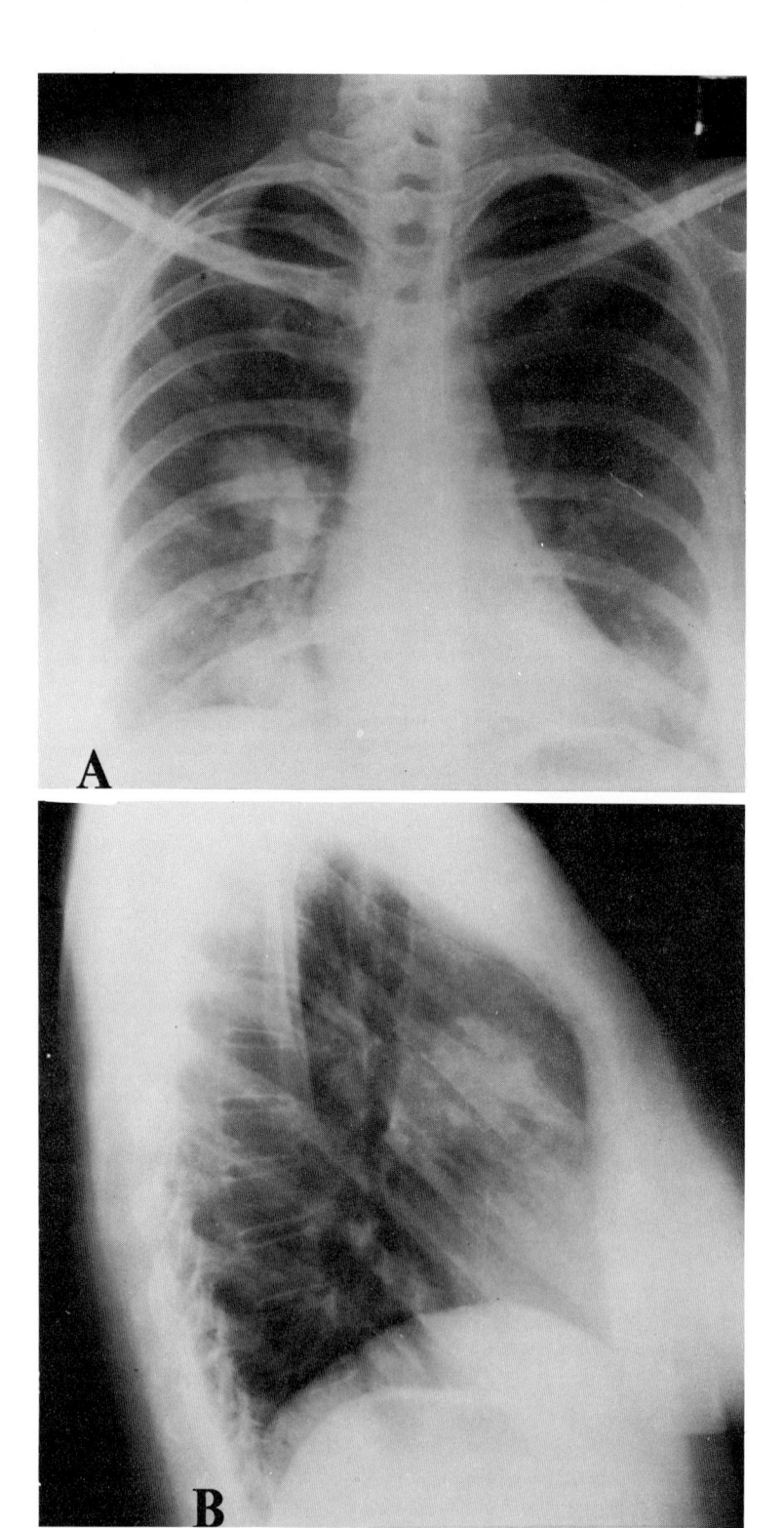

B

yet completely known. Hahn et al. (9) showed that *in vitro* and *in vivo* treatment of mouse mammary tumor cells with a combination of elevated temperature (42 to 43°C) and adriamycin increased cell death irrespective of the duration of the combined treatment. Further experiments (10) on Chinese hamster cells exposed to simultaneous hyperthermia (43°C) and adriamycin showed that the cells initially were sensitized to the cytotoxic agent. If the duration of combined treatment exceeded about 30 min, however, the cells became refractory to additional destruction by adriamycin. If heat was applied before exposure to adriamycin, the cells could also be rendered insensitive.

As far as we know, the only trials on man that have been carried out using combined whole-body hyperthermia and adriamycin are our own. It is our impression that, under the experimental clinical conditions described above, the hyperthermia increases the therapeutic effect of adriamycin, because the majority of responders to combined therapy had previously been unsuccessfully treated with adriamycin. We have not observed any increase of toxicity of the drugs used, so this is probably not modified by heating.

A particular problem is that of patients with malignant intracranial neoplasms. To the author's knowledge, the literature contains no case reports on whole-body hyperthermia in combination with chemotherapy. The patient whom we treated received cortisone and mannitol in order to prevent the possible acute elevation of intracranial pressure. It is noteworthy, even though this is only one case, that this patient has not shown particular disturbances, and that he demonstrated favorable response.

Although none of our patients exhibited fatal complications such as disseminated intravascular coagulation (DIC), this problem must be kept in mind (16). Cancer and DIC may be induced by different stimuli. The most important parameters to be evaluated regarding possible fatal complications seem to be the degree of liver involvement, the tumor mass, and the thermosensitivity of the tumor. Liver damage by high temperature is generally slight and reversible under 42.0°C. Over this limit, jaundice may appear. Moreover, some antiblastic drugs have liver toxicity. Therefore, if considerable liver involvement exists and if the tumor is highly thermosensitive, the residual functional parenchyma cannot detoxify the large amount of toxic product brought into the circulation following tumor necrosis.

The results obtained in our series of patients are in agreement with those of Pettigrew (18). He treated 82 patients with hyperthermia using molten paraffin wax as the source of heat. Sixty-four patients had hyperthermia alone, 15 had combined hyperthermia and cytotoxic drugs, and 3 had hyper-

---

←

FIG. 4A. Chest X-ray of the same patient after treatment (6 weeks): frontal view.
B. Chest X-ray of the same patient after treatment (6 weeks): lateral view.

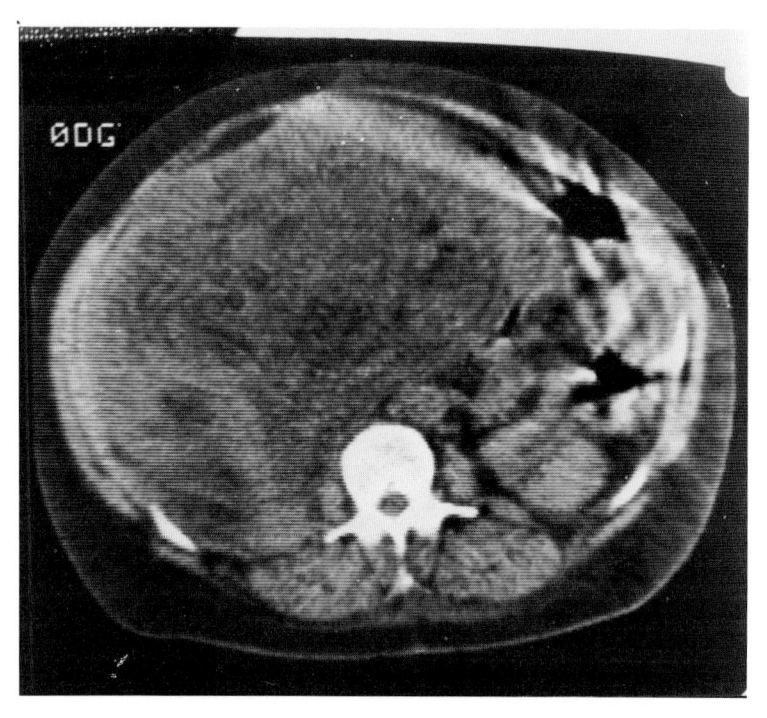

FIG. 5. Abdominal computerized axial tomography (CAT) showing a large mass occupying the right hemi-abdomen (retroperitoneal fibrosarcoma before treatment).

thermia in combination with local radiotherapy. The best results were observed in soft-tissue sarcomas and in tumors of gastrointestinal origin, whereas breast cancers did not respond well to hyperthermia alone but only to thermochemotherapy.

It is of particular interest that pancreatic and gastric carcinomas, which generally have a poor prognosis because of their poor response to the currently available treatments, have shown favorable response. Although the small number of patients treated does not permit the drawing of definite conclusions, further controlled clinical trials are justified.

Another point that should be discussed concerns the possible enhancement of immunologic defenses produced by heating. Since our first clinical experiments with regional hyperthermic perfusion for the treatment of tumors of the limbs (4), the best results have been obtained when amputation or tumor excision was performed some time after hyperthermic perfusion and not immediately afterward. This led us to conclude that the presence of the heated tumor acts as an antigenic source for immunization of the host against metastases even if whole-body hyperthermia can be quite different, from this point of view, from local hyperthermia by perfusion. Experimental work on this subject is underway in our laboratory.

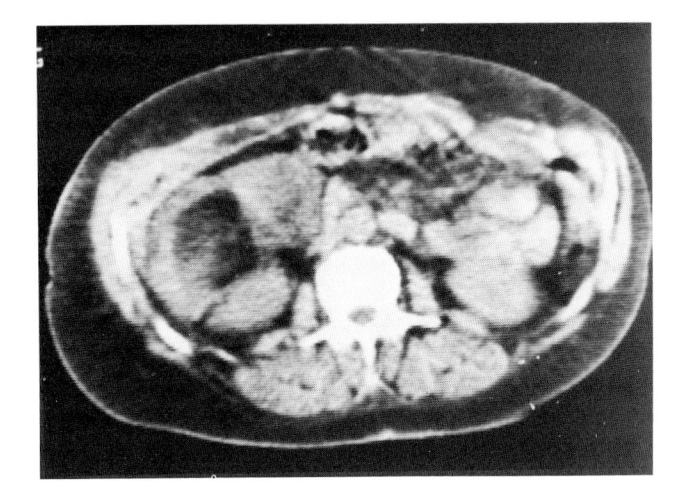

FIG. 6. Abdominal CAT of the same patient after treatment (7 weeks).

The problem of treating tumors using thermochemotherapy has certainly not been resolved. It can, however, be said that the technique is, in any event, valid in view of the success achieved in obtaining pain-relief.

REFERENCES

1. Bruns, P. (1887): Die Heilwirkung des Erpsipels auf Geschwulste. *Beitr. Klin. Chir.,* 3:443–446.
2. Busch, W. (1866): Über den Einfluss, welchen heftigere Erysipelan zuweilen auf organisierte Neubildungen austuben. *Verh. Naturh. Preuss. Rhein. Westphal.,* 23:28–30.
3. Cavaliere, R., Ciocatto, E. C., Giovannella, B. C., Heindelberger, C., Johnson, R. O., Margottini, M., Mondovi, B., Moricca, G., and Rossi Fanelli, A. (1967): Selective heat sensitivity of cancer cells. *Cancer,* 20:1351–1381.
4. Cavaliere, R., Moricca, G., and Caputo, A. (1975): Regional hyperthermia by perfusion. In: *Proceedings of the International Symposium on Cancer Therapy by Hyperthermia and Radiation.* Washington, April 28–30.
5. Coley, W. R. (1893): The treatment of malignant tumors by repeated inoculations of erysipelas, with a report of ten original cases. *Am. J. Sci.,* 105:487–511.
6. Dietzel, F., Seibert, G., and Klobe, G. (1975): Der Einfluss einer Hochfrequenz-hyper-thermie auf den Verlauf des Ehrlich Ascites Karzinoms der Maus. *Strahlentherapie,* 149:105–107.
7. Giovannella, B. C., Lohman, W. A., and Heidelberger, C. (1970): Effects of elevated temperatures and drugs on the viability of L1210 leukemia cells. *Cancer Res.,* 30:1623–1631.
8. Goss, P., and Parsons, P. G. (1977): The effect of hyperthermia and melphalan on survival of human fibroblast strains and melanoma cell lines. *Cancer Res.,* 37(1):152–156.
9. Hahn, G. M., Braun, J., and Har-Kedar, I. (1975): Thermochemotherapy: Synergism between hyperthermia (42–43°C) and adriamycin (or bleomycin) in mammalian cell inactivation. *Proc. Natl. Acad. Sci. USA,* 72:937–940.
10. Hahn, G. M., and Strande, D. P. (1976): Cytotoxic effects of hyperthermia and adriamycin on Chinese hamster cells. *J. Natl. Cancer Inst.,* 57(5):1063–1067.

11. Johnson, H. J. (1940): The action of short radio waves on tissues-III. A comparison of the thermal sensitivities of transplantable tumors *in vivo* and *in vitro*. *Am. J. Cancer,* 38:533.
12. Kirsch, R., and Schmidt, D. (1966): Erste Experimentelle und Klinische Erfahrungen mit der Ganzkorper-Extrem-Hyperthermie. In: *Aktuelle Probleme aus dem Gebiet der Cancerologie,* edited by W. Doerr, F. Linder, and G. Wagner, pp. 53–70. Springer-Verlag, Heidelberg.
13. Mackenzie, A., McLeod, K., Cassels-Smith, A. J., and Dickson, J. A. (1975): Total body hyperthermia: Techniques and patient management. In: *Proceedings of the International Symposium on Cancer Therapy by Hyperthermia and Radiation.* Washington, April 28–30.
14. Moricca, G., Cavaliere, R., Caputo, A. Bigotti, A., and Colistro, F. (1977): Hyperthermic treatment of tumors. Experimental and clinical applications. *Recent Results Cancer Res.,* 59:112–152.
15. Nauts, H. L., Fowler, G. A., and Bogatko, F. A. (1953): A review of the influence of bacterial infections and bacterial products (Coley's toxins) on malignant tumors in man. *Acta Med. Scand.,* 145: suppl. 276.
16. Peck, S. D., and Reiquam, C. W. (1973): Disseminated intravascular coagulation in cancer patients: Supportive evidence. *Cancer,* 31:1114–1119.
17. Percy, J. F. (1916): Heat in the treatment of carcinomas of the uterus. *Surg. Gynecol. Obstet.,* 22:77–79.
18. Pettigrew, R. T. (1975): Cancer therapy by whole body heating. In: *Proceedings of the International Symposium on Cancer Therapy by Hyperthermia and Radiation.* Washington, April 28–30.
19. Pettigrew, R. T., Galt, J. M., Ludgate, C. M., Horn, D. B., and Smith, A. W. (1974): Circulatory and biochemical effects of whole body hyperthermia. *Br. J. Surg.,* 61:727–730.
20. Pettigrew, R. T., Galt, J. M., Ludgate, C. M., and Smith, A. N. (1974): Clinical effects of whole body hyperthermia in advanced malignancy. *Br. Med. J.,* 4:679–682.
21. Preclinical Brochure (1967): Sandoz Compound VM-26, Sandoz Pharmaceuticals. Hanover, New Jersey.
22. Schramberg, J. F., and Tseng, H. W. (1927): Experiments on the therapeutic value of hot baths with special reference to the treatment of syphilis: Physiologic observations. *Am. J. Syph.,* 11:337–397.
23. Stehlin, J. S., Jr. (1969): Hyperthermic perfusion with chemotherapy for cancer of the extremities. *Surg. Gynecol. Obstet.,* 129:305–308.
24. Suryanarayan, C. R. (1966): Certain interesting observations during and after hydrohyperthermic chemotherapy in advanced malignancies (preliminary survey). *Indian J. Cancer,* 3:176–181.
25. Vidal, E. (1911): *Travaux de la Deuxieme Conference Internationale pour l'Étude du Cancer,* p. 160. Paris.
26. Von Ardenne, M. (1972): Selective multiphase cancer therapy: Conceptual aspects and experimental basis. *Adv. Pharmacol. Chemother.,* 10:339–380.
27. Warren, S. L. (1935): Preliminary study of the effects of artificial fever upon hopeless tumor cases. *Am. J. Roentgenol ,* 33:75–87.
28. Westermark, F. (1898): Ueber die Behandlung des ulzerierenden Cervix Karzinomes mittels konstanter Warme. *Zentralbl. Gynaekol., pp.* 1336–1339.

Discussion

Part II. Management of Pain of Advanced Cancer: Anticancer Modalities

D. Fink (Moderator)

Questioner: Dr. Bonadonna, do *in vitro* tests of sensitivity to antitumorogens constitute a useful guide to therapy?

Bonadonna (Milano): No.

Questioner: Dr. Pannuti, what are possible side effects associated with MAP treatment given at the high doses discussed in your paper?

Pannuti (Bologna): As I've stated, since 1973, we have used high doses of MAP. The toxic profile of high doses of MAP is known and has also been verified by other authors. Local intolerance is the only limiting factor, because its intramuscular injection leads to 10 to 15% of abscesses. As for the systemic toxicity at the hematochemical level, the only parameter significantly verified is potassium level, which is significantly increased but is still within normal limits. There is an increase of the alpha-2-globuline level, but it also stays within normal limits. Furthermore, one should notice a statistically significant increase of the white cells and platelets, but such effects have already been shown by using MAP even in low doses. As for the other side effects of high doses of MAP, some new findings must be reported as regards low doses:

1. cramps in the legs at night beginning usually after 10 to 15 days and lasting 4 to 5 days.
2. tremors lasting no more than 20 days after the MAP treatment has ended, and
3. night sweats.

Gaining weight has also to be associated with these effects; patients can gain even 10 to 12 kilos. This weight increase is real, and it is due to an anabolic effect. It is not associated with fluid retention or with significant electrolytic alterations. We have also demonstrated this in animals in collaboration with the Pharmacological Institute of our University. In animals, doses such as 4 gr orally or intramuscular produce a significant increase of the anus elevator, which is the best test for deciding whether or not these animals have undergone an anabolic effect. There are no other side effects. We have already begun studies that have also given us the opportunity to use doses higher than the 3 or 4 gr orally for 1 month of treatment with 200 to 280 gr given also as maintenance treatment, showing no significant toxicologic effects.

Questioner: Has MAP been used in other centers?

Pannuti: Dr. Martino's study has compared the administration of 1500 mg MAP for 1 month with the hypophysiolysis achieved by the infusion into the hypophysis of ethanol. Thus, a group of patients has been treated with hypophysiolysis and high doses of MAP. The use of MAP gives pain remission in a larger number of cases than the hypophysiolysis alone. Relief intervenes, as we have already reported, after 3 or 4 weeks and is slower than the hypophysiolysis, but it lasts longer. The average duration of the pain remission is, in our studies, approximately 6 months. It is very important that the administration of high doses of MAP gives not only pain remission in a significantly larger number of patients but also an objective remission of advanced breast carcinoma.

Ricci (Genova): Can a second treatment by radiotherapy for lung cancer be given at the same site as radiotherapy given in the past for control of pain?

Pannuti: For lung cancer, it can be in the same site or in the contiguous site.

Ricci: What is the effect of radiotherapy on pain when given at a dose of 800 to 1000 rads?

Pannuti: This kind of application has been widely used in other institutes but much less in ours, mainly at the level of secondary lesions, of the nervous system, and in or near the bone marrow. Results are not better than the ones achieved with the usual administration of 200 rad instead of 800 rad.

Questioner: Drs. Bonadonna and Basso Ricci, after giving a single, high dose of cyclophosphamide 1,500/2,000 mg or radiation 1,000/1,500 rads to patients with metastasis from Ewing sarcoma or breast cancer, the severe pain is reduced or disappears in a day. How do you explain the mechanism of the relief of pain even though there is not time for reduction in the number of tumor cells?

Bonadonna: If you give treatment with an alkylating agent in susceptible patients, cells are killed within a few hours.

Questioner: Dr. Cavaliere, has hyperthermia been attempted with ultrahigh frequencies?

Cavaliere (Rome): Yes, but mainly at a systemic and not a regional level. We should remember the problems of establishing the temperature we reach, which cannot always be monitored because the thermometers we use are metallic and cannot be kept inside the tumor during the high-frequency heating. Furthermore, the high-frequency heating does not seem really homogeneous, so it is difficult to keep all the tumoral cells exposed at a given temperature and for a given period of time.

Moricca (Rome): Dr. Lopez, does total-body hyperthermia induce intratumoral hemorrhage?

Lopez (Rome): Cases of massive necrosis in various metastatic areas have been reported.

Questioner: What is the relationship of your hyperthermia technique with that described in Germany a few years ago?

Lopez: The technique we used was not substantially different from the Von Norden one.

Questioner: Was the patient with the brain tumor treated with hyperthermia checked with computerized axial tomography before and after the treatment?

Lopez: Computerized axial tomography showed a reduction of the volume of the brain neoplastic growth. But there was also an objective evaluation, because the protrusion of the neoplasm through the residual operative window was not observed anymore after hyperthermia.

Questioner: Is there information about the effect of ovariectomy performed at the time of breast resection in young, still-menstruating women?

Pannuti: The ovariectomy problem in breast cancer is still open. As for us, we do not believe in the use of prophylactic ovariectomy, but only in its therapeutic use. Our present experience is the one also common in the literature, i.e., a remission rate of approximately 40%.

Questioner: Dr. Basso Ricci, in some institutes, multiple bony metastases are submitted to polyirradiation with 850 rad in 2 days. What do you think?

Basso Ricci (Milano): In our opinion, the localized treatment at a lower dose for each metastasis is better.

Questioner: Dr. Pannuti, how useful is calcitonin in bony metastases?

Pannuti: The use of calcitonin in bony metastases, particularly in breast cancer, has not yet been studied in a controlled way. In the terminal stages with hypercalcemia, my personal experience is very disappointing.

Questioner: Why not have a maintenance treatment with MAP after the initial 1-month cycle?

Pannuti: This is a question we have already asked ourselves. As we did not know what side effects could be expected in the future with such high doses, we limited them to the first month. As soon as we verified that there were no dangerous side effects, we used the maintenance treatment that we use now, which is as follows: 1-month treatment, 15 days interruption, and then again high doses, 1 or 2 g for 15 days every month. We have already administered to many patients doses higher than 200 g without their showing any systemic side effects.

Questioner: In your experiments on the MAP analgesic effects, do you consider useful the use of such a general codification of the pain symptom by levels according to the kind of analgesic administered?

Pannuti: This is a very important problem concerning the codification of the pain. When I used the terms *signal tumor* and *signal symptom,* I meant a pain symptom generating from the tumor location. This is the signal symptom definition and its value is established according to the treatment. A pain is defined as being of first degree when a patient is in moderate pain and does not take more than one analgesic. Obviously, if a patient takes only one dose of morphine, he is in a very different position from the one who takes only one aspirin. The patient taking morphine will have more intense pain. The definition of pain is very difficult because different factors have to be investigated: the semantics, the pain quality, and the emotional, psychological, and social connotations of the patient himself.

Psychologic and Psychiatric Techniques for the Relief of Advanced Cancer Pain

M. R. Bond

Department of Psychological Medicine, Southern General Hospital, Glasgow, G51 4TF Scotland

At the outset it must be emphasised that pain is a *symptom* of illness and, as such, must be taken as an integral part of that illness. Indeed, in many instances where pain is part of a chronic and potentially fatal illness of the cancer group, success in treatment will not be gained unless this approach is adopted. Consideration of the whole illness also means more than attending solely to physical symptoms, because it means taking account of a patient's emotional problems and the effects of changes caused by his illness in the family in terms of their own emotions and social activities. Thus, management of cancer patients, with or without pain, entails the use of a team of trained individuals—doctors, nurses, social workers, nonmedical therapists of various kinds and, where appropriate, ministers of religion—in such a way that a continuum of care is available at all times between hospital and home.

One of the problems posed by this counsel of perfection is that we know relatively little about the detailed nature of services required for cancer patients in the community other than those of a physical nature, and it is only within recent times that attempts have been made to examine patterns of care needed by patients with chronic, painful diseases who are not in a hospital. In other words there is currently a discrepancy between psychologic and social services needed by cancer patients and their families and the care available (9,10). This is partly due to failure of the medical and social services to recognize and treat emotional and social problems. It is also due to the reluctance of patients to report their needs in this regard, because they see doctors as being concerned with their physical health only and fear being regarded as weak should they complain. This is an unfortunate consequence of the British attitude toward illness and suffering.

In order to comment specifically upon the use of psychiatric and psychologic techniques in pain-relief for cancer patients, it is first necessary to examine the nature of the emotional and social problems raised by various stages of the illness, when pain is present and when it is absent.

THE EMOTIONAL CONSEQUENCES OF CANCER FOR PATIENT AND FAMILY

The diagnosis of cancer is often withheld from patients in Britain, although relatives are told of it at an early stage. The family are quite naturally very distressed by what has been revealed to them, because the illness presents the threat of loss of a loved one, loss of income, and loss of social status. They are often forced by the doctor into a "conspiracy of silence" because of the lack of his or her willingness or inability to tell the patient the true nature of the illness. Moreover, the stress imposed by this knowledge among relatives poses a heavy burden, especially if psychologic support is not offered, as is often the case. Thus, until the chronicity of the disease and the failure of doctors to check its progress becomes evident, or except where fear of cancer appears at the outset as in the case of a woman who develops a breast lump, the level of emotional disturbance may be quite low initially.

In practice, however, patients often become aware through unspoken clues from doctors and relatives or friends that their illness is more serious than they first believed. However, sooner or later overt anxiety develops as a patient faces a series of stresses including uncertainty of the outcome of the illness, threat of loss of identity, self-esteem, and life. Regarding the last point, unspoken awareness of impending death is present in as many as three-quarters of those within 6 months of the end of their lives (5). The chronically ill person, especially when in pain, becomes increasingly withdrawn and introspective, mobility is reduced, social contacts are lost; and preoccupation with physical symptoms, anxiety, and especially depression, are the hallmarks of the mental state. It has been suggested that depression develops out of a sense of helplessness, of being at the mercy of an uncontrollable malignant process; and of hopelessness because others are unable to provide a cure or even satisfactory relief from pain. For some this seems to be a punishment for real or fantasied misdeeds in the past, and to others it is a useless and disturbing experience which produces extreme feelings of loneliness (2).

Pain heightens emotional responses already evoked by illness, and this process increases if the patient feels that doctors have lost control of the disease and have reached the limit of their therapeutic powers. It is a situation with which some doctors cannot cope and causes their withdrawal from close contact with the patient because of personal feelings of inadequacy, or the fact that they see the patient's decline as a failure and a threat to their professional role as a healer. The daily work is then left to others often more junior and less experienced, though perhaps more compassionate. The use of increasingly powerful drugs and surgical treatment bring unpleasant side effects too, including reduced awareness and powers of concentration, anesthesia, dysesthesias, failure of bladder control, dyspnea, nausea, and vomiting, which add yet further to the general level of misery and discomfort.

Cancer patients are said to pass through four stages in their responses to the progress of a fatal illness, and their relatives are said to experience them too, though not necessarily at the same time. In practice all four reactions may occur in the space of hours, may be repeated, and may appear in several different sequences. They are illustrated by the following case history of a 56-year-old housewife who discovered that she had bladder cancer and who survived for a period of 7 months afterward.

Having been told of her cancer after a cystoscopy, performed after two severe episodes of hematuria, the patient appeared to accept the diagnosis with an unusual degree of cheerfulness and apparent lack of concern. At this stage she was reticent to accept major surgery but was persuaded to undergo a course of radiation therapy. It was felt at this time she was coping with the overwhelming anxiety imposed by the nature and the extent of the illness by operating the mental mechanism of denial (Stage 1). Initially the illness was not painful. However, radiation therapy produced severe cystitis and excruciating pain only partially controlled by narcotics. The patient became very depressed (Stage 2), her feelings were mixed with anger, and the comment, "Why should this have happened to me?" was made frequently. Considerable blame was placed on the various doctors for their negligence in not having reached the diagnosis sooner—for which there was some justification (Stage 3). Although the pain was never fully controlled from that time onward the level of depression fell, perhaps because of the use of psychotropic drugs. Although the patient did not mention her impending death, it became obvious about a month beforehand that she had accepted it as inevitable. She became quite composed, cheerful, and reasonably constructive with her remaining weeks of life (Stage 4). About 10 days before she died she asked us if death would be painful, a common fear among cancer patients. After discussing the issue she did not refer to the matter again but became quiet and clearly resigned to her fate. Throughout the illness her husband, with whom she had had a close relationship all their marital life, remained unnaturally cheerful and optimistic in her presence, and yet elsewhere showed extreme agitation, depression with frequent weeping, and expressions of despair. Despite their long and close life together, spoken communication in the final illness was strained. This strained relation clearly would have been improved if an experienced doctor could have become involved in psychotherapy with both the patient and her husband.

The sequence of events described is by no means unique, but it highlights common physical and emotional problems with which doctors and nurses must cope. Examination of studies which have looked at pretreatment and posttreatment levels of emotional disturbance are of interest. A search of the literature did not reveal references referring specifically to cancer patients in pain, but Lee and Maguire (7) who investigated 400 women attending a breast clinic found that anxiety levels were high in all patients and remained so among those admitted for biopsy. It was noted that levels of distress were also high in patients' husbands, and that the surgeons tended to ignore the latter's distress if it were not put into words. Lumps in the breast are greatly feared by virtually all women, and by many they are thought of as malignant until proved otherwise. The findings of Lee and Maguire draw attention to the fact that the patient's need to cope with emotional distress begins, though to a varying degree, at the time of initial consultation with a doctor.

In a more recent paper on breast cancer patients (10), it was reported that many patients have emotional disorders long after surgery at a time when surgeons regard them as having completed treatment. For example, 1 year later a quarter of their patients had anxiety, depression, or both, requiring treatment, and a third had moderate to severe sexual difficulties. However, only a very small proportion (8 of 75) of patients sought help for their emotional problems, and only 2 felt they were given appropriate support. Pain was not a feature of patients in this study, but the point is made that the trials posed by the illness and its treatment are potent causes of psychiatric illness. Undoubtedly if pain had been present, the patient who suffered it would have experienced even more mental distress. Maguire (9) likens the response to mastectomy, as others have done in the case of different mutilating operations, for example surgery for rectal cancer (3), and limb amputation (11), to a bereavement reaction incorporating the following sequence of events: (a) initial shock and disbelief; (b) sadness and weeping; (c) some preoccupation that the individual has become physically unattractive; (d) resentment and hostility revealed in complaints about others, or different aspects of the environment; (e) some loss of self-confidence and self-esteem. It is clear that the reactions described are also those experienced by many patients with a progressive and ultimately fatal disease.

THE TREATMENT OF EMOTIONAL DISTURBANCES AND PAIN

From what has been written it is obvious that an understanding of, and ability to deal with, the emotional consequences of cancer pain are essential if the emotional well-being of patients is to be supported, and relatives' problems are to be resolved. Psychiatrists, psychologists, and social workers are by virtue of their training more able to deal with this aspect of illness than others and have certain methods of special treatment at their disposal including psychotropic drugs, psychotherapies, and social manipulation. However, it should not be thought that this area of work is the sole prerogative of those with a specific training in psychiatry and allied disciplines. Surgeons, radiotherapists, nurses, and others should also acquire and develop some measure of skill.

Kraft (6) recommends that the surgeon should never condemn patients' behavior when it is driven by necessary mental defense mechanisms which he may regard as "neurotic" and that he should produce an empathic response to patients' expressions of anxiety and their need for a sense of control in the face of helplessness. Kraft advocates ready, simple, and direct communications with the patient and the maintenance of compassion at all times, preferably in an environment as free as possible from the complex and perhaps frightening paraphernalia found in certain hospital wards. The surgeon should also remember that the patient's view of him is governed by inner needs for security and safe deliverance rather than by objective facts and that he or she almost always places child-like trust in the surgeon and other doctors directly concerned with treatments, including pain-control. Such dependency demands a warm and comforting approach which will satisfy emotional needs and reduce levels of anxiety and depression.

Psychotropic Drugs

Bearing in mind that the most common disorders of emotion in chronically ill patients with pain are anxiety and depression, it is clear that anxiolytic and antidepressant drugs have their uses. Unfortunately there is surprisingly little reliable information about well-conducted trials of these drugs in the literature. In order to deal with anxiety, and much of this is based in reality and connected with the nature of the illness and apprehensions about treatment, the use of drugs should be carefully controlled. Preferably they should be used in association with counseling designed to remove as much anxiety as possible. This approach has been shown to reduce anticipatory preoperative anxiety substantially and, as a consequence, postoperative pain (4). An alternative, namely the use of benzodiazepines alone, as described by Battelli et al. (1) in the treatment of cancer patients, is less acceptable because they were not combined with counseling.

Patients with cancer may become very depressed (14). Therefore the use of antidepressant drugs is indicated in such instances for those who are deeply depressed, and these are usually easily distinguished from those with lesser degrees of emotional disturbance. It should be remembered that many patients are sad rather than depressed. Consequently, occasionally it is difficult to decide upon the depth of depression because many of the normal biologic features of the malignant disease process simulate organic changes associated with depression in psychiatric patients, e.g., weight loss, anergia, and poor sleep. Thus, care must be taken to avoid unnecessary use of antidepressants, for they have unpleasant side effects. Where the patient is depressed, tense, and anxious, and the medicine preferred is a tricyclic antidepressant, amitriptyline is recommended; and where apathy predominates imipramine is of value as it has an energizing effect.

Psychotropic drugs are commonly and quite properly used as adjuncts to analgesic therapy. Chlorpromazine in doses above 25 mg potentiates analgesics; and some advocate the use of tricyclic antidepressants too, because over and above their ability to reduce depression they also appear to have analgesic properties. The use of chlorpromazine and an antidepressant together has been advocated because chlorpromazine may increase feelings of depression. There are many different tranquilizers and antidepressants available. It is this writer's recommendation that those who wish to use them should select one or two drugs and become familiar with their use, effects, advantages, and disadvantages, for we believe that there is little to choose between different preparations of similar compounds.

Psychotherapy

It has been reported by Maguire (9) that the patients often regard doctors as too busy to listen to them and see them as uninterested in their emotional problems. Many see doctors as individuals who are dealing with their physical symptoms and not people to whom they should take their emotional difficulties (12). However, the mainstay of a psychiatrist's treatment is a psychotherapeutic approach, and although this is not a subject which can be dealt with at length in this paper, several comments about its use are relevant. Firstly, patients with organic illnesses may feel angry and resentful at being interviewed by a psychiatrist. His presence threatens already weakened self-esteem and feelings of self-control, bringing the implications of inability to cope to the bedside. Secondly, patients may feel that doctors engaged in their physical therapy have given up hope and that they have become untreatable. Thirdly, patients may believe they are being troublesome in some way by letting "their nerves get the better of them." These issues must be dealt with at the outset by emphasizing that the physical illness remains a major concern but that inevitably it brings with it both personal and interpersonal difficulties. Most patients recognize and accept this view and come to welcome the psychiatrist's visit.

The main purpose of therapy is to help the patient accept the reality of the threat his or her illness poses in a positive way and to encourage the living of a full emotional life with new and limited but obtainable goals in the remaining weeks or months. Le Shan and Gassmann (8) commented that fear of death, which must be dealt with eventually, is often a reflection of guilt about not having really lived earlier in life and that this may be overcome by engaging the patient in the process of living for the day, for, as Le Shan and Gassmann emphasize (and this can be pointed out with confidence), "no human being has assurances about the future." Thus physical, social, and emotional goals for the day are set and discussed and then adjusted to suit each individual's level of physical and emotional well-being. It should be appreciated that the approach is empathic and that direct expressions of sympathy for the patient are *not* encouraged, for they may be detrimental in causing him or her to focus upon the hopeless aspects of the situation and thus worsen feelings of depression.

The reduction of anxiety associated with psychotherapy and the feeling patients develop that they have not been deserted is often associated with reduction in feelings of futility, hopelessness, and depression. Pain levels often fall too, and the need for analgesic drugs may be reduced or even abolished. Two other major emotional difficulties may be present, and they represent crises in the relationship between the patient and his or her doctor centered upon the failure of the latter to bring expected relief from suffering, or the actual or anticipated rejection of the patient by the physician (13). These conflicts arouse much anxiety, which generally remains unformulated because of the serious threat such feelings pose for the emotional integrity of both doctor and patient. However, they may become manifest in anger and frustration with the doctor, who in turn may react with threats of abandonment or other more subtle forms of punishment—an unpleasant situation which psychiatrists are not infrequently called upon to disentangle.

It should be remembered that psychotherapy is arduous for the therapist as well as the patient. He or she may develop feelings of futility or hopelessness too as a result of working with a dying patient. The therapist must work through this, remembering that the task on hand is helping the patient to achieve a fuller emotional life, which may bring with it relief of physical symptoms and even lengthened life. Nevertheless, the death of the patient when it occurs is a severe blow, and irrational feelings of failure may develop. It is for this reason that the therapist should be protected by being a member of a team caring for the patient. Anxieties are shared and discussed among members of the team with the purpose of resolving feelings of pain and disappointment among colleagues, as well as planning and executing different stages of physical treatment.

Group and Family Therapy

Group therapy may be carried out with patients and has very definite benefits. The function and composition of groups vary from place to place, but in most cases their basic goals are the gaining of emotional support by one patient from another in controlled surroundings and discussion of practical difficulties arising out of pain and disability. The sense of loneliness which tends to afflict patients is removed by sharing difficult experiences with others who have similar problems.

Family therapy is a growing area in psychiatry and also has much to offer in the world of physical disease. All too often physicians, surgeons, and family doctors, confine their interests to the patient, because for many the complexity and taxing nature of the work demanded by relatives is beyond their personal skill and interests (15).

There are three basic steps in family therapy: first, the analysis of emotional interactions between family members with emphasis upon methods they can adopt for coping with stress. Next, the provision of a setting in which previously unspoken fears and feelings can be expressed in a controlled and "safe" fashion. Lastly, the provision of a situation in which correct information about the illness can be delivered to avoid misunderstanding and anxiety in the patient's family. The feeling that the patient's physical and emotional welfare is being controlled is usually a great source of comfort. Eventually members achieve a realistic understanding of the illness and its treatment and improve upon their own ability to cope with personal feelings and therefore those of the stricken family member.

REFERENCES

1. Battelli, T., Bonsignori, M., Manocchi, P., and Rossi, G. (1976): Anxiety therapy in neoplastic patients. *Curr. Med. Res. Opin.,* 4:185–188.
2. Bodley, P. O., Jones, H. V. R., and Mather, M. D. (1974): Pre-operation anxiety: A qualitative analysis. *J. Neurol. Neurosurg. Psychiatry,* 37:230–239.
3. Devlin, H. B., Plant, J. A., and Griffin, M. (1971): Aftermath of surgery for rectal cancer. *Br. Med. J.,* 3:413–418.
4. Egbert, L. D., Battit, G. E., Welch, C. E., and Bartlett, M. K. (1964): Reduction of postoperative pain by encouragement and instruction of patients. *New Engl. J. Med.,* 270:825–827.
5. Hinton, J. M. (1963): The physical and mental distress of the dying. *Quart. J. Med.,* 32:1.
6. Kraft, I. A. (1976): The surgeon's psychological management of his patient. In: *Modern Perspectives in the Psychiatric Aspects of Surgery,* edited by J. G. Howells, pp. 637–658. Brunner Mazel, New York.
7. Lee, E. G., and Maguire, P. (1975): Proceedings: Emotional distress in patients attending a breast clinic. *Br. J. Surg.,* 62:162.
8. Le Shan, L., and Gassmann, M. L. (1958): Some observations on psychotherapy with patients suffering from neoplastic disease. *Am. J. Psychother.,* 12:723–734.
9. Maguire, P. (1976): The psychological and social sequelae of mastectomy. In: *Modern Perspectives in the Psychiatric Aspects of Surgery,* edited by J. G. Howells, pp. 390–422. Brunner Mazel, New York.
10. Maguire, P., Lee, E. G., Bevington, D. J., Küchemann, C. S., Crabtree, R. J., and Cornell, C. E. (1978): Psychiatric problems in the first year after mastectomy. *Br. Med. J.,* 1:963–966.
11. Murray Parkes, C., and Napier, M. M. (1975): Psychiatric sequelae of amputation. In: *Contemporary Psychiatry,* edited by T. Silverstone and B. Barraclough, pp. 429–440. Headley Bros., London.
12. Peck, A., and Boland, J. (1977): Emotional reactions to radiation treatment. *Cancer,* 40:180–184.
13. Pinsky, J. J. (1975): Psychodynamics and psychotherapy in the treatment of patients with chronic intractable pain. In: *Pain Research and Treatment,* edited by B. L. Crue, pp. 383–398. Academic Press, New York.
14. Woodforde, J. M., and Merskey, H. (1972): Personality traits of patients with chronic pain. *J. Psychosom. Res.,* 16:167–172.
15. Worby, C. M., and Babineau, F. (1974): The family interview: Helping patient and family cope with metastatic disease. *Geriatrics,* 29(6):83–90.

Hypnotherapy in Pain of Advanced Cancer

Basil Finer

Department of Anaesthesiology, Samariterhemmes, Box 609, S-75125 Uppsala 1, Sweden

> This you shall know:
> Dull ache wants company
> Sharp pain does not want to be alone
> So do not go to bed
> You may not lie comfortably
> even if you can
> For then it will be tyrant over your loneliness
>
> No, you shall sit up
> You shall rock to and fro
> You shall lean in all directions
> You shall keep your own company
> You shall write letters to someone
> if there is someone, otherwise to no one
> as I do now
> You shall move things and objects
> from place to place
> You shall do things in the kitchen
> if you have one and can walk
> You shall think thoughts if you can
> or do some handwork, knit a sock
> with a foot miles long. You shall keep company
> with your ache, you shall entertain it
> the whole time until the grey morning.
>
> Gunnar Ekelöf (1907–1968)
> *Partitur: Posthumous Poems,* 1969
> (Own translation—by permission)

The Swedish poet wrote this 3 months before his death from larynx cancer.

It was 440 years ago that the far-sighted rulers in the enlightened government of Venice placed Andreas Vesalius in the chair of Surgery with care of Anatomy in their University of Padua. Five years later was published *Fabrica Humani Corporis,* the beginning not only of modern anatomy but of modern physiology, in as much as Vesalius was the distinct forerunner of Harvey. For Harvey's great exposition of the circulation of the blood did for physiology what Vesalius' *Fabrica* did for anatomy: It first rendered true progress possible. And Harvey's great work was the direct outcome of Vesalius' teaching and yet, one reached by successive steps, steps taken by men of the Italian school, of which Vesalius was the founder and father (11). In Uppsala, there is a copy of the anatomy theatre from Padua in the Gustavianum.

We are all involved in trying to alleviate an intolerable situation for our patients, and no one method can as yet suffice. We need to know the best of each other's methods, so that we can administer the most efficient combination.

The method I will discuss, hypnotherapy, is well known and has been used for more than 200 years, but repeated exaggerated claims for its usefulness, followed by the skepticism of repeated disappointment in its failures have cast an unwarranted shadow over the method. I should like to compare hypnotherapy with nitrous oxide–oxygen anesthesia. Both methods alone are rather weak, and it was a long time before scientific research could be used to investigate their physiologic, pharmacologic, and psychologic mechanisms of action. This research is only in its infancy and both nitrous oxide–oxygen anesthesia and hypnotherapy are still best used in combination with other complementary methods, which they can greatly enhance.

As you began to listen to this lecture, you probably went through various procedures. You chose somewhere that was comfortable, warm, and quiet, with suitable lighting. You more or less consciously shook off your previous thoughts and feelings, while your curiosity and interest in the subject motivated a concentrated effort to take in the words of the speaker. As long as the subject matter captures your attention, you forget your surroundings, but as soon as the subject matter becomes boring, or you get tired, or other matters impinge on your consciousness, your concentration wavers. If you can shake off these interruptions, it may be possible to recapture your interest in the lecture, but otherwise you give up and wait to see the lecture in print later on. The brain functions so that it is difficult or impossible to concentrate strongly on more than one thing at a time. If such strong concentration is possible, it usually implies that there is a simultaneous detachment from other stimuli. Concentration and detachment are like two sides of a mirror, which always exist together. Hypnosis is a way of strengthening these qualities.

FEAR OF CANCER

Cancer is usually a frightening condition. Just the word, *cancer,* is often filled with negative associations—in the first place, its literal meaning of "crab." Nowadays, we are very clever at diagnosing cancer early and removing it totally or subtotally. This means that cancer patients often survive much longer these days than they used to and are usually aware of the diagnosis. There is thus plenty of time to develop a state of chronic fear of cancer. It can imply pain, anxiety, stress, suffering, loss of human dignity, hopelessness, total dependency, guilt, ugliness, jealousy, hate, loneliness, and fear of loss of support from family, friends, and hospital staff. There is a possibility of a prolonged, tortured process of dying. Fear of death is usually greatest for the time preceding it; sometimes the fear is for death itself or even for possible suffering after death. All of these factors increase fear, and fear always increases pain. Anything which counteracts the fear-provoking negative associations to cancer has great value in a comprehensive treatment plan for cancer pain. Hypnotherapy is one contribution among several for counteracting these negative associations (5).

HYPNOSIS

Hypnosis is an altered state of consciousness (12), arising during a specific trusting relationship (13) between one or more "teachers" and one or more "pupils." There are various methods of developing this state; mine is by a modified progressive relaxation and training of the imagination (5). In this state, the patient (pupil) is able to develop a selective increase in concentration, e.g., on maximal enjoyment of the life-time that remains, and a selective increase in detachment, e.g., from fear and pain. This ability can be increased to some extent by training. If the teacher is needed to produce this state, it is called *heterohypnosis,* but if the pupil can continue producing the state alone, it is called *autohypnosis*. Both methods can be used on different occasions. The role of teacher in heterohypnosis can be transferred to another member of staff, family, or friend. In addition, the hypnosis-induction program can be recorded on tape, so that the pupil can recapture the heterohypnosis at will, even when no living teacher or stand-in is available. This increases the pupil's independence.

Physiology

Recent work shows that there is a basic normal plasticity of the central nervous system, which can be mobilized under various circumstances, including hypnosis (12). Reflex responses to pain include spinal segmental reflexes with short latency times, slightly susceptible to hypnosis, and suprasegmental (brainstem) reflexes with longer latency times, markedly susceptible to hypnotic influence. Thus, one effect of hypnosis on pain is a conditioned block of reflex, relieving learned pain. Other recent work has shown that in some chronic limb pain, blood-flow changes in skin and muscle can vary with the pain experience. Finer and Graf (7,8) found that the changes were normalized when pain was relieved both by hypnosis and by beta-sympathetic blockade. Furthermore, during an operation for varicose veins with stripping under hypnosis, there was no change in blood pressure, pulse, or catecholamine excretion attributable to the surgical procedure (9). Thus, another effect of hypnosis on pain is a sympathetic block, relieving the autonomic responses and the anxiety component of pain.

Technique

The various factors and mental manipulations of the technique I use are shown schematically in Fig. 1. The pupils are trained in modified progressive relaxation in a permissive manner, preferably in groups. Sometimes it is difficult for a pupil to start in a group, and individual training can be begun until group work is possible. During relaxation, the pupil is encouraged to imagine pleasant scenes or music. This ability is trained, so that the pupil can concentrate on pleasant things at any time. While in this positive state, the pupil is encouraged to tolerate fear and pain in the imagination. This is called *symptomatic desensitization* and results in a greater ability to tolerate fear and pain in reality. Also in this positive state, the pupil can be encouraged to live fully for the moment, no longer comparing the present with the past and not thinking of the future (16,18).

Thus strengthened, the pupil can begin to imagine unpleasant things. Most patients with pain of advanced cancer have many unpleasant emotions bottled up inside, which they readily release while in the hypnotic state. Thus the pupil reduces tension and consequently pain is diminished. The patient can also be encouraged to accept reality as it is, tolerating and enduring the change in attitude to life and death which this entails. While concentrating on these things, the pupil can be trained to detach from anxiety, stress, and pain.

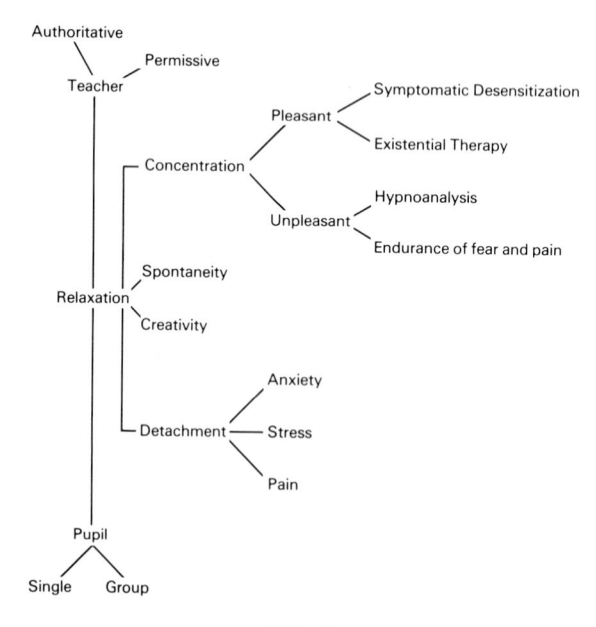

FIG. 1.

The pupil can be encouraged to develop spontaneity and creativity, taking responsibility for himself during the life that remains.

HYPNOTHERAPY FOR THE MANAGEMENT OF CANCER PAIN

The patient with pain of advanced cancer needs: (a) pain reduction with as little mental clouding as possible; (b) emotional support with training in maximal independence. Hypnotherapy is a system of treatment, in which patients and staff interact to produce maximal placebo effects, together with detachment from symptoms (19). My own clinical experience is fairly similar to that of other workers in the field of chronic pain, and especially cancer pain, including Crasilneck and Hall (2), Erickson (4), Kroger (15), LaBaw et al. (17), Sacerdote (21), and particularly Hilgard and Hilgard (14).

Hypnotherapy in the comprehensive management of advanced cancer pain is of value for patient, family, friends, and hospital staff. Patients are easier to work with when they have less pain and are more conscious through less need for narcotics. Where possible, the patients are trained in groups, encouraging and helping each other. The program can be recorded on tape to suit individual patients, so that they can play back at any time night and day and recollect the warm, encouraging atmosphere of the groups. This contact can even be transmitted by telephone when direct contact is delayed and distances are long. Sleep is improved: Patients fall asleep more easily, sleep is calmer and more restful, and they wake more refreshed. Appetite is improved, food and drink better retained. It is easier to perform unpleasant diagnostic and therapeutic procedures and anticipatory fear is reduced. At the same time the patients become more independent, helping themselves and each other in the group to make the remaining life-time more worth-while (20). The efficacy of hypnotherapy in cancer pain can be increased if the patient is trained before the symptoms become severe. Sometimes small operative procedures can be performed under hypnotic analgesia, e.g., on small skin or gland metastases, as shown in my film (6).

Advantages

Hypnotherapy is a comparatively simple method for helping patients with advanced cancer pain. Contrary to popular misconception, it is not particularly time-consuming, especially when compared with other procedures routinely used. In addition, time is greatly reduced by group treatment, the patients helping each other, while the stress and fatigue in the therapist, reported by Butler (1) is eased by the sharing of responsibility. The method is not at all exclusive, being usefully combined with other psychotherapeutic and routine physical and pharmacologic methods. Finally, hypnosis lends itself readily to physiologic and psychologic research analysis in the laboratory and clinic.

Disadvantages

The main disadvantage is the variability in patients' susceptibility to hypnosis, so that it is difficult to know in advance how much the method will help until it is tried. Intelligent use of the method requires adequate training of the whole staff, and this necessitates an educational program to counteract misunderstanding and scepticism.

Deficiencies

The main deficiency is the variability in effectivity, so that an expectant attitude is necessary. While many patients can be helped to some extent and some can be helped very much, the staff must be positive in their attitudes, for skepticism and misunderstanding weaken the method.

RECOMMENDATIONS

The whole staff should be trained in hypnotherapy. They can be trained by the therapist, then train on each other, and finally take part in therapy with patients. Associate therapists are welcome, and the staff will have a much more positive attitude to the therapy.

It is suggested that the therapist should go into therapy too, and particularly go into a supervisory group. Being a therapist to patients close to death arouses much anxiety, and it is important to have help in coping with one's own problems. This will also help to reduce the fatigue and stress described by Butler (1).

The efficacy of hypnosis can be increased by adjuvants. A pilot study by Finer et al. (10) suggested that small concentrations of nitrous oxide–oxygen have this effect. Further research is indicated and indeed necessary. In general, research on hypnosis and hypnotherapy must be expanded, parallel with research in other areas of pain, e.g., acupuncture and endomorphines.

It is increasingly clear that patients with pain of advanced cancer have the right to expect the help that hypnotherapy can give in any effective plan of treatment. It is the duty of the professions involved in the care of patients with pain of advanced cancer to train themselves in this method and to further develop hypnotherapy as an integral part of the comprehensive management of these patients.

ACKNOWLEDGMENTS

I should like to express my sincere thanks to my colleagues, medical, nursing, auxiliary, and secretarial at Samariterhemmes for their support and help. Dr. Elisabet Olander has continuously encouraged me in my work. My debt to her is great.

I should also like to express my appreciation to the Floriani Foundation of Milan and the Scientific Program Committee for organizing this International Symposium on the Management of Pain of Advanced Cancer.

REFERENCES

1. Butler, B. (1954): The use of hypnosis in the care of the cancer patient. *Cancer*, 7:1–14.
2. Crasilneck, H. B., and Hall, J. A. (1975): *Clinical Hypnosis*. Grune & Stratton, New York.
3. Ekelöf, G. (1971): *En självbiografi*. Albert Bonniers Förlag, Stockholm.
4. Erickson, M. H. (1967): An introduction to the study and application of hypnosis for pain control. In: *Hypnosis and Psychosomatic Medicine,* edited by J. Lassner, pp. 83–90. Springer-Verlag, Berlin.
5. Finer, B. L. (1974): Clinical use of hypnosis in pain management. In: *Advances in Neurology, Vol. 4: International Symposium on Pain,* edited by J. J. Bonica, pp. 573–579. Raven Press, New York.
6. Finer, B. L. (1975): Hypnotherapy in cancer pain. Paper read at the International Symposium on Cancer Pain, Florence, Italy.
7. Finer, B. L., and Graf, K. (1968): Circulatory changes accompanying hypnotic imagination of hyperalgesia and hypoalgesia in causalgic limbs. *Z. Ges. Exp. Med.*, 146:97–114.
8. Finer, B. L., and Graf, K. (1968): Mechanisms of circulatory changes accompanying hypnotic imagination of hyperalgesia and hypoalgesia in causalgic limbs. *Z. Ges. Exp. Med.*, 148:1–21.
9. Finer, B. L., Jonzon, A., Sedin, G., and Sjöstrand, U. (1973): Some physiological changes during minor surgery under hypnotic analgesia. *Acta Anaesthesiol. Scand.* [Suppl.], 53:94–96.
10. Finer, B. L., Lundberg, M., and Wigh, G. (1975): *Research Report,* Psychological Institute, Uppsala University.
11. Foster, Sir M. (1970): *Lectures on the History of Physiology*. Dover Publications, Inc., New York.
12. Hagbarth, K.-E., and Finer, B. L. (1963): The plasticity of human withdrawal reflexes to noxious skin stimuli in lower limbs. *Prog. Brain Res.*, 1:65–78.
13. Haley, J. (1963): *Strategies of Psychotherapy*. Grune & Stratton, New York.
14. Hilgard, E. R., and Hilgard, J. R. (1975): *Hypnosis in the Relief of Pain*. William Kaufmann, Inc., Los Altos, California.
15. Kroger, W. S. (1963): *Clinical and Experimental Hypnosis*. Lippincott, Philadelphia.
16. Kurosawa, A. (1952): "Ikiru." Film.
17. LaBaw, W., Holton, C., Tewell, K., and Eccles, D. (1975): The use of self-hypnosis by children with cancer. *Am. J. Clin. Hypnosis*. 17:233–238.
18. LeShan, L. (1964): Mobilizing the life-force: An approach to the problem of arousing the sick patient's will to live. In: *Psychosomatic Aspects of Neoplastic Disease,* edited by D. Kissen and L. LeShan, pp. 109–120. Lippincott, New York.
19. Orne, M. T. (1974): Pain suppression by hypnosis and related phenomena. In: *Advances in Neurology, Vol. 4: International Symposium on Pain,* edited by J. J. Bonica, pp. 563–572. Raven Press, New York.
20. Pirsig, R. (1976): *Zen and the Art of Motor Cycle Maintenance*. Corgi Books, London.
21. Sacerdote, P. (1968): Involvement and communication with the terminally ill patient. *Am. J. Clin. Hypnosis,* 10:244–248.
22. Tart, C. (1975): *States of Consciousness*. E. P. Dutton and Co., Inc., New York.

Psychophysiologic Control of Cancer Pain

Sophia S. Fotopoulos, Charles Graham, and Mary R. Cook

Midwest Research Institute, Kansas City, Missouri 64110

The etiology and underlying mechanisms of pain associated with carcinoma are complex and difficult to delineate (2,6). Theoretical models of pain generally assume that activation of higher neural substrates, such as integrative functions of the cerebral cortex or the brainstem reticular formation, forms the basis of sensory responding and perception of pain. With pain related to carcinoma, structural and functional physiologic factors combine with psychologic factors to play a crucial role in the pain experienced. In the past, psychologic factors have been classified under the heading of suffering, and were considered merely subjective "feelings" separate from underlying neural mechanisms. Experimental evidence, however, indicates that these reactive components of the pain experience have, to some degree, a conditioned physiologic basis and are related to the neural substrate through complex mechanisms (6). Consequently, traditional stimulus-response models of pain, which assume that pain is a specific sensation reflecting a direct correlation between intensity and extent of tissue damage, are inadequate to characterize chronic pain states. Pain is influenced by cognitive variables, attention, suggestion, motivation, and affective factors, as well as stimulus, organizational, and interpretive functions of the brain and central nervous system.

This model suggests that techniques that alter the decision-making aspects of the pain experience, the affective factors associated with pain, or the conditional responses associated with intense stimulation could be effective in reducing pain without stress, central nervous system (CNS) and autonomic nervous system (ANS) side effects, or danger of diminishing effectiveness. They would leave the individual fully alert and in control of his or her life and death.

Behavioral modification approaches to the reduction of pain attempt to induce change in overt as well as physiologic behavior. Operant conditioning techniques, which entail reinforcement of an emitted response, and its subsequent learning and perpetuation, use strategies for establishing contingencies such as lack of complaining about pain for a specified time and for reinforcement produced by attention by a loved one, going out to dinner, etc. Maladaptive behaviors often tend to intensify pain and frequently lead to affective disturbances, such as depression, which negatively affect the patient's network of family and friends. Behavior-modification techniques can be effective in decreasing secondary gain and in reducing the frequency of behaviors developed as a consequence of the pain syndrome. Operant behavioral techniques are minimally effective in decreasing the pain itself. More appropriate behavioral techniques are classical conditioning, hypnosis, or biofeedback, which are more closely linked to both sensory and affective physiologic sensory processes.

A previous report made at the 1975 International Symposium on Cancer Pain by Fotopoulos et al. (3) described the clinical use of biofeedback in the treatment of 12 cancer-pain patients. Electroencephalographic (EEG) feedback of 8 to 12 Hz activity (alpha) appeared to have little effect on pain. Electromyographic (EMG) feedback had more positive effects, but pain-relief was brief. Significant pain reduction was observed, however, when EMG feedback was presented in combination with EEG feedback of 4 to 8 Hz activity (theta). This type of combined feedback resulted in a state of low physiologic arousal, often accompanied by pain reduction, vivid imagery, and increased feelings of well-being and physical relaxation. While little work has been reported with theta feedback, Beatty (1) has presented evidence suggesting that individuals can learn to suppress theta activity. Stoyva et al. (9) and Graham et al. (5) have reported the enhancement of theta activity with biofeedback techniques and also observed concomitant increases in relaxation and feelings of well-being. The combination of EMG and EEG theta feedback seemed, therefore, to hold great promise for the management of cancer pain.

The findings reported by Fotopoulos et al. (3) were obtained under clinical treatment conditions where psychotherapeutic techniques were employed, in addition to the use of EEG and EMG biofeedback. It was important, therefore, to submit this apparently effective biofeedback procedure to controlled laboratory evaluation. As part of a larger experimental program, the therapeutic effectiveness of a biofeedback technique was evaluated in ambulatory cancer-pain patients. The therapeutic goal was not the total elimination of pain; rather it was to reduce chronic pain to a level which would allow more normal daily function, both psychologically and physiologically. The biofeedback procedure focused on the alleviation of reactive pain components and reduction of physiologic pain concomitants. The hypothesis that providing combined EEG/EMG biofeedback would result in a physiologic state of low autonomic activation, accompanied by a subjective state of well-being and comfort, was tested. The evaluation included: (a) extensive pre- and posttreatment physiologic and psychologic assessments; (b) multiple measures of physiologic activation obtained during biofeedback sessions; (c) assessment of pain parameters and concomitants in the laboratory and at home; and (d) evaluation of the relationship between therapeutic success and the degree of physiologic control achieved.

EXPERIMENTAL METHODS AND PROCEDURES

The overall experimental program called for separate evaluation of the use of biofeedback or self-hypnosis in the treatment of cancer pain. Participation in the program was voluntary. Criteria for participation included: medical diagnosis involving carcinoma; current medical treatment specifically for pain; and ambulatory condition. When subjects completed the pretreatment assessment procedures described below, they were assigned on a pseudo-random basis to receive either biofeedback or self-hypnosis. Material presented here focuses on those subjects who were assigned to the biofeedback treatment condition. Where such information is either not generally available in regard to cancer-pain patients, or may be of interest to other investigators in the area, data from hypnosis subjects are included.

The subject population consisted of 10 females and 7 males between the ages of 31 and 68. The most common diagnoses were carcinoma of the bladder, breast, and lung. Subjects had been in pain an average of 15.7 months and were using both narcotic ($\bar{X} = 10.04$ mg morphine equivalent per day) and nonnarcotic analgesics ($\bar{X} = 1,204$ mg aspirin equivalent per day). Of these 17 subjects, 7 were assigned to the experimental biofeedback treatment group.

PRETREATMENT MEASURES

Psychologic and Demographic Measures

The initial interview included a sociodemographic inventory (age, sex, race, ethnic origin, and background) and a detailed pain history. In the second assessment session, a psychologic test battery was administered and consisted of: Eysenck Personality Inventory (EPI), Repression-Sensitization Scale (RS), Ego-Strength (ES), Locus of Control (LOC), and the McGill Pain Questionnaire (MPQ).

Psychophysiologic Battery

A psychophysiologic assessment examines the interaction between a particular individual's physiologic responsivity and a variety of standardized situations varied for physical, cognitive, and affective demands. The dynamic base line allows examination of possible changes in these relationships before and after treatment. This information provides understanding of the effects of biofeedback treatment, as well as information concerning physiologic responsivity over time in individuals in pain. To evaluate individual response patterns, it was necessary to record a variety of autonomic functions continuously during diverse stress and performance situations. The measures and experimental procedures are summarized in Table 1.

TABLE 1. *Procedures for psychophysiologic battery*

I. Physiologic measures

Measure	Recording Site	Purpose
Electroencephalograph (EEG)	Left occipital Right occipital Right central	Allow examination of EEG amplitude and percent time at various frequencies
Electromyograph (EMG)	Frontalis area Muscle associated with pain site Stress site	Allow evaluation of patterns of skeletal muscle response to various stressors
Heart rate (HR)	Clavicle vs. 3rd intercostal space	Evaluate base levels and responsivity from a variety of autonomic variables
Skin conductance level (SCL)	2nd and 4th fingers of nondominant hand	
Photoplethysmograph (ppg)	3rd finger of nondominant hand	
Temperature (Temp.)	Oral Skin	Evaluate metabolic and homeostatic lability
Blood pressure (B.P.)	Nondominant arm	Determine suitability for stressors
Respiration (R)	Halfway between umbilicus and xyphoid process	Allow evaluation of relationship between respiratory changes and autonomic changes

II. Experimental conditions

Class	Task	Duration
Physiologic base lines	Uninstructed relaxation	2 min
	Instructed "eyes open" (EO)	2 min
	Instructed "eyes closed" (EC)	2 min
Physical stressors	Valsalva's maneuver	varies
	Arm-lift	varies
	Cold-pressor	varies
Cognitive stressors	Serial subtraction of 7's	2 min
	Name nouns beginning with "Y"	2 min
Affective stressors	Word-association to neutral, personally relevant, and disease-relevant stimuli	varies
Instructed relaxation	Zen breathing exercise	5 min
	Pleasant fantasy	5 min

Hypnotic Susceptibility

As a final pretreatment measure, all subjects were individually administered a standardized hypnotic-susceptibility scale [Stanford Scale of Hypnotic Susceptibility, Form C: Weitzenhoffer and Hilgard (10)].

Biofeedback Procedures

The original study protocol called for 20 treatment sessions to be given over a 9-week period. During the first week there were to be daily 2-hr sessions; subsequently, the interval between sessions was to be gradually increased so that the last three sessions were held on a weekly basis. The physical condition of the subjects often made it impossible to adhere to this schedule.

Prior to each biofeedback session, the subject rated his pain, and measures of weight, oral temperature, blood pressure, pulse, and respiration rate were obtained. Electrodes were then attached precisely as for the psychophysiologic battery, and three 2-min physiologic base-line measures obtained: sitting quietly with eyes open, then with eyes closed, followed by a volitional control period during which the subject was asked to relax as deeply as possible without feedback. Each session of biofeedback began with three 5-min periods of EMG training.

Feedback was alternated among the three EMG sites, so that each session began with the muscle showing the highest level of activity, and continued until that muscle group was no longer highest. The highest site was again selected, feedback given from that site, and so forth. An operant shaping procedure was employed to reinforce reduction of muscle activity at each EMG site. Specified levels of EMG activity, relative to base-line EMG activity, were selected. The subject was required to produce EMG activity below this specified microvolt threshold 50% of the time in order to hear the biofeedback tone. Based on this criterion, the threshold was changed at 1-min intervals.

EEG feedback from C_2 followed the EMG biofeedback conditioning procedure. The object of this was to teach subjects to emit EEG activity in the 4 to 8 Hz range (theta). The frequency filter was set initially at 4 to 12 Hz, with the lower amplitude cutoff at 10 μv. When the subject emitted EEG activity within this range, he received the audio biofeedback signal. If EEG activity was in the range selected for a period of time equal to 50% of a 1-min trial, the upper frequency limit was lowered to 11 Hz. This process continued until activity in the theta range was continuously produced as recorded both in polygraphic record and in the digital displays. Once activity was predominantly in the theta range, the lower level of the amplitude cutoff was gradually raised in order to enhance the amplitude of theta bursts.

Combined feedback was then given. During this period the subject had to maintain both EMG and EEG levels within the selected ranges in order to receive feedback. There were three 5-min trials with 30-sec pause periods interspersed, during each session. The three 2-min base-line periods (eyes closed, eyes open, and volitional control) were repeated at the end of each session, followed by oral temperature, blood pressure, and subjective pain ratings. The electrodes were removed, and the day's session discussed with the subject.

Posttreatment and Outcome Measures

After the 20 biofeedback sessions were completed, the protocol called for the psychophysiologic battery and the psychologic test battery to be administered again, and a posttreatment interview conducted. Death or hospitalization of the subjects often made it impossible to adhere to this schedule.

A variety of measures was used to evaluate treatment outcome: subjective pain report, changes in physiologic reactivity to stimuli, changes in use of analgesic medication, and changes in psychologic factors.

PRELIMINARY RESULTS

Pretreatment Characteristics of the Subjects

Because few data on the cancer pain patient are available, pretreatment measures were analyzed for all 17 subjects.

Psychologic Tests

Pretreatment scores were summarized (see Table 2) and compared with appropriate standardization samples or samples of hospitalized patients who did not have a diagnosis of carcinoma. Cancer-pain patients showed significantly lower ego-strength scores ($p < .01$) than either normative or

TABLE 2. Psychologic test data summary

		ES	RS	EPI E	EPI N	EPI L	SRI	McGill Sensory	McGill Affective	McGill Evaluative
Males	$\bar{X}$	35.2	65.6	12.9	13.4	2.4	10.6	17.4	5.1	3.1
	S.D.	6.4	17.2	4.8	5.3	1.3	2.4	8.6	3.7	1.1
	N	5	5	7	7	7	7	7	7	7
Females	$\bar{X}$	33.2	51.0	10.9	11.1	4.3	10.6	18.5	4.5	3.3
	S.D.	7.1	22.8	5.1	4.7	1.6	4.3	9.1	3.9	1.5
	N	10	10	10	10	10	10	10	10	10
Total	$\bar{X}$	33.9	55.9	11.7	12.1	3.5	10.6	18.1	4.8	3.2
	S.D.	6.7	21.6	4.9	4.9	1.7	3.6	8.6	3.7	1.3
	N	15	15	17	17	17	17	17	17	17

Legend: EPI = Eysenck Personality Inventory; ES = Ego-Strength; RS = Repression-Sensitization Scale; E = Extraversion; N = Neuroticism; SRI = Social Reaction Inventory (Rotter Internal-External Control Scale).

hospitalized patients with tuberculosis. The neuroticism (N) scale on the EPI resulted in significantly higher N scores for cancer patients compared to normal samples ($p < .05$). On the Locus of Control Scale, male cancer-pain patients were more "internal" ($p < .05$) than college undergraduate males; no such difference was found for the female patients. Cancer patients did not differ from normative samples on Extraversion or Repression-Sensitization.

Pain Ratings

Multiple measures of pretreatment pain were employed: physicians' ratings of subject pain using a scale of 0 to 100, with 100 indicating intolerable, intractable pain; the subject's mean pretreatment pain rating using the same scale; the rating of present pain intensity from the McGill Pain Questionnaire (MPQ); the Sensory, Affective, and Evaluative scores from the MPQ. These data are summarized in Table 3. An experimental cold-pressor, pain task measure from the psychophysiologic battery was also employed where the subject's physical condition allowed.

Significant agreement was found among the various pain measures as indicated by Kendall's $W = .59$, $p < .001$. A correlation matrix using Spearman's rho was also computed. Of particular interest are the findings that: (a) the sensory, affective, and evaluative scales of the MPQ were highly correlated; (b) the subject's mean pretreatment pain ratings did not correlate significantly with the sensory scale of the MPQ; and (c) the physicians' ratings were highly correlated with all subjects' self-report measures except the evaluative and global MPQ scale scores.

Subjects were divided into high- and low-pain groups using a median split of their pretreatment pain ratings. A correlational analysis showed higher pain levels to be associated with more external control (higher external scores on the LOC) and lower Extraversion scores ($p < .05$). High- and low-pain groups did not differ with regard to age, sex, tumor site, time since diagnosis, or occurrence of metastases. Of particular interest is the observation that the two groups did not differ on the 12 variables assessed during the base-line portion of the pretreatment psychophysiologic battery (see Table 4).

TABLE 3. *Summary of pain data*

Measure	Mean	Standard deviation
Physician rating	55.5	28.7
Subjects' base-line rating	42.9	26.7
MPQ "Now"	33.1	26.0
MPQ Sensory	18.1	8.6
MPQ Affective	4.8	3.7
MPQ Evaluative	3.2	1.3

TABLE 4. *Comparison of base-line physiologic measures for high- and low-pain report groups*[a,b]

Variable	N (H/L)	Group $\bar{X}$ High	Group $\bar{X}$ Low	t	dF	p
EMG: pain site	5/7	3.196	3.219	0.022	10	ns
stress site	3/9	4.892	3.123	1.562	10	ns
frontalis	5/9	5.126	9.33	1.509	12	ns
EEG: amplitude	5/9	12.72	12.217	0.201	12	ns
% time θ	5/9	35.99	40.27	0.658	12	ns
Heart rate	5/8	87.08	88.25	0.134	11	ns
Skin conductance level	4/7	9.35	15.72	0.867	9	ns
Respiration rate	5/8	4.0	4.75	0.941	11	ns
Weight	4/8	154.75	143.12	0.496	10	ns
Systolic blood pressure	5/9	133.80	131.89	0.151	12	ns
Diastolic blood pressure		81.69	81.56	0.006	12	ns
Oral temperature	5/9	98.46	98.49	0.074	12	ns
Pain site rating[c]	4/9	50.0	33.33	0.954	11	ns
Total pain rating[c]	5/8	190.8	48.13	2.82	11	.05

[a] All psychophysiologic measures obtained from first EC period of pre-battery.
[b] High- and low-pain groups defined as above or below the median of base-line period ratings.
[c] Pain site and total pain ratings taken from pain picture data collected at beginning of pre-battery session.

Psychophysiologic Battery

Physiologic data obtained during the eyes-closed (EC) base line of the pretreatment psychophysiologic battery are presented in Table 5. As previously mentioned, the population consisted of men and women who differed as to primary tumor site, chemotherapy, and radiation therapies. Overall the

TABLE 5. *Pretreatment physiologic measures*

Measure	Mean	S.D.
EMG: pain site	3.25 μv	1.59
stress site	3.61 μv	1.74
frontalis	7.71 μv	5.06
EEG: amplitude in range (4–8 Hz)	12.22 μv	4.21
% time in range	42.7%	38.5%
Heart rate	87.8 bpm	14.1
Skin conductance level	14.5 μMho	11.7 μMho
Respiration rate	14.4	2.94
Weight	146.5 lb	35.4
Oral temperature	98.4°F	0.67
Systolic blood pressure	132 mm Hg	21.2
Diastolic blood pressure	81 mm Hg	11.6

patients' physiology did not differ markedly from that observed in a normal adult sample, except that theta amplitude and percent time were elevated.

Results of Experimental Biofeedback Treatment

Subjective Pain

Pain ratings obtained before and after each biofeedback session were compared by separate t-tests for each subject. All subjects showed pain-relief after biofeedback sessions, with significance levels ranging from $p < .05$ to $p < .001$. Complete daily home ratings were available for 5 of the 7 subjects and showed mixed results. Four subjects did not show any significant reduction in home pain ratings. However, 1 of these 4 subjects (No. 03) completely ceased use of opiates, and her pain ratings increased minimally. The remaining subject (No. 14) showed significant decrease ($p < .01$) on the daily measures. In summary, the pain-relief obtained in the laboratory appeared to generalize to the home situation for 2 of the 7 subjects.

It was not possible to statistically evaluate changes on the McGill Pain Questionnaire as 4 of the 7 subjects died or were hospitalized before the final test battery. Of the remaining subjects, MPQ scores indicated that pain was greatly alleviated for 1 subject, increased for another, and the final subject's affective pain was better, while the sensory and evaluative pain factors were worse.

Physiologic Changes

It was expected that learned EMG decreases and EEG theta increases would be associated with reduced autonomic responsivity and concomitant pain reduction. Biofeedback-session data were therefore examined to determine whether learning occurred, whether the expected "relaxation response" was observed, and the relationship to pain reduction.

Learning. Three learning criteria were defined: (a) better control of a physiologic variable when feedback was being provided compared to when it was not; (b) better control of EEG/EMG activity during feedback than during EC base line; and (c) a significant rank-order correlation between time in feedback and level of physiologic activity (positive for EEG, negative for EMG). A subject was designated a learner only if two out of three of these criteria were met. Based on this operational definition of learning, two subjects (Nos. 03 and 14) were designated EMG learners; only subject 03 met any of the criteria for learned control of EEG activity.

Autonomic responsivity. Only subjects 03 and 14 met the dual criterion of decreasing autonomic arousal during feedback and lower levels of arousal after feedback. The response was stronger for subject 14, but not significantly so.

Relationship with pain reduction. It was pointed out above that only subjects 03 and 14 showed pain-relief which generalized to the home environment. These two subjects also learned EMG control and showed decreased autonomic responsivity during biofeedback sessions.

Psychophysiologic Battery

Comparisons of pretreatment versus posttreatment changes in the psychophysiology battery focused on two autonomic indicators, heart rate (HR) and skin conductance level (SCL). Because of the great variance among subjects, nonparametric tests were used. Results are shown graphically in Fig. 1. Despite marked increases in SCL during the posttreatment EC base

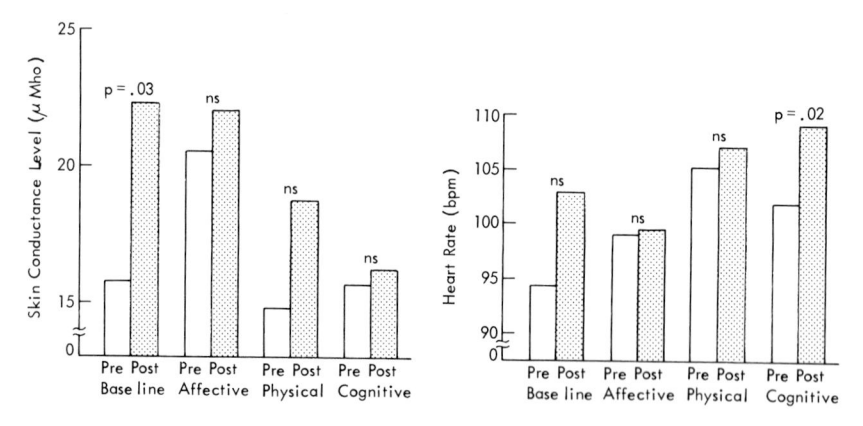

FIG. 1. Skin conductance and heart rate during pre- and posttreatment psychophysiologic batteries for various stress tasks.

line, no significant differences were observed for the affective, physical, or cognitive stress tasks.

DISCUSSION

Significant pain-relief was obtained during biofeedback sessions for all subjects; however, only two of the subjects (29%) were able to generalize this pain-relief to the home environment. These two subjects also were successful in learning EMG control and responded during the biofeedback sessions with decreased autonomic arousal. These results are encouraging in that they partially support the hypothesis being tested, and clearly indicate the importance of further work in the area. Such further work should take into account the complexities of physiologic learning, as well as the difficulties encountered because of the physical state of the subjects.

Conditioning of physiologic parameters is not a simple process. The physiologic variables chosen for conditioning should be closely linked to the disease process(es) itself. In attempting to develop techniques to decrease pain related to cancer, the lack of specific knowledge as to etiology and exacerbation of pain confuses the issue.

From a theoretical standpoint, and on the basis of our previous experience with cancer patients (3) and opiate addicts (4), we expected that simulating the CNS and/or cortical effects of opiates (increased 4 to 10 Hz activity with elevated amplitude) would result in decreased pain. Because of the low levels of physiologic learning observed in the present study, this question remains unanswered. It is possible, however, that the use of lower EEG frequencies as a feedback parameter is not the best choice for pain reduction. Previous research (8) on the production of alpha and theta in normal subjects has frequently reported distortions in time-perception (time-slowing). Such time-distortion associated with low-frequency EEG activity might lead to increased attention to, or perception of, pain because of the perceptual elongation of the sensory and/or reactive components of pain. Alternatively, pain itself might increase the occurrence of cortical responses related to attention or orienting, such as the contingent negative variation (CNV), and increase pain perception. If so, such cortical responses might be subject to deconditioning or extinction. These are speculations, but issues which need to be addressed.

Regardless of the appropriateness of the feedback variables chosen, the low level of learning observed suggests that the biofeedback procedures were not optimal. Because of instrumentation limitations, the feedback procedure was not ideally time-linked to the subject's physiology. Shaping consisted of establishing a set threshold for EEG (decreased by specified degrees) of the immediate dominant frequency emitted during the trial period. Additionally, the most appropriate shaping procedures and reinforcement schedules for the enhancement of theta activity are not known. Progress is being made, however, and systematic controlled experiments are continuing. Appropriate feedback parameters and appropriate conditioning procedures (shaping limits, schedules of reinforcement, etc.), be they operant, classical, or combinations, need to be delineated. Experiments concentrating on the specific sensory or affective components of pain as well as placebo aspects of pain-relief also need to be further examined.

Such experiments are particularly difficult to perform in pain populations suffering from a disease process which is often unpredictable and progressive. Changes in metabolic functioning and other aspects of the disease as well as changes in medical regimens markedly influence pain perception, sensory aspects, ANS and CNS changes, motivation, participation ability, pre-post comparisons, and generalization of treatment effects. Ideally, changes in chemotherapy treatment, other medications, etc., would be controlled experimental variables; however, the patient's health is always foremost, and this degree of control is seldom possible. Such factors should be taken into account in designing future studies of experimental treatment for cancer-related pain.

The work reported here suggested a somewhat different approach to the use of biofeedback techniques for pain reduction. Subjects currently receive biofeedback for both EMG and skin conductance level. Skin conductance level was selected because it is directly related to levels of autonomic arousal. An alternating treatment-base line-treatment design (ABA) with multiple base lines and reduced treatment time is now employed in an attempt to deal with the progressive physical deterioration often associated with cancer. Specific techniques for generalization of pain-relief to the home environment are also included in the protocol.

It is important to note that the cancer-pain patients who entered the current research program had been in continuous pain for 15 months and were in poor psychologic and physiologic health. They had been referred only after other sources of pain management proved unsuccessful. For many of them, biofeedback represented a "treatment of last resort." It is significant that under these circumstances any pain-relief at all was observed. The fact that all patients obtained relief during the sessions and some patients were able to extend this relief to the home environment indicates that biofeedback holds definite promise. Whether the physiologic parameters of choice for conditioning should be cortical, autonomic, or a combination is yet to be determined. The effectiveness of this approach to pain management if applied early in the pain/disease process is also a question of importance. Pain and associated effects such as energy-depletion and suffering are devastating to both the person with cancer and to his or her family. Our efforts are worthwhile so long as there is hope that increasing numbers of patients will experience some freedom from their continuing anguish.

ACKNOWLEDGMENT

This investigation was supported, in part, by Grant No. 5R18 CA17936–03 CCG, awarded by the National Cancer Institute DHEW, and, in part, by Midwest Research Institute. We wish to thank Harvey D. Cohen, Theodore M. Knapp, Susan S. Bond, and Whitney P. Sunderland for their research contributions, and Florence I. Metz for her critical review of the manuscript.

REFERENCES

1. Beatty, J. (1974): Theta feedback, attention, and performance. Paper presented at the Biofeedback Research Society Annual Meeting.
2. Bonica, J. J. (1973): Fundamental considerations of chronic pain therapy. *Postgrad. Med.,* 53:81–85.
3. Fotopoulos, S., Graham, C., and Cook, M. R. (1977): Biofeedback and cancer pain. Unpublished manuscript. Paper presented at the International Symposium on Cancer Pain, Florence, Italy, 1975.
4. Graham, C., Cook, M. R., and Fotopoulos, S. (1976): Studies on the use of bio-

feedback techniques with opiate addicts. Final Report, Contract No. ADM–45–74–139, National Institute on Drug Abuse.
5. Graham, C., Cook, M. R., and Fotopoulos, S. (1976): Studies on the use of biofeedback techniques with opiate addicts. Final Report (Addendum), Contract No. ADM–45–74–139, National Institute on Drug Abuse.
6. Liebeskind, J. C. (1977): Psychological and physiological mechanisms of pain. *Annu. Rev. Psychol.,* 28:41–60.
7. Pos, R. (1974): Psychological assessment of factors affecting pain. *CMA J.,* 111:1213–1215.
8. Stoyva, J., and Budzynski, T. (1974): Cultivated low arousal—An anti-stress response? In: *Limbic and Autonomic Nervous System Research,* edited by L. DiCara, pp. 265–290. Plenum Press, New York.
9. Stoyva, J., Budzynski, T., Sittenfeld, P., and Yaroush, R. (1974): A two-phase biofeedback approach to sleep onset insomnia. Paper presented at the Biofeedback Research Society Annual Meeting.
10. Weitzenhoffer, A. M., and Hilgard, E. R. (1962): *Stanford Hypnotic Susceptibility Scale, Form C.* Consulting Psychological Press, Palo Alto, California.

Psychosocial and Nursing Technique

Ada G. Rogers

Analgesic Studies Section, Sloan-Kettering Institute for Cancer Research, New York, New York 10021

In caring for patients with pain due to advanced cancer, we must consider all the ramifications of the illness. To achieve this goal the most important thing is to communicate with the patient. Developing effective communications will open avenues of good rapport between the patients and those caring for him. Although the physician is primarily responsible for the patient's care, it seems unreasonable to expect him to attend to all aspects of the care of the patient. Part of this responsibility must, by necessity, be transferred to other health-care professionals.

In recent years, it has been recognized that the best care given to the patient has been accomplished through a multidisciplinary team approach. Each discipline has its own specialized techniques that may contribute to the ultimate goal of enabling the patient to function as normally as possible under the circumstances. It should be understood that full cooperation among these specialists is essential to achieve this goal. There are some health-care professionals who may be reluctant to relinquish part of the patient's care to others in fear of losing "control" over the patient. Although not all patients with advanced cancer will require the services of these specialists, these services should always be available to the patients who require them and the patients should be informed of these services.

ROLE OF HEALTH PROFESSIONALS

Although all cancer patients may be depressed and at times may find it difficult to cope with the many aspects of his or her illness, this may not mean he or she will need a psychiatrist. However, there are patients with prior psychiatric problems, patients with suicidal tendencies, patients in an acute psychotic episode due to the aftermath of surgery or medications (e.g., steroids), sudden death of a member of the family, diagnosis of advanced disease, age and pain, who will need crisis intervention. Other situations not so acute may warrant help from the psychiatric service. Unfortunately, in many of these cases, the patient may be reluctant to see a psychiatrist. His reaction may be, "I'm not crazy—why do I *need* a psychiatrist?" In this instance a good rapport with the patient is most essential. An approach, that at times has been successful, has been to indicate to the patient that he or she may need a medication that will help him or her to relax or help his or her depression and the only person who could decide the right kind of medication would be a psychiatrist. The patient may also agree to see a psychiatrist if a member of the staff that he has confidence in will be present at the interviews.

The patient may not be the only one who is having difficulty in communicating and coping with pain of advanced cancer: the family and hospital staff may also be under pressure. In many hospitals, psychiatrists or psychologists have weekly meetings with nurses, social workers, families, and medical staff to enable these members to interact, ventilate their feelings and frustrations, and establish better communication. The feeling should be that all are in this together, and together we can promote better living for the patients, their families, and the health team.

The role of the psychologist parallels that of the psychiatrist except that the psychologist may be interested in gaining more information about the patient, family, and other members of the team through the use of psychologic testing and studies. Some of the tests used are the Rorschach Test (2), the Minnesota Multiphasic Personality Inventory (MMPI) (8), Symptom Check List (SCL-90) (6), Verbal Rating Scale and the Visual Analogue Scale (10) to name a few.

For some time the social service worker's role has been in the area of specific social problems that relate to relationships within the family, parent-child tensions, personal relationships outside the family, household management, health care, use of community resources, and public relief if needed (7). Social service workers have meetings with family members on a one-to-one basis or in groups. Many have teamed up with nurses, physical therapists, and physicians on a weekly basis to discuss various problems. Some social service workers have meetings with patients and families to discuss discharge planning. They have been involved in the education of other social service workers by conducting programs and institutes.

The social service worker is responsible for investigating and planning for financial aid, assistance with employment problems, nursing services outside the hospital, such as nursing homes or terminal care facilities, visiting nurse service, private-duty nursing in the home, transportation, equipment, household help, and self-help groups. The patient should be encouraged to utilize the services of the social worker and contact should be made with them as early as possible during the course of the patient's illness. This may help to eliminate or minimize some of the anxieties that may arise from certain types of problems. One patient tried to commit suicide because she did not want her husband to mortgage their house in order to pay for her many hospitalizations. Another dying patient was concerned about her mentally retarded daughter and who would care for her. In both cases, the social service worker was able to find solutions to these problems.

REHABILITATION PROGRAMS FOR CANCER PATIENTS

Rehabilitation programs involve the physical therapist, occupational therapist, speech therapist, and volunteer, as well as the social service worker, nurse, and physician. The programs available in many comprehensive cancer centers include: (a) *Laryngectomee:* Members of the International Association of Laryngectomees, who teach these patients esophogeal speech and/or use of the electro-larynx. Speech therapists have had an effective role with patients with facial paralysis and/or partial removal of any of the oral articulators. (b) *Mastectomy—Reach to Recovery Programs:* These are intended to aid women who have had surgery for breast cancer to adjust psychologically and physiologically. (c) *Ostomy Program:* This program was designed to assist the colostomy and urinary ostomy patients, but now includes ileostomy. The program includes training of enterostomal therapists (ET), a new category of allied health professionals. Since 1970, 500 ETs have been trained. The training takes 6 weeks, and these therapists are prepared to assist in the total rehabilitation of ostomates (1). In most hospitals ostomy care is provided by registered nurses.

A new program established at Memorial Sloan-Kettering Cancer Center is a preoperative teaching program for the thoracotomy patient. This involves a nurse, a social worker, and a physical therapist. Its purpose is to teach perioperative care regimes and to emphasize the importance of these regimes by explaining the underlying physiologic rationale to the patient and the family.

Physical therapists are involved in the rehabilitation of all types of patients, pre- and post-surgery, in ambulation, which includes the proper way to move and turn, get out of bed into a chair, use a walker, adjust properly to crutches and prosthesis, and in passive and active exercises. These techniques are also useful in patients with muscle-wasting and pain. Some patients may need an overhead trapeze to facilitate moving in bed. Patients have to be taught how to breathe and cough to avoid pulmonary complications at any time during their illness. Today, in many hospitals, this function is conducted by respiratory therapist.

Occupational therapists can help the patient by teaching and aiding in the recovery of patients through interesting occupations and pastimes. The idea behind occupational therapy dates back to Galen (7) who said "Employment is nature's best medicine and essential to human happiness." Many occupational therapists have artistic and creative abilities, and they are able to teach patients how to knit, crochet, sew, paint, and how to do ceramics, wood-carving, metalwork, weaving, etc. The occupational therapist may teach the patient who has lost an upper extremity the use of the other arm and hand in eating, dressing himself, and writing. If a hospital does not have occupational therapists, these activities may fall under the direction of the Recreational Department.

SOCIAL ACTIVITIES

Patients are encouraged to participate in any social activity that is available in the hospital or in their communities. These are techniques that are used to distract the patient, diminish the feeling of isolation and, in general, help him back into a social setting. Many hospitals have hours set for movies, bingo, Las Vegas nights, and live entertainment performed by well-known artists. Women patients always feel better if they can get their hair washed, cut, and set. These services should be provided for both men and women.

In a long hospitalization, a day or weekend pass perhaps will help to decrease the feeling of isolation that so often is a part of depression and hostility. This is especially true during holidays, when all family members will be missed. Patients with small children are particularly affected. If a pass is not feasible, arrangements should be made to allow children under-age to see their parents. Brown (3) has said, "To deprive a mother or father when sick of even a glimpse of what may be most dear and important in life runs counter to the current philosophy of the therapeutic value of meeting patients' psychological needs. To prevent a child from seeing his parents . . . to whom he is psychologically tied, may do him severe damage."

DIETARY ASPECTS

In some cancer patients and their families, eating is synonymous with survival. Unfortunately, many aspects of the patient's illness and treatment may inhibit the patient's ability to eat, as in cases of nausea, vomiting, intestinal obstruction, esophagitis, stomatitis, and loss of appetite. The dieticians, or as they now are called "nutritionists," play an important role. Patients may be on special diets, have food allergies, religious restrictions, and at certain times certain foods may not appeal to them.

Although this may not be the best way, patients usually are given menus to fill out a few days ahead, and the set hours for the delivery of the meals may not be at the time that the patient is hungry. Unfortunately, the routine of most hospitals demands this. However, there are times when the dietician may be able to substitute something more suitable for the patient or the patient's tray may be held for a short period of time. At Memorial Sloan-Kettering Cancer Center, a new computerized system is being considered whereby the patient will be able to select the meals for the day in the same morning. In some hospitals, a dining room facility is provided for patients on each floor, and this allows ambulatory patients to eat and socialize in a more congenial fashion. When a patient's intake decreases, i.v. feedings can be substituted, or in patients with consistent weight loss and/or malabsorption, total parenteral nutrition (TPN) can be started. In some cases, patients may have to be discharged on TPN. Patients are taught how to mix the formula and how to care for the equipment.

ROLE OF THE CLERGY

In recent years, the clergy has been taking a more active role as members of the group of counseling services. Their education has been expanded to include all aspects of the patient's care. Priests, ministers, and rabbis are members of hospital committees, group therapy programs, as well as being involved in educational symposia and workshops. Their input is an important part of the team approach. There are some religious beliefs that are based on superstition rather than doctrine, and these beliefs may be detrimental to the patient who is ill. The clergy may be helpful in changing these misconceptions. The religious patient may feel that his or her church representative is the only person whom he or she can communicate with, who will understand about his or her suffering, or whom he or she will talk to about death and dying. The clergy have had to reexamine their own feelings about death and dying, and as one minister reminded us, even Jesus Christ said as he was dying on the cross, "Oh Father, why have you forsaken me?"

ROLE OF VOLUNTEERS

Volunteers have always been important in time of need and illness. Some volunteers get close to the patients; others prefer to be behind the scenes. In times of disasters such as blackouts, snowstorms, and strikes, it is the volunteers who will replace many of the employees who are unable to get to work. Many volunteers are also former patients and are used in self-help modality in patient-visitors programs.

A "self-help" group can be defined as a group of people sharing common needs and experiences who organize action-oriented programs to help others with the same problems, usually because traditional systems cannot meet their needs. Cancer patients commonly report that almost immediately following their diagnosis a wall of silence begins to grow between them and their families, friends, clergy, and physicians with whom they had shared their anxieties, fears, and concerns. With the progression of the disease and its complications, all communications may stop. Members of the self-help group may be able to break down these barriers by sharing mutual experiences. The visitor—former patient is a vivid demonstration that life goes on in the face of death. The visual impact of the socially active visitor restores the patient's confidence in his or her ability to cope with the continuing trauma of cancer. At some comprehensive cancer centers, this type of volunteer has helped the patient to realize that his pain can be controlled, by informing the patient that there is a group available to deal with pain problems.

VISITORS

Visitors are welcomed by family members. The family can express fears, misunderstandings, or distorted communications, and may ask questions that they would be reluctant to impose on the patient, the nurses, or the physician. Professional resistance to using lay counselors has been a major impediment to the success of self-help programs. Resistance stems from the lack of volunteer accountability and supervision, and the failure to seek direct professional intervention when necessary. Professional health-care givers may fear that this group will either deliberately or unwittingly damage the relationship between the patient and the health-care professionals. Granting lay persons access to patients implies approval, and many professionals may feel that volunteers are not adequately educated or supervised (9).

THE ROLE OF THE NURSE

Traditionally, the nurse has been the liaison between the patient and the physician. She not only spends more time with the patient, but she is administering to many of the patient's basic needs. If the patient has confidence in the nurse, he will likely relate his problems to her. When the problem is understood, then the nurse can be instrumental in applying, obtaining, or suggesting the appropriate means of dealing with the problem. Unfortunately, for many years nursing care has been fragmented because of the team approach. Instead of having a nurse responsible for the patient's total basic care, the care was administered by dividing the responsibility so that there was a medication nurse, a treatment-room nurse, an i.v. nurse, and other specialized nursing duties. This system confused the patient; the patient did not know whom to ask for what and this contributed to delay, duplication of effort, and inefficiency.

Today, the primary care approach is being started in many hospitals, but in one institution in New York, it has been in effect since 1969 (4). Their philosophy of nursing is based upon the thesis that the relationships among the human beings who are members of the health team are, at all times, dynamic and collaborative and not limited by the walls of the hospital temporarily surrounding the patients. The members of the team are the patient, his or her family, nurses, doctors, social workers, and other members of the hospital organization. The end result sought by the members of the team is the attainment of a satisfactory resolution of the patient's health problem. In order to implement this philosophy, it is essential that the primary nursing model be the structure within which the nursing process takes place. Moreover, nurses must be free from involvement with nonnursing functions, which should be the responsibility of Unit Service Management. Human beings have inalienable rights to be respected at all times and to pursue happiness, and the nurse has a major role in assisting the patient in the attainment of these rights.

In this milieu the nursing process is defined simply as the sum of the activities jointly performed by the patient and the nurse. The sum of these activities can be divided into a three-part problem-solving approach: (a) assessment (includes nursing history and nursing diagnosis); (b) intervention (includes nursing orders and nursing care plan); and (c) evaluation (includes nursing prognosis) (5). Moreover, the special sheet for nurses' notes has been eliminated, and instead, along with other members of the health team, the nurses chart their observations in the progress sheets. This chronologic data gathered by all who are caring for the patient can be used by them in assessing the patient's problems and tailoring their care to fulfill the patient's needs.

Nursing History

The nursing history is obtained by the nurse who is admitting the patient, and she greets, orients, and interviews the patient and his family. Certain prerequisite information such as vital signs, dentures, allergies, diet, and medication are specifically elicited. Additional information includes the nurse's observation of the physical status of the patient, his reaction to his illness and the hospital, his social, occupational, and educational history, recreational activities, and additional pertinent information. These data are based on the nurse's knowledge of human behavior in health and sickness. The process of diagnosis is identification of the patient's needs in order to begin a plan of nursing care. The nursing history is included in and becomes a part of the patient's permanent record.

Nurses Order Sheet

The Nurses Order Sheet, also known as the Nursing Care Plan, is inserted in the Doctor's Order Book, and it becomes a part of the patient's chart. Orders are written by the nurse who admitted the patient, and these orders are followed by the nurses on all other shifts. This ensures continuity of care. Orders are written according to the problems identified on a Master Problem List (5). Some orders for a patient with advanced lung cancer and pain may read:

1. *Problem of depression*
   a. Elicit the patient's and family's understanding of the reason for this hospitalization.
   b. Encourage verbalization.
   c. Explain any diagnostic procedures that have been ordered.
   d. Obtain any available information about proposed definitive therapy and review with patient.
2. *Relief of pain*
   a. Assessment of the patient's pain, onset, site, character, what makes it worse or better.
   b. Assessment of analgesics, prior to admission.

      c. Explain to patient PRN orders, time interval, route of administration, name of drug.
      d. Medicate patient for relief of pain as per M.D. and assess the effectiveness of medication, onset of action, degree of relief, duration of effect, side effects (11).
3. *Discharge planning*
      a. Refer patient to social service worker (this should be done early in patient's care).
      b. Discuss family situation and home environment.
4. *Immediate care*
      a. Demonstrate and encourage the patient to practice techniques for coughing and deep breathing.
      b. Explain machines that may be used for pulmonary problem.
      c. Explain the role of the respiratory therapist.
      d. Check intake and output.
      e. Constipation should be avoided. Make sure orders are written for stool softness, laxatives, and/or enema.
      f. Health teaching about diet and medication other than analgesics.

These orders are transcribed onto the Kardex just as doctors' orders are transcribed by the unit receptionist. The Kardex is kept in pencil and as nursing orders change, the Kardex is changed, but there is always a permanent record of nursing intervention on the patient's nursing order sheet.

Centers with this type of philosophy and services by nurses usually have lists of nurse specialists available for consultation. Unfortunately, in most institutions the list does not include a nurse who can be consulted for pain problems.

The above primary care approach will enable the nurse to become better acquainted with the patient and the patient's needs. It will give the patient a feeling of security, a feeling that someone really cares about all of him, and he will be able to relate to the nurse. These nurses will be reliable and trustworthy, and the genuine interest will inspire confidence.

Regardless of the kind of nursing-care approach used, the nurse must apply psychologic, biologic, and social knowledge to the understanding of the individual as a member of a family and of a specific social group. The nurse must examine her unconscious as well as conscious motivation, prejudices, and objective and subjective reasons for her feelings and behavior toward a particular patient. Every bit of information is important. The nurse has preconceived attitudes and misconceptions learned through education and experience, and she can not assume that her attitude is correct. She should refrain from imposing these judgments on the patient. Accusatory questions or those with hostile implications arouse fear, suspicion, or anger and do not inspire confidence. This is particularly true of the patient who has pain due to cancer. The patient needs to know that the nurse believes he has pain and that she will do something about it. There should be a mutual feeling of confidence, trust, respect, and empathy. The nurse may use gestures to enhance such optimal relationships by holding the patient's hand or stroking the forehead. She should use sympathetic facial expressions, her voice should have a warm tone and quality, and she should use words of encouragement and avoid arguing. Patients often find pep talks to be depressing and patronizing. Schedules of physical activity must be planned with common sense. Patients may be unable to reach goals set by the nursing team, and this causes mutual frustration. The nurse can be most effective when she recognizes that her role and the role of other health-care givers is to help the patient understand his or her life processes so that he or she can better control and cope with the illness (5). Our guidelines should be: Stop, look, and above all, listen.

ACKNOWLEDGMENTS

Supported in part by grants awarded by the National Institute on Drug Abuse (DA 01707–02).

I wish to thank Miss Julie Franchi and Mr. George Heidrich, R.N., B.S.N., for their assistance in the literature search and Miss Natalie M. Rogers for her assistance in the preparation of the manuscript.

REFERENCES

1. American Cancer Society (1978): *Cancer Facts and Figures.* American Cancer Society, New York.
2. Beck, S. J. (1949): *Rorschach Test,* Vols. I, II, and III. Grune & Stratton, New York.
3. Brown, E. L. (1961): *Newer Dimensions of Patient Care,* Part I, pp. 64–84. Russell Sage Foundation, New York.
4. Carlson, S. (1969): An experiment in self-determined patient care. *Nurs. Clin. North Am.,* 4(3):495–506.
5. Carlson, S. (1972): A practical approach to the nursing process. *Am. J. Nurs.,* 72(9):1589–1591.
6. Derogatis, L. R. (1976): The SLC-90 and the MMPI: A step in the validation of a new self-report scale. *Br. J. Psychiatry,* 128:280–289.
7. Hardy, R. E., and Cull, J. G. (1975): *Counseling and Rehabilitating the Cancer Patient, No. 964: American Lecture Series.* Charles C Thomas, Springfield, Ill.
8. Hathaway, S. R., and McKinley, J. C. (1951): *The Minnesota Multiphasic Personality Inventory,* Rev. ed. Psychological Corporation, New York.
9. Mantell, J. E. (1976): Social work and self-help group. *Health and Social Work,* 1(1):86–100.
10. Ohnhaus, E. E., and Adler, R. (1975): Methodological problems in the measurement of pain: A comparison between the Verbal Rating Scale and the Visual Analogue Scale. *Pain,* 1(4):379–384.
11. Rogers, A. (1977): *Drugs for Pain: Proceedings of the Second Nursing Conference on Cancer Nursing,* pp. 39–43. American Cancer Society, New York.

Nonnarcotic Analgesics

H. U. Gerbershagen

Institut für Anaesthesiologie, Klinikum, Johannes Gutenberg-Universität Mainz Postfach 3960, Langenbeckstrasse 1, 6500 Mainz, West Germany

This chapter will discuss the role of nonnarcotic analgesics in the management of cancer pain. First, some factors important to drug treatment have to be considered.

BASIC CONSIDERATIONS

In considering the use of drugs for cancer pain it is essential to appreciate the placebo effect. Clinical studies show that a placebo drug will be effective in pain in some 30 to 40% of patients (1,4,5). It is our experience that in cancer pain this effectivity is reduced to some 20% and that the effect is limited to a period of 2 to 3 weeks. Moreover, it is necessary to appreciate that outpatients will take not only the prescribed drugs, but also other medication.

The aim of responsible treatment for physicians and patients alike is the reduction of pain to a tolerable degree. Painlessness or complete freedom from pain is difficult and in some patients impossible to achieve with current therapeutic modalities. Narcotic drugs, including morphine and its derivatives will produce ample pain-relief only in about 75 to 80% of patients, provided that large doses are administered.

Stage of disease. In cancer pain the stage of the neoplastic disease plays an important role. Nevertheless, the psychophysiology of pain is such that the physician cannot adopt the view that terminal cancer pain is more severe than that of the earlier stages. At the same time there is no basis for assuming that a severe pain necessarily demands a narcotic analgesic. The quality, the type, and localization of pain and the attendant circumstances often matter most. Many patients with advanced cancer can be managed by nonnarcotic analgesics.

Mental state of the patient. The psychologic, emotional, and behavioral aspects of pain and the reactions to pain have been reviewed and emphasized by Bond and Chapman (*this volume*). It is important to adopt a qualitative rather than a quantitative viewpoint in such a complex psychophysiologic problem as cancer pain.

PHARMACOLOGIC CONSIDERATIONS

For the rational use of nonnarcotic analgesics an understanding of the basic principles of drug action and a knowledge of the pharmacologic effects are essential. Nonnarcotic analgesics constitute a heterogeneous group of substances with divergent chemical structures and various pharmacologic actions.

Nonnarcotic analgesics most often are derivatives of salicylic acid, p-aminophenol, pyrazolone, dioxopyrazolidine, indole, anthranylic acid, phenylpropionic acid, malonic acid, and nicotinic acid.

In addition to their analgesic property, p-aminophenol, pyrazolone, and salicylic acid derivates display a central nervous system (CNS)–mediated antipyretic effect. Pyrazolone, indole, anthranylic and phenylpropionic acid

TABLE 1. *The main effects of nonnarcotic analgesics*

	Analgesic[a]	Antipyretic	Anti-inflammatory	Adverse
Acetylsalicylic acid	++	++	++	++
Paracetamol	++	++	0	+
Metamizol	+++	+++	+++	+
Phenylbutazone	+	++	+++	+++
Indomethacin	++	+++	++	+++
Mefenamic acid	++	++	++	++
Ibuprofen	++	++	+	+
Naproxen	+	+++	++	+
Nefopam	+++	0	0	+

Legend: +++ = high; ++ = medium; + = low; 0 = none.
[a] In cancer pain.

derivates, and salicylates are potent anti-inflammatory agents as well (Table 1).

Salicylates

Salicylates in particular reduce pain arising from muscles, ligaments, tendons, and bone. Visceral pain is usually said to be poorly influenced (23). In my experience, pain of pancreatic neoplasms is often partially, and in a few instances, completely controlled for weeks and months.

Acetylsalicylic acid is the most frequently used drug of the salicylate group. Numerous alternative compounds have been synthesized in the hope of obtaining a more rapid onset, greater peak analgesic action, prolonged duration of analgesia, and a reduced incidence of side effects. No study has proved the superiority of these compounds.

Soluble, buffered, enteric-coated, and sustained-release acetylsalicylic acid formations have been introduced, but it has not been possible to demonstrate improved analgesic activity or reduced adverse effects. *Injectable* acetylsalicylic acid should be thought of if the patient is already receiving intravenous nutrition or other drugs. *Salicylamide* contained in many analgesic mixtures has no proven analgesic effect.

Para-aminophenol Derivates

Phenacetin and one of its metabolites, paracetamol (N-acetyl-*p*-aminophenol), are equieffective alternatives to aspirin (21). The para-aminophenols can relieve moderate pain arising from integumental and musculoskeletal structures (9).

Many reports have linked chronic consumption of phenacetin-containing drugs with renal papillary necrosis and renal cancer (22). Well-controlled studies are lacking. Nevertheless many countries prohibit the use of phenacetin. Paracetamol does not cause nephropathy and gastrointestinal hemorrhage. It has the advantage of producing less gastric irritation than acetylsalicylic acid and is a good alternative to acetylsalicylic acid in spite of its lacking anti-inflammatory activity.

Pyrazolone and Dioxopyrazolidine Derivates (20)

Aminophenazon (aminopyrine), *noramido-pyrinmethansulfonate-sodium* (metamizol), and *phenylbutazone* are the commonly used drugs of this group (14,15). Aminophenazone can induce fatal agranulocytosis and will form dimethyl-nitrosamine, a very potent cancerogenic, in the stomach and should therefore no longer be administered (3).

Metamizol, a good analgesic and smooth muscle relaxant fell into disrepute because of poorly controlled reports by Discombe (3) and Huguley (11,12) in which they stated that a high incidence (0.5 to 1%) of agranulocytosis is associated with its use. Worldwide surveys show that agranulocytosis may be induced in some 0.001% of cases (10). There is no nitrosamine formation by this drug. Metamizol can be administered orally, intramuscularly, and intravenously.

Phenylbutazone is a drug for muscle and skeletal pain. Because of its frequent and marked side-effects, it should only be used for periods up to 8 days. *Oxyphenbutazone,* a metabolite of phenylbutazone, should also only be used for severe pain states.

Indole, Anthranylic Acid and Phenylpropionic Acid Derivates

The compounds of these groups are about as potent as the groups already mentioned. We feel that they are especially advantageous because they allow a frequent rotation to different analgesic groups. For the past 10 years we have rotated nonnarcotic analgesics every 6 to 8 weeks in order to reduce side effects and abuse liability. In spite of employing larger doses in moderate and severe cancer pain than usually recommended, we have never observed any serious side effects.

Nefopam

Nefopam, a benzoxacine derivate, is a centrally acting, nonnarcotic analgesic and has no antipyretic and anti-inflammatory effects (8). It is approximately one-third as potent as morphine in its parenteral application form. This drug has a mild cardiovascular stimulating action. Respiratory mechanics and pulmonary gas exchange are not influenced (7). This compound, like most nonnarcotic analgesics, does not cause mood alterations or sedation, so that in cancer pain the simultaneous administration of a neuroleptic drug is advisable. Nefopam should not be given with paracetamol because of possible drug interaction causing hepatotoxicity.

ADVERSE EFFECTS OF NONNARCOTIC ANALGESICS

The adverse effects, listed in Table 2, are very similar with all groups, differing only in degree and frequency. Provided that the contraindications (Table 3) and drug-rotation scheme are considered, adverse side effects are infrequent and mild with all compounds.

TABLE 2. *Adverse effects of nonnarcotic analgesics*

Derivates of	Adverse side effects
Salicylic acid	Damage to gastrointestinal tract (bleeding, ulceration), allergic reactions (skin rash, angioedema, asthma)
p-Aminophenol	Methemoglobinemia, hemolytic anemia, nephrotoxicity, headache
Pyrazolon	Skin rash, leukopenia, agranulocytosis (0.001%)
Pyrazolidine	Gastrointestinal bleeding and ulcer, leukopenia, agranulocytosis, renal-function disturbances (sodium and water retention), dizziness, headache
Indole	Gastrointestinal bleeding and ulcer, fatigue, mental confusion, depression
Anthranylic acid	Diarrhea, gastrointestinal bleeding, allergy, fatigue
Phenylpropionic acid, phenylformic acid	Gastrointestinal disturbance, ulcer
Malonic acid	Gastrointestinal disturbance, skin rash
Benzoxacine	Sweating

TABLE 3. Contraindications for nonnarcotic analgesics

Derivates of	Contraindications
Salicylic acid	History of gastrointestinal ulcers
p-Aminophenol	Anemia, liver disease, severe pulmonary disease
Pyrazol, pyrazolidine	History of gastrointestinal ulcers, myocardial insufficiency, reduced renal function, porphyria, granulocytopenia
Indole	Parkinsonism, epilepsy, psychosis
Anthranylic acid	History of gastrointestinal ulcers
Benzoxacine	Elevated pulmonary-artery pressure

SITE AND MODE OF ACTION OF NONNARCOTIC ANALGESICS

Several hypotheses have been advanced to explain the actions of nonnarcotic and nonsteroid anti-inflammatory agents. These include stabilization of lyosomal membranes (13), inhibition of lyosomal enzymes (13,19), hyperpolarization of neuronal membranes (16), the displacement of an endogenous anti-inflammatory peptide from plasma protein (17,18), interference with the migration of leukocytes (2), and interference with phosphorylation (24). One of several possible modes of action is the inhibition of the biosynthesis of prostaglandins and precursors and similar substances in inflamed and traumatized tissues (6,19). Thus, the prevention of prostaglandin release reduces or prevents the sensitization of pain receptors to nociceptive stimuli. There is also the possibility that acetylsalicylic acid and p-aminophenols involve central mechanisms. Nefopam acts on CNS pain mechanisms (26).

EFFICACY OF NONNARCOTIC ANALGESICS

The analgesic efficacy of nonnarcotic analgesics is usually underrated. This may partly be due to the general availability, the general use in mild discomforts, and low susceptibility of experimental pain, and numerous papers published by pharmacologists not involved in patient-care. Unfortunately, the various groups have been defined as weak or minor analgesics for several decades. The nonnarcotic analgesics are potent analgesics if dose-effect relationships are considered. Most often it is ineffective to treat cancer pain, for instance, with single doses of 200 to 500 mg of acetylsalicylic acid.

Nonnarcotic analgesics must be administered in larger doses than usually prescribed. Table 4 gives the dosage required to achieve effective concentrations at their site of action. This brings up the problem of analgesic mixtures. Analgesic mixtures have been compounded in the belief that a synergistic or better-than-additive effect could be obtained, and that adverse effects could be reduced. There is no proven synergistic potency, and the side effects are

TABLE 4. *Effective doses of nonnarcotic analgesics for control of cancer pain*

Generic name	Dose (mg)	Interval of administration during day
Acetylsalicylic acid	750–1250	q. 3 hr
Salicylamide	750–1000	q. 3 hr
Phenacetin	400–600	q. 3 hr
Paracetamol	600–800	q. 3 hr
Acetylaminosalol	400–800	q. 3 hr
Phenazon	500–1000	q. 3 hr
Propyphenazon	450–800	q. 3 hr
4-Aminophenazon	450–800	q. 3 hr
Aminophenazon	450–800	q. 3 hr
Noramidopyrin methansulfonate-sodium (metamizol)	750–1000	q. 3 hr
Mofebutazon		
monophenylbutazon	200–400	q. 4 hr
phenylbutazon	200–400	q. 4 hr
oxyphenbutazone	100–200	q. 4 hr
Mefenamic acid	500	q. 3 hr
Flufenamic acid	200	q. 4 hr
Indomethacin	50–75	q. 4 hr
Benzydamin	100	q. 4 hr
Ibufenac		q. 4 hr
Ibuprofen	200–400	q. 3 hr
Naproxen	250–500	q. 3–4 hr
Niflumic acid	250–500	q. 3–4 hr
Bumadizon	220	q. 4 hr
Alclofenac	500–1000	q. 4 hr
Nefopam	60–120	q. 3 hr

not lessened. They are only different and therefore more dangerous. Owing to drug interactions between nonsteroid anti-inflammatory agents (19) the effectiveness might even be reduced. There are only few analgesic mixtures that contain adequate dosage of analgesics. Therefore, individual drugs should be administered.

Reasonable mixtures of analgesics might contain an analgesic with a chiefly peripheral action and an analgesic with a central site of action, e.g., acetylsalicylic acid plus nefopam or dextropropoxyphene. In most instances the full dose of each drug must be given.

Caffeine, local anesthetics, vitamins, barbiturates, and many other ingredients of compounded analgesic drugs do not increase the analgesic potency (9). Vitamins, in particular, have no potentiating effect and are not analgesics. Perhaps, it may be assumed that the placebo effect of vitamin-containing drugs is slightly greater than with other mixtures. Barbiturates, tranquilizers, and neuroleptics are usually contained in doses which are insufficiently large to produce a clinical effect. However, the dosage is sufficient to induce dependence, and since these compounded drugs are ineffective and also produce side effects, they should *not* be prescribed. If sedative, anxiolytic, or mood-elevating effects are desired, they can be achieved by using an adequate dosage of sedative or psychotropic drug. Drugs containing barbiturates, phenacetin, or ergotamine may induce pain, for instance, headache (25).

In treating cancer pain it is important to differentiate between pain caused by tumor infiltration, by metastatic disease, by complications of cancer therapy, and by problems unrelated to cancer (see Foley, *this volume*). Thus, it is often realized that positive feedback mechanisms, causing motor and sympathetic nervous system hyperactivity, are active. The reflex sympathetic disturbances are often amenable to nonsteroid anti-inflammatory agents and neuroleptic drugs. The painful reflex muscular hypertonicity can be controlled with nonnarcotic analgesics and centrally acting muscle relaxants, such as orphenadrine citrate or chlormezanon.

Antipyretic anti-inflammatory analgesics (with the exception of metamizol) relieve pain of visceral spasm poorly. Therefore, smooth muscle relaxants, e.g., butopromide, should simultaneously be given.

Most nonnarcotic analgesics do not cause subjective effects and do not influence psychoreactive processes of pain. Therefore, it has been our policy for the past decade to simultaneously give nonnarcotic analgesics and neuroleptics. In the treatment of cancer pain only low doses of neuroleptics, far below the so-called "neuroleptic threshold," are required. Some 15 to 20% of our cancer-pain patients, managed with nonnarcotic analgesics and neuroleptics also need small doses of a tricyclic antidepressant. This drug combination often delays the usage of narcotic analgesics.

The timing of drug administration is important. Most nonnarcotic analgesics have an effective duration of some 3 to 5 hr. Therefore, they are regularly given at 3-hr intervals. In cancer patients the pharmacologic considerations are as important as behavioral aspects.

Drug treatment of cancer pain, at any stage of the disease, should begin with nonnarcotic analgesics and neuroleptics. Therapy has to provide ample pain-relief; the patient should be comfortable. If this aim is not achieved by the treatment outlined, narcotic analgesics have to be administered without delay.

REFERENCES

1. Beecher, H. K. (1970): *Research and the Individual Human Studies.* Oxford Press, New York.
2. Di Rosa, M., Papadimitriou, J. M., and Willoughby, D. A. (1971): A histopathological and pharmacological analysis of the mode of action of nonsteroidal anti-inflammatory drugs. *J. Pathol.,* 105:239–256.

3. Discombe, G. (1952): Agranulocytosis caused by aminopyrine. *Br. Med. J.,* 1:1270.
4. Evans, F. J. (1974): The placebo response in pain reduction. *Adv. Neurol.,* 4:289–296.
5. Feather, B. W., Chapman, C. R., and Fisher, S. B. (1972): The effect of a placebo on the perception of painful radiant heat stimuli. *Psychosom. Med.,* 34:290–294.
6. Ferreira, S. H., and Vane, J. R. (1974): New aspects of the mode of action of nonsteroid anti-inflammatory drugs. *Annu. Rev. Pharmacol.,* 14:57–73.
7. Gerbershagen, H. U., and Schaffner, E. (1978): Das Verhalten der Atmung nach intravenöser Verabreichung von Nefopam-HCl und Pentazocin bei Lungengesunden. In: *Nefopam, ein potentes Analgetikum,* edited by H. U. Gerbershagen and G. E. Cronheim. Fischer, Stuttgart, New York.
8. Gerbershagen, H. U., and Cronheim, G. E. (editors) (1978): *Nefopam, ein potentes Analgetikum.* Fischer, Stuttgart, New York.
9. Goodman, L. S., and Gilman, A. (1975): *The Pharmacological Basis of Therapeutics.* Macmillan, New York.
10. Hoechst, Comp. (1977): *Dipyron, eine Übersicht 1977.* Fa. Hoechst AG, Frankfurt (Main).
11. Huguley, C. M. (1964): Agranulocytosis induced by dipyrone, a hazardous antipyretic and analgesic. *JAMA,* 189:938–941.
12. Huguley, C. M. (1964): Drug-induced blood dyscrasias. *JAMA,* 188:817–818.
13. Ignarro, J. L., and Colombo, C. (1972): Enzyme release from guinea-pig polymorphonuclear leucocyte lysosomes inhibited *in vitro* by anti-inflammatory drugs. *Nature New Biol.,* 239:155–157.
14. Krohs, W., Hensel, O. (1961): *Pyrazolone und Dioxopyrazolidine.* Edito Cantor, Aulendorf, Württ.
15. Krohs, W. (1965): Pyrazole derivates. In: *Analgesics,* edited by G. de Stevens. Academic Press, New York.
16. Levitan, H., and Barker, J. L. (1972): Effect of non-narcotic analgesics on membrane permeability of molluscan neurones. *Nature New Biol.,* 239:55–57.
17. McArthur, J. N., Dawkins, P. D., Smith, M. J. H., and Hamilton, E. B. D. (1971): Mode of action of antirheumatic drugs. *Br. Med. J.,* 2:677–679.
18. McArthur, J. N., Dawkins, P. D., and Smith, M. J. H. (1971): The displacement of L-tryptophan and dipeptides from bovine albumin *in vitro* and from human plasma *in vivo* by antirheumatic drugs. *J. Pharm. Pharmacol.,* 23:393–398.
19. Paulus, H. E., and Whitehouse, M. W. (1973): Nonsteroid anti-inflammatory agents. *Annu. Rev. Pharmacol.,* 13:107–125.
20. Roth, H. J. (1978): Pyrazolone und Nitrosamine. *Pharmaz. Z.,* 123:625–633.
21. Shelley, J. H. (1967): Phenacetin, through the looking glass. *Clin. Pharmacol. Ther.,* 8:427–471.
22. Smith, P. K. (1958): *Acetophenetidin: A Critical Bibliographic Review.* Interscience Publ., New York.
23. Smith, M. J. H. (1967): *The Salicylates.* Wyley, London.
24. Whitehouse, M. W., and Haslam, J. M. (1962): Ability of some antirheumatic drugs to uncouple oxidative phosphorylation. *Nature,* 196:1323–1324.
25. Wörz, R., Baar, H., Draf, W., Gerbershagen, H. U., Gross, D., Magin, F., Ritter, K., Scheifele, J., and Scholl, W. (1975): Kopfschmerz in Abhängigkeit von Analgetika-Mischpräparaten. *Münchn. Med. Wschr.* 117:457–462.
26. Zimmermann, M. (1978): Neurophysiologische Untersuchungen über einen spinalen Wirkungsort von Nefopam. In: *Nefopam, ein potentes Analgetikum,* edited by H. U. Gerbershagen and G. E. Cronheim. Fischer, Stuttgart, New York.

Systemic Analgesics and Related Drugs: Narcotic Analgesics

Raymond W. Houde

Department of Medicine, Memorial Sloan-Kettering Cancer Center, New York, New York 10021

NARCOTIC ANALGESICS

The narcotic analgesics are, without doubt, the most efficacious of the drugs employed for the relief of intractable pain and suffering due to advanced or terminal cancer. The narcotics have long been recognized to be singularly capable of modifying both the perception of, and reaction to, pain, as well as of inducing a sense of calm indifference to other physical and psychologic stresses not uncommonly experienced by the dying patient and the patient with cancer (12,20). Ironically, the capacity to induce a sense of well-being, or euphoria, is a property of the narcotics which we have been making a great effort to eliminate from the so-called "ideal analgesic" of our aspirations (1). This unfortunate paradox has been the result of an association of euphoria with drug abuse and with the popular misconception that drugs with this capability enslave, demoralize, and lead the unwitting patient down the primrose path to addiction (16).

There has, in fact, been a trend to substitute the term *addictive analgesics* (5) as a more specific designation for what we have traditionally called the *narcotic analgesics*. For the purpose of this presentation, however, we shall adhere to the older term. The drugs about which we shall be speaking are morphine and its surrogates, and their agonist-antagonist congeners, which have been employed for the treatment of pain due to cancer.

INDICATIONS

The major indication for the administration of a narcotic is severe or intractable pain. Customarily, the narcotics are not administered for chronic pain, even in advanced cancer, unless the milder, simple analgesics have been found wanting in being able to relieve the patient of suffering. There are times, however, when we should resort directly to narcotics, for not all pain due to cancer is the same, and it is better to be governed by the demands of the particular clinical situation than by dogma.

Like the mild analgesics, the narcotics are generally readily available and require no special facilities or technical skills to administer them. Because they act centrally to relieve pain, the effects of narcotics are less likely to be influenced by the site or source of pain—which may be an important consideration in a patient with widely disseminated cancer. Not infrequently, the effects of narcotics will also relieve suffering from other causes than pain (8).

Most narcotic analgesics can be given by any of the commonly employed routes of administration, whereas most analgesics of the antipyretic–anti-inflammatory class can only be given by mouth or by rectum. Because the narcotics are much more potent than the simple analgesics, there is a greater risk of acute dose-related toxicity. However, specific antagonists are available (such as naloxone) which can promptly counteract or reverse those effects. Paradoxically, the antipyretic–anti-inflammatory type analgesics are more hazardous, for their more serious acute toxic manifestations, such as gastrointestinal hemorrhage and agranulocytosis, are less predictable but just as formidable as the acute side effects of narcotics. Moreover, the acute hepatic necrosis and "analgesic nephropathy" associated with the overuse of the mild analgesics are far more serious and irreversible than any form of chronic toxicity due to narcotics. There are no specific nonnarcotic drug antagonists (21).

The chronic administration of narcotics can, of course, produce a number of familiar, undesired central nervous system, gastrointestinal, and genitourinary side effects. Tolerance to the analgesic and sedative effects of narcotics appears to develop more rapidly than tolerance to their constipating and sphincteric effects, so that reliance on the use of narcotics for analgesia over long periods of time can complicate the management of the patient with advanced cancer. Unfortunately, many physicians also equate tolerance with drug addiction and believe that the patient will become refractory to all drugs and other methods of relieving pain when in the throes of terminal illness. In keeping with this viewpoint, the caveat that, "The physician should use morphine only as a miser spends his gold," (4) has been the prevailing doctrine of American physicians.

CLINICAL PHARMACOLOGY

The narcotic analgesics are comprised of drugs of several different origins and chemical classes which share, at least in part, the properties of the classic narcotic agonist, morphine. The major groupings are the *opiates* and the *opioids*. The former are comprised of the naturally occurring opium alkaloids and their semisynthetic derivatives; the latter are comprised of a number of purely synthetic classes of drugs of which the most important are the *morphinan* series, the *benzomorphan* series, the *phenylpiperidine* (meperidine) series, and the *diphenylpropylamine* (methadone) series. There are literally hundreds of derivatives of these compounds, as well as a few other purely synthetic narcotics such as the benzimidazoles, thiambutenes, and phenampromide series. Most of the latter have either not been released for clinical use or have not been used to any appreciable extent in the management of pain due to advanced cancer.

For the purpose of our discussion, we shall speak of the individual, clinically important drugs as being of one of three types. The first type would be those drugs which are most similar to morphine in their pharmacologic properties; the second, those which more closely resemble codeine; and the third, those which resemble nalorphine. Codeine, which is simply 3-methyl morphine is very similar to morphine in its pharmacologic actions except that it is less potent and more commonly administered by the oral route, primarily because it is less subject to first-pass effects than morphine. Nalorphine, on the other hand, is both a narcotic agonist and an antagonist, and it differs appreciably in its pharmacologic profile from both morphine and codeine. Although, currently, nalorphine is *not* employed clinically as an analgesic, it is the prototype of the series of which the drug best known as an analgesic is pentazocine (Talwin®). The distinguishing features of the mixed agonist-antagonist analgesics are that they do not produce physical dependence of the morphine type, that tolerance develops more slowly to their repeated administration, and their dominant agonist or antagonist effects are largely determined by whether they are administered before or after a patient has developed physical dependence to narcotics (14).

CHOICE OF ANALGESIC

The choice of an appropriate analgesic and its proper dose should be based on what is known of the nature and the character of the pain and an understanding of the patient and his disease. Virtually all kinds and intensities of pain may be encountered in advanced cancer, and treatment is likely to be most successful if the drug, dose, and route of administration are tailored to fit that individual patient's needs. This requires that we exercise some clinical judgment based on our past experiences with patients in similar circumstances. Reports of pain intensity, in themselves, are not always reliable, particularly if one does not know the patient well. However, it is usually possible to reach a reasonable decision based on physical and laboratory findings and what is known of the extent of the disease and its probable course. The initial goal should be to provide *relief promptly* but not at the expense of inducing adverse side effects. If it were felt that this could be accomplished by the use of a simple analgesic, such as aspirin or acetaminophen, we should surely try that first. After those drugs have been tried in adequate doses, then it is time to take the next step.

Table 1 is a list of relative potencies of analgesics commonly employed for severe pain, expressed in terms of the intramuscular and oral doses approxi-

TABLE 1. *Relative potencies of analgesics commonly employed for severe pain, expressed in terms of the intramuscular (i.m.) and oral (p.o.) doses approximately equivalent in total effect to a 10-mg i.m. dose of morphine*

	i.m. (mg)	p.o. (mg)	Major differences from morphine
Oxymorphone (Numorphan®)	1	6	None
Hydromorphone (Dilaudid®)	1.5	7.5	Shorter-acting.
Levorphanol (Levo-Dromoran®)	2	4	Relatively high p.o. to i.m. potency.
Phenazocine (Prinadol®)	3	15	None
Metopon	3	18	None
Heroin	4		Shorter-acting.
Dextromoramide (Palfium®)	7.5	10	High p.o. to i.m. potency.
Piminodine (Alvodine®)	7.5		None
Methadone (Dolophine®)	10	20	Relatively high p.o. to i.m. potency.
Morphine	10	60	
Oxycodone	15	30	Shorter-acting. Relatively high p.o. to i.m. potency.
Dipipanone (Pipadone®)	20		None
Methotrimeprazine (Levoprome®, Nozinan®)	20		Phenothiazine—unlike morphine.
Anileridine (Leritine®)	30	50	Relatively high p.o. to i.m. potency.
Alphaprodine (Nisentil®)	45		Very short-acting.
Pentazocine (Talwin®)	60	180	Narcotic antagonist analgesic.
Meperidine (pethidine, Demerol®)	75	300	None
Codeine	130	200	Relatively high p.o. to i.m. potency. Relatively more toxic in higher doses.
Dextroproxyphene (Darvon®)	240		Similar to codeine but more toxic in high doses.

Relative potencies of analgesics employed orally for less severe pain, expressed in terms of doses approximately equivalent in total effect to 650 mg of aspirin

	p.o. (mg)	Salient features
Pentazocine (Talwin®)	30	Weak narcotic—narcotic antagonist, high analgesic potential,[a] low addiction liability.
Codeine	32	Weak narcotic, high analgesic potential, relatively low addiction liability.
Meperidine (Demerol®)	50	Narcotic, high analgesic potential, high addiction liability.
Propoxyphene (Darvon®)	65	Weak narcotic, low analgesic potential, low addiction liability.
Aminopyrine (Pyramidon®)	600	Nonnarcotic, low analgesic potential, no addiction liability, risk of agranulocytosis.
Aspirin (ASA)	650	Nonnarcotic, anti-inflammatory, low analgesic potential, no addiction liability or tolerance.
Phenacetin (acetophenetidin)	650	Similar to aspirin but with limited anti-inflammatory properties.
Acetaminophen (paracetamol)	650	Similar to phenacetin, less potential renal toxicity.
Sodium salicylate	1000	Similar to aspirin.

[a] "Analgesic potential" refers to level of analgesia attainable by increasing dose to point of limiting side effects.

mately equianalgesic in total effect to a 10-mg intramuscular dose of morphine. Where both the intramuscular and the oral equianalgesic doses are stated, that has been based on a double-blind crossover comparison within the same patients of the same drug by two different routes of administration (7). In the lower portion of the table, the relative potencies of analgesics employed orally for less severe pain are expressed in terms of the doses approximately equivalent in total effect to 650 mg of aspirin. It has been our experience (15) that doses in excess of 650 mg of either aspirin or acetaminophen are not as likely to provide the desired increment in analgesia that we could more easily achieve by giving an equianalgesic dose of a weak narcotic analgesic such as codeine or pentazocine along with the aspirin or acetaminophen (10). If this were not sufficient, the dose of the narcotic in the combination should be increased.

There is no single standard dose of any narcotic for all clinical situations. Only after our initially chosen drug and dose have been observed to be ineffective *and* produced adverse effects, should we consider changing to another without titrating either up or down. All too frequently, physicians tend to switch prematurely to another medication simply because they started with the wrong dose of a drug which was otherwise appropriate for the circumstances. Switching from an inappropriate dose of one drug to an equianalgesic but equi-inappropriate dose of another drug really does not help matters. On the basis of our studies, there are no significant differences in side effects at the equianalgesic doses stated (9).

Differences among Analgesics

The terms *potency* and *relative potency* appear to be interpreted in quite different ways by clinicians and pharmacologists. To a clinician, the statement that drug "A" is more potent than drug "B" generally conveys to him the impression that drug "A" is capable of producing a greater effect than drug "B." The pharmacologist would merely conclude that it takes a smaller dose of drug "A" to produce the *same effect* as drug "B," and that it does not follow that either drug is capable of producing a greater effect than the other. The analgesic potencies of narcotic drugs in man differ by as much as several hundred-fold, and yet there is no substantial evidence that even the extremely potent drugs, such as etorphine (an oripavine derivative of thebaine), etonitazine (a substituted benzimidazole), and azidomorphine are any more effective than morphine when all drugs are given in their maximal tolerated doses. Whether or not there are any differences in ceiling effects of the morphine-type analgesics has been the subject of some controversy. When the dose is increased on a logarithmic scale, the increment effect appears to be linear, virtually to the point of loss of consciousness. However, before that level is reached, other undesired pharmacologic effects of the drug become manifest;

and we have observed that the level at which this occurs for different drugs can differ appreciably.

Route of Administration

The narcotic analgesics may differ in other ways. Some (alphaprodine, fentanyl, azidomorphine) have very prompt but short durations of action, whereas others (methadone, buprenorphine) do not act so quickly but have relatively long durations of action. Moreover, some drugs, such as morphine, have a relatively low oral/parenteral potency ratio, whereas others, such as methadone and dextromoramide, have relatively high ones. Thus, if we were to choose an oral narcotic equal in effect to a 10-mg intramuscular dose of morphine, methadone would be a better choice than oral morphine, if only because the patient would probably find swallowing two tablets at a time more acceptable than six.

As patients become tolerant, the dose-effect curves shift to the right, so that one has to give a larger dose to achieve the same effect. In these circumstances, if the patient were receiving a parenteral medication, questions of solubility of the drug and of the concentrations in which it is available may become important considerations. In America, most parenteral narcotics come in fixed concentrations, usually the amount contained in 1 ml of solution being the equianalgesic dose of 10 mg of morphine. The drug with which we are provided the widest latitude is morphine, for it is available in concentrations as high as 30 mg/ml. For that reason, many of us in America tend to reserve morphine for the last, if our patients are expected to need large doses of narcotics by injection. Although morphine sulfate is actually soluble in water to the extent of about 65 mg/ml, it is only about one-eighth as soluble as diamorphine (heroin). Since diamorphine is also 2 to 3 times as potent as morphine by intramuscular injection, diamorphine provides physicians in those countries in which its use is permitted (U.K. and Belgium) even greater dose flexibility in treating terminal cancer patients requiring parenteral analgesics (18).

Insofar as possible, oral medications should be employed rather than injections, for they are usually easier to administer and less likely to cause complications. Tolerance and physical dependence can, of course, develop on the repeated administration of even an orally administered narcotic, and this is a predictable dose-related phenomenon. However, pain due to cancer does not always remain the same or, necessarily, continue to get worse. It is, therefore, incumbent on the physician to monitor the patient closely, and it is just as important to recognize when to titrate downward as when to titrate upward in the course of events. When possible, it is usually advisable to give an antipyretic-type analgesic together with the narcotic, since there is little reason to believe that tolerance develops to that class of drugs, and the added analgesic effect which it provides will help stay the rapid development of tolerance.

Pain Behavior and Drug Dependence

In any consideration of the treatment of pain, we must never lose sight of what might be causing the pain. If there is any chance that some definitive measure—such as radiation therapy, steroids, chemotherapy, or even surgery —is feasible and capable of removing the cause for pain, then, obviously, this is probably the most effective way of preventing or delaying the development of analgesic tolerance and physical dependence.

The prescription governing when the patient can take or receive narcotics may also influence the degree and rate of development of tolerance and physical dependence. Twycross (17) maintains that by administering narcotics *by-the-clock* in amounts sufficient to prevent the patient from having pain, the daily amount of narcotic is less than if the patient were requesting it on-demand. We have little reason to doubt this from our observations, since the more severe that pain is allowed to become, the more difficult it seems to be to control. The conventional way in which analgesics are prescribed is p.r.n. This *on-demand* method of administering drugs has been implicated in the acquisition of what is known as "pain behavior"—which generally means that the patient uses the complaint of pain as a means of manipulating others (2,3). The narcotics are felt to be a prime cause or reinforcer of this behavior and, in addition, the patient is often suspected of being addicted or of getting some vicarious pleasure from the drug. We have not seen any outward signs of elation in our cancer patients receiving on-demand narcotics. However, these patients do frequently develop tolerance to narcotics. Physicians and nurses often speak of such patients as being "clock-watchers" or "addicts" when, in fact, they have simply failed to recognize that one of the cardinal signs of developing tolerance is shortening of the duration of effect. We would assume that Dr. Twycross' patients do not develop pain behavior, for his patients are assured of receiving large enough doses of narcotics regularly to prevent pain from recurring. Whether we should consider those patients addicted will depend on how one wishes to define "addiction." The term *addict* connotes opprobrium. Applying this epithet to a sick and dying patient becomes a matter for one's conscience.

The by-the-clock method of prescribing narcotics with the intention of preventing pain may not always be the wisest course to follow in some cancer patients. When the patient is not being closely monitored, as is the case for most outpatients or home-care patients who are being seen only periodically, potentially serious complications which are commonly heralded by pain could be masked just long enough for there to be disastrous consequences for the patient. By the same token, patients whose pains tend to be intermittent and unpredictable, or are likely to lessen in response to definitive therapy, could be exposed to larger amounts of narcotics than they may actually need and, consequently, experience unwanted dose-related side effects. However, the customarily employed *pro re nata* approach is, itself, not without limitations, some of which have been mentioned above. More importantly, the on-demand prescription forces the patient to re-experience pain before taking or requesting medication, which can be very damaging to the morale of many patients.

NARCOTIC AGONISTS-ANTAGONISTS

In the quarter of a century since the discovery that nalorphine had significant analgesic activity (13), it has been well established that the classic properties of narcotics, their ability to relieve pain, and their capacity for inducing physical dependence, are not inseparable. Since then, a large number and variety of narcotic congeners with mixed agonist-antagonist properties have been developed. Although very few have thus far been introduced into medical practice as analgesics, they have had appreciable impact on how narcotic analgesics are employed.

Pentazocine, the only one of these currently marked for use in the United States, has enjoyed some popularity in the management of severe chronic pain despite its limitations, for the drug is a relatively short-acting analgesic, and it can precipitate some rather disturbing, though transitory, psychotomimetic reactions. Although pentazocine is not free of potential for abuse, it is not listed as a controlled substance in our country. That it is used so much in spite of its shortcomings is, perhaps, an indication of the importance many physicians give to what is construed as addiction liability in their choice of analgesics for the management of chronic pain. The prospects for the future, however, are more promising, for there are now several new drugs of this class under investigation which appear not only to be more potent and to have longer durations of action, but also to produce fewer of the undesired side effects of pentazocine (11).

The narcotic agonist-antagonists vary appreciably in their relative agonist and antagonist properties. Consequently, there are more substantial differences in the pharmacologic profiles of drugs of this type than there are among the typical morphine surrogates. However, they do share in common the property of increased antagonistic potency in the presence of physical dependence. Thus, if pentazocine or any of the newer drugs of this class were to be employed, the best time to do so would be before the patient is first placed on a narcotic analgesic. Drugs of this type act centrally, and they are always used to best advantage when they are given together with the simple analgesics of the antipyretic–anti-inflammatory type. Pentazocine, currently available as an analgesic, is also marketed as a compound mixture with aspirin. Propiram, a phenampromid analog, and tilidine, which has some structural relationship to meperidine, are two agonist-antagonists with very weak antagonist properties. Both of these drugs are marketed in Europe and, at this time, are investigational drugs in the United States. Three agonist-antagonists with more potent antagonist properties are nalbuphine, an analog of naloxone; butorphanol, a morphinan; and buprenorphine, an oripavine. All of these are still investigational drugs that have proven to be very effective analgesics which are felt to have low abuse-potential.

LOW-POTENCY NARCOTICS

The weaker or low-potency narcotic agonists consist of propoxyphene, a methadone analog; meperidine, the prototype of its class; and codeine, a natural opium alkaloid. Both codeine and propoxyphene have good oral/parenteral potency ratios so that, in effect, they are low-potency agonists even when given parenterally. Meperidine, on the other hand, is only about one-quarter as potent by mouth as it is by intramuscular injection (19), so that it is considered with the weaker narcotics when given by mouth and with the potent narcotics when given by injection. When administered by mouth, all of these drugs are best used in combination with other simple analgesics and, in fact, all are marketed in mixtures containing either aspirin, acetaminophen, or APC (aspirin, phenacetin, and caffeine).

HIGH-POTENCY NARCOTICS

Oxycodone, which bears the same chemical structural relationship to oxymorphone as codeine does to morphine, is a potent narcotic agonist which is available to us in America only in fixed-dose combinations with either APC (Percodan®) or acetaminophen (Percocet®). In these formulations, the highest unit dose of oxycodone is 5 mg, which is approximately equivalent to 60 mg of oral codeine.

Other potent narcotics which have relatively high oral/parenteral potency ratios and are not commonly marketed as mixtures include levorphanol, methadone, anileridine, and dextromoramide. The latter drug is not available in the United States but is marketed in Europe. Like oxycodone, all of these drugs are what are considered Schedule II drugs in the United States, a designation applied to drugs with recognized medical uses but high addiction liability. The pharmacologic profiles of virtually all of these drugs are quite similar to morphine, except that morphine has a poor oral/parenteral potency ratio. However, many hospitals and institutions in the United States are now administering morphine orally in some variation of the British Euphoriant Elixir. Diamorphine (heroin), which is more commonly used in the mixture in the U.K., is, of course, illegal in the United States. To my knowledge, the only systematic study of this combination is that reported by Twycross (18), who found that morphine substituted well for diamorphine if added to the solution in a dose 1½ times that of diamorphine.

As usually employed in British hospices, the Brompton Cocktail consists of an orally administered mixture of cocaine, ethyl alcohol, chloroform water, and varying amounts of diamorphine, ranging from 5 to 100 mg, tailored to fit the patients' needs for analgesia. This Elixir is generally administered on a regular 4-hr schedule around-the-clock. Comparable mixtures containing morphine and methadone are generally being administered in the same manner to patients with terminal cancer in the United States and Canada.

SUMMARY

In summary, the use of narcotic analgesics plays an essential role in the effective management of pain due to advanced or terminal cancer. These drugs are the most efficacious of all the systemic analgesics and are capable of relieving virtually all types of pain regardless of site or sites of origin. However, there is no single drug, dose, or route of administration which is appropriate for all patients with advanced cancer. Important to success in controlling pain is titrating the dose within the limits of tolerable side effects before deciding to change to another drug. Pain due to advanced cancer is not static. These patients require continuous monitoring for indicated modifications of their analgesic regimens. The narcotic agonist-antagonists are best employed before the patient has had appreciable exposure to pure narcotic agonists. There are several drugs of this class which appear to have substantial advantages over the presently available pentazocine. An orally administered by-the-clock regimen designed to keep the patient from experiencing pain has many advantages if it can be closely monitored. In the final analysis, successful management of pain in the patient with advanced cancer will, in large measure, depend on understanding the patient, the underlying disease, and the reason for the patient's having pain (6).

ACKNOWLEDGMENT

Supported in part by a grant from the National Institute on Drug Abuse, No. DA-01707.

REFERENCES

1. Eddy, N. B., Halbach, H., and Braenden, O. J. (1957): Synthetic substances with morphine-like effect. Clinical experience: side effects, addiction liability. *Bull. W.H.O.*, 17:569–863.
2. Fordyce, W. E. (1974): Pain viewed as learned behavior. In: *Advances in Neurology, Vol. 4: International Symposium on Pain*, edited by J. J. Bonica, pp. 415–422. Raven Press, New York.
3. Fordyce, W. E. (1974): Treating pain by contingency management. In: *Advances in Neurology, Vol. 4: International Symposium on Pain*, edited by J. J. Bonica, pp. 583–589. Raven Press, New York.

4. Goodman, L. S., and Gilman, A., editors (1941, 1955): *The Pharmacological Basis of Therapeutics,* 1st and 2nd editions, Macmillan, New York.
5. Halpern, L. M., and Bonica, J. J. (1976): Analgesics. In: *Drugs of Choice,* edited by W. Modell, pp. 195–232. C. V. Mosby, St. Louis.
6. Houde, R. W. (1956): Pain and the patient with cancer. In: *The Medical Clinics of North America—Symposium on the Medical Aspects of Cancer,* edited by D. A. Karnofsky and R. W. Rawson, pp. 687–703. W. B. Saunders Co., Philadelphia and London.
7. Houde, R. W. (1974): Medical treatment of oncological pain. In: *Recent Advances on Pain: Pathophysiology and Clinical Aspects,* edited by J. J. Bonica, P. Procacci, C. A. Pagni, pp. 168–188, Charles C. Thomas, Springfield, Ill.
8. Houde, R. W. (1974): The use and misuse of narcotics in the treatment of chronic pain. In: *Advances in Neurology, Vol. 4: International Symposium on Pain,* edited by J. J. Bonica, pp. 527–536. Raven Press, New York.
9. Houde, R. W., Wallenstein, S. L., and Beaver, W. T. (1965): Clinical measurement of pain. In: *Analgetics,* edited by G. de Stevens, pp. 75–122. Academic Press, New York.
10. Houde, R. W., Wallenstein, S. L., and Beaver, W. T. (1966): Evaluation of analgesics in patients with cancer pain. In: *International Encyclopedia of Pharmacology and Therapeutics, Section 6, Volume I: Clinical Pharmacology,* edited by L. Lasagna, pp. 59–97. Pergamon Press Ltd., Oxford.
11. Houde, R. W., Wallenstein, S. L., Rogers, A., and Kaiko, R. F. (1976): Annual report of the Analgesic Studies Section of the Memorial Sloan-Kettering Cancer Center. *Proceedings of the Thirty-eighth Annual Scientific Meeting of the Committee on Problems of Drug Dependence,* National Academy of Sciences, pp. 149–168.
12. Krueger, H., Eddy, N. B., and Sumwalt, M. (1941): *The Pharmacology of Opium Alkaloids, Part 1, Suppl. No. 165 to the Public Health Reports,* pp. 26–29. U.S. Gov't. Printing Office, Washington, D.C.
13. Lasagna, L., and Beecher, H. K. (1954): The analgesic effectiveness of nalorphine and nalorphine-morphine combinations in man. *J. Pharmacol.,* 112:356–363.
14. Martin, W. R. (1967): Opioid antagonists. *Pharmacol. Rev.,* 19:463–521.
15. Modell, W., and Houde, R. W. (1958): Factors influencing clinical evaluation of drugs. *JAMA,* 167:2190–2198.
16. Terry, C. E., and Pellens, M. (1928): *The Opium Problem,* pp. 94–136. Bureau of Social Hygiene, Inc., New York.
17. Twycross, R. G. (1975): Relief of terminal pain. *Br. Med. J.,* 4:212–214.
18. Twycross, R. G. (1977): Choice of strong analgesic in terminal cancer: Diamorphine or morphine? *Pain,* 3:93–104.
19. Wallenstein, S. L., and Houde, R. W. (1959): Relative oral and parenteral potencies of anileridine and meperidine. *Fed. Proc.,* 18:456.
20. Wikler, A. (1950): Sites and mechanisms of action of morphine and related drugs in the central nervous system. *Pharmacol. Rev.,* 2:435–506.
21. Woodbury, D. M., and Fingl, E. (1975): Analgesic-antipyretics, anti-inflammatory agents, and drugs employed in the therapy of gout. In: *The Pharmacological Basis of Therapeutics,* 5th ed., edited by L. S. Goodman and A. Gilman, pp. 325–358. Macmillan, New York.

Psychotropics, Ataractics, and Related Drugs

Lawrence M. Halpern

Department of Pharmacology, University of Washington School of Medicine, Seattle, Washington 98195

Recent advances in our understanding of central factors which play roles in the perception of pain and its modulation emphasize the need to parcel out and separately treat various psychologic factors which can intensify or decrease pain experiences in cancer patients. Depression as a temporary mood state, i.e., normal depression or grief states, depression secondary to psychiatric or medical disorders or chronicity of illness, and primary depression or melancholia, may exacerbate pain or make preexisting pain worse. Elation, excitement, or mania may relieve or ameliorate pain. Anxiety may be responsible for *de novo* pain or may make preexisting pain considerably worse. It is now a generally accepted principle that the psychologic circumstances described above may centrally modulate pain arising from nociceptive sources and may even give rise to pain in the absence of nociceptor input.

The last 10 years of progress in the area of chronic pain management have renewed our interest in the actions of psychotropic drugs as "pain medications." Psychotropic agents have been employed to reduce anxiety, provide nighttime sedation, elevate mood, block emesis, or produce analgesia. These alternative uses for psychotropic drugs have emerged empirically as a result of clinical experience with these agents and careful clinical observation by individuals interested in the newly emerging field of chronic pain management. Unfortunately, there are very few studies in the literature which could qualify as good clinical pharmacology. In a recent survey of the cancer-treatment literature this author was able to find few studies of the effects of psychotropic drugs done using reasonable parametric techniques. This is at once surprising and shocking when one considers that the frequency of occurrence of painful malignancy requiring palliative therapy with analgesic and other drugs is reasonably high.

INDICATIONS

Treatment of moderate and severe terminal-cancer pain syndrome is frequently complicated by inappropriate drug selection, inadequate dosage, and in the case of the narcotic analgesics, the development of dependence. Failure

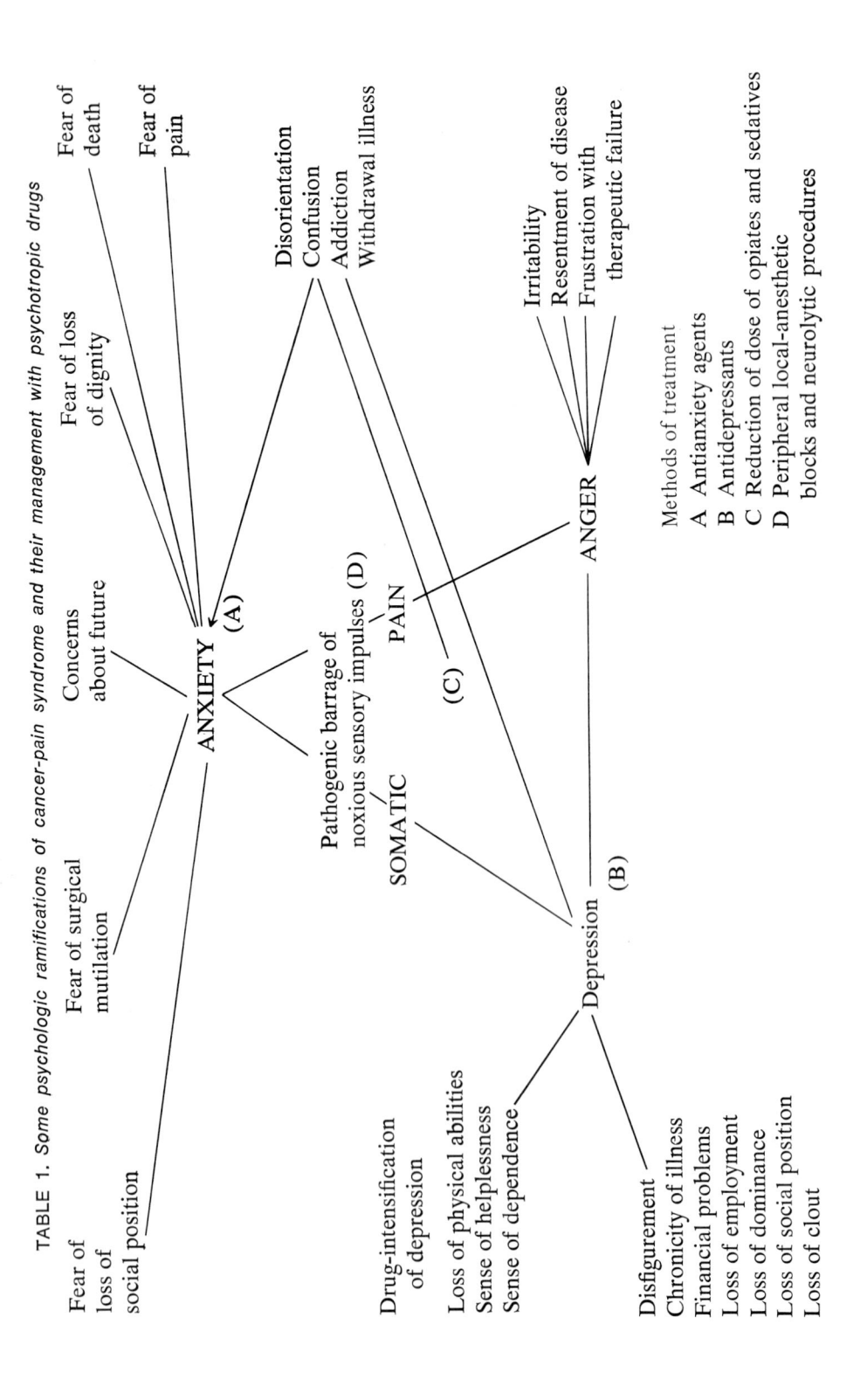

TABLE 1. *Some psychologic ramifications of cancer-pain syndrome and their management with psychotropic drugs*

Fear of loss of social position — Fear of surgical mutilation — Concerns about future — Fear of loss of dignity — Fear of death — Fear of pain

→ ANXIETY (A)

Disorientation, Confusion, Addiction, Withdrawal illness

Pathogenic barrage of noxious sensory impulses (D)

SOMATIC PAIN (C)

Irritability, Resentment of disease, Frustration with therapeutic failure

→ ANGER

Depression (B)

Drug-intensification of depression, Loss of physical abilities, Sense of helplessness, Sense of dependence

Disfigurement, Chronicity of illness, Financial problems, Loss of employment, Loss of dominance, Loss of social position, Loss of clout

Methods of treatment
A Antianxiety agents
B Antidepressants
C Reduction of dose of opiates and sedatives
D Peripheral local-anesthetic blocks and neurolytic procedures

to recognize and appropriately treat the narcotic-analgesic–tolerant individual results in the patient not only receiving inadequate pain-relief, but also having to deal with the unpleasantness of unsupported opiate withdrawal. Narcotics dependence *per se* is not a problem so long as attention to the rising intake levels prevents the patient from discomfort. Once dependence on narcotics is involved, personality change, drug-induced intensification of depression, uncomfortable constipation, and emotional consequences some patients have difficulties dealing with, and reduction in activities outside of maintenance of adequate narcotics dosage severely limit the interactions of the patient with his/her former activities. For these reasons methods of pain control involving psychotropic drugs have begun to appear and are becoming more common as our collective experience with them grows.

Reduction of anxiety with psychotherapy, reassurance, progressive muscular relaxation techniques, transcendental meditation, or drugs; reversal of depression with psychotherapy or drugs; use of selected phenothiazines, sympathomimetic amines, sedative antihistamines, cannabis and its derivatives, and even psychodysleptic agents such as LSD have been used to modify psychologic variables in the management of terminal pain.

Chapman's model for pain associated with advanced cancer (*this volume*) describes many of the psychologic variables which form the rationale for psychotropic drug selection for the management of terminal pain syndrome in advanced cancer (Table 1). While it is true that narcotic analgesic drugs and their potentiators and antianxiety drugs are probably the most frequently used agents for the management of cancer pain, these agents add yet another dimension to the variables in Chapman's model.

As a result of chronic cancer pain and its management with opiates and antianxiety agents, the cancer patient has to deal with the additional burden of chronic drug-induced disorientation, excessive sedation alternating with withdrawal illness, and in some cases uncomfortable feelings of almost a sexual nature which some patients find disquieting. In addition drug-induced intensification of depression may increase fear, anger, and frustration levels and even pain itself. Family members are sensitive to and quick to note progressive personality changes centering around isolation and withdrawal from family members due to drug use. The patient's main preoccupation becomes an involvement with pain medication. Medication is used in anticipation of pain. Inappropriate doses of analgesic drugs are used in attempts to calm anxiety, reduce fear, prevent uncomfortable drug withdrawal symptoms, and to achieve excessive sedation.

TECHNIQUES OF MANAGING PAIN IN THE ADVANCED CANCER PATIENT

Because of the concerns discussed above, our experience has centered around two basic alterations in the usual strategy for providing pain-relief for the terminally ill patient. First, orally active doses of long-acting drugs are used whenever possible, i.e., methadone or levo dromoran, phenobarbital or chlordiazepoxide. Secondly, attempts are made to minimize the dose and duration of usage of narcotics and sedatives by prolonging the time before it becomes necessary to administer them. This is accomplished by use of appropriate psychotropic medications, systematic partial or total detoxification, and the use of local-anesthetic nerve block and peripheral neurolytic procedures where appropriate.

Long-acting drugs prevent euphoria-withdrawal swings, medication in anticipation of pain, and inappropriate use of narcotics for the treatment of anxiety. This allows reduction in opiate and sedative dosage, and as a consequence of lowered dosage, disorientation and withdrawal illness are reduced. In many cases, reversal of chronic drug-induced intensification of depression results in better pain control as a result of lessened depression. Reduction in sedative dosage seems to lessen anger-agitation and emotional lability resulting in a calmer, less-upset patient.

Substitution-withdrawal using long-acting opiates and sedatives (6) allows for reduction of drug-induced effects as described above. Tricyclic antidepressant drugs, usually amitryptiline or doxepine, are started immediately and maintained at 150 mg for the duration of pain treatment. Anxiety and agitation and emotional lability decrease as a consequence of reduction of barbiturate-diazepam dosage. Sedation and an antianxiety effect can be achieved with doses of sedative antihistamines, i.e., diphenhydramine or hydroxyzine, and by taking advantage of the sedative qualities of the antidepressants given H.S. This medication technique permits stable pain-control. As pain reappears during opiate-dosage reduction, the dose of long-acting opiate is held constant at levels which do not completely obliterate pain.

Diagnostic local-anesthetic blocks are done, and if the results show promise, permanent peripheral neurolytic procedures may be employed. Should the peripheral neurolytic procedure provide adequate relief of pain, the dosage of methadone or other long-acting opiates can be reduced even further. In many cases the patient becomes much more active, personalities change toward their former direction, and patients and their families are more comfortable with the dying process.

SYMPATHOMIMETIC AMINES

Amphetamine has recently been shown to potentiate the action of narcotic analgesic drugs (5), 5 mg and 10 mg P.O. produce 1.5 and 2 times the analgesia for a given dose of morphine. Because of the rapid development of tolerance to sympathomimetic amines, this agent should not be used for long periods of time, but is quite useful for short periods where its use can brighten up an excessively sedated patient and provide increased analgesia. This agent antagonizes phenothiazine sedation and is itself antagonized by

TABLE 2. *Psychotropic drugs useful in the management of chronic pain*

Action	Example

Sympathomimetic amines
  Elevate mood
  Potentiate analgesia
  Prevent withdrawal
	D-Amphetamine
	Methylphenidate

Antidepressants
  Elevate mood
  Increase sedation
  Potentiate analgesia
  Analgesic action
	Amitryptiline
	Doxepine

Phenothiazines
  Confusion
  Delirium
  Psychotic manifestations
  Increase sedation
  Analgesic action
	Levomepromazine
	Perphenazine
	Chlorpromazine

Sedative antihistamines
  Antianxiety
  Sedative hypnotic
  Analgesic action
	Diphenhydramine
	Hydroxyzine

Benzodiazepines	Clonazepam

Cannabis derivatives
  Antianxiety
  Antinauseant
  Antidepressant
	Marihuana
	Nabilone

phenothiazine. Methylphenidate (Ritalin®) has been used for this purpose and reportedly can substitute for meperidine, maintaining good analgesia and preventing opiate withdrawal after discontinuation of meperidine (14).

COCAINE

Cocaine was first used in combination with morphine by Snow (13), who claimed that this substance helped to "sustain vitality." It is a relatively brief, amphetamine-like agent, and its use in fixed-dose combinations with an opiate cannot be recommended. Appropriate dosage of antidepressant drugs, i.e., amitryptiline and doxepine pushed to adequate levels not only serve to brighten the patient but may also have an analgesic action of their own.

TRICYCLIC ANTIDEPRESSANTS

Amitryptiline and doxepine have been used successfully in the management of cancer pain. Prior to the use of narcotic analgesics these agents may be used alone or in combination with the phenothiazines levomepromazine or perphenazine. Levomepromazine is a phenothiazine with analgesic potency (8); when used alone or in combination with an antidepressant, narcotic-like analgesia results without the development of physical-dependence–withdrawal concerns which interfere with narcotic analgesic therapy. One must exert care that excessive sedation does not develop and that the orthostatic hypotension occurring as a result of use of the phenothiazine does not result in falling and further injury to the patient. It is recommended that patients being started on this psychotropic combination be at bed rest until tolerance to these symptoms and appropriate dosages are achieved. Maintenance of patients without narcotic analgesics, or with low doses of narcotic analgesics potentiated with appropriate psychoactive agents, prolongs the patient's ability to interact with family and friends, and may even keep the patient alert and active enough to maintain a job or participate in other outside activities.

Once narcotics have been started, the antidepressants may potentiate narcotic analgesia, have an analgesic action of their own (10), or reduce pain by elevating mood. In any case, the presence of antidepressant drug permits overall reduction in the dosage of narcotics while maintaining adequate analgesia.

The combination of amitryptiline and perphenazine (15) or doxepine and perphenazine is frequently used in the management of post-herpetic neuralgia, which can plague already uncomfortable cancer victims. This is thought to occur as a consequence of supression of immune responses as a result of radiotherapy or chemotherapy. In this situation, the antidepressant is administered at doses of 50 mg H.S. for 3 days, 100 mg H.D. for 3 days and up to 150 mg H.S. thereafter. The perphenazine is started at 1 mg and the dosage increases at 5-day intervals, until doses of 5 to 6 mg/day have been reached.

PHENOTHIAZINES

Methotrimeprazine (Levomepromazine, Levoprome) is a phenothiazine derivative possessing many of the pharmacologic characteristics of the group. Levomepromazine has no antitussive properties, and less respiratory depression occurs as compared with the narcotics. It does not produce psychologic or physical dependence, nor does it suppress the symptoms of morphine withdrawal. It produces narcotic-like analgesia and seems to be half as potent as morphine on a milligram basis (2). Equianalgesic doses for 15 mg of mephotrimeprazine are 10 mg morphine and 75 to 100 mg meperidine. The onset of action of this agent is as rapid as morphine, with a similar duration of analgesic action. As with all phenothiazines, orthostatic hypotension develops, which may outlast the duration of the analgesia produced by this drug. Dizziness, blurred vision, disorientation, and marked sedation are all undesirable side effects which may tend to limit the use of this drug to nonambulatory patients in whom addiction to narcotics is to be avoided. Thus, its major use in the management of cancer patients is to provide full analgesia during the period prior to the introduction of narcotic analgesics. The drug has successfully been combined with amitryptiline and doxepine to provide potentiated analgesia at doses low enough to provide for some careful ambulation while not producing excessive sedation.

Phenergan

Phenergan potentiates the sedation produced by narcotic analgesic drugs while antagonizing the analgesia they produce (4). Thus phenergan is a poor choice of psychotropic agents to be used in the management of cancer pain.

Chlorpromazine

Chlorpromazine is an early member of the group of phenothiazine tranquilizers and is useful for potentiating sedation from narcotic analgesic drugs as well as dealing with confusion, delirium, and psychotic manifestations, should these occur.

SEDATIVE ANTIHISTAMINES

The diphenylmethane antihistaminics diphenhydramine and hydroxyzine have been found to be helpful in the management of chronic pain, and especially cancer pain. An interesting question is raised as to whether the beneficial effect of the agents is due to their antianxiety effect or because these agents have some additional analgesic effect. Beaver (1) has demonstrated an analgesic effect similar to that of morphine, i.e., 100 mg hydroxyzine i.m. is equivalent to 8 mg of morphine sulfate. Kantor (7) was unable to demonstrate analgesic activity for hydroxyzine after doses of 100 mg P.O.

The beneficial effect in cancer patients may be due to a wholly different mechanism. It has been our experience that cancer patients on elevated doses of sedative hypnotic agents, such as diazepam, are likely to have moodswings which include spontaneous crying for no apparent reason that the patient can describe. Substitution-withdrawal from diazepam or other sedative and the use of diphenhydramine or hydroxyzine eliminates mood-swings and spontaneous crying.

The use of diphenhydramine 100 mg P.O., H.S., or hydroxyzine 100 mg P.O., H.S., often eliminates the need for additional nighttime sedation. When antidepressants are used, the sedative effect of the antihistamines is enhanced, and this combination can be used to good advantage in most patients. Hydroxyzine offers some advantages over diphenhydramine in that maximum daily dosage tolerated without potentially dangerous central side effects is greater.

BENZODIAZEPINES

As a group, the benzodiazepines have not been valuable in the management of cancer pain because of problems associated with physical dependence after chronic use. Barbiturates and meprobamate have been shown to have antianalgesic properties. While there is no clear demonstration as yet, at least after chronic use the benzodiazepines may indeed possess antianalgesic properties. Clonazepam has been recently reported to differ from other members of the benzodiazepine group. This agent has been described to possess valuable intrinsic analgesic activity and has been described as useful in the treatment of neuralgias, atypical facial pain, and other resistant conditions of the head and neck (3).

CANNABIS DERIVATIVES

Studies of delta-9-tetrahydrocannabinol have demonstrated that it possesses euphoriant, analgesic, appetite-stimulant, and antiemetic effects. These effects may have use in the management of the despondency, weight loss, and pain which pose difficult problems, since other psychotropic agents currently in use prove inadequate (12). Studies of these effects in cancer patients suggest that delta-9-THC has value as an antidepressant and can be of value in the management of both inpatient and outpatient cancer patients, provided that somnolence, dizziness, and depersonalization do not result in early discontinuation.

NABILONE

Nabilone is a new THC homologue (9) which has antianxiety properties (11) and is currently being evaluated for use as a substitute. Should this agent prove to be of value, it would simplify problems currently encountered in the administration of marihuana or delta-9-tetrahydrocannibinol, since nabilone is reportedly water-soluble and parenterally injectable.

REFERENCES

1. Beaver, W. T., and Geise, G. (1975): Comparison of the analgesic effects of morphine, hydroxyzine and their combination in patients with post-operative pain. In: *Advances in Pain Research and Therapy, Vol. 1: Proceedings of the First World Congress on Pain,* edited by J. J. Bonica and D. Albe-Fessard. Raven Press, New York.
2. Beaver, W. T. (1976): Comparison of morphine, hydroxyzine and morphine plus hydroxyzine in postoperative pain. *Hosp. Prac.* (Special Edition) p. 19.
3. Budd, K. (1978): Psychotropic drugs in the management of chronic pain. *Anesthesiology,* 33:531–534.
4. Dundee, J. W., Love, W. J., and Moore, J. (1963): Alterations in response to somatic pain associated with analgesia and further studies with phenothiazine derivatives and similar drugs. *Br. J. Anesth.,* 35:597–609.

5. Forrest, W. H., Brown, L. R., Mahler, D. L., Katz, J., Schroff, P., Defalque, R., and Brown, B. (1973): The evaluation of morphine and desamphetamine combination for analgesia. *Clin. Pharmacol. Ther.,* 14:132.
6. Halpern, L. M. (1977): Analgesic drugs in the management of pain. *Arch. Surg.,* 112:861–869.
7. Kantor, T. G., and Steinberg, F. P. (1975): Studies of tranquilizing agents and meperidine in clinical pain. Hydroxyzine and Meprobamate. In: *Advances in Pain Research and Therapy, Vol. 1: Proceedings of the First World Congress on Pain,* edited by J. J. Bonica and D. Albe-Fessard, p. 567. Raven Press, New York.
8. Lasagna, L., and DeKornfeld, T. J. (1961): Mephotrimeprazine: A new phenothiazine derivative with analgesic properties. *JAMA,* 178:827.
9. Lemberger, L., and Rowe, H. (1975): Clinical pharmacology of nabilone, a cannibinol derivative. *Clin. Pharmacol. Ther.,* 18:720–726.
10. Merskey, H., and Hester, R. A. (1972): The treatment of chronic pain with psychoactive drugs. *Postgrad. Med. J.,* 58:594–598.
11. Nakano, S., Gillespie, H. K., and Hollister, L. E. (1978): Nabilone and diazepam. *Clin. Pharmacol. Ther.* 23:51–62.
12. Regelson, W., Butler, J. R., Schulz, J., Kiek, J., Peek, L., Green, M. L., and Zalis, M. O. (1976): Delta-9-tetrahydrocannabinol as an effective antidepressant and appetite-stimulating agent in advanced cancer patients. In: *The Pharmacology of Marihuana,* edited by M. C. Braude and S. Szara. Raven Press, New York.
13. Snow, H. (1897): The opium cocaine treatment of malignant disease. *Br. Med. J.,* 1:1019–1020.
14. Stambaugh, J. E.: Personal communication.
15. Taub, A., and Collins, W. F., Jr. (1974): Observations on treatment of denervation dysesthesia with psychotropic drugs: Post-herpetic neuralgia, anesthesia dolorosa, peripheral neuropathy. In: *Advances in Neurology, Vol. 4: International Symposium on Pain,* edited by J. J. Bonica, pp. 309–315. Raven Press, New York.

The Use of Psychotropic Drugs in the Treatment of Cancer Pain

R. Kocher

Psychiatrische Universitätsklinik Basel, Neurologischer Dienst und EEG-Station, 4025 Basel, Switzerland

Since the introduction of psychotropic drugs, especially thymoleptics and neuroleptics, the treatment of all chronic and severe pain including cancer pain has been decisively improved. Shortly after the introduction of neuroleptics (1951 to 1952) and of thymoleptics (1957) in medicine, the first reports of their effective analgesic actions were published. Furthermore, an analgesic potentiating action and a narcotic analgesic-sparing effect were described. These reports suggested to us that we treat the patients of chronic pain including cancer pain with a combination of drugs of both groups. In this report we briefly summarized the results obtained in our clinic and those reported by others.

CLINICAL MATERIAL

Personal Experience

We have been using combinations of drugs of both groups for chronic pain therapy for over a decade. In a previous report (8) we summarized the results of psychotropic drug combinations in patients with a variety of chronic pain syndromes including cancer pain. The results were rated as follows: *very good to excellent* when patients had complete relief of pain and were able to terminate narcotic analgesics; *good to fair* when there was significant (but not total) pain-relief and narcotic analgesic intake could be reduced significantly; and *no improvement* when there was no change in the pain and it was impossible to reduce the dosage of analgesics the patient had been taking. In a group of 91 patients who received the drug combination, 22 (24%) had excellent results; 60 (66%) derived fair to good results; and 9 (10%) had no improvement. The failures occurred in patients with degenerative disk disease and other serious musculoskeletal problems. Among the small group of patients who had moderate to severe cancer pain, all derived good results. During the subsequent 2 years we have continued to use this drug-combination therapy for patients with pain of advanced cancer as well as other chronic pain syndromes with similar results.

Dosage Schedule

As a result of our experience, a clear-cut dosage schedule has been established for inpatients and outpatients. A therapy based on these guidelines has been shown to be without relevant side effects. For outpatients the best combination consists of chlorimipramine 25 mg by mouth 3 times daily and haloperidol beginning with 0.5 mg 2 times daily and then carefully increasing the dosage to 1 mg given 2 or 3 times each day.

For inpatients the best dosage schedule is as follows: chlorimipramine given via an intravenous infusion containing 25 to 50 mg of the drug in 250 ml of 5% glucose solution administered over the course of 2 to 3 hr daily. After 1 week this is changed to 25 mg given by mouth 3 times daily. At the same time, haloperidol is given in initial doses of 0.5 mg 2 times daily and then carefully increasing the dosage to 1 mg 2 to 3 times each day. It is important that in elderly, debilitated persons the daily dosage of haloperidol should not exceed 1.5 mg daily.

Results Reported by Others

Review of the literature reveals that it is difficult to compare the therapeutic results of one group with those of others. This is because there is

TABLE 1. *The analgesic efficacy of psychotropic drugs for cancer pain*

Author	Drug used	No. of pts.	Cause of pain	Improvement of pain
Thymoleptics				
Daxelmüller (5)	Imipramine	40	Neurol. pat. incl. cancer	80%
Gebhardt et al. (7)	Chlorimipramine	52	Cancer	67%
Mönkemeier and Steffen (9)	Imipramine	20	Cancer	75%
Adjan (1)	Imipramine	31	Cancer	80%
Adjan (1)	Chlorimipramine	50	Cancer	90%
Barjou (2)	Imipramine	30	Surg. pat. incl. cancer	70%
Deutschmann (6)	Imipramine	44	Cancer	80%
Neuroleptics				
Bloomfield (4)	Laevomepromazine	18	Cancer and arthritis	>50%
Combinations				
Bernard and Scheurer (3)	Chlorimipramine + laevomepromazine or haloperidol	83	Inoperable cancer (ENT)	87%
Put (10)	Fluanxol and dixeran	17	Visceral cancer	67%

TABLE 2. Results with use of psychotropic drugs in the treatment of cancer pain

	No. of pts.	Psychotropic drugs[a]	Improvement in %
Germany			
Duisburg	100	T, N, A	10
Göttingen	250	T, N, A	41
Berlin	300	T, N	30
Austria			
Vienna (2. Med.)	50	A, N	70
Switzerland			
Zürich	134	A, N	30
St. Gallen	1500	A, N	80
Basel	100	T, N, A	30
Neuchâtel	20	T, A	75

[a] T, tranquilizer; N, neuroleptic; A, antidepressant.

usually a lack of uniformity of experimental design of clinical trials and significant variation in the clinical measurement of pain and pain-relief. Despite these reservations of mine, I have listed the results obtained by other clinicians who have used various psychotropic drugs for the management of patients with cancer pain. Review of the data in Table 1 reveals that although the number of patients reported by each writer or group of writers is relatively small, an average of about 80% of the patients had improvement reflected by decrease of the severity of the pain and reduction of narcotic analgesic requirements.

In order to obtain additional data, we carried out a survey of various cancer centers of the German-speaking countries. A questionnaire was sent to the important cancer centers in Austria, Germany and Switzerland. Of 39 questionnaires sent out, 20 were returned consisting of 11 from Germany, 3 from Austria, and 6 from Switzerland. Of these 20 centers, 4 reported no experience with these drugs; in each of 3 other centers, only 1 patient had been treated; and in the reports of 5 centers some of the data were lacking. Table 2 lists the results reported by the remaining 8 centers.

DISCUSSION

The results obtained in the literature, as well as our own personal results, indicated that psychotropic drugs are useful and effective in managing patients with pain of advanced cancer. In general, one can expect improvement in the form of partial or complete pain-relief and reduction or complete elimination of narcotic drugs in about 60 to 80% of the patients, depending on the drug combination used.

In contrast, the results obtained from the survey of some of the cancer centers in the three German-speaking countries strongly suggest that: (a) in general, the use of psychotropic drugs for the treatment of pain of advanced cancer is not well known in these centers. This lack of knowledge should be eliminated by more intense efforts in diffusing information, including all publications on the subject; and (b) the percentage of patients who experience improvement varied greatly among the different centers, which is somewhat in contrast to the publications found in the literature. This suggests that each center should carry out a prospective study in the future in order to ascertain the efficacy of the drug and the best combination of drugs and doses of each agent.

The advantages in using psychotropic drugs for the treatment of cancer pain (as well as other chronic pain syndromes) include: (a) they improve the general emotional condition of patients by their action as antidepressants; (b) they appear to be effective in patients who have developed tolerance to established treatment with narcotic analgesics; (c) properly used, these drugs are associated with few, if any, harmful side effects; and (d) there is evidence that they potentiate the analgesic efficacy of narcotics.

Drug combinations, but particularly the administration of neuroleptics and thymoleptics concomitantly, offer the following additional advantages: (a) a smaller dose of each drug is usually sufficient, and consequently, we can minimize incidence and severity of troublesome side effects; (b) combined thymoleptic and neuroleptic effects are valuable because one of them may be missing or insufficient when a drug of one group alone is given; and (c) the spectrum of pharmacologic action is broadened.

Mode of Action

The generally favorable results for relief obtained with psychotropic drugs, especially when a combination of thymoleptics and neuroleptics is used in the treatment of pain, suggests that these drugs do not have only one but a variety of pharmacologic actions which, as previously mentioned, is greatly broadened when a combined therapy is used. It is now believed that psychotropic drugs have both central and peripheral pharmacologic action. In regard to their *peripheral action,* one thinks immediately of the pain-producing substances. It is possible that psychotropic drugs have their peripheral effect by interfering in some way with these pain-producing substances such as prostaglandins. This is merely a speculation, because evidence to support such a hypothesis is lacking.

Central action. Psychotropic drugs, especially when both thymoleptics and neuroleptics are given, alter pain perception and pain sensation. The drugs effect a "depersonalization of the pain" or a "pain distancing." Many patients have said: "I still have the pain, but it no longer hurts" or "I still have the pain, but it is far away." In addition, thymoleptics and neuroleptics are able to interrupt or prevent the vicious circle: pain→anxiety→depression→pain and so on. In states of anxiety and depression, which often accompany cancer pain, the probability of an interruption or prevention of this vicious circle is greater with a combination therapy than with thymoleptics or neuroleptics alone.

REFERENCES

1. Adjan, M. (1970): Zur therapeutischen Beeinflussung des Schmerzsymptoms bei unheilbaren Tumorkranken. *Ther. Gegenw.,* 109:1620–1627.
2. Barjou, B. (1971): Étude du Tofranil sur les douleurs en chirurgia. *Revue med. Tours,* 6:473–482.
3. Bernard, P., and Scheurer, H. (1972): Action de la Chlorimipramine (Anafranil) sur la douleur des cancers en pathologie cervicofaciale. *ORL,* 21:723–729.
4. Bloomfield, S., Simard-Savoie, S., Bernier, J., and Tetrault, L. (1964): Comparative analgesic activity of leavomepromazine and morphine in patients with chronic pain. *Can. Med. Assoc. J.,* 90:1156–1159.
5. Daxelmüller, L. (1966): Zur Therapie schwerer Schmerzzustande mit Tofranil. *Med. Welt.,* 43:2339–2340.
6. Deutschmann, W. (1971): Tofranil in der Schmerzbehandlung bei Krebskranken. *Med. Welt.,* 22:1346–1347.
7. Gebhardt, K. H., Beller, J., and Nischk, R. (1969): Behandlung des Karzinomschmerzes mit Chlorimipramin (Anafranil). *Med. Klin.,* 64:751–756.
8. Kocher, R. (1976): Use of psychotropic drugs for the treatment of chronic severe pain. In: *Advances in Pain Research and Therapy, Vol. 1: Proceedings of the First World Congress on Pain,* edited by J. J. Bonica and D. Albe-Fessard, pp. 579–582. Raven Press, New York.
9. Mönkemeier, D., and Steffen, U. (1970): Zur Behandlung von Schmerz mit Imipramin bei Krebserkrankungen. *Med. Klin.,* 65:213–215.
10. Put, I. R. (1974): Traitment des douleurs rebelles a l'aide du flupenthixol et du melitracene. *Ars. Medici,* 29:1401–1413.

The Brompton Cocktail

Robert G. Twycross

The Churchill Hospital, Headington, Oxford, England

INTRODUCTION

For many centuries opium has held a unique place in the physician's armoury on account of its ability to relieve severe pain without undue sedation. With the extraction and purification of opium alkaloids in the 19th century, morphine was increasingly substituted for opium. In 1896, Snow, a surgeon at the Cancer Hospital (now the Royal Marsden Hospital, London), reported the combined use of morphine and cocaine in advanced cancer, though subsequently he stopped adding cocaine because of the cost (6,7). Some 30 years later, however, it was re-introduced by Roberts, a surgeon at the Brompton Hospital, who used a morphine-cocaine elixir as a post-thoracotomy analgesic (2). At other hospitals, similar elixirs were used in advanced malignant or terminal respiratory disease. These were known by a variety of names, such as *Mistura pro moribundo, Mistura pro euthanasia,* and *Mistura euphoriens*. It was not until 1952, when the Brompton Hospital produced its own supplement to the National Formulary, that the composition of a morphine-cocaine elixir appeared in print; in this supplement it was called *Haustus E* and contained:

Morphine hydrochloride	¼ grain	(15 mg)
Cocaine hydrochloride	⅙ grain	(10 mg)
Alcohol 90%	30 minims	(2 ml)
Syrup	60 minims	(4 ml)
Chloroform water to	½ fl. oz.	(15 ml)

This was a modification of the pre-war Brompton formulation which contained gin and honey instead of alcohol and syrup. It appeared subsequently in Martindale's *Extra Pharmacopoeia* (4) together with three variant formulations. In recent years, diamorphine (diacetylmorphine, heroin) has commonly been used instead of morphine as the analgesic component in such elixirs, now generally known as the *Brompton Cocktail*. The correct method of use is summarized in Table 1.

There is, however, a tendency to endow the Brompton Cocktail with almost mystical properties and to regard it as the panacea for terminal cancer

TABLE 1. *Use of the Brompton Cocktail in cancer pain compared with the use of injected morphine for acute severe pain*

	Brompton cocktail (cancer pain)	Injected morphine (acute pain)
Aim	Pain-relief	Pain-relief
Sedation	Usually undesirable	Often desirable
Desired duration of effect	As long as possible	2–4 hr
Timing	Every 4 hr regularly (in anticipation)	Every 2–6 hr as required (on demand)
Dose	Individually determined (5–100 mg)	Usually standard (10 mg)
Route	By mouth	Injection
Adjuvant medication	Common	Uncommon

pain. Experience at St. Christopher's Hospice, London, and similar units specializing in symptom control in far-advanced cancer, while testifying to the cocktail's general usefulness, emphasizes that to obtain the best results, the cocktail must be used within a comprehensive pattern of total patient care (5,10).

It does, however, contain four substances all of which have a side-effect potential and which, on occasion, have led to noncompliance by the patient and continued unrelieved pain. In view of this, it is necessary to examine in the light of present knowledge and experience whether such a mixture is a prerequisite of success or whether a simple solution of morphine or diamorphine would be equally effective.

DIAMORPHINE OR MORPHINE

A randomized, controlled trial of orally administered diamorphine and morphine when given every 4 hr in individually optimized doses to advanced cancer patients has recently been completed at St. Christopher's Hospice, London (9). The primary aim was to compare the incidence and severity of the side-effects of the two preparations when prescribed at the effective analgesic dose for each patient (Fig. 1). Patients, stratified for sex, were randomly allocated to receive either diamorphine or morphine by mouth as first treatment. All the patients received a phenothiazine; other medication was prescribed when indicated clinically. There were 699 patients, of median age 67 years, who entered the trial, of whom 146 were well enough to cross over. Of these, 89 remained on an unchanged dose of "diamorphine equivalent" and did not have their adjuvant medication modified during the 5-day period

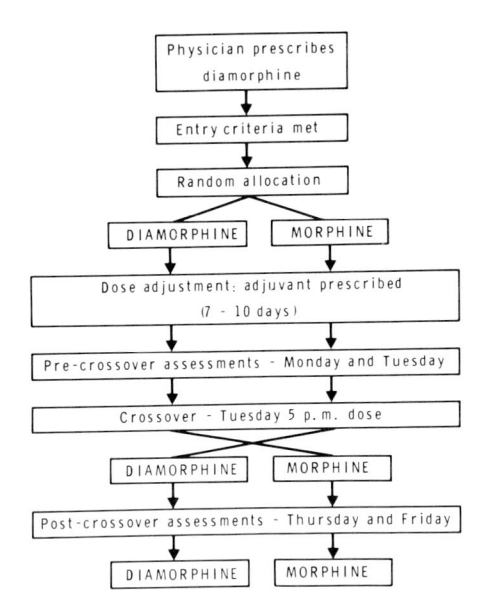

FIG. 1. Flow diagram describing method of diamorphine/morphine trial.

of observation. A potency ratio for orally administered diamorphine and morphine of 1.5:1 was assumed on the basis of a pilot trial.

In the 51 satisfactory female crossover patients, no statistically significant difference was noted in relation either to pain or the other symptoms evaluated. On the other hand, 38 satisfactory male crossover patients experienced significantly more pain and were significantly more depressed, while receiving diamorphine. In these, the potency ratio of diamorphine to morphine appeared to be less than 1.5:1. If this is allowed for, then the difference in mood is probably not significant. The patients who did not cross over appeared to do equally well on either opiate (Fig. 2).

It was concluded that, provided allowance is made for the potency difference between the two opiates, diamorphine and morphine are equally efficacious when given in a solution *by mouth* every 4 hr in individually optimized doses with a fixed dose of cocaine hydrochloride (10 mg) and in association with a phenothiazine such as prochlorperazine or chlorpromazine. (The oral/parenteral potency ratio of morphine when used in *solution* in this way appears to be of the order of 1:3, though this has not been tested formally.)

In a parallel study of urinary excretion of morphine in patients receiving diamorphine or morphine regularly, the results indicated that diamorphine is completely absorbed by the gastrointestinal tract but that morphine is only some two-thirds absorbed (11). This suggests that the potency ratio of orally administered diamorphine and morphine merely reflects the alimentary absorption ratio of the two preparations. This accords with the view of Way and his associates (13,14), based largely on studies using organ homogenates

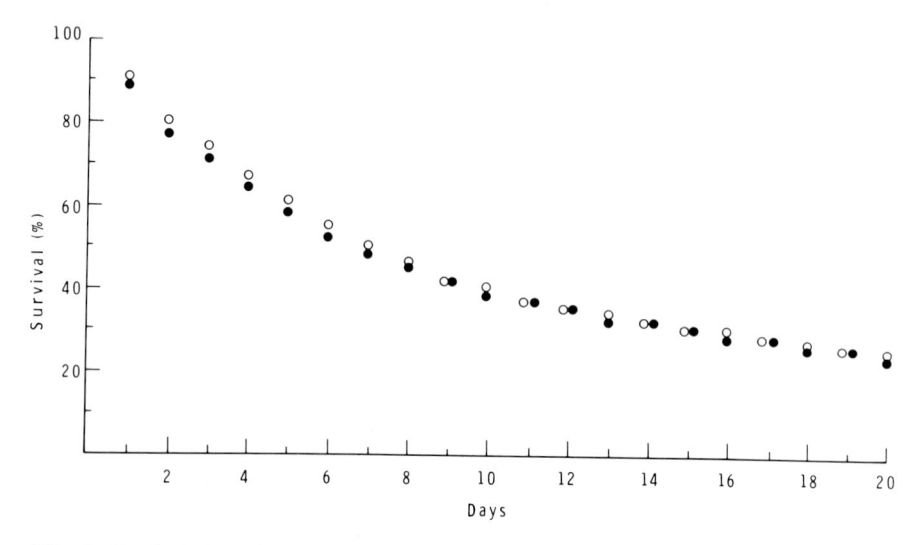

FIG. 2. Survival chart for 350 diamorphine-receiving patients (open circles) and 349 morphine-receiving patients (filled circles).

from both animals and man, that diamorphine is so rapidly deacetylated *in vivo* to O^6-monoacetylmorphine and morphine that it has only a transient pharmacological action of its own even after intravenous injection, its effects being almost entirely mediated via its two biotransformation products.

COCAINE

Cocaine was first used with morphine by Snow at the end of the last century on the grounds that it helped "sustain vitality" (6). More recently it has been claimed that the addition of cocaine enhances the mood of the patient: "The euphoria renders the patient comparatively cheerful, and relieves his mental and physical distress" (3). On the other hand it has been reported that the longer an opiate-cocaine elixir is administered, the greater is the likelihood that the patient will become depressed (12).

In order to clarify matters a randomized, controlled trial of morphine and diamorphine elixirs with and without cocaine was undertaken, again at St. Christopher's Hospice (8). After stabilization on an individually determined 4-hourly regimen only 61 out of 400 patients were well enough to cross over. Surprisingly, it was found that although introducing cocaine (10 mg/dose) resulted in a small, statistically significant increase in alertness, stopping cocaine had no detectable effect. Although debatable, it was considered that these findings could be explained if, in this dose, cocaine was of borderline efficacy and that tolerance to this borderline effect occurred within a few days. That tolerance does not always readily occur, however, is indicated by the occasional phenomenon—not seen in this trial—of the patient who becomes restless, agitated, confused, or hallucinated when prescribed cocaine and whose symptoms abate only when cocaine is withdrawn.

As a result of the trial, cocaine is no longer used routinely at St. Christopher's Hospice or at Sir Michael Sobell House. Cocaine is added only if a patient remains drowsy after 3 or 4 days on a steady dose of morphine. Even then my policy is to give a test dose of dexamphetamine or methylphenidate in order to help determine whether the addition of cocaine is likely to be of benefit. I have, in fact, used cerebral stimulants in only 2 patients out of some 200 during the past year. It is a matter of regret, therefore, that the current British National Formulary includes both morphine- and diamorphine-cocaine elixirs, since inclusion lends official blessing to the efficacy of such combinations. More regrettable is the inclusion of variant mixtures containing chlorpromazine. I would suggest that, given their respective doses, any stimulant action of cocaine will be antagonized by the chlorpromazine.

It should be mentioned that, by and large, it is standard practice in those British hospices where cocaine is still administered with diamorphine or morphine to use a standard 10 mg of cocaine hydrochloride. Occasional prescribers of the Brompton Cocktail not infrequently use a higher dose of cocaine and, moreover, commonly vary the dose of the opiate by varying the volume rather than the strength of the mixture. This means the dose of cocaine is increased in parallel with that of the opiate. This is true of its use in a number of American centers. It is perhaps not surprising that, at one center known to the author, hallucinations are so common a concomitant of the use of the Brompton Cocktail, that patients are warned to expect them and are taught to accept them as the necessary price to pay for pain-relief.

FORMULATION

In 1972, a survey of more than 90 teaching and district general hospitals throughout the United Kingdom confirmed that such elixirs were still in widespread use and also demonstrated considerable variation in composition (Twycross, *unpublished observations*). Differences existed both in the active constituents and in the vehicle in which they were dissolved. In addition to morphine or diamorphine, the majority included cocaine. A number also contained a phenothiazine (chlorpromazine or prochlorperazine) and, in some, morphine and diamorphine were both included. The variation in the vehicle was even greater; for example, the alcohol content ranged from 0 to 40% and was frequently replaced by gin, whisky, or brandy. The syrup content varied from 0 to 50% and honey was often substituted for sucrose. In the light of this, the introduction of standard diamorphine- and morphine-cocaine elixirs is welcome (11). Even with these, however, some patients complain about the "sickliness" of such mixtures, while other dislike the alcoholic "bite." As a result it is now my practice to dispense morphine in water alone, the patient adding blackcurrant juice or other flavoring as desired. If dispensed in combination with prochlorperazine or chlorpromazine, the incorporation of one of the flavored proprietary syrups usually circumvents the need for additional flavoring.

SIDE EFFECTS

Most patients with terminal cancer have more than one symptom. Nausea and vomiting are both common, and the use of a narcotic analgesic tends to precipitate or exacerbate these symptoms, particularly if the patient is ambulant. Patients prescribed the Brompton Cocktail should be questioned about nausea and vomiting and either have an antiemetic prescribed simultaneously or the need for such reviewed 2 or 3 days later. A patient will not continue to take an analgesic if it results in nausea or vomiting. At St. Christopher's Hospice a phenothiazine (generally prochlorperazine) is prescribed routinely. It acts not only as an antiemetic but also supplements the sedative effect of the narcotic analgesic. This is often replaced by chlorpromazine or, occasionally, methotrimeprazine in patients with an appreciable psychological component to their pain—for example, the patient with lung cancer experiencing both pain and dyspnea and who fears death by suffocation, or the woman who feels that her fungating breast cancer is jeopardizing her relationship with her husband. Chlorpromazine or promazine are also used to control confusion, delirium, or psychotic manifestations. Because many patients are both elderly and debilitated, it is wise to prescribe not more than 12.5 mg of chlorpromazine initially, to be administered every 4 hr with the (dia)morphine.

Some patients require an additional antiemetic such as cyclizine or metoclopramide. Constipation often occurs and requires an appropriate regimen of diet, laxatives, suppositories, and/or enemas.

A quarter of the patients at St. Christopher's Hospice are also prescribed either a tricyclic antidepressant or a benzodiazepine tranquilizer. Generally speaking, the latter are used for short periods to help patients at times of severe anxiety, whereas the former are used for longer periods if the patient becomes depressed. This occurs more frequently in patients who have a prolonged terminal phase.

Physicians not used to prescribing oral (dia)morphine are often concerned about the possibility of drowsiness. In fact, no study to determine whether there is a relationship between dose administered and drowsiness has yet been reported. In practice, it is generally found that the initial drowsiness experienced by some patients when prescribed (dia)morphine and a phenothiazine diminishes after a day or two. Persistent drowsiness is unusual and is possibly related more to advanced physical debility than to (dia)morphine itself.

As stated above, persistent drowsiness unrelated to debility is so infrequent that the author has prescribed a cerebral stimulant in only 1% of patients prescribed oral morphine during the past year. Inactivity or boredom drowsiness does persist in the majority of patients, but this does not prevent normal activity. In fact, the ability of many patients to "cat nap" when alone or resting is generally seen as an advantage in that it helps to pass the time during what often seems a long 16 hr between getting up in the morning and retiring to bed at night.

CONCLUSIONS

The Brompton Cocktail is, therefore, merely a traditional way of prescribing oral (dia)morphine. It is not the panacea nor does it possess magical properties. The results are best when the cocktail is used within the context of general emotional support for the patient and his family (5). Attention to the several other symptoms the patient is likely to be suffering from is also important. In practice a combination of drug, nondrug, and common-sense measures are necessary to achieve maximum benefit (10).

Although the median 4-hourly dose of oral diamorphine is 10 mg (Fig. 3) and that of morphine 15 to 20 mg, *the effective analgesic doses of both range from as little as 2.5 mg to more than 100 mg.* It is important not to transfer the concept of a "maximum dose" from acute parenteral use to the relatively long-term *oral* use in patients with advanced cancer. Not only does

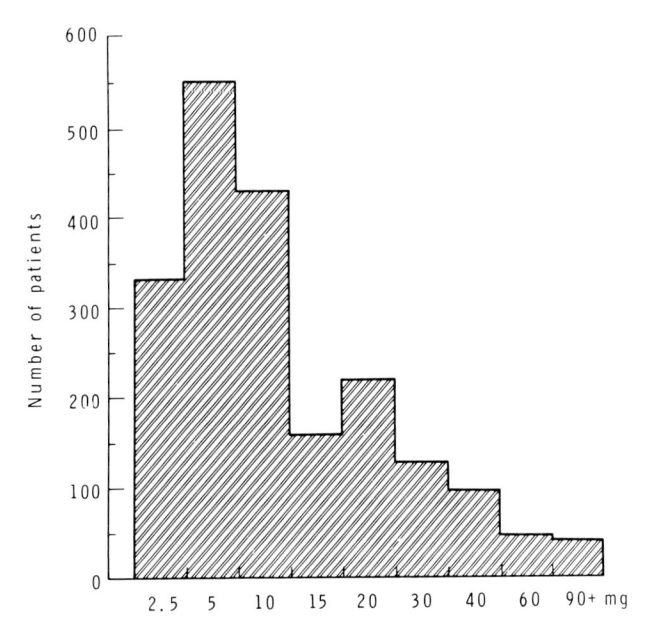

FIG. 3. Histogram of maximum 4-hr doses of diamorphine given to 2,000 patients admitted to St. Christopher's Hospice, 1972–1975 inclusive.

the effective dose vary considerably, but problems associated with continuous parenteral use, such as tolerance, are minimal (12).

Whether or not a physician prescribes the Brompton Cocktail or, simply, morphine in tap water will probably depend on personal inclination. Provided, however, the physician appreciates that each of the four constituents has a side-effect potential and enquires of his patients about untoward effects, including unpleasant taste and a burning sensation in the throat, there is no reason for his not continuing to use the cocktail. On the other hand, he should be aware that it is simpler for the pharmacist, cheaper for the patient, and easier for the physician to manipulate opiate doses if a simple solution of morphine hydrochloride or sulphate is used.

SUMMARY

The use of the Brompton Cocktail, an opiate-cocaine elixir, for the relief of pain in far-advanced cancer is recorded. Results from a comparative trial of diamorphine (diacetylmorphine, heroin) and morphine are summarized. These indicate that, by mouth, both opiates are equally efficacious, though diamorphine is about 1.5 times more potent than morphine. The value of cocaine is questioned, as is the automatic inclusion of alcohol and syrup. The place of antiemetics, laxatives, and other adjuvant medication is discussed. It is emphasized that the Brompton Cocktail is no more than a traditional British way of administering oral morphine to cancer patients in pain. Moreover, if prescribed, it should be used within the context of a comprehensive pattern of patient care, and as one prong of a broad-spectrum approach to the relief of pain.

ACKNOWLEDGMENT

I thank Dr. Cicely Saunders, Medical Director, St. Christopher's Hospice, London, for her continued encouragement and support. The studies reported were carried out at St. Christopher's on patients under her care between 1971 and 1976.

ADDENDUM

Pain-Relief in Advanced Cancer—General Principles

Aim: To keep the patient both free of pain and fully alert.

Assessment

1. *Treatment* varies according to the cause of the pain; use *body chart* to record sites of pain and their probable mechanism.

2. Because a person has cancer, it does not mean that the malignant process is necessarily the cause of the pain.

Choice of Analgesics
1. Establish a simple, practical *analgesic "league table"*
    a. *Non-narcotic*—aspirin (alt. acetominophen)
    b. *Weak narcotic*—codeine (alt. DHC, *d*-propoxyphene)
    c. *Strong narcotic*—morphine (alt. papaveretum, diamorphine)
2. *Avoid* pentazocine, meperidine, and dextromoramide (Palfium®).
3. *Methadone* should be used with caution, particularly in the elderly and debilitated.
4. The use of a narcotic analgesic is dictated by intensity of pain and not by brevity of prognosis.
   "Morphine exists to be given, not merely to be withheld."

Use of Analgesics
1. *Oral medication* is normally possible. When injections are necessary, use freeze-dried ampoules of diamorphine.
2. *Persistent pain requires preventive therapy.* This means that analgesics should be given regularly and prophylactically: "as required" medication is both irrational and inhumane.
3. Doses should be determined on an *individual basis;* the right dose is that which gives relief for at least 3, preferably 4 or more hr.
4. Adjuvant medication is the rule rather than the exception. *Laxatives* are almost always necessary, an *antiemetic* commonly so.
5. If very anxious, an *anxiolytic* such as diazepam should be tried; if depressed, an *antidepressive*.
6. The perception of pain requires both attention and consciousness. *Diversional therapy*—people to talk to, activities to attend, etc.—is of great value.
7. *Tolerance* is not usually a practical problem.
8. Rightly used, *psychological dependence* (addiction) does not occur.
9. *Physical dependence* does not prevent the downward adjustment of the dose of a narcotic analgesic should the pain ameliorate.
10. Neither diamorphine nor morphine is the panacea for terminal pain. Their use does not guarantee automatic success, particularly if the psychological component of pain is ignored.

Reassessment
1. *Relief of pain* should be assessed in relation to comfort achieved
    a. during the night,
    b. in the daytime at rest,
    c. on movement.
2. Reassessment remains a continuing necessity; old pains may get worse and new ones may develop.
   REVIEW. REVIEW. REVIEW. REVIEW. REVIEW.

REFERENCES

1. British Pharmaceutical Codex (1973): Pharmaceutical Press, London. p. 669.
2. Kerrane, T. A. (1975): The Brompton Cocktail. *Nursing Mirror,* 140:59.
3. Love, M. (1962): Management of advanced cancer. *Br. Med. J.,* 2, 1192.
4. Martindale (1958): *Extra Pharmacopoeia* (24th ed.), p. 911. Pharmaceutical Press, London.
5. Melzack, R., Ofiesh, J. G., and Mount, B. M. (1976): The Brompton mixture: Effects on pain in cancer patients. *Can. Med. Assoc. J.,* 115:125–129.
6. Snow, H. (1896): Opium and cocaine in the treatment of cancerous disease. *Br. Med. J.,* 2:718–719.
7. Snow, H. (1897): The opium-cocaine treatment of malignant disease. *Br. Med. J.,* 1:1019–1020.
8. Twycross, R. G. (1976): *Studies on the Use of Diamorphine in Advanced Malignant Disease.* D. M. Thesis, University of Oxford.
9. Twycross, R. G. (1977): Choice of strong analgesic in terminal cancer: Diamorphine or morphine? *Pain,* 3:93–104.
10. Twycross, R. G. (1978): Bone pain in advanced cancer. *Topics in Therapeutics 4,* edited by D. W. Vere, pp. 94–110. Pitman Medical, Tunbridge Wells.
11. Twycross, R. G., Fry, D. E., and Wills, P. D. (1974): The alimentary absorption of diamorphine and morphine in man as indicated by urinary excretion studies. *Br. J. Clin. Pharmacol.,* 1:491–494.
12. Twycross, R. G., and Wald, S. J. (1976): Long-term use of diamorphine in advanced cancer. *Advances in Pain Research and Therapy, Vol. 1: Proceedings of the First World Congress on Pain,* edited by J. J. Bonica and D. Albe-Fessard, pp. 653–661. Raven Press, New York.
13. Way, E. L., Kemp, J. W., Young, J. M., and Grassetti, D. R. (1960): The pharmacologic effects of heroin in relationship to its rate of biotransformation. *J. Pharmacol. Exp. Ther.,* 129:144–154.
14. Way, E. L., Young, J. M., and Kemp, J. W. (1965): Metabolism of heroin and its pharmacological implications. *Bull. Narcot.,* 17(1):25–33.

Discussion

Part II. Management of Pain of Advanced Cancer: Systemic Analgesics and Related Drugs

R. Houde and B. R. Fink (Moderators)

Moricca (Rome): Dr. Twycross, can you make a short comment on the use of addictive drugs for the relief of pain in advanced cancer patients for the doctor?

Twycross (Oxford): I don't talk about addictive drugs; it's as alien to me as referring to, let's say, aspirin as a drug which induces deafness.

Hildebrandt (Göttingen): Dr. Kocher, is haloperidol useful as a neuroleptic agent for the treatment of pain?

Kocher (Basel): I think so. At first we began with neuroleptic caevomepromazine (nozinan) and the analgesic effect was better, but we had too many side effects. Now we use haloperidol because you have practically no side effects, and for me, it has the same analgesic effect.

Gerbershagen (Mainz): One should always use these drugs. If you want to have anxiolytics, you would not use that. But if you want to have a sleeping effect, then you would use haloperidol.

Procacci (Florence): Dr. Houde, I have found that atarax has been effective in the treatment of postoperative pain. Has your experience in cancer pain been similar?

Houde (New York): We have not evaluated hydroxyzine in a controlled study, but we do use it clinically, and we have found it to be an effective adjuvant when given along with morphine, generally from 25 to 50 mg.

Iacono (Ragusa): Dr. Twycross, how do you reduce the gastrointestinal effect of analgesics? Which analgesics do you use in patients affected by peptic ulcer?

Twycross: First of all, I tend to give the aspirin with alkali or milk or after food. Most patients seem to be able to tolerate that. In fact, the main reason for stopping aspirin in my ordinary cancer patients has been deafness when I have been using it in doses of 4 g or more a day. But if there is obvious gastric upset, then I may try enteric-coated phenabutizone, which was a favorite; I would tend to use phelebepropane now. What do I do if the patient has a peptic ulcer? So far, I haven't had the combination of a patient with active advanced cancer and active peptic ulcer. Maybe that will happen next week. Until I do, I tend to avoid soluble aspirin if there is a strong history of peptic ulcer, and I tend to use one of these alternatives.

Sapio (Taranto): Dr. Gerbershagen, what is the analgesic effect of cortisone derivatives and the relevant dosage? What is the analgesic effect of local anesthetics by intravenous and relevant dosage?

Gerbershagen: There are many effects of cortisone derivatives. I think the most important effect, besides, of course, the antiproliferative effect, is the antiedema effect. Local anesthetics are mainly used in South America and in some hospitals in Germany, but in South America they are used even for anesthesia in large doses; 1, 2, 3 g of procaine for instance. I think we use it only if there is itching—one type of pain—and then we give i.v. tetracine, about 200 mg in ½ liter of normal saline, and then the itch is usually gone for about a day or two and sometimes it stays away.

Twycross: As regards prednisolone, I agree that we are using it for the antiedema effect and, therefore, perhaps we could list three or four common situations where I find it useful: (a) Headache due to raised intracranial pressure. Often we use dexomethazone, the far more potent corticosteroid, starting at a dosage of 4 mg t.i.d. or q.i.d., and reducing down to about 2 mg t.i.d. subsequently. But sometimes prednisolone is adequate. (b) In patients with head and neck cancer, you get extensive soft-tissue infiltration and secondary edema, and the drug can be remarkable in easing the pain associated with that. (c) For nerve compression pain, it is always worth treating with a combination of morphine and prednisolone initially, perhaps in a dose of 10 mg t.i.d., reducing to 5 mg t.i.d. before you call your anesthetist for a nerve block. (d) The pelvic cancer patient where, again, you have extensive pelvic malignancy with extensive soft-tissue infiltration and secondary edema; and here again, the use of morphine plus prednisolone and often aspirin or other anti-inflammatory drugs together produce very good results when on their own you don't get more than 50/60% relief.

Hildebrandt: Dr. Houde, what do you think of Tiladine®?

Houde: Tiladine is a drug that has narcotic agonist and very weak antagonist properties, like morphine. I realize it is abused quite a bit in Germany. We found it about $\frac{1}{25}$ or $\frac{1}{24}$ as potent as prophine by injection. It is a little more effective orally, about $\frac{1}{15}$ as potent as morphine—not too promising.

Tommasi Morgano (Torino): What do you think of physical and psychological drug dependence from morphine and heroin?

Houde: The question is directed to what the relative physical and psychological dependence potentials are of morphine and heroin. The physical dependence potentials of the drugs are very similar. Whether one has a greater psychological dependence-producing potential than the other is unresolved. The general opinion today is that there is very little to choose between them.

Netti (Conversano): Which measures do you adopt to avoid dependence and tolerance development of narcotic analgesics? How do you evaluate when a patient has developed tolerance when instead there is an insufficient dosage?

Houde: Tolerance development and physical dependence development are dose-related phenomena; we know that. The way of avoiding it is to use drugs in low enough doses or in combinations such that you do not too rapidly escalate the dose. But these are properties of narcotics. They are not important if you adjust your doses. Remember that though patients can gain tolerance and physical dependence, they can also lose it, particularly if you also pay attention to definitive means of treating or removing the cause of pain.

Twycross: When morphine or diamorphine (heroin) is used in an individually determined dosage in association with other treatments, then in those controlled circumstances, associated with attention to other symptoms and emotional support of family and patient, tolerance is not a practical problem. Please get away from all that you have learned from basic pharmacologists and from the addiction center of Lexington. In advanced cancer, tolerance is not a practical problem; physical dependence may occur but doesn't prevent the progressive downward adjustment of dose should the pain ameliorate. A craving for the drug does not occur if the drug is administered prophylactically. (Houde does not agree with all that but will discuss it later.)

Introduction to Nerve Blocks

John J. Bonica

Department of Anesthesiology, University of Washington School of Medicine, Seattle, Washington 98195

Nerve blocks, or analgesic block, whereby a local anesthetic or a neurolytic agent is injected near or into a nerve or nerves, have been used to relieve the pain of cancer for over a century (2). Personal experience during the past 35 years and experience reported by many others suggests that, skillfully administered in properly selected patients, nerve blocks are among the most effective methods of relieving cancer pain (1,3,4,5,6,7). On the other hand, improperly applied, these procedures often result in failures and, at times, serious complications. Despite the long use of the procedures, there is still some serious misconception about their role in managing chronic pain in general and cancer pain in particular. The objective of the chapters in this section is to evaluate the efficacy, indications, and advantages, as well as the limitations, disadvantages, and complications of various nerve-block techniques used to relieve cancer pain. I will introduce the discussion by briefly giving a historical perspective, discussing the bases and indications for the application of nerve blocks, emphasizing certain conditions and requisites that must be met in order to obtain optimal results, and giving a brief overview of the various agents and techniques that are used.

HISTORICAL PERSPECTIVE

The first recorded use of analgesic blocks to relieve cancer pain occurred in 1875 when Fauvel (9), Collins, Taglia and others (30) applied cocaine to the larynx in patients with severe cancer pain. This was 9 years before Karl Koller (12) gave the first clinical demonstration of the local anesthetic properties of cocaine for eye surgery, an event considered to be a milestone in the history of anesthesia, because it ushered in the widespread use of local and regional anesthesia for surgery. In 1894, Corning (7), an American neurologist, wrote what was probably the first book devoted to the use of regional analgesia for the relief of pain. In this little-known monograph Corning mentioned the use of cocaine injection into the subarachnoid space and near nerves to relieve neuralgia and other forms of chronic pain including cancer pain. However, the widespread use of nerve blocks for definitive control of cancer pain did not really begin until sometime after 1900, when Schlosser (26) began experimenting with the injection of alcohol near and into nerves for the treatment of neuralgia with particular emphasis on trigeminal neuralgia. The numerous reports of the successful use of alcohol block for trigeminal neuralgia prompted other clinicians to use it for the relief of cancer pain (11,13,20). Similarly, the report of Lewy (14) in 1911, in which he described the successful use of alcohol block of the superior laryngeal nerve to relieve the pain of tuberculosis, led Lukens (16) and, subsequently, Swetlow (29) to apply this technique for the relief of cancer pain.

Another technique which was developed right after the turn of the century was paravertebral block, which entails the injection of spinal nerves as they emerge from the intervertebral foramen (2). Although this technique was first used in surgical anesthesia, it soon became applied as a diagnostic tool to ascertain visceral pain pathways and, subsequently, it was used for the therapy of severe intractable pain. In 1926, Mandl (18) reported the successful use of paravertebral block with procaine to relieve severe pain of cancer of the pancreas. In the same year, Swetlow (29) reported the use of paravertebral alcohol block for a variety of painful conditions including the pain of cancer.

One of the most important events in the history of analgesic block for the relief of cancer pain is the report by Dogliotti (8) in 1931, describing the successful use of the injection of alcohol into the subarachnoid space to achieve chemical rhizotomy. This technique was promptly used widely, and in the ensuing decade, dozens of reports were published attesting to the efficacy of the procedure in relieving cancer pain (10,22,24,25). Five years later, Putnam and Hampton (23) published the first report on the use of aqueous phenol as a neurolytic agent for gasserian ganglion block. About a decade later, phenol was used by Mandl (18a) and others to achieve chemical sympathectomy.

The report by Maher (17) in 1955, in which he described the injection of hyperbaric phenol into the subarachnoid space to produce chemical rhizotomy for the relief of cancer pain must be considered another milestone in the history of the use of nerve block for this purpose. This report had the same type of impact as the report by Dogliotti about alcohol. Consequently, many, many reports have been published attesting to the efficacy of this technique (15,19,21,27,28,31). Since the history of subarachnoid neurolysis will be discussed in detail by Dr. Swerdlow and Professor Papo and others in this volume, I will make no further comments. A detailed discussion of the use of nerve blocks for cancer therapy can be found elsewhere (2,3,6,32).

BASES AND INDICATIONS

The basis for the efficacy and utility of nerve blocks to relieve cancer pain is the interruption of specific sensory, and particularly nociceptive or pain pathways and, in certain circumstances, block of the sympathetic nerves. Sensory block relieves pain and interrupts the afferent limb of any abnormal reflex mechanisms that may be contributing to the physiopathology of the pain and associated phenomena. By using low concentrations of local anesthetics, it is possible to block the small, myelinated A-delta fibers and the unmyelinated C-fibers, some of which are involved in nociception, without significant impairment of motor function. As will be discussed by Professor Gerbershagen, in many instances, block with local anesthetics produces pain-relief which outlasts the pharmacologic action of the drug by hours, days, and sometimes weeks. The exact mechanism for this almost enigmatic phenomenon is not definitely known. It has been suggested that the block of sensory input for several hours brings about a cessation of the self-sustaining activity of the neuron pools in the neuraxis which are considered to be responsible for some chronic pain states (5). Alcohol and phenol produce prolonged pain-relief by destruction of nociceptive pathways. These procedures may be used as diagnostic and prognostic tools, as well as for the definitive therapy of pain.

DIAGNOSTIC BLOCKS

Properly applied and skillfully executed, nerve blocks may be used effectively as diagnostic tools to: (a) help to ascertain the specific nociceptive or pain pathways; (b) help to define the mechanisms of the cancer pain; and (c) aid in differential diagnosis of the site of the pain. For example, nerve blocks help to define the nociceptive pathways in patients with pain in the angle of the jaw, which can be caused by involvement either of the trigeminal nerve or the glossopharyngeal and vagal nerves. Moreover, nerve blocks are useful to differentiate pain due to involvement of viscera from the pain of somatic origin. Examples are patients complaining of chest pain, epigastric pain, or suprapubic pain. Block of those intercostal nerves which supply the area of the chest wall where pain is felt will completely relieve pain due to somatic tissue or chest wall involvement by the cancer, but will have little or no effect on pain from the thoracic viscera. Similarly, pain in the suprapubic region which is relieved by block of the lower two thoracic and first and second lumbar spinal nerves suggests that its cause is in the abdominal wall rather than its being a referred pain from pelvic viscera, which are supplied by the middle three sacral segments.

Prognostic Blocks

Prognostic blocks are useful to predict the effects resulting from prolonged interruption, either by injection of a neurolytic agent or by neurosurgical operation. Moreover, prognostic blocks afford the patient an opportunity to experience the numbness and other side effects that follow surgical section on neurolytic block and thus help the patient decide whether or not to have the procedure.

Therapeutic Blocks

Therapeutic blocks can be achieved with either a local anesthetic or a neurolytic agent. Local anesthetic blocks are very useful in the temporary relief of very severe pain due to cancer in the chest, abdomen, pelvis, and lower limbs. Although various techniques may be used for this purpose, continuous segmental epidural block permits the repeated injection of local anesthetics at intervals to produce continuous pain-relief. In addition to blocking the nociceptive pathways, the local anesthetic eliminates reflex muscle spasm and reflex sympathetic mechanisms which may be acting as positive feedback mechanisms to contribute to the nociceptive input. Thus, for example, in patients with cancer of the pancreas, continuous epidural block limited to the fifth to tenth thoracic segments will provide complete relief of pain which can be continued for several days and as long as a week. As will be emphasized by Professor Gerbershagen, repeated single injection with long-lasting local anesthetics may also prove effective in producing prolonged pain-relief in many patients with cancer.

Neurolytic blocks achieved by the injection of alcohol or phenol involve the intentional destruction of the nerve or nerves for a period of time to produce prolonged pain-relief. If the neurolytic agent is injected into the subarachnoid space, it should, theoretically, destroy the nociceptive fibers in the dorsal root proximal to the spinal ganglion and thus produce permanent interruption of some or all of the affected axons and thus simulate surgical rhizotomy. Similarly, injection of alcohol into the gasserian ganglion should destroy many or all of the nerve cell bodies and, consequently, produce permanent interruption. The efficacy and duration of analgesia are dependent on the completeness of the destruction of the nerve roots or ganglion cells by the neurolytic agent. It deserves reemphasis that neurolytic blocks should be limited to control of pain due to inoperable or recurrent cancer.

GENERAL CONSIDERATIONS

Skillfully administered in properly selected patients, nerve blocks are among the most effective methods of relieving cancer pain. These procedures are especially indicated in patients with moderate to severe pain of advanced cancer whose physical and emotional conditions place them at risk and may contraindicate neurosurgery and whose life-expectancy is less than 6 months. In contrast to narcotics and other systemic drugs, nerve blocks usually produce complete relief of pain without the side effects of systemic drugs. Nerve blocks do not tax the physiologic and emotional resources of the patient to the same extent as neurosurgery. Moreover, since they require short hospitalization, they impose less financial strain on the patient and family. By relieving the pain, they facilitate improved nutrition and enhance the physical and emotional condition of the patient to permit radiation therapy or other oncologic treatments and even neurosurgery. Since the nerves to any part of the body can be blocked, nerve blocks are applicable to relieve the pain of virtually any type of cancer.

REQUISITES FOR OPTIMAL RESULTS

To obtain optimal results for nerve blocks it is essential to adhere to certain basic principles which I originally developed a quarter-century ago and whose importance I have repeatedly emphasized since then (1,4,5). The first is that the physician using this method must be willing to devote the necessary time to evaluate the patient thoroughly. Experience has shown that this is essential even if the patient has already been evaluated by a highly competent colleague. A detailed history and thorough physical examination not only provide additional information but also afford the opportunity for the physician to become acquainted with the patient, to investigate his or her personality, and most important to establish rapport and win the confidence of the patient. A careful neurologic examination not only provides useful information, but will constitute a base line in evaluating the effects of the block. It is also essential to determine the presence of cardiovascular or vesical dysfunctions prior to initiating the procedure.

Another requisite is that the physician must be highly skilled in carrying out the most appropriate nerve block procedure and know thoroughly the immediate and long-term effects. Patients with cancer pain are not good subjects on whom to practice nerve blocks. The skill should be acquired in the application of nerve blocks for surgical anesthesia and in patients with nonmalignant chronic pain. Moreover, nerve blocks must be performed carefully, with meticulous attention to anatomic detail and with utmost gentleness.

In order to select the best nerve block procedure in each particular case it is essential that the physician know well the distribution of the pain, its etiology and mechanisms, the nociceptive pathways involved, the type of neoplasm, its grade of differentiation and possible extension, and the structures it might invade, and all of the other issues I mentioned in my introductory remarks to the management of the problem (pp. 115–130).

An obviously important requisite is to prepare the patient carefully for the procedure. This includes informing the patient and his family of what is going to be done, how it will be done, and what is to be accomplished with the procedure. If the patient and family do not realize beforehand that the diagnostic or prognostic block is only to gain information and will provide only temporary relief, he or she may be disappointed prematurely and become bitter. Moreover, the patient and the family must be made to realize that since the intractable pain of cancer is a difficult problem to manage and complete relief is not always obtained in the first treatment, it may be necessary to do several blocks. If this is explained beforehand, the patient is much less likely to become discouraged before treatment is completed. In addition, it is important to inform the patient and his family, and even the referring physician, of the possible complications because, although these patients often express a desire for relief at almost any price before the procedure, they may become bitter if urinary disturbances or rectal incontinence occur or the extremities become weakened or paralyzed as a result of the block. When the patient is cognizant of the true status of the disease, he or she should be made to understand clearly that the nerve block procedure itself is palliative and not curative. Finally, the patient should receive pharmacologic preparation for the block procedures in the form of sedatives/analgesics.

If the block procedures are to be done for diagnostic or prognostic purposes prior to permanent interruption, it is essential to localize exactly and precisely the involved nerve or nerves. This can be accomplished by eliciting paresthesia, by checking the position of the needle with X-ray with or without prior injection of a contrast medium, or by the use of a nerve stimulator. Moreover, in using diagnostic or prognostic blocks, three essential principles must be adhered to: (a) The injection should entail only small amounts of local anesthetic solution to avoid diffusion to adjacent segments and thus preclude misleading information; (b) no decision should be made until two or three blocks produce consistent responses; and (c) it is best to use local anesthetics of different duration for each of the procedures so that the duration of block can be correlated with the duration of subjective pain-relief.

During and following the block it is essential to assess carefully the results. Observation of the reaction of the patient to the insertion of small needles, the formation of intracutaneous wheals and other parts of the procedure help in evaluating the patient's reactions to noxious stimuli. Following the block, it is essential to ascertain whether the appropriate nociceptive pathways have been interrupted by repeating the neurologic examination.

Once it is established that the procedure has interrupted the intended nociceptive pathways, the effects of the procedure in relieving the pain must be carefully assessed. This usually requires observation for from a few hours to several days or weeks. The amount, type, and duration of relief obtained should be carefully noted and recorded on the patient's chart. In addition to observation by the physician, the results should be evaluated by the patient and his or her family, if they are available, and, most importantly, by the nursing staff.

It is important that all concerned fully appreciate the fact that nerve blocks have certain limitations and should be integrated with other therapeutic measures. It deserves reemphasis that the pain of cancer not only involves nociceptive input, but the emotional, psychologic, and affective responses thereto. While nerve blocks and neurosurgical operation may eliminate the nociceptive input, they do nothing for the other aspects of the cancer pain and, therefore, other therapeutic modalities need to be used.

Finally, it is also essential that the patient and the physicians realize two important disadvantages of these techniques: (a) pain-relief may be incomplete or, if it is complete, may not last until the patient's death. Fortunately, since the block can be extended or repeated several times, these are only minor disadvantages. (b) More importantly, side effects and serious complications can occur during or after the block. The most important of these are orthostatic hypotension from extensive sympathetic interruption, paresthesia and dysesthesia, limb-muscle weakness or dysfunction of vesical or rectal sphincter, or a combination of these. It is the responsibility of the administrator to carry out all prophylactic measures against these undesirable side effects and complications.

REFERENCES

1. Bonica, J. J. (1952): Management of intractable pain with analgesic blocks. *JAMA*, 150:1581–1586.
2. Bonica, J. J. (1953): *The Management of Pain*. Lea & Febiger, Philadelphia.
3. Bonica, J. J. (1954): The management of cancer pain. *GP (American Academy of General Practice)*, 10:34–43.
4. Bonica, J. J. (1955): Teaching residents diagnostic and therapeutic nerve blocks. *Anesth. Analg.*, 34:202–213.
5. Bonica, J. J. (1974): Current role of nerve blocks in diagnosis and therapy of pain. In: *Advances in Neurology, Vol. 4: International Symposium on Pain,* edited by J. J. Bonica, pp. 433–453. Raven Press, New York.
6. Bonica, J. J. (1954): The management of pain of malignant disease with nerve blocks. *Anesthesiology*, 15:(March) 134 and (May) 280–301.
7. Corning, J. L. (1894): *Pain in Its Neuropathologic, Diagnostic and Neurotherapeutic Relations*. J. B. Lippincott, Philadelphia.
8. Dogliotti, A. M. (1931): Traitment des syndromes douloureux de la peripherie par l'alcoholisation sub-arachnoidienne. *Presse Med.*, 67:11.
9. Fauvel, H. (1884): De l'anesthesie produite par le chlorhydrate de cocaine sur la muquese pharyngienne et laryngienne. *Gas des hop.*, Nr., 134, S. 1067.
10. Greenhill, J. P. (1935): Intraspinal (subarachnoid) injection of alcohol for pain associated with malignant conditions of the female genitalia. *JAMA*, 105:406.
11. Hartel, F. (1914): Über die intracranielle injections behandlung der trigeminus neuralgie mit intrakraniellen alkoholeinspritzungen. *Deutsche. Ztschr. f. Chir.*, 126:429.
12. Koller, C. (1884): Vorläufige Mittheilung über local Anästhesirung am Aug. *Klin. Monatsb. f. Augenh.*, 22, Beilagenheft, p. 60.
13. Levy, F., and Baudouin, A. (1906): Les injections profondes dans le traitment de la neuralgia facial rebelle. *Presse Med.*, 13:108.
14. Lewy, A. P. (1911): Analgesia of the larynx by alcohol injection of the internal branch of the superior laryngeal nerve. *Laryngoscope*, 21:9.
15. Lifschitz, S., Debacker, L. J., and Buchsbaum, H. J. (1976): Subarachnoid phenol block for pain relief in gynecologic malignancy. *Obstet. Gynecol.*, 48:316–320.
16. Lukens, R. McD. (1918): Dysphagia in tuberculous laryngitis. *N.Y. State J. Med.*, 107:353.
17. Maher, R. M. (1955): Relief of pain in incurable cancer. *Lancet*, 1:18–20.
18. Mandl, F. (1925): Die anwendungsbreite der paravertebralen injektion. *Klin. Schnschr.*, 4:49.
18a. Mandl, F. (1950): Phenol as a substitute for alcohol in sympathetic block. *J. Int. Coll. Surg.*, 13:566–568.
19. Nathan, P. W. (1972): Pain in cancer: Comparison of results of cordotomy and

chemical rhizotomy. In: *Present Limits of Neurosurgery,* edited by I. Fusek and Z. Kung, pp. 513–516. Excerpta Medica, Amsterdam.
20. Ostwald, F. (1905): Traitment des neuralgies rebelles par les injections profondes d'alcohol. *Presse Med.,* 12:812.
21. Papo, I., and Visca, A. (1974): Phenol rhizotomy in the treatment of cancer pain. *Anesth. Analg.,* 53:993–997.
22. Poppen, J. L. (1936): Subarachnoid alcohol injection: Indication, contraindications, technique and results in 82 patients. *Surg. Clin. North Am.,* 16:1663.
23. Putnam, T. J., and Hampton, A. O. (1936): A technique of injection into the Gasserian ganglion under roentgenographic control. *Arch. Neurol. Psychiatry,* (Chicago), 35:92–98.
24. Russell, W. R. (1937): *Intraspinal Injection of Alcohol for Intractable Pain.* M. J. May, Edinburgh.
25. Saltzstein, H. C. (1934): Intraspinal (subarachnoid) injection of absolute alcohol for the control of pain of advanced malignant growths. *JAMA,* 103:242.
26. Schlosser, H. (1907): Erfahrungen in der neuralgiebehandlung mit alkoholeinspritzungen. *Verhandl. d. Cong. f. innere Med.,* 24:49.
27. Stovner, J., and Enrenen, R. (1972): Intrathecal phenol for cancer pain. *Acta Anaesthesiol. Scand.* 16:17–21.
28. Swerdlow, M. (1973): Intrathecal chlorocresol. A comparison with phenol in the treatment of intractable pain. *Anaesthesia,* 28:297–301.
29. Swetlow, G. I. (1925): Injection of the superior laryngeal nerve with alcohol for the relief of pain in laryngeal tuberculosis. *Am. Rev. Tuberc.,* 12:189.
30. Taglia, S. Cited by Bonica, J. J. (1953): *The Management of Pain.* Lea & Febiger, Philadelphia.
31. Wilkinson, H. A., Mark, V. H., and White, J. C. (1964): Further experiences with intrathecal phenol for the relief of pain. *J. Chron. Dis.,* 17:1055–1059.
32. Wood, K. (1978): The use of phenol as a neurolytic agent: A review. *Pain,* 5:205–229.

Blocks with Local Anesthetics in the Treatment of Cancer Pain

H. U. Gerbershagen

Department of Anesthesiology and Interdisciplinary Pain Clinic, Johannes Gutenberg University, Mainz, West Germany

Regional block procedures for the relief of cancer pain are usually performed with neurolytic substances such as alcohol or phenol. There are, however, pain states associated with neoplastic disease which do not require destructive nerve blocks with their inherent side effects and complications. Local anesthetic blocks useful for cancer pain include sympathetic block, somatic nerve block, and extradural block.

SYMPATHETIC NERVE BLOCKADE

Cancer pain amenable to local anesthetic blocks is characterized by symptomatology of so-called carcinomatous (or sarcomatous) neuritis, which is identical to the signs and symptoms of reflex sympathetic dystrophy. These include: (a) pain; (b) hyperpathia (hyperesthesia and/or hyperalgesia); (c) neurovascular instability (vasoconstriction with cyanosis and edema or vasodilatation); (d) sudomotor disturbances (hyper-, hypo-, or anhidrosis); and (e) pilomotor changes.

The quality of pain is burning, throbbing, dull, and in some cases even sharp and stabbing (21). Characteristically, the pattern of distribution of this constant pain and of the hyperpathic area does not correspond to segmental or peripheral nerve innervation. Therefore, physicians who are not familiar with these pain syndromes do not accept the patient's symptom-report and search for neurotic or hysterical traits. Nonrecognition and nontreatment of these conditions almost regularly result in trophic tissue changes which eventually become irreversible. It is therefore essential to initiate treatment with sympathetic blocks promptly after the onset of pain and related symptomatology.

In the initial state of tumor-induced reflex sympathetic dystrophy, which usually occurs 6 to 10 months after radical and effective tumor surgery, objective signs of tumor recurrence are lacking (3). However, in many instances carefully performed *sweat tests* (16,21) are helpful, because tumor infiltration of the cervicothoracic and lumbar sympathetic chains results quite early in hypohidroses or anhidroses in the upper and lower limbs respectively (10,22). These changes, which precede any X-ray evidence of tumor recurrence by months and sometimes years, are particularly likely to occur with lymphogenous spread of Pancoast, breast, urogenital, and rectal tumors (5,6,9).

Another distinct clinical entity frequently observed with cancer pain can be ascribed to reflex sympathetic dystrophy: the quadrant syndrome or vascular zone disturbance described by Gross (12), Laux (14), and Pette (19). These conditions present with burning, dull pain; nonsegmental sensory disturbances; vasomotor, sudomotor, and pilomotor changes; and a special quality of pain which can be detected on careful physical examination. These patients will either indicate a latency between a nociceptive stimulus with a pinprick and pain perception *or* immediately feel a sharp pain on stimulation followed by a dull, severe burning pain.

The distribution of the pain is the typical sympathetic vascular innervation pattern. Thus, the pain distribution can correspond (a) to one or more quadrants of the body in accordance with the sympathetic nervous system

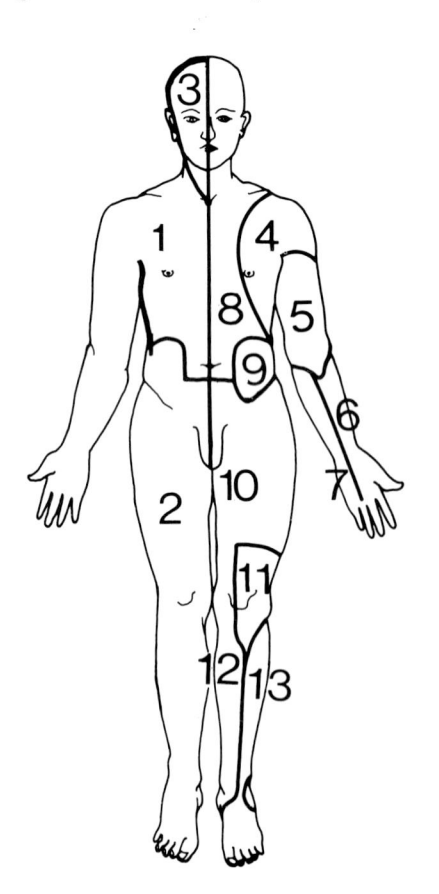

FIG. 1. Arterial supply of the skin (front). The identity of each artery by number is given on page 313.

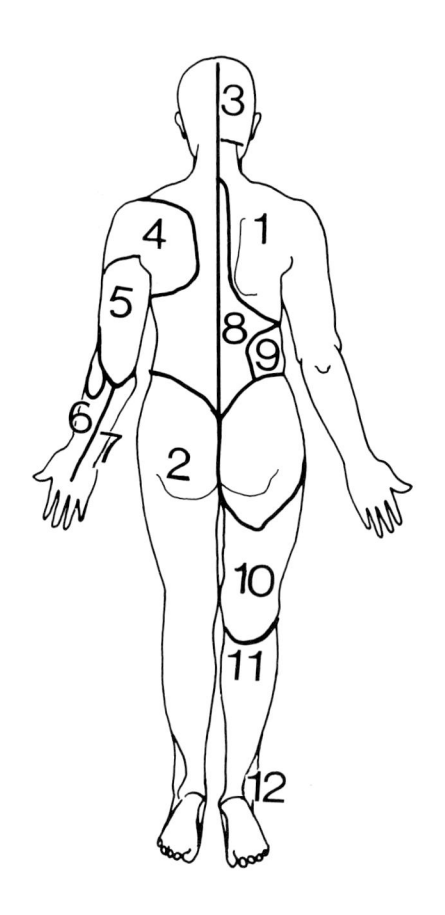

FIG. 2. Arterial supply of the skin (back). See below for identity of each artery.

distribution of subclavian and iliac arteries (Fig. 1) or (b) to the vascular zone of one arterial branch such as the axillary or external carotid arteries (Fig. 2).

Arterial Supply of the Skin

Topographically abnormal sensory disturbances, such as hyper- or hypoalgesia, frequently accompany peripheral nerve and vascular injuries. These nonsegmentally distributed sensory disturbances do not correspond to the innervation of peripheral nerves but can be traced to a typical sympathetic vascular innervation pattern. Gross (12)—and our clinical findings endorse his topographical findings—ascribes the skin areas to the following vascular innervation: (1) subclavian artery = right cervicothoracic trunk outflow = upper quadrant of the body; (2) iliac arteries = right lumbar sympathetic outflow = lower quadrant of the body; and subdivisions of these major trunks; (3) common carotid artery; (4) axillary artery; (5) brachial artery; (6) radial artery; (7) ulnar artery; (8) thoracic aorta; (9) abdominal aorta;

(10) femoral artery; (11) popliteal artery; (12) posterior tibial artery; (13) anterior tibial artery.

About 10 years ago we observed that one diagnostic sympathetic block with a local anesthetic prior to planned neurolytic injections relieved the burning cancer pain and the often-associated muscle-tension pain for days and even weeks. This unexpectedly long effective duration of a local anesthetic block is explained by the following actions of local anesthetics on pain mechanisms. The local anesthetic: (a) blocks pain receptors (nociceptors) and thus prevents transformation and coding of nociceptive impulses in these specialized nerve endings; (b) blocks nociceptive impulse-

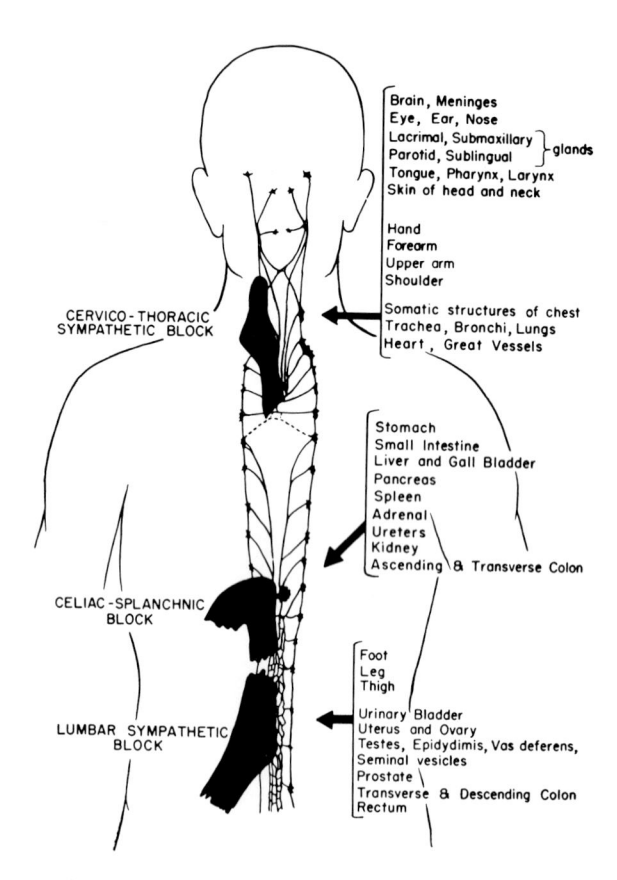

FIG. 3. Diagram illustrating the three "critical sites" which may be employed to interrupt the peripheral sympathetic nervous system. On the reader's left the diagram shows the pattern of diffusion (black) of local anesthetic solutions injected in the vicinity of the cervicothoracic (stellate) ganglion, celiac plexus, and lumbar sympathetic ganglia. On the reader's right are the names of the structures affected with each block. (After F. A. D. Alexander, courtesy of J. J. Bonica, *Clinical Applications of Diagnostic and Therapeutic Nerve Blocks,* Charles C Thomas, Springfield, Ill., 1959).

transmission in those efferent fibers associated with sympathetic fibers and thus prevents such impulses from reaching the central nervous system; (c) blocks sympathetic pathways and thus interrupts sympathetic reflex mechanisms, which act as positive feedback mechanisms and which are usually active in painful conditions (Zimmermann, *this volume*), (d) reduces or eliminates the increased skeletal muscle activity, which contributes to the sustenance of the vicious circle of pain; and (e) regional anesthetic blocks possibly influence higher cortical functions, altering mental constitutional conditions (more directness, spontaneity, integrative tendencies, higher distinctivity, clarity, availability of mental functions) (24).

The pain-relieving effects of regional anesthetic blocks often outlast the pharmacologic impulse-blocking effect of the local anesthetic (11,12). This prolonged analgesic effect, which is obtained even in neoplastic disease, is presumably due to interruption of the aforementioned vicious circle. In treatment of pain, the goal of regional analgesia is interruption of C- and A-delta fibers and of efferent sympathetic fibers (7). This requires only low concentrations of local anesthetics such as 0.5% lidocaine or mepivacaine, or 0.125 to 0.25% bupivacaine. Because of the long duration of action of bupivacaine, an almost-continuous, small-fiber blockade can be achieved with blocks performed once daily (11,17). Our experience clearly has demonstrated that best results with regional analgesic block will be achieved if a series of 6 to 8 blocks are performed at 1- or 2-day intervals. The results achieved with local anesthetics in tumor-induced reflex sympathetic dystrophy are comparable with those attained with neurolytic blocks, i.e., 4 to 6 months of pain relief (11), for interrupting the sympathetic chain and its branches as depicted in the three critical sites (Fig. 3).

Stellate ganglion and cervicothoracic sympathetic blocks are performed for burning cancer pain of the face, head, and neck and celiac plexus blocks, for upper abdominal pain. The following is a brief description of these techniques.

Stellate Ganglion Block

The stellate ganglion, usually a fusion of the inferior cervical and first thoracic ganglia, is located between the anterolateral surface of the seventh cervical vertebral body and the neck of the first rib. Although several methods of blocking the stellate ganglion have been described, the anterior paratracheal technique is the simplest and most widely used (Fig. 4).

The patient lies in the dorsal recumbent position with a pillow under his shoulder and his head slightly hyperextended. A thin, 4- to 5-cm-long needle is inserted 3 cm above the sternoclavicular joint of the side ipsilateral to the block and passed horizontally between trachea and carotid artery to contact the base of the sixth (or seventh) cervical transverse process. (The top of the sixth transverse process (Chassaigniac's tubercle) is easily palpated at the level of the cricoid cartilage.) After the needle is withdrawn 0.5 cm, the needle point lies in the tissue plane anterior to the prevertebral fascia where the stellate ganglion lies. Figure 4 points out that the paravertebral sympathetic chain is enclosed by a fascial sheath. Thus, any solution injected into the correct fascial plane will achieve a *volume-dependent* sympathetic block distribution. Two ml of local anesthetic solution will produce a stellate ganglion block and thus interrupt sympathetic fibers to face and head; 10 ml will interrupt cervicothoracic sympathetic outflow to the upper extremity, intrathoracic organs, and the chest (2,4).

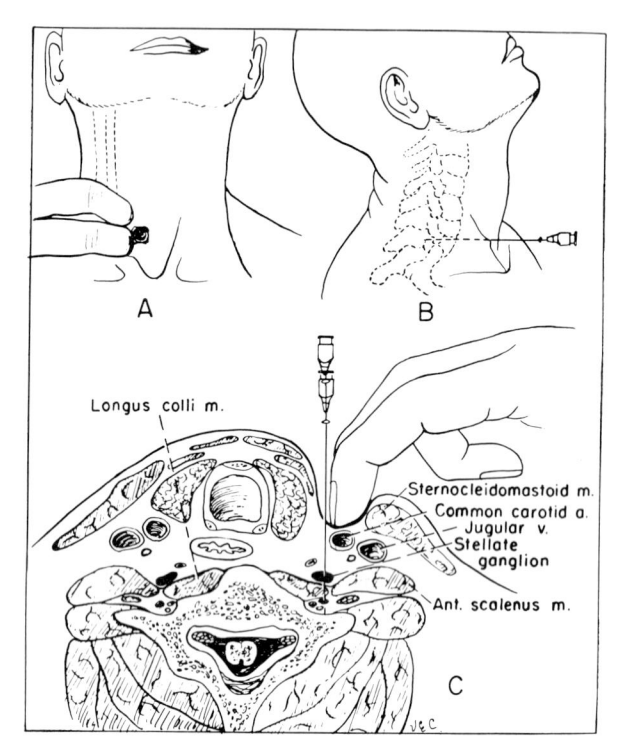

FIG. 4. Technique of stellate ganglion block by the anterior (paratracheal) approach. **A:** Anterior view, showing the maneuver of retracting the large vessels laterally and placing the needle medial to the fingers. **B:** Lateral view showing the needle in place with its tip on the base of the transverse process of the 6th cervical vertebra. **C:** Cross-section depicting the technique. Note the relationship of the fingers to the common carotid and jugular vein and these to the stellate ganglion. After contact with the bone, the needle is withdrawn about 5 mm until its point is anterior to the longus colli muscles and in the same fascial plane as the stellate ganglion. Injection of the solution in this fascial plane permits its diffusion cephalad to involve the lower portion of the cervical sympathetic chain and caudad to affect the upper portion of the upper thoracic chain. Should the needle not be withdrawn and the injection made into the muscle, the diffusion of drug will be limited. (From J. J. Bonica, *Clinical Applications of Diagnostic and Therapeutic Nerve Blocks,* Charles C Thomas, Springfield, Ill., 1959).

Lumbar Sympathetic Block

Technique of lumbar sympathetic block. The lumbar sympathetic ganglia lie along the anterolateral surface of the vertebral bodies and medial to the psoas muscle (Fig. 5). The patient lies in the lateral position on the side opposite the one to be blocked. A 10-cm-long needle is inserted perpendic-

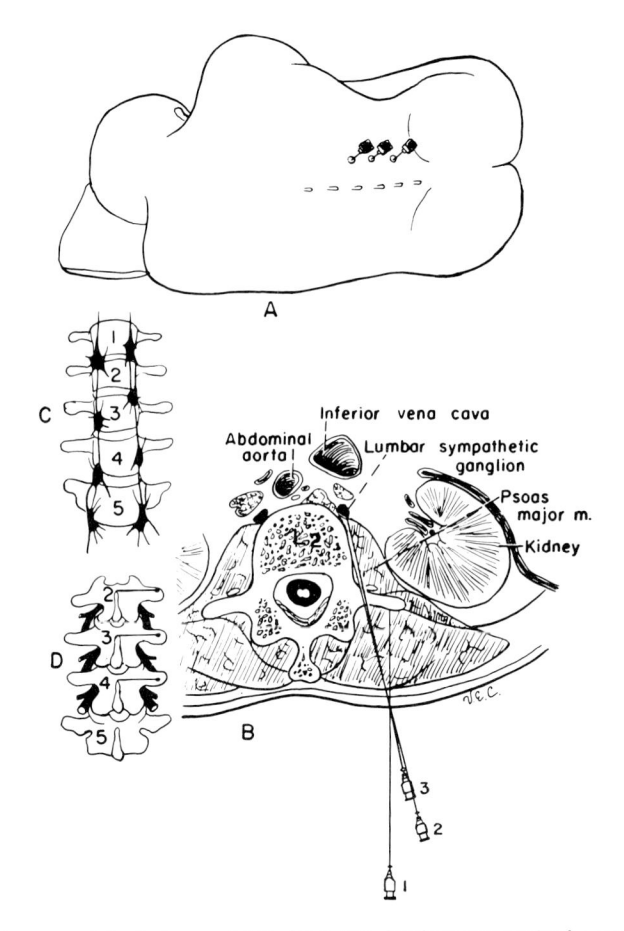

FIG. 5. Anatomy and technique of blocking the lumbar sympathetic ganglia by the paravertebral approach. **A:** Position of the patient for unilateral block. Note the skin wheals are opposite the upper edge of the spinous processes of the 2nd, 3rd, and 4th lumbar vertebra. **C:** Cross-section showing details of technique. The ganglia are on the anterolateral surface of the vertebra anterior to the margin of the psoas major muscle and posterior to the large vessels and abdominal viscera. In the diagram, needle 1, depicting the first step of the procedure, impinges the transverse process; needle 2, the lateral surface of the vertebra; and needle 3, with its point in the proximity of the lumbar sympathetic chain. **C:** Anterior, and **D:** posterior view of the vertebral column showing relation of sympathetic chain. The lines in **D** indicate the landmarks used on the overlying skin. (From J. J. Bonica, *The Management of Pain,* Lea & Febiger, Philadelphia, 1953.)

ularly to the skin surface 4 cm lateral from the middle of the second or third lumbar spinous process. The needle is then advanced until the transverse process is contacted (usually at a depth of 4 cm). The needle point is withdrawn to the subcutaneous tissue, then directed cranially and slightly medially to pass between the transverse process and make contact with the anterolateral aspect of the vertebral body. The correct position of the needle point can fairly well be tested by injection of 2 ml air. If the needle is well placed, there will be no resistance to the air injection; if the needle point is within the psoas muscle or subperiostally a resistance to air-injection will be obvious. After negative aspiration tests, 10 ml of local anesthetic are injected. The lumbar sympathetic block will interrupt sympathetic innervation of the lower ipsilateral extremity and part of the pelvic viscera (1,4,13).

Celiac Plexus Block

Block of the celiac plexus with a local anesthetic can be used as a diagnostic or prognostic aid or for temporary relief of upper abdominal visceral cancer pain. The technique we use is similar to that described by Moore (*this volume*).

Somatic Nerve Block

Since 1972, we have most often interrupted sympathetic and afferent C-fiber impulse-transmission within *somatic plexus* and the *peridural space* instead of performing standard sympathetic-block procedures. Thus, we have used axillary nerve blocks with low concentrations of local anesthetic instead of cervicothoracic sympathetic blocks for the treatment of pain and functional disturbances (such as lymphedema) of the upper extremity and caudal blocks and 3-in-1 blocks instead of lumbar sympathetic blocks for pain states of the pelvis and lower extremities (26). Studies in volunteers (21,23) and pain patients (11) proved that the sympathetic-fiber blockade was comparable and that patient's acceptance of these block types was better than with series of classic sympathetic-block procedures.

Caudal Block

The signs and symptoms of reflex sympathetic dystrophies, especially those of the lower half of the body, often have a bilateral distribution. Therefore, a bilateral sympathetic nerve blockade is necessary to obtain good pain-relief and reduction of functional disturbances. Lymphangiographic studies in our department have shown that bilateral sympathetic blockade produced with caudal block achieved with 30 ml of 0.125 to 0.25% bupivacaine is very effective in reducing edema and in improving lymph drainage from para-aortic and pelvic lymph nodes within a period of 4 to 5 days.

Technique of caudal block. The local anesthetic is injected through the sacral hiatus into the peridural space. The patient is asked to assume the prone position. The posterosuperior iliac spines are palpated, marked, and a connecting line drawn. On this base line an equilateral triangle is drawn, the apex of which usually overlies the sacral cornua. A 3- to 4-cm-long, thin needle inserted in a slightly cranial direction, will palpably pierce the sacrococcygeal ligament. Thirty ml of local anesthetic (low concentration!) is injected. Sympathetic and C-fibers of the lower extremities and the pelvis will be interrupted in some 20 min. (10).

Axillary Block

Burning pain due to tumor infiltration into the supraclavicular fossa can be controlled for several months by performing axillary nerve blocks with 30 ml of 0.25% bupivacaine or cervicothoracic sympathetic blockade achieved by injecting 10 ml of bupivacaine using the standard paratracheal stellate ganglion block technique. In the proximal third of the shaved axilla the axillary artery is palpated and a short, thin needle (23 g) is inserted directly lateral to the artery to a depth of 1.0 to 1.5 cm. After a negative aspiration test, 20 to 25 ml of local anesthetic is injected. With this paravascular technique it is unnecessary to elicit paresthesias, since artery, vein, and nerves are contained in a neurovascular sheath.

Pain and dysfunction in the upper abdomen due to lymphogenous spread of tumors can also be controlled for several weeks with local anesthetic blocks of the celiac ganglion. In these cases, however, we feel that a celiac plexus block with small volumes (15 ml) of 50% alcohol is relatively harmless and a preferable procedure (see Moore, *this volume*).

In comparison of neurolytic nerve blocks, local anesthetic blocks have minimal side effects and no permanent complications if good block techniques are employed (11). The block can be repeated without significantly increasing the risk.

SOMATIC NERVE BLOCKS

Somatic nerve blocks, which include block of A-delta and C afferent and sympathetic fibers, are employed advantageously in patients with acute, severe cancer pain, such as develops with pathologic fractures (rib, femur) or severe pain associated with a radiculopathy caused by tumor compression. These blocks are performed to keep the patient comfortable until more definite therapeutic measures are carried out. For these blocks, it is advisable to use higher-concentration local anesthetics such as 0.5% bupivacaine in order to achieve a more profound and long-lasting nerve block. More often, paravertebral somatic blocks are performed (Fig. 6).

We block paravertebral somatic nerves according to a technique described

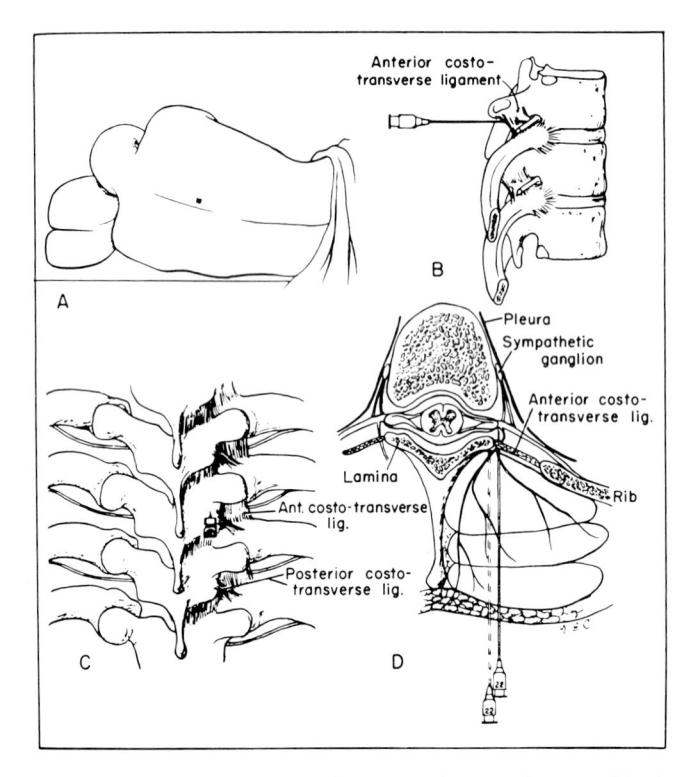

FIG. 6. Technique of paravertebral thoracic somatic nerve block.

by Fervers (8) and reintroduced by Shaw (20) and Bonica (1a) (Fig. 6). It is the only technique described which prevents the needle point from entering the vertebral canal. A 5- to 6-cm-long needle is inserted perpendicular to the skin surface 1 to 1.5 cm lateral of the spinal process and advanced until contact is made with the vertebral lamina. The needle point is withdrawn to subcutaneous tissue and skin moved laterally ½ cm, and the needle point is aimed at the lateral margin of the lamina. After one or two corrections, the needle point will palpably slip off the lamina. The needle is advanced 0.5 cm, an aspiration test performed, and 5 ml of local anesthetic solution injected.

CATHETER TECHNIQUES

In hospitalized patients, *catheter technique* is often preferable. Although the results of this continuous fiber blockade do not differ from the daily, single-injection technique, the catheter technique is advantageous in irritable and aggressive patients and in patients in poor general health.

There is another small group of patients who can benefit from local anesthetic blocks. Patients suffering from cancer pain which cannot be con-

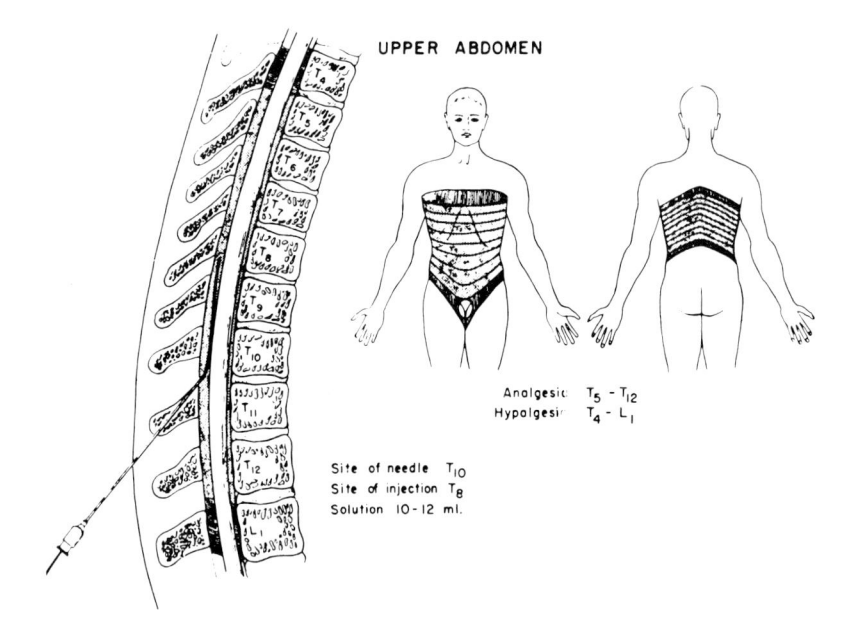

FIG. 7. Pattern of analgesia and hypalgesia produced by means of continuous epidural block to control pain in the upper abdomen, as occurs with acute pancreatitis. (From J. J. Bonica, *Clinical Applications of Diagnostic and Therapeutic Nerve Blocks.* Charles C Thomas, Springfield, Ill., 1959).

trolled by narcotic analgesics and other systemic drugs during their terminal 2 to 3 weeks of life can receive complete pain-relief by continuous nerve blocks via catheters. In most such cases, the catheters are introduced into the epidural space to effect continuous segmental epidural analgesia (2,11) (Fig. 7). These patients are usually dependent on narcotics and should continue to receive these drugs to keep them comfortable. We feel strongly that no dying patient should have to suffer pain, but should spend the last few weeks of life in relative comfort.

Disadvantages

A disadvantage of local anesthetic blockade is the need to repeat the block daily or every other day, which is inconvenient as it subjects the patient to repeated needling. However, taking into consideration that prior to neurolytic block a diagnostic block with local anesthetic should be performed, and that in many patients neurolytic blocks have to be repeated, the aforementioned disadvantage of local anesthetic blocks is not so great. Another significant disadvantage of block with local anesthetic is that in about 10 to 20% the procedure only produces transient relief of pain and the related symptomatology. In these patients neurolytic blocks should then be performed.

REFERENCES

1. Bonica, J. J. (1968): Autonomic innervation of the viscera in relation to nerve block. *Anesthesiology,* 29:793.
1a. Bonica, J. J. (1959): *Clinical Applications of Diagnostic and Therapeutic Blocks.* Charles C Thomas, Springfield, Ill.
2. Bonica, J. J. (1953): *The Management of Pain.* Lea & Febiger, Philadelphia.
3. Bues, E. (1954): Gezielte Grenzstrangresektion. Höhendiagnostik des Sympathikusgrenzstranges und ihre chirurgische Bedeutung. *Chirurg.,* 25:443.
4. Challenger, J. H. (1974): Sympathetic nervous system blocking in pain relief. In: *Relief of Intractable Pain,* edited by M. Swerdlow. Excerpta Medica, Amsterdam.
5. Chiappa, S., Bonadonna, G., Uslenghi, C., and Veronesi, U. (1967): Lymphangiography in the diagnosis of retroperitoneal node metastasis in rectal cancer. *Br. J. Radiol.,* 40:584.
6. Dargent, M. (1948): Role of the sympathetic nerve in cancerous pain; inquiry into 300 cases. *Br. Med. J.,* 1:440.
7. de Jong, R. (1963): Theoretical aspects of pain: Bizarre pain phenomena during low spinal anesthesia. *Anesthesiology,* 24:628.
8. Fervers, C. (1929): Eine vereinfachte Technik der paravertebralen Anästhesie und ihre Anwendung. *Zentralbl. Chir.,* 37:2318.
9. Fuchs, W. A. (1969): *Lymphangiography in Cancer.* Springer, Heidelberg, New York.
10. Gerbershagen, H. U. (1973): Behandlung chronischer Schmerzzustände mit Nervenblockaden. In: *Lokalanästhesie und Lokalanästhetika,* edited by H. Killian. Thieme, Stuttgart.
11. Gerbershagen, H. U., Panhans, C., and Schwarz, R., editors (1978): *Regionalanästhesie in Schmerzdiagnostik und -therapie.* Acron, Berlin.
12. Gross, D. (1972): *Therapeutische Lokalanästhesie.* Hippokrates Verlag, Stuttgart.
13. Haugen, F. P. (1968): The autonomic nervous system and pain. *Anesthesiology,* 29:785.
14. Laux, W. (1958): *Über Quadrantensyndrome. Ein Beitrag zu Klinik und Pathogenese der "Vegetativen Körperviertelstörungen" als Grundlage Chronischer Schmerzzustände.* Karger, Basel, New York.
15. Mandl, F. (1947): *Paravertebral Block in Diagnosis, Prognosis and Therapy.* Grune & Stratton, New York.
16. Moberg, E. (1958): Objective methods for determining the functional value of sensibility in the hand. *J. Bone Jt. Surg.,* 3:454.
17. Nolte, H., Meyer, J., Köpf, B., and Renz, M. (1974): Klinische und elektrophysiologische Parameter zur Differenzierung der Wirkung von Lokalanästhetika. *Anaesthesist,* 23:165.
18. Oeser, H., Taenzer, V., and Behrendt, C. (1971): Das Syndrom nach Rektumamputation (Postproktektomie-Syndrom). *Dtsch. Med. Wochenschr.,* 23:973.
19. Pette, H. (1927): Das Problem der wechselseitigen Beziehungen zwischen Sympathicis und Sensibilität. *Dtsch. Z. Nervenkh.,* 100:143.
20. Shaw, W. W. (1952): Medial approach for paravertebral somatic nerve block. *JAMA,* 148:742.
21. Schenk, C. (1978): *Objektivierung sympathischer Blockaden.* PhD. Thesis, Johannes Gutenberg-Universität, Mainz, West Germany.
22. Schliack, H., and Schiffer, R. (1971): Anhidrose der Fuss-sohle: Symptom retroperitonealer Tumorinvasion. *Dtsch. Med. Wochenschr.,* 96:977.
23. Theiss, D., Robbel, G., Theiss, M., and Gerbershagen, H. U. (1977): Experimentalle Bestimmung einer optimalen Elektrodenanordung zur elektrischen Nervenlokalisation. *Anaesthesist,* 26:411.
24. Türk, H., Frey, R., and Gerbershagen, H. U. (1975): Regional anesthesia as a psychotherapeutic method: A new approach to the psychic system (an experimental study). Paper read at the First World Congress on Pain, Florence, Italy, September 5–8, 1975.

25. White, J. C., and Smithwick, R. H. (1944): *The Autonomic Nervous System.* Kimpton, London.
26. Winnie, A. P., Rammamurthy, S., and Durrani, Z. (1973): The inguinal paravascular technic of lumbar plexus anesthesia: The 3-in-1 block. *Anesth. Analg.,* 52:989.

Subarachnoid and Extradural Neurolytic Blocks

M. Swerdlow

Regional Pain Relief Centre, University of Manchester School of Medicine, Salford, M6 8HD, Lancashire, England

It is nearly 50 years since a neurolytic agent (alcohol) was first injected into the theca deliberately to produce pain-relief (7). Strangely enough, although Dogliotti introduced the procedure for noncancer pain, most of the subsequent use has been for relief of cancer pain. The method has seen many changes in frequency of use in the intervening years. In the early decades after Dogliotti's reports, inadequate techniques of asepsis rendered intrathecal injections somewhat hazardous. By the late 1950s this problem had been solved, and the introduction of phenol gave a new impetus to the use of the method (26). During this period, the extradural injection of neurolytic agents to relieve cancer pain was also initiated. Apart from chlorocresol, which Maher (24) introduced in 1963, no important new neurolytic agents have appeared.

During the 1960s neurosurgeons were exploring new surgical techniques of interrupting central nervous system pain transmission and during the present decade percutaneous cordotomy, chemical hypophysectomy, and cytotoxic drugs have been shown to have important roles to play in the treatment of intractable cancer pain. It is the purpose of this report to provide a comprehensive, albeit concise, review of neurolytic subarachnoid and extradural block within the framework of other therapeutic modalities currently used for the control of pain of advanced cancer.

SUBARACHNOID NEUROLYSIS

What is the present position of the intrathecal neurolysis? I believe that it still has an important place in the total spectrum of methods of relieving cancer pain for the following reasons: (a) When properly employed it provides good quality pain-relief in a reasonable proportion of patients; (b) it could easily be made available to all patients with cancer pain; (c) it requires only brief hospitalization; (d) it provides an adequate duration of relief for many of the patients and can be repeated if necessary; (e) it can be applied to the old and very ill; and (f) complications are usually absent or slight.

Pathologic studies have shown that neurolytic solutions injected intrathecally affect large and small fibers indiscriminately (38). The degree of block produced depends on the number rather than the type of fibers destroyed, and this in turn is related to the quantity and concentration of solution employed (41). However, as Papo and Visca (32) point out, the extent of parenchymal damage is not always directly related to the success of the block.

Subarachnoid Phenol and Alcohol

In the early years phenol was often used dissolved in iophendylate. It has been subsequently shown that phenol solutions in iophendylate are less active than those in glycerine, and there is now a consensus that iophendylate is only indicated when it is necessary to have radiological control of the injection (30).

Nathan et al. (31) consider that phenol has a biphasic action—an almost immediate but temporary local anesthetic action and a permanent destructive action on the blocked fibers. According to Gonsette and Andre-Balisaux (9) chlorocresol has only a slight anesthetic action, a fact which is obvious in clinical practice. The destructive effects of alcohol are more intense (41) and less localized (14) than those of phenol.

Technical Considerations

The technique of intrathecal neurolytic injection is now well established. For injections of hyperbaric solutions the patient is positioned with the pain-

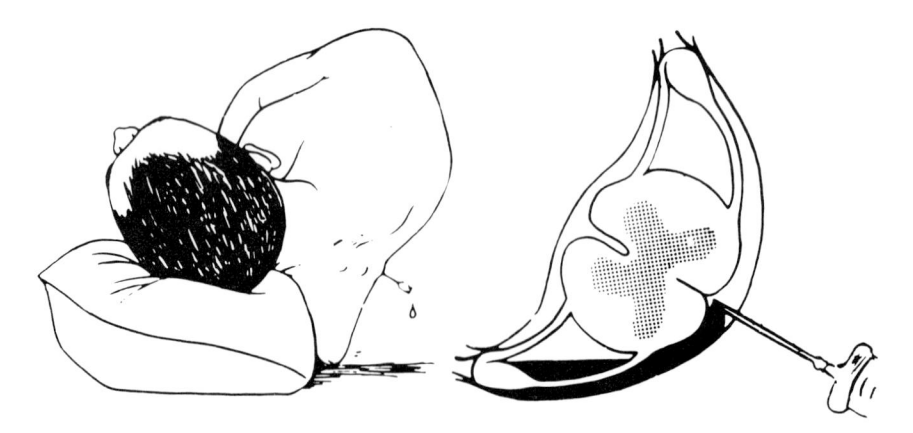

FIG. 1. Subarachnoid injection of hyperbaric neurolytic solution (hyperbaric phenol) to interrupt the posterior rootlets of spinal nerves. The subarachnoid puncture is made with the patient on his side with the affected side underneath. Once subarachnoid fluid emerges from the hub of the needle, the upper part is displaced posteriorly so that the posterior surface of the back makes an angle of 45° with the superior surface of the table. This will place the posterior (sensory core) rootlets of the nerves involved in conducting the pain lowermost. (Courtesy of J. J. Bonica.)

ful side underneath, and the spinal puncture is made at a level such that the neurolytic solution will fall onto the appropriate posterior nerve roots (Fig. 1). When alcohol is being injected, the patient is placed with the painful side upward (Fig. 2). The patient should be retained in the injection position for about 20 min to allow the neurolytic agent to become "fixed" to the nerve roots.

In my opinion, proper siting of the needle is more important than tilting in obtaining good localization of the solution. I also believe that it is important to avoid excessive dosage. Occasionally, with hyperbaric solutions the patient's report of symptoms on the upper side signals that the bevel of the needle is not pointing downward as it ought to be. Judging from published reports (32,45) and personal enquiries, phenol is now the most widely used agent for this purpose; the optimum concentration appears to be 5 to 7%. As will be seen below, I have found that chlorocresol in a concentration of 1:40 or 1:50 is slightly more efficacious than phenol, but side effects are liable

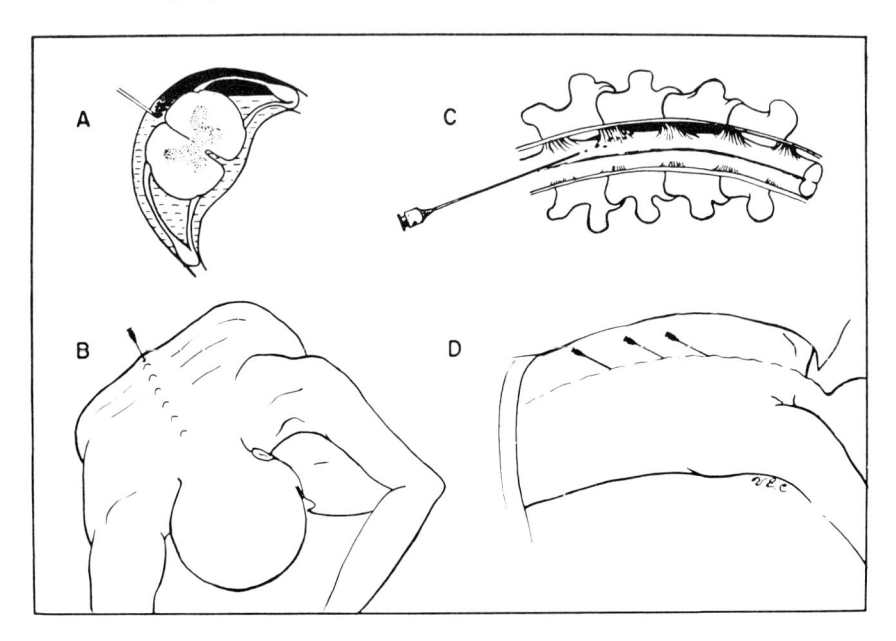

FIG. 2. Diagram showing the position of the patient for subarachnoid alcohol block in the thoracic position. Note that the patient is placed in the lateral-prone position so that the posterior surface of the back makes an angle of 45° with the superior surface of the table. **B:** One or two pillows are placed under the region to be blocked and the table flexed so as to produce a scoliosis of the spine with a maximum curve corresponding to the nerve roots conveying the pain. This will place the posterior (sensory) nerve roots involved in conducting pain uppermost **(A)** with the head and extremities lower than the point of injection. **C:** Longitudinal section showing diffusion of the hypobaric alcohol to involve the uppermost sensory roots. **D:** Note that three needles are used in order to permit the injection of small volumes of solution and thus minimize complications. (Courtesy of J. J. Bonica, *Clinical Applications of Diagnostic and Therapeutic Nerve Blocks,* Charles C Thomas, Springfield, Ill., 1959.)

to be longer-lasting with chlorocresol. Furthermore it has the disadvantage of not causing localizing symptoms at the time of injection, so that it is more difficult to assess exactly which nerve roots are being affected. In order to obtain some of the advantages of chlorocresol whilst avoiding its disadvantages, some workers (27,32) use a mixture of the two agents.

Indications

Subarachnoid neurolysis is particularly appropriate in patients with fairly localized pain. When there is widespread pain and especially in those in whom pain arises early in the course of the disease, a percutaneous cordotomy (or in appropriate cases pituitary adenolysis) would offer a better chance of long-term relief. In patients with bilateral multifocal pain, however, many workers consider that the serious risks of bilateral cordotomy should be avoided by performing cordotomy only on the worse side and applying subarachnoid neurolysis on the other side (47). In patients who are unfit, unwilling, or unable to have a cordotomy, an intrathecal neurolysis is usually the best therapy.

Although techniques of blocking both sides at one injection have been described both with alcohol and phenol, the consensus of opinion favors the two sides' being injected on separate occasions (29).

There is little to choose between the results of alcohol and phenol in expert hands. The choice usually depends on the operator's training and experience, but sometimes the state of the patient, (e.g., marked dyspnea in the Trendelenburg position, inability to lie on the painful side) will dictate whether hypobaric (alcohol) or a hyperbaric (phenol) solution is used. In my opinion the method of choice is to use phenol for blocks in the lumbosacral segments and chlorocresol at higher spinal levels. In view of the superior results reported (15,16) when alcohol rather than phenol was used in the cervicothoracic region, it would seem that alcohol should be given a trial in cases of shoulder and neck pain. At any spinal level it is worthwhile giving a second injection if the first is unsatisfactory; but if two injections fail, there is little chance of a third's being effective and there is an increased risk of complications.

Results

One of the most contentious aspects of intrathecal neurolysis is the nature of the results. This is not surprising when we consider the differences among the patients being treated and the variations in assessment and reporting of results (45). There are a great number of factors involved in the pain of patients with malignant disease: the condition at the time of the injection; the rapidity of growth of tumor; the tissues involved in the production of pain; the type of tumor and part of the cord affected; whether there is sheltering of nerve roots by secondary tumor cells; whether there has been radiotherapy to the cord region or a previous intrathecal injection, both of which can affect results; how long the patient has been suffering pain at the time of the block and how widespread the pain. Moreover, following treatment, growth of the tumor or the advent of new secondary deposits can cause new pain which may make it difficult to assess whether the effects of the block have worn off. Furthermore, in many cases the general condition deteriorates rapidly, or the patient is put on medication which makes pain assessment difficult. Finally, different reports adopt different standards of what is a "good," "moderate," or "poor" result. In general "good" relief implies a high degree of freedom from pain with little curtailment of activity and little need to take analgesic drugs, whereas "moderate" relief implies that the pain level is reduced but that pain may still be causing some curtailment of activities and some analgesic supplementation may be necessary. Tables 1 and 2 are compiled from results reported by different workers with alcohol and phenol respectively.

To date, I have treated over 300 patients with cancer pain with intrathecal neurolysis. The earlier ones were followed up for 3 months (or until death if that occurred earlier), and those results have already been reported (47). Of that group, 44% obtained good relief, 30% had moderate relief, and 26% had little or no relief. It will be seen that further experience has resulted in a rather higher success rate.

The more recently treated patients have, as far as possible, been followed up until death. Analysis of the cases of 130 patients treated shows 69 received phenol and 61 chlorocresol. Of the 130 patients, 79 received one injection, 39 were given two injections, 9 received three, 2 were given four injections and 1 patient received six. Table 3 shows the duration of effectiveness of the block (or time from injection date to death if analgesia was still effective at death) in all single-dose cases or bilateral-dose cases, and also the duration of the first dose in patients who later had more than one therapy.

TABLE 1. *Results with subarachnoid alcohol block for relief of cancer pain*

Author(s)	No. of patients	Efficacy of therapy (% of patients)		
		Good relief	Fair relief	Little or no relief
Kuzucu et al. (16)	322	58	26	16
Hay (11)	252	46	32	22
Dogliotti (7)	150	59	25	16
Greenhill (10)	100	60	10	30
Bonica (2)	182	53	29	18
Perese (35)	95	57	32	11
Stern (40)	50	63	27	10
Total/Average	1151	56	27	17

TABLE 2. *Results with subarachnoid phenol block for relief of cancer pain*

Author(s)	No. of patients	Efficacy of therapy (% of patients)		
		Good relief	Fair relief	Little or no relief
Maher (23)	433	62	6	32
Papo & Visca (32)	282	40	35	25
Ciocatto et al. (5)	207	78	11	11
Swerdlow (46)	200	56	19	25
Stovner & Endreson (42)	151	77%		23
Brown (3)	114	68	5	27
Total/Average	1387	61	15	24

Among this group, 27 patients died within 1 month and 62 within 3 months of the subarachnoid injection.

Pain-relief of more than 1 year's duration is somewhat exceptional, although such cases have been reported by a number of workers. Wilkinson et al. (50) and White and Sweet (49) had patients with analgesia lasting over 2 years and Papo and Visca (32) have reported analgesia lasting 2 to 3 years in several patients. Brown (4) and Lassner (17) have also reported long-lasting relief.

The type of cancer involved is detailed in Table 4. Analysis of the results shows that the type of cancer and the stage at which the patient was presented for treatment play a greater part in determining the duration of relief

TABLE 3. *Analysis of results in 130 patients given subarachnoid neurolysis*

Duration of relief	Agent administered					
	Phenol			Chlorocresol		
	Result of treatment			Result of treatment		
	Good	Moderate	Poor	Good	Moderate	Poor
Less than 1 month	11	5	6	14	6	3
1–2 months	6	3	2	7	4	2
2–3 months	7	1	3	3	2	1
3–4 months	3	1	2	2	2	1
4–5 months	8		1	1		1
6–8 months	6	1		8	1	
8–10 months	1			1		
10–12 months	1					
Over 1 year	1					
Over 2 years				1	1	
Total	44	11	14	37	16	8
%	64	16	20	61	26	13

TABLE 4. *Type of cancer in the author's latest 130 patients*

Disease	No. of patients
Ca Rectum	31
Ca Bronchus	30
Ca Cervix	24
Ca Breast	9
Ca Pancreas	7
Ca Colon	5
Ca Stomach	3
Ca Bladder	3
Ca Ovary	2
Ca Kidney	2
Others	14
Total	130

than the nature of the neurolytic solution. Pain-relief lasting 3 to 6 months occurred in the following number of patients with the various lesions: cervix, 7; rectum, 5; breast, 3; colon, 2; bronchus, 1; pancreas, 1; and stomach, 1. Relief lasting 6 months or more was derived by 10 patients with carcinoma of the rectum, 4 with carcinoma of the breast, 3 with lesions of the bronchus, and 3 with lesions of the cervix.

Complications

The easy accessibility of the nerve roots to subarachnoid neurolytic agents sometimes results in complications, some of which are due to involvement of unintended nerves or even vessels, whereas others (such as headache) are unrelated to effect of the neurolytic agent. Furthermore, neurolysis may sometimes aggravate a preexisting deficit such as paresis or dysuria. A comprehensive list of complications of intrathecal neurolysis has been given elsewhere (44). Table 5 lists complications lasting more than 7 days.

The complications are usually transient, but some persist and cause difficulties in patient-management. Headache, paresthesias, and numbness are common, give little trouble, and are unpredictable. Less common and much

TABLE 5. *Complications lasting longer than 7 days in 300 patients.*

Drug(s)	No. of patients	Bladder paresis	Bowel paresis	Muscle paresis	Headache	Paresthesia	Numbness
Phenol	145	7	1	4	—	1	4
Chlorocresol	138	10	1	7	1	1	4
Phenol and chlorocresol	17	3	1	—	1	—	1

TABLE 6. *Duration of complications*

Duration of complications	No. of patients
Lasting more than 3 days	48
Lasting more than 1 week	28
Lasting more than 2 weeks	19
Lasting more than 1 month	10
Total no. of patients	300
Total no. of injections given	453

more serious are muscular pareses and interference with rectal and vesical sphincter action. These complications are to some extent predictable; there is very little risk of interference with rectal or vesical action except when a neurolytic agent is being applied for the first time to the lumbosacral nerves. Likewise, there is a very small risk of significant muscular weakness except when the lumbar or the cervicothoracic outflow are being blocked. Table 6 shows the duration of complications in my series of 300 patients.

It is not generally realized that there are dangers from the effects of neurolytic agents on the blood supply to the cord, although these have been demonstrated by pathologic studies (14,51). There have been few clinical publications of such complications, although anecdotal and medicolegal reports suggest the incidence is not negligible. A recent case report by Superville-Sovak and her colleagues (43) is of interest. These workers report a case in which a subarachnoid injection of 6% phenol in glycerine at the level of T5–6 was followed by temporary respiratory arrest and subsequent weakness and sensory loss in the right upper limb. Respiratory infection led to death 5 weeks after the intrathecal injection, and post-mortem examination showed lesions of many small arteries supplying the posterolateral aspect of the cord.

Intrathecal neurolysis may fail to produce relief. Sometimes this is due to the sheltering action of neoplastic infiltration of the nerve roots (1,25) or of previous radiotherapy. On the other hand, Pellegrini et al. (34) have found gross meylin and axon damage in patients in whom treatment failed altogether. Papo and Visca (32) consider that in chronic cases, failure may be due to development of central summation and that a good result on pain of recent onset is due more to the fact that central changes have not yet developed rather than to absence of sheltering. Nathan (28) found that 32 of 112 patients with cancer pain were not relieved by intrathecal phenol and required anterolateral cordotomy. An adequate explanation is not easy to find.

Conclusion

There is a need to provide the training which will enable subarachnoid neurolysis to be made more widely available. The rapidly increasing spread of worthwhile pain-relief centers should in due course be able to satisfy this need. More should be done to inform doctors providing primary treatment for cancer of the methods which are now available for relief of cancer pain so that more patients are referred earlier for pain-relief therapy. Finally, there is a need to discover a more effective neurolytic agent—an agent with better penetrative and destructive ability, even though such an agent would result in a longer duration of complications. There is also a need to investigate the reasons why intrathecal neurolysis is sometimes totally ineffective.

Intrathecal Saline

Hitchcock (12) and subsequent workers have shown that saline can produce a certain amount of neurolysis that results in pain-relief when injected into the subararchnoid space. The effects appear to be due to the hypertonicity of the saline rather than its temperature (18). However, the injection causes painful twitching, paresthesias, confusion, and a rise in blood pressure and is therefore done under sedation or general anesthesia (47). The method has been used mostly for pain due to malignant disease, but some workers have employed it in such conditions as causalgia and postherpetic neuralgia (6).

Technique

The patient lies on his side with the painful side underneath, the table being tilted foot down for pain in the lower half of the body and head down for pain in the upper half. After lumbar puncture is performed and some cerebrospinal fluid is removed, 20 ml of 7.5% to 15% saline is injected rapidly, and the needle is then removed. For bilateral pain the patient is now placed supine; for unilateral pain he is kept lying on the painful side.

Results

The results are often disappointing. In Hitchcock's series (13) fewer than half the patients obtained more than 1 month's relief. Furthermore the method is unfortunately not so free from complications as was originally hoped; Lucas et al. (21) reported an 11% incidence of temporary complications with 1% incidence of serious sequelae. Subarachnoid saline is probably better reserved for terminal cases, particularly those with widespread pain from metastases.

More recently barbotage of the cerebrospinal fluid has been experimented with as a method of producing pain-relief (19). The barbotage is performed via a Tuohy needle inserted at the spinal level of the pain. The duration of relief is usually unsatisfactorily brief and it cannot be recommended for clinical use.

EPIDURAL NEUROLYSIS

Now for a few words about epidural neurolysis. Although the epidural route avoids the risks of meningeal irritation and allows good localization of the neurolytic solution, the method is not widely used for relief of intractable pain. Moreover, there does not appear to have been increased usage parallel with the contemporary popularity of epidural block for both surgical and obstetric analgesia. One reason may be that at the time of injection it is not so easy to gauge the response and effectiveness as it is with subarachnoid injection.

Patterson and Marcello (33) and Spaetz and Wagner (39) claimed good results with extradural alcohol, but the injection is often painful and may be followed by postinjection neuropathy with neuralgia. Phenol appears to be a more promising agent for epidural use. A number of workers employ extradural phenol for pain in the cervical and higher thoracic segments to avoid the risks of subarachnoid neurolytics at this level (20).

Results

Lourie and Vanasupa (20) claim pain-relief of more than 9 months with 6% phenol, but Madrid (22) although finding the method successful could only achieve 2 to 4 weeks relief with 7½% phenol in glycerine. Sometimes I use extradural 7 to 10% phenol for neck and shoulder pain of malignancy, especially when subarachnoid injection proves impossible or unsuccessful. Raftery (37) has reported the use of intermittent, small doses of 6% aqueous phenol via an indwelling epidural catheter. The technique was used at all levels of the spinal cord and was often found to give good relief. Extradural phenol has also been used by Doughty (8) to relieve attacks of tenesmus and burning pain which occur with rectal cancer.

Complications

Muscular palsy has been reported by Usubiaga (48) after lumbar epidural injection of both phenol and alcohol for cancer pain; recovery occurred after a period of time. Hypertonic saline has been administered via the epidural route, but it is not yet clear whether this is a worthwhile procedure. Reports suggest that unfortunately it is not without risk (48).

Continuous Epidural Analgesia

Finally, the extradural route can be used to provide useful pain-relief in terminal care. In patients who have widespread pain and are too ill for more major pain-relieving procedures and in whom analgesic drugs are proving unsatisfactory, good relief can be achieved by intermittent injection of a dilute, local anesthetic solution through an appropriately positioned epidural catheter. Such a catheter can be retained for several weeks and can even be used in patients at home. A recent modification of this method is described by Pilon and Baker (36), who connected to the epidural catheter a small reservoir which was then implanted under the skin. Injections of local anesthetic were made percutaneously into the reservoir, pressure on which would "inject" a dose into the catheter. The equipment was maintained *in situ* and gave effective relief for 4½ months.

REFERENCES

1. Berry, K., and Olszewski, J. (1963): Pathology of intrathecal injection in man. *Neurology,* 13:152.
2. Bonica, J. J. (1958): Diagnostic and therapeutic blocks: A reappraisal based on 15 years experience. *Anesth. Analg. Curr. Res.,* 37:58.
3. Brown, A. S. (1976): Pain relief in malignant disease. Symposium on malignant disease. *Roy. Coll. Phys. Edin.,* Publication No. 47.
4. Brown, A. S. (1961): Treatment of intractable pain by nerve block with phenol. *Proc. 2nd Int. Cong. Neurol. Surg. Int. Cong., Series 36.* Excerpta Medica, Amsterdam.
5. Ciocatto, E., Moricca, G., and Cavaliere, R. (1967): L'infiltration sous arachnoïdienne antalgique. *Cahiers Anesth.,* 15:747.
6. Collins, J. R., Duras, E. P., Van Housen, R. J., and Spruell, L. (1969): Intrathecal cool saline solution: A new approach to pain evaluation. *Anesth. Analg. Curr. Res.,* 48:816.
7. Dogliotti, A. M. (1931): Traitement des syndromes douloureux de la peripherie par l'alcolisation sub-arachnoïdienne. *Presse Med.,* 67:11.
8. Doughty, A. (1972): In: *A Practice of Anaesthesia,* edited by W. D. Wylie and H. Churchill-Davidson. Lloyd Luke, London.
9. Gonsette, R., and Andre-Valisaux, G. (1964): Resultats éloignés dans le traitement neurochirurgical de la spasticité des membres inferieurs dans la sclerose en plaques. *Acta Neurol. Belg.,* 64:481.
10. Greenhill, J. P. (1947): Sympathectomy and intraspinal alcohol injections for relief of pelvic pain. *Br. Med. J.,* 2:859.
11. Hay, R. C. (1962): Subarachnoid alcohol block in the control of intractable pain. *Anesth. Analg. Curr. Res.,* 41:12.
12. Hitchcock, E. (1967): Hypothermic subarachnoid irrigation for intractable pain. *Lancet* 1:965.
13. Hitchcock, E. (1976): The treatment of intractable pain with subarachnoid saline infusion. In: *Current Controversies in Neurosurgery,* edited by T. P. Morley. Saunders, Philadelphia.
14. Hughes, J. T. (1966): Pathological findings following intrathecal injection of ethyl alcohol in man. *Paraplegia,* 4:1671.
15. Katz, J. (1975): Subarachnoid alcohol injections for the management of chronic pain. In: *Recent Progress in Anaesthesiology and Resuscitation.* Excerpta Medica, Amsterdam.
16. Kuzucu, E. Y., Derrick, W. S., and Wilber, S. A. (1966): Control of intractable pain with subarachnoid alcohol block. *JAMA,* 195:133.
17. Lassner, J. (1962): L'analgesie prolongée par l'alcolisation sous-arachnoïdienne. *Anesth. Analg.,* 19:5.
18. Lipton, S. (1976): Pain relief. In: *Recent Advances in Anaesthesia and Analgesia,* 12th ed., edited by C. L. Hewer and R. S. Atkinson, p. 239. Churchill Livingstone, Edinburgh.

19. Lloyd, J. W., Hughes, J. T., and Davies-Jones, G. A. B. (1972): Relief of severe intractable pain by barbotage of the C.S.F. *Lancet,* 1:354.
20. Lourie, H., and Vanasupa, P. (1963): Comments on the use of intraspinal phenol-pantopaque for relief of pain and spasticity. *J. Neurosurg.,* 20:60.
21. Lucas, J. T., Ducker, T. B., and Perot, P. L. (1975): Adverse reactions to intrathecal saline for control of pain. *J. Neurosurg.,* 42:557.
22. Madrid, J. (1975): Proceedings of Symposium on Cancer Pain, Florence, Italy.
23. Maher, R. M. (1960): Further experiences with intrathecal and subdural phenol. Observations on two forms of pain. *Lancet,* 1:895.
24. Maher, R. M. (1963): Intrathecal chlorocresol in the treatment of pain in cancer. *Lancet,* 1:965.
25. Maher, R. M. (1957): Neuroma section in relief of pain. Further experience with intrathecal injections. *Lancet,* 1:16.
26. Maher, R. M. (1955): Relief of pain in incurable cancer. *Lancet,* 1:18.
27. Mehta, M. (1973): *Intractable Pain.* Saunders, London.
28. Nathan, P. W. (1963): Results of antero-lateral cordotomy for pain in cancer. *J. Neurol. Neurosurg. Psychiatry,* 26:353.
29. Nathan, P. W. (1970): Treatment of intractable pain by chemical rhizotomy with phenol solution. In: *Gillingham Clinical Surgery. Neurosurgery,* edited by J. F. Gillingham. Butterworths, London.
30. Nathan, P. W., and Sears, T. A. (1961): Some factors concerned in differential nerve block by local anaesthetics. *J. Physiol. (Lond.),* 157:565.
31. Nathan, P. W., Sears, T. A., and Smith, M. (1965): Effects of phenol on the nerve roots of the cat. An electrophysiological and histological study. *J. Neurol. Sci.,* 2:7.
32. Papo, I., and Visca, A. (1976): Intrathecal phenol in the treatment of pain and spasticity. *Prog. Neur. Surg.,* 7:56.
33. Patterson, A., and Marcello, M. (1963): Cited by F. A. D. Alexander and L. W. Lewis (1963): In: *Anesthesiology,* edited by D. E. Hale, p. 801. Blackwell, Oxford.
34. Pellegrini, G., Visca, A., and Papo, I. (1969): Considerazioni sul meccanismo d'azione antalgica delle soluzioni di fenolo intratecali. *Acta Neurol. (Bari),* 24:85.
35. Perese, D. M. (1958): Subarachnoid alcohol block in management of pain of malignant disease. *Arch. Surg.,* 76:347.
36. Pilon, R. N., and Baker, A. R. (1976): Chronic pain control by means of an epidural catheter. *Cancer,* 37:903.
37. Raftery, H. (1977): *Proceedings of the Intractable Pain Society of Great Britain.*
38. Smith, M. C. (1963): Histological findings following intrathecal injections of phenol solutions for relief of pain. *Br. J. Anaesth.,* 36:387.
39. Spaetz, . . and Wagner, . . (1963): Cited by F. A. D. Alexander and L. W. Lewis (1963): In: *Anesthesiology,* edited by D. E. Hale, p. 801. Blackwell, Oxford.
40. Stern, E. L. (1937): Dangers of intraspinal (subarachnoid) injection of alcohol. Their avoidance and contraindications. *Am. J. Surg.,* 35:99.
41. Stewart, W. A., and Lourie, H. (1963): An experimental evaluation of the effects of subarachnoid injections of phenol-pantopaque in cats: A histological study. *J. Neurosurg.,* 20:64.
42. Stovner, J., and Endresen, R. (1972): Intrathecal phenol for cancer pain. *Acta Anaesth. Scand.,* 16:17.
43. Superville-Sovak, B., Rasminsky, M., and Finlayson, M. H. (1975): Complications of phenol neurolysis. *Arch. Neurol. (Chicago),* 32:226.
44. Swerdlow, M. (1979): Complications of neurolytic blocks. In: *Neural Blockade,* edited by M. Cousins and P. Bridenbaugh. Lippincott, New York.
45. Swerdlow, M. (1978): Current views on intrathecal neurolysis. *Anaesth.,* 33:733.
46. Swerdlow, M. (1975): Proceedings of Symposium on Cancer Pain, Florence, Italy.
47. Swerdlow, M. (1978): *Relief of Intractable Pain,* 2nd ed. Excerpta Medica, Amsterdam.
48. Usubiaga, J. E. (1975): *Neurological Complications Following Epidural Anesthesia.* Little, Brown & Co., Boston.

49. White, J. C., and Sweet, W. H. (1969): *Pain and the Neurosurgeon.* Charles C Thomas, Springfield, Ill.
50. Wilkinson, H. A., Mark, V. H., and White, J. C. (1964): Further experiences with intrathecal phenol for the relief of pain. *J. Chron. Dis.,* 17:1055.
51. Wolman, L. (1966): The neuropathological effects resulting from the intrathecal injection of chemical substances. *Paraplegia,* 4:97.

Phenol Subarachnoid Rhizotomy for the Treatment of Cancer Pain: A Personal Account on 290 Cases

I. Papo and A. Visca

Neurosurgery Division, Regional General Hospital, 60100 Ancona, Italy

Inasmuch as we have recently surveyed the literature in previous papers (10,11,12), and Dr. Swerdlow has already updated the basic knowledge of subarachnoid and extradural neurolytic techniques, in this brief report we shall deal only with our personal experience with intrathecal phenol in the treatment of cancer pain.

Over the past 18 years we have used phenol rhizotomy on 290 patients. We should distinguish two different phases in our experience. At the beginning we were very impressed with the results reported by Maher (4,5,7) and Brown (1), and we thought that intrathecal phenol would be the most suitable procedure for cancer pain, whereby it would be possible to avoid cordotomy and other conventional surgical procedures in most cancer patients. On these grounds, for about 3 years all patients complaining of painful syndromes from advanced cancer underwent phenol rhizotomy at different levels. During this phase, surgical operations were carried out only in patients in whom chemical rhizotomy had previously failed.

After the clinical experience during this first phase, we realized that the high hopes aroused by previous reports on subarachnoid neurolysis were not entirely justified, because not-negligible failures and complications had been observed. Consequently, we revised our criteria and attempted to outline the specific indications for intrathecal phenol and to establish well-defined guidelines for the future clinical management of these patients. As a consequence of these steps, the overall number of phenol rhizotomies dropped abruptly, but at the same time the rate of good results rose significantly.

RESULTS

Overall we have treated 290 patients with the following major categories of neoplastic lesions: (a) gynecologic tumors, 92; (b) rectal tumors, 44; (c) tumors of abdominal organs, 49; (d) tumors of lung, pleura, and mediastinum, 46; (e) primary and metastatic bone tumors, 52; and (f) kidney and bladder tumors, 7; with a total of 290.

TABLE 1. *Summary of overall therapeutic results*

Neoplastic disease	No. of pts.	Good No.	Good %	Fair No.	Fair %	Failure No.	Failure %
Gynecologic cancer	92	37	40.2	30	32.6	25	27.2
Rectal cancer	44	21	47.7	15	34.1	8	18.2
Abdominal cancer	49	23	46.9	17	34.7	9	18.4
Tumors of lung, pleura, mediastinum	46	10	21.8	20	43.4	16	34.8
Primary and secondary bone tumors	52	23	44.2	16	30.8	13	25
Kidney and bladder tumors	7	3	42.8	2	28.6	2	28.6
Total/Average	290	117	40	100	35	73	25

In assessing the results we have accepted the criteria suggested by Mark et al. (8). A result is classed as "good" if the patient is pain-free until death; as "fair" if pain-relief is sufficient to allow a significant decrease in the amount of analgesic medication required to keep the patient comfortable for a prolonged period or if pain is completely relieved for over 3 weeks. The overall results are summarized in Table 1. In Table 2 the results are analyzed in detail according to the localization and type of pain. Complications are listed in Table 3.

DISCUSSION

If we look at the overall results we see that we succeeded in relieving pain satisfactorily in about 40% of patients. In most of these patients the average duration of the analgesia was 2 to 4 months, which was long enough to keep the patient pain-free until death. Moreover, several patients who lived longer than 3 or 4 months died pain-free at 6 to 12 months, and some of these up to 2 or 3 years without recurrence of pain.

The overall rate of *good results* is not very high. However, it must be borne in mind that in this overall series the highest rate of failures occurred in the patients treated in the first phase of our experience when the proper indications of phenol rhizotomy were still not well defined. The *fair results* deserve further explanation. Whereas in patients who lived for a short period they can be considered as very worthwhile (good) because the patient was painfree until death, when survival was longer very often the pain, though relieved for a short period, recurred and further analgesic treatment was required. Recurrence took place mostly in patients with chest and/or upper limb pain from lung and breast cancer that invaded the chest wall and the brachial plexus. Also, pain in lower limb due to nervous compression from

TABLE 2. *Therapeutic results in different types and locations of pain*

Neoplastic disease	No. of pts.	Good No.	Good %	Fair No.	Fair %	Failure No.	Failure %
Gynecologic cancer							
Lower limb pain	45	—	—	22	49	23	51
Groin hemiabdomen, and thigh pain (survival 3 months)	9	4	44	4	44	1	12
Visceral pain (plexalgia pelvica)	8	3	38	3	38	2	24
Abdominal and lumbar pain (somatic)	14	14	100	—	—	—	—
Saddle pain	16	16	100	—	—	—	—
Rectal cancer							
Saddle pain	28	16	57	8	29	4	14
Sciatic pain	7	1	14	2	29	4	57
Sciatic and saddle pain (only saddle pain relieved)	5	—	—	5	100	—	—
Abdominal pain	4	4	100	—	—	—	—
Abdominal cancer (abdominal and lumbar pain)							
Stomach	16	10	63	5	31	1	6
Pancreas (girdle pain)	14	5	36	4	28	5	36
Colon	12	7	58	2	17	3	25
Liver and peritoneal carcinosis	7	1	14	6	86	—	—
Tumors of lungs, pleura, and mediastinum							
Apical and upper chest pain	21	3	14	9	43	9	43
Upper chest pain (above T_6)	8	1	12	6	75	1	13
Lower chest pain (below T_6)	17	6	35	5	30	6	35
Primary and secondary bone tumors							
Bone pain	25	16	64	6	24	3	12
Radicular pain (only the pain from thoracic roots compression was relieved)	27	7	26	10	37	10	37
Kidney and bladder cancer							
Lumbar, abdominal, and hypogastric pain	7	3	42.8	2	28.6	2	28.6

TABLE 3. *Complications*

	Mild and/or transient No.	Mild and/or transient %	Severe No.	Severe %
Lower limb weakness	9	3	11	3.8
Upper limb weakness	4	1.4	1	0.3
Bladder function disturbance	Transient		Permanent	
Urine retention	9	3	5	1.7
Urinary incontinence	2	0.7	—	—

pelvic and vertebral cancer often recurred. Therefore, from a rigid viewpoint, it would seem logical that one should consider only good results in assessing the practical value of phenol rhizotomy and in identifying the proper indications of this procedure. With fair results, though useful to the patients because they reflect good pain-relief for a time, the fact that the pain recurs makes their interpretation less reliable.

The proper range of applications on intrathecal phenol can be derived from the data in Table 2. The efficacy, advantages, limitations, and complications in the therapy of the different types of pain will be briefly discussed.

Saddle Pain

Saddle pain, including superficial and deep sacrococcygeal and perineal pain. Many other authors (2,3,5,6,8,9,13,14) have reported similar results. Small amounts of the neurolytic agent (about 0.5 ml phenol in glycerin) usually relieve saddle pain. Altogether we have treated 49 patients: 16 were suffering from gynecologic cancer (carcinoma of the cervix) and 33 from rectal cancer. Of these, 32 patients obtained good relief of pain and 8 patients improved significantly so that the amounts of systemic analgesics could be reduced until their death.

In 5 patients with rectal cancer, phenol was ineffective. In 5 patients who complained of perineal and sciatic pain, phenol abolished the saddle component; but a spinothalamic cordotomy was necessary to control the sciatic pain, which was not modified by phenol rhizotomy. Four patients underwent sacral surgical rhizotomy, in 3 of whom phenol had failed to relieve the pain at all and in the other pain recurred 3 months after the injection and further introduction of phenol proved ineffective.

Complications consisted of permanent urinary retention in 5 males in whom vesical function was presumably already impaired.

Abdominal, Lumbar, and Inguinal Somatic Pain

A total of 67 patients complaining of these types of pain from different cancers were treated. Pain from pelvic cancer (cervix or rectal carcinoma) was satisfactorily relieved in all 18 patients. In patients with intraperitoneal carcinomas, in whom pain was more protean with a visceral component in several cases, the rate of good results was lower. However, complete relief was achieved in 23 patients out of 49. Fair results were obtained in an additional 17 patients. In 9 patients the treatment was ineffective.

Girdle pain from pancreatic carcinoma was the most refractory (5 failures among 14 patients) so that the highest doses had to be used. Visceral pain seems to be much less affected by subarachnoid phenol neurolysis. The technique may produce good results in some patients with pelvic plexus pain, but is completely ineffective in relieving pain from smooth muscle dyskinesia and subocclusive crisis, as Maher (4) noted long ago.

Bone Pain

Of 25 patients with typical bone pain without root compression, 16 were satisfactorily relieved and in 6 others the pain was significantly reduced. Conversely, radicular pain from bone metastases is seldom abolished. Of 27 patients, only 7 had any significant benefit from chemical rhizotomy. All of them had radicular compression at the thoracic level; therefore high doses could be introduced to produce extensive destruction of sensory fibers with no risk of damaging motor or sphincter fibers. In the remaining patients the results obtained can be considered less than gratifying.

As most of these painful syndromes which are relieved by phenol rhizotomy are bilateral, the advantages of a method that can avoid the well-known disadvantage of bilateral cordotomy become evident. Moreover, although myelotomy has also been advocated for the treatment of bilateral abdominal and saddle pain, these can be managed effectively with the much simpler and less traumatic procedure of chemical rhizotomy. On the other hand, we believe that subarachnoid phenol neurolysis should not be attempted for the relief of lower limb pain except typical bone pain.

Lower Limb Pain

In patients with lower limb pain from root compression and massive edema, the results are usually disappointing and the incidence of complications is high. In fact, in about 25% of our patients treated for lower limb pain, chemical rhizotomy, even using small doses that never exceeded 1 ml of 5% phenol in glycerin, made the ipsilateral lower limb weak. The motor loss was mild and/or transient in 9 patients, but severe and permanent in 11. Muscles innervated by L_2, L_3, and L_4 were selectively involved, with serious functional disability. In contrast, motor disturbances in musculature innervated by the sciatic nerve were seldom observed.

For many years we have not performed chemical rhizotomies for lower limb pain except for bone pain: instead we have been carrying out spinothalamic cordotomy at the outset, especially in all patients expected to survive more than 3 months.

Upper Chest and Upper Limb Pain

The overall results with intrathecal phenol were likewise poor in upper chest and/or upper limb pain from lung and breast cancer. Only lower thoracic pain (below T_6) was permanently relieved in a significant percentage of patients (6 out of 17). In the latter instances we feel that phenol rhizotomy is a valuable procedure which produces beneficial effects similar to surgical rhizotomy provided that high doses are used, so as to produce massive destruction of sensory fibers without impairing motor and sphincter function. For this reason, abdominal, lumbar, and groin pain are usually very well controlled, with no residual neurologic disorders. Oddly enough, thoracic pain from lung cancer is much more refractory even though high amounts of phenol are introduced.

MECHANISM OF THERAPEUTIC ACTION

It is also noteworthy that in nearly all cases no definite cutaneous analgesia is produced. As Maher first pointed out (5), it seems as though the nerve roots were sheltered from the action of the neurolytic agent. The therapeutic effect of phenol on saddle pain is even more difficult to explain. Small doses produce very little, if any, sensory loss, and yet the procedure abolishes even the most severe pain. We speculate that the mechanism of this peripheral somatic pain involves only small branches and terminal arborizations of the lumbosacral nerves and these are effectively interrupted by small doses of neurolytic agent. However, when major nerve roots and plexuses are affected by more invasive neoplasias, the analgesic effects are much less even for sacrococcygeal and perineal pain, and hence more complete surgical procedures should be used.

CONCLUSIONS

We would like to reemphasize that phenol rhizotomy is by no means the last resort for severe pain of terminal cancer in which more effective surgical procedures would not be warranted. The main criteria for the proper selection of patients for subarachnoid neurolysis are the site, type, and extent of the pain. The patient's condition usually plays a minor role in making the decision for this modality. In fact, if intrathecal phenol is likely to be ineffective, as in lower limb pain from major nerve compression and massive edema, it should not be considered whatever the condition of the patient. Although the use of large doses may increase the chance of success, the procedure should be used with caution, if at all, because of the high risk of complications and incomplete relief of pain.

On the other hand, when it is indicated, phenol rhizotomy should be used early. The argument that the effects of chemical rhizotomy are of too short duration to be considered of real clinical value is not valid. In actual fact, the mean duration of the therapeutic action of phenol rhizotomy is 2 to 4 months, and this is enough to keep most patients pain-free until death. Furthermore, on some occasions, particularly when high dosages can be used (e.g., trunk) in patients who survive for a long period, pain-relief may last as long as 8 to 12 months and even longer. In this regard, it is relevant to point out that the problem of long survivals often arises in patients in whom phenol rhizotomy is not indicated, such as in patients with pain from lung tumors or lower limb pain from pelvic malignancies. Moreover, in patients with saddle pain from rectal or cervical carcinoma, phenol rhizotomy usually produces effective relief long enough to keep the patients pain-free until death. Since intraperitoneal cancers which produce abdominal, lumbar, and/or inguinal pain usually run a rather rapid course, surgical procedures are seldom indicated and chemical rhizotomy should be used.

On the basis of our experience we believe that phenol rhizotomy still retains an appreciable range of applications. It is especially indicated in abdominal, lumbar, inguinal, saddle, and bone pains. Properly executed, this technique produces good pain-relief in about 70 to 75% of patients complaining of these painful syndromes. Of course, if doubtful indications are included, the overall results will be less satisfactory. In patients for whom chemical rhizotomy is indicated, we never perform surgical operations before trying subarachnoid neurolysis. In the event two injections fail to modify the pain or if it recurs quickly, within a few hours or days, it is most likely that further injections will prove ineffective, and other forms of treatment must be attempted without wasting time.

In conclusion, although we feel that phenol rhizotomy is not effective in as many patients suffering from cancer pain as was previously believed, nonetheless it remains a valuable weapon in our armamentarium against pain and enables us to avoid more major procedures. If subarachnoid neurolysis has been given up by many workers and neglected in the past few years, it is likely due to failures and complications caused by wrong selection of patients.

REFERENCES

1. Brown, A. S. (1958): Treatment of intractable pain by subarachnoid injections of carbolic acid. *Lancet,* 2:975–978.
2. Kuhner, A. (1976): La valeur des interventions sur les racines sacrées dans le traitement des syndromes douloureux du bassin. *Neuro-Chirurgie,* 22:429–436.
3. Kuhner, A., and Assmus, H. (1975): Intrathecal applications of phenol in the treatment of intractable pain. In: *Advances in Neurosurgery, Vol. 3,* edited by H. Penzholz, M. Brock, J. Hamer, M. Kunger, and O. Spoerri, pp. 256–263. Springer, Berlin.
4. Maher, R. M. (1960): Further experiences with intrathecal and subdural phenol. Observations on two forms of pain. *Lancet,* 1:895–899.
5. Maher, R. M. (1957): Neurone selection in relief of pain. Further experiences with intrathecal injections. *Lancet,* 1:16–19.
6. Maher, R. M. (1966): Phenol for pain and spasticity. Pain. *Henry Ford International Symposium,* pp. 335–343. Little, Brown, Boston.
7. Maher, R. M. (1955): Relief of pain in incurable cancer. *Lancet,* 1:18–20.
8. Mark, V. H., White, J. C., Zervas, N. T., Ervin, F. R., and Richardson, E. P. (1962): Intrathecal use of phenol for the relief of chronic severe pain. *N. Engl. J. Med.,* 267:589–593.
9. Mullan, S. (1971): The surgical relief of pain. *Clin. Neurosurg.,* 18:208–224.

10. Papo, I., and Visca, A. (1973): Intrathecal phenol in the treatment of cancer pain. *J. Neurosurg. Sci.*, 12:146–156.
11. Papo, I., and Visca, A. (1976): Intrathecal phenol in the treatment of pain and spasticity. *Progress in Neurological Surgery*, Vol. 7, pp. 56–130. Karger, Basel.
12. Papo, I., and Visca, A. (1974): Phenol rhizotomy in the treatment of cancer pain. *Anesth. Analg.*, 53:993–997.
13. Robbie, D. S. (1969): General management of intractable pain in advanced carcinoma of the rectum. *Proc. R. Soc. Med.*, 62:1225.
14. Tank, T. M., Dohn, D. F., and Gardner, W. J. (1963): Intrathecal injections of alcohol or phenol for relief of intractable pain. *Cleveland Clin. Q.*, 30:111–117.

Cranial Nerve Blocks

Jose L. Madrid and John J. Bonica

Department of Anesthesiology and Pain Clinic, Ciudad Sanitaria "10 de Octubre," Madrid, Spain; and *Department of Anesthesiology, University of Washington, School of Medicine, Seattle, Washington 98195

The head and neck frequently are sites of malignant tumors, which in their terminal stages are often accompanied by pain. In many instances the pain is severe, persistent, and continuous, interfering with the patient's nutrition and sleep and thus rapidly sapping the sufferer's strength and morale. Relief of pain in such patients is a matter of urgent necessity and the primary objective of management. In such patients the symptomatic management of pain is influenced to a great extent by the physical and emotional condition and the life-expectancy of the patient. Although many patients can be managed with narcotic analgesics, in many, if not most instances, it is far better to interrupt pain pathways by either chemical or surgical means. If a patient's condition is good, then surgical interruption should be considered. Unfortunately, however, in many instances these patients are not likely to tolerate a major operation and nerve block should be used. The success of nerve block depends in part on how early it is performed. Unfortunately there is a misconception among colleagues about the efficacy of these procedures, for most of them do not refer patients with severe pain for this type of treatment until the patient has had pain not adequately relieved with systemic analgesics and the lesion is so far advanced that it presents technical difficulties in carrying out the nerve block.

Proper provision for nerve blocks requires a thorough study of the course of the lesion and the location and the nature of the pain, a thorough knowledge of the structures supplied by the various cranial nerves and the upper four cervical nerves and, of course, skill in carrying out the various techniques.

ANATOMIC CONSIDERATIONS

It may be recalled that the trigeminal nerves supply sensory fibers to the anterior two-thirds of the head, including the skin of the face, and anterior two-thirds of the scalp, the mucous membranes of the cheek, the upper and lower teeth, gums and hard palate, the anterior two-thirds of the tongue, the anterior pillar of the tonsil, the mucous membranes of the nose, the eyelids and orbit, the maxillary, frontal, ethmoid, and sphenoid sinuses. (See

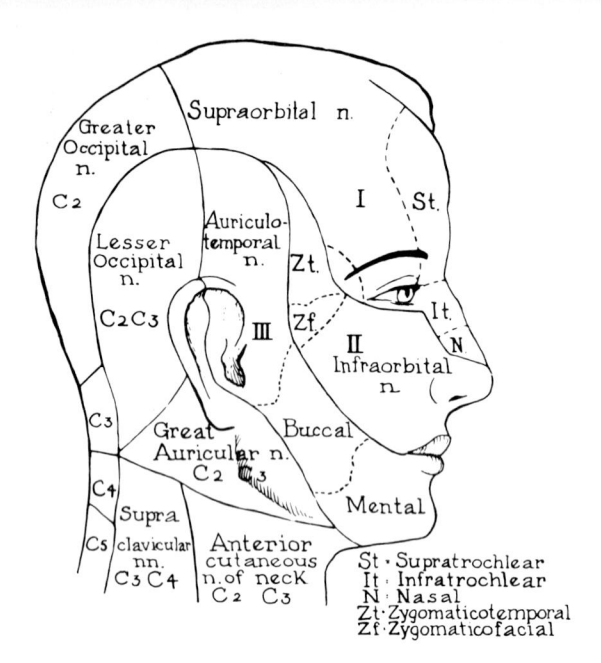

FIG. 1. The cutaneous distribution of the trigeminal nerve and its branches. (Courtesy of J. J. Bonica, *The Management of Pain,* Philadelphia, Lea & Febiger, 1953).

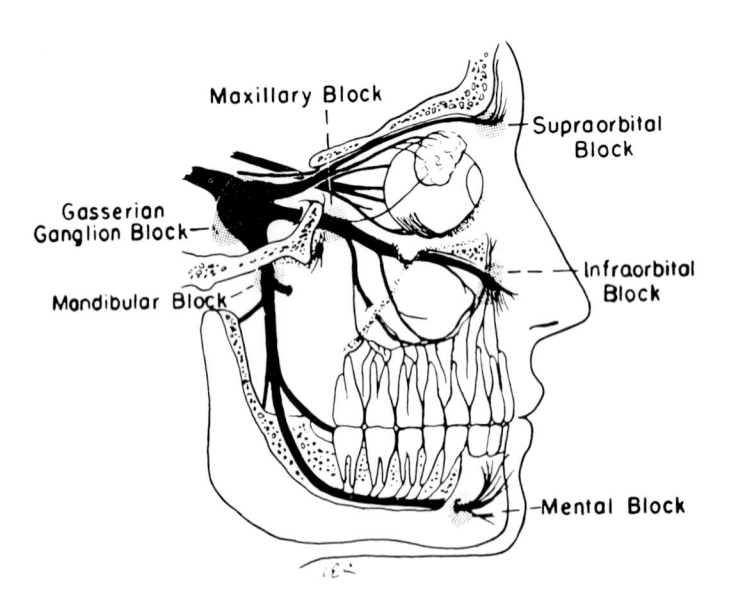

FIG. 2. Diagram showing the anatomy and distribution of the trigeminal nerve and the optimal sites of injecting it (stippled areas). Gasserian ganglion block is accomplished by passing a needle through the foramen ovale and into the gasserian ganglion; maxillary nerve block is accomplished in the pterygopalatine fossa just after the nerve passes through the formen rotundum; mandibular block is accomplished just below the foramen ovale; supraorbital block is accomplished at the supraorbital ridge; infraorbital block is accomplished at the infraorbital foramen or canal, and mental block at the mental foramen. (Courtesy of J. J. Bonica, *Clinical Applications of Diagnostic and Therapeutic Nerve Blocks,* Charles C Thomas, Springfield, Ill., 1959.)

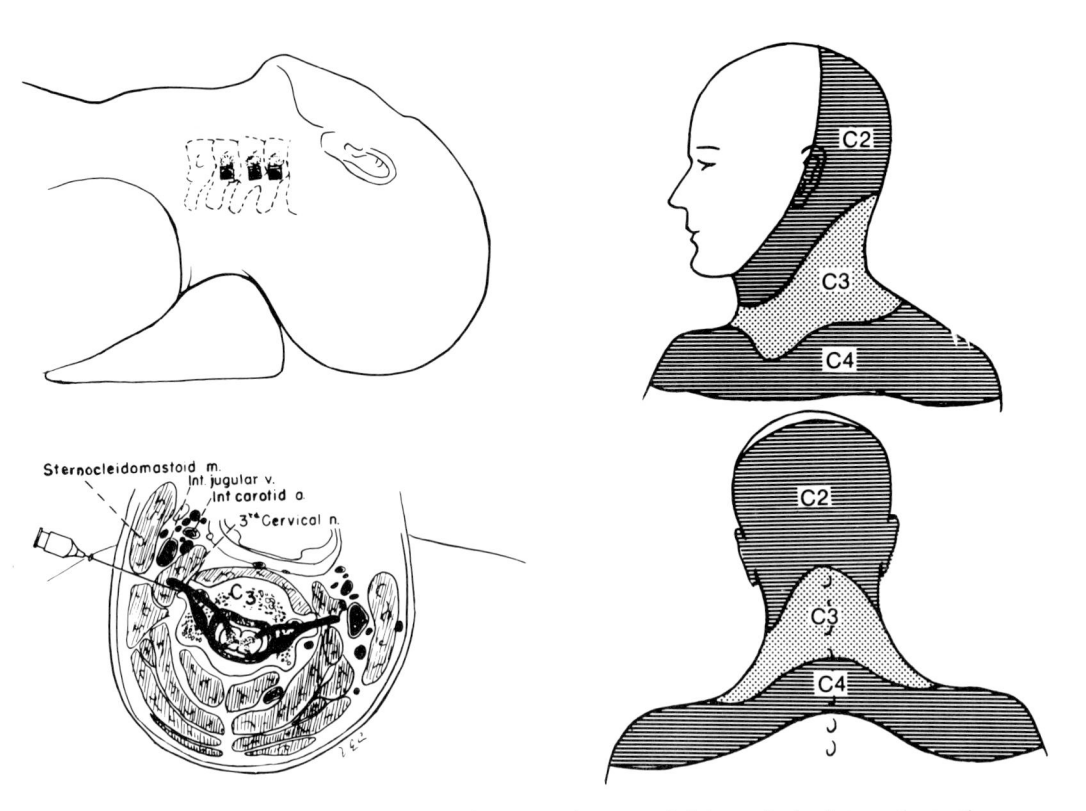

FIG. 3. Anatomy and technique of injecting the superficial cervical plexus. Area of anesthesia resulting from injecting the cervical plexus shown on the right. (Courtesy of J. J. Bonica, *The Management of Pain*, Lea & Febiger, Philadelphia, 1953).

Figs. 1 and 2.) It also contributes sensory fibers to the soft palate, uvula, and tonsils, which also receive fibers from other nerves.

The sensory area of the glossopharyngeal nerve comprises the nasopharynx, the eustachian tube, soft palate, uvula, tonsil, tonsillar pillar base of the tongue, and the pharynx as far as the epiglottis and possibly below it. It contributes fibers to the external auditory canal. The vagus nerve contributes sensory fibers to the ear, the external auditory canal, and the tympanic membrane, and supplies the larynx. The second, third, and fourth cervical nerves supply the neck, the posterior portion of the scalp, the ear, and the skin over the angle and lower portion of the mandible, as shown in Fig. 3. Sympathetic fibers supply the entire region by accompanying somatic nerves and the blood vessels.

CLINICAL CONSIDERATIONS

Chemical section is particularly applicable to cancer pain within the distribution of the trigeminal nerve, and all such cases should be first treated with this method, because experience shows that alcohol injections produce analgesia for 6 to 18 months, sufficiently long to afford relief until death in most patients with cancer pain. Moreover, if pain returns either because the chemical interruption has disappeared or because the tumor has spread beyond the confines of the anesthesia, the injection can be repeated. In some patients block of one of the major divisions of the trigeminal nerve (e.g., maxillary or mandibular) is sufficient but in most instances it is far better to carry out a gasserian ganglion block to produce widespread analgesia because probably the disease will spread if the patient lives sufficiently long. Although gasserian ganglion block is inherent in the risk of keratitis, the problem is quite different than when dealing with patients with tic douloureux in whom life-expectancy is long and where a corneal ulcer would be a serious complication.

Obtaining radiographs prior to the block may be of great importance in some cases. If, for example, a block of the trigeminal nerve at the level of the gasserian ganglion in Meckel's cave is planned, a radiographic plate of the base of the skull is required in order to ascertain the presence of the foramen ovale. In patients with carcinoma of the nasopharynx and the floor of the mouth, the tumor may destroy bone structures of the base of the skull, making it impossible to identify the foramen ovale. In these cases it will be necessary to adopt a different approach for the block or a different procedure. Alcohol diffuses very poorly in tissues so that, if the block is to be effective, exact positioning of the needle in the nerve or nerves is necessary. This is one of the main reasons for the use of radiologic control when these blocks are undertaken (4). Another reason is to obtain objective evidence of the position of the needles at the time of the injection of the neurolytic agent. Moreover, the use of X-ray control allows even the beginner to ensure the exact positioning of the needles in the correct anatomic region so that the solution achieves the desired effect.

TECHNIQUE OF BLOCKING THE GASSERIAN GANGLION

The following brief description of the technique of blocking the gasserian ganglion is included. For a more detailed description, the reader is referred to Bonica's book (1). The most frequently used and best technique of blocking the gasserian ganglion (and also the mandibular nerve) is by the anterolateral (Härtel) approach. The needle is inserted through a skin wheal which is on the skin overlying the 2nd upper molar tooth and advanced in a direction so that when it is viewed from the side its point is directed to the midpoint of the zygomatic arch, and when viewed from the front it is directed to the pupil of the ipsilateral eye. It is advanced until it contacts the infratemporal plate lateral to the base of the pterygoid process just anterior to the foramen ovale. The depth mark is then set 1.5 cm from the skin surface, the needle withdrawn until its point is in the subcutaneous tissue and then reinserted so that its point will eventually go through the foramen.

For the injection, the patient is made to lie in the supine position looking straight ahead. The skin overlying the midpoint of the zygomatic arch and the skin overlying the articular tubercle are marked with a pencil. These points act as a guide to the infratemporal plate and the foramen ovale, respectively. A wheal is made with a local anesthetic in the skin of the cheek 3 cm lateral to the angle of the mouth at the level of the 2nd upper molar tooth. A 10-cm, 22-gauge needle threaded with a depth marker is introduced through this wheal and is advanced in a posteromedial and superior direction, so that when it is viewed from the side, its axis points to the midpoint of the zygomatic arch, and when it is viewed from in front, the axis of the needle points to the pupil (Fig. 4). After piercing the skin, the needle progressively passes through the buccinator muscle, then beneath the mucous membrane between the mandibular ramus and tuberosity of the maxilla, and finally through the external pterygoid muscle before it makes contact with the infratemporal plate lateral to the base of the pterygoid process and just anterior to the foramen. As soon as this contact is made, usually at a depth of about 5 cm, the depth marker is set 1.5 cm from the skin surface, the needle is withdrawn until its point is in the subcutaneous tissue, and it is then reinserted so that its point will eventually go through the foramen. During this second insertion, the axis of the needle, when viewed from the side, points to the articular tubercle, while when viewed from the front, it still points to the pupil. Usually when the needle has been inserted to a depth just 1 cm short of the rubber marker, its point makes contact with the mandibular nerve, causing paresthesia along the course of the latter. These

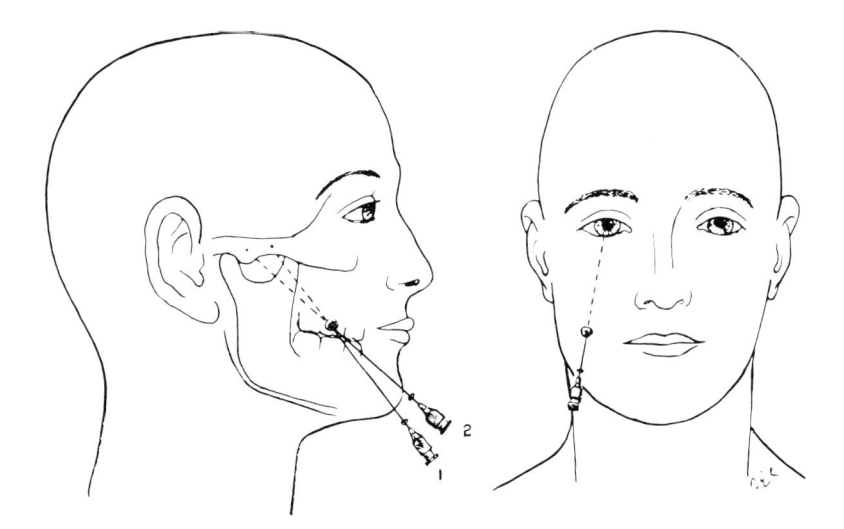

FIG. 4. Gasserian ganglion and mandibular nerve block by the anterolateral technique (Härtel). Note the relationship of the skin wheal to the second upper molar and the direction of the needle in relation to the zygomatic arch (*lateral view*) and to the pupil of the eye (*anterior view*). (Courtesy of J. J. Bonica, *The Management of Pain,* Lea & Febiger, Philadelphia, 1953).

lancinating sensations, usually radiating to the lower jaw and ear, indicate that the point of the needle is in the right position at the inferior entrance of the foramen. The needle is then advanced until the marker is flush with the skin, and presumably its point lies within Meckel's cave or within the ganglion itself. Lack of paresthesia indicates that the needle has been improperly placed, and it should be withdrawn and reinserted correctly. Once the needle is in place, 0.5 ml of local anesthetic is injected to ascertain its correct position. This should produce some analgesia in the region of the Gasserian ganglion. Subsequently, 1 ml of alcohol is injected slowly in increments of 0.2 ml at a time.

The complications of this technique include hematoma of the cheek and herpetic eruptions on the face several days following the injection. Keratitis and corneal ulcers may occur if the eye is not properly cared for. Accidental subarachnoid injection may cause unconsciousness and subsequent involvement of several of the cranial nerves.

TECHNIQUES OF BLOCKING THE MAXILLARY AND MANDIBULAR NERVES

The maxillary and mandibular nerves are best approached by the lateral extra-oral route shown in Fig. 5. The figure on the left indicates the point of entrance into the skin just below the midpoint of the zygomatic arch where a skin wheal is formed for the local anesthetic. For the average patient a 8 cm long 22-gauge security needle is used. The needle is inserted perpendicular to the skin and advanced slowly until the lateral pterygoid plate is contacted. To carry out maxillary nerve block, the needle is withdrawn until its point is in the subcutaneous region; it is then reinserted so that it will pass slightly anteriorly and superiorly and advance until its point enters the pterygopalatine fossa and contacts the maxillary nerve therein (needle 2). In carrying out mandibular nerve block, needle 1 is withdrawn and reinserted in a direction slightly posterior. It is advanced until its point contacts the mandibular nerve just below the foramen ovale (needle 3). It is best to inject 0.5 to 0.75 ml. of alcohol intraneurally to produce complete destruction of the nerves.

TECHNIQUE OF BLOCKING THE GLOSSOPHARYNGEAL AND VAGUS NERVES

Figure 6 depicts the technique of blocking the glossopharyngeal and vagus nerves. The figure on the left shows the site where the skin wheal is formed, approximately midway between the posterior border of the mandible and tip of the mastoid process. The needle is inserted perpendicular to the skin and advanced until its point impinges on the styloid process, as depicted by

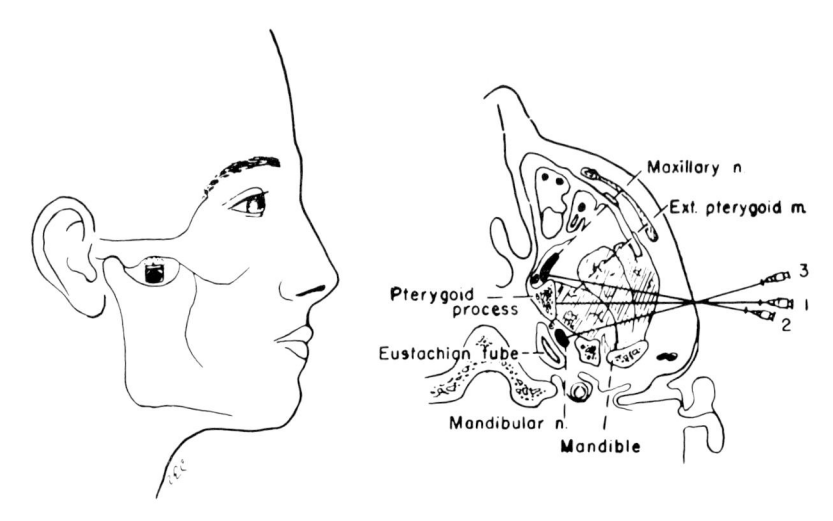

FIG. 5. Diagram depicting the technique of maxillary and mandibular nerve block by the lateral extra-oral route. **Left:** The point of entrance into the skin is just below the midpoint of the zygomatic arch. **Right:** A schematic cross-section. The point of the needle (needle 1) is impinging on the lateral pterygoid plate. To carry out maxillary nerve block, the needle is withdrawn until its point is in the subcutaneous region and then reinserted so that it will pass slightly anteriorly and superiorly, and advance until its point enters the pterygopalatine fossa and contacts the maxillary nerve therein (needle 2). In carrying out mandibular nerve block, needle 1 is withdrawn and reinserted in a direction slightly posterior. It is advanced until its point contacts the mandibular nerve just below the foramen ovale (needle 3). After contacting each nerve and eliciting paresthesia, 1 to 2 ml of solution is injected. (Courtesy of J. J. Bonica, *Clinical Applications of Diagnostic and Therapeutic Nerve Blocks,* Charles C Thomas, Springfield, Ill., 1959.)

needle 1 in the cross-sectional diagram on the right. The needle is then withdrawn and redirected so that it will pass anterior to the styloid process and slightly deeper until its point is in contact with the glossopharyngeal nerve (needle 2). The vagus nerve is blocked by passing the needle posterior to the styloid process and advancing it about 1 cm deeper than the bone (needle 3). Injection of 3 to 5 ml of solution is sufficient.

RESULTS

Table 1 lists the neurolytic cranial nerve blocks performed during the past 11 years by the senior author in patients with malignant tumors localized in the areas innervated by the trigeminal nerve. As may be noted, most of the procedures have involved the gasserian ganglion block, which was carried out in a total of 371 patients representing 41% of all the cranial nerve block procedures done. For blocking the branches of the trigeminal nerve we have used exclusively absolute alcohol. On blocking the gasserian ganglion we used alcohol in 267 cases. Phenol in glycerine 7.5% solution has been in-

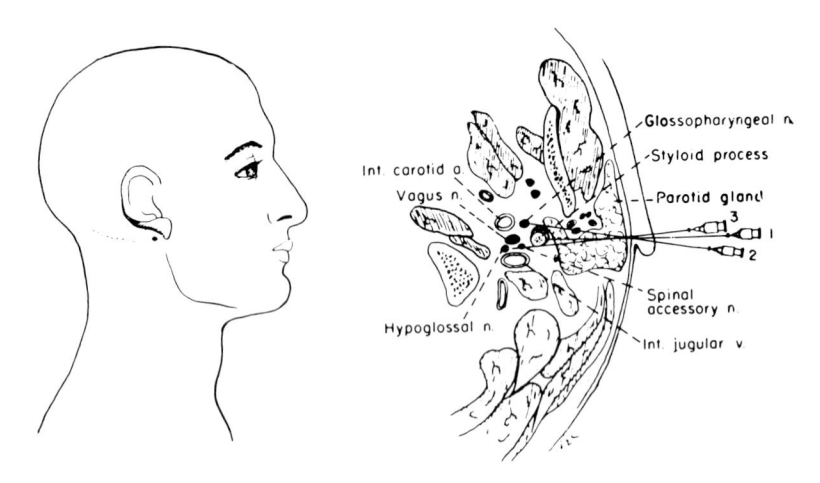

FIG. 6. Technique of blocking the glossopharyngeal and vagus nerves. **Left:** The site where the skin wheal is formed, approximately midway between the posterior border of the mandible and tip of the mastoid process. The needle is inserted perpendicular to the skin and advanced until its point impinges on the styloid process, as depicted by needle 1 in the cross-sectional diagram on the right. The needle is then withdrawn and redirected so that it will pass anterior to the styloid process and slightly deeper until its point is in contact with the glossopharyngeal nerve (needle 2). The vagus nerve is blocked by passing the needle posterior to the styloid process and advancing it about 1 cm deeper than the bone (needle 3). Injection of 3 to 5 ml of solution is sufficient. (Courtesy of J. J. Bonica, *Clinical Applications of Diagnostic and Therapeutic Nerve Blocks,* Charles C Thomas, Springfield, Ill., 1959.)

jected in 82 patients. Early in our series we carried out 22 gasserian ganglion blocks with hypertonic saline, but we have given it up due to poor results. Phenol in glycerine for blocking the gasserian ganglion is well tolerated by the patient, and its injection is painless. The only disadvantage is the need of a larger needle, usually a 20-gauge needle; otherwise, it is difficult to inject the phenol. With a larger needle there is risk of hemorrhage and/or fistula along the path of the needle.

TABLE 1. *Neurolytic cranial nerve blocks (July, 1966 to July, 1977)*

Type of block	Absolute alcohol	Phenol in glycerine	Hypertonic saline	Total
Gasserian ganglion	267	82	22	371 (41%)
Supraorbital	89			89 (9.8%)
Maxillary	57			57 (6.3%)
Infraorbital	198			198 (21.8%)
Mandibular	101			101 (11.2%)
Lingual	12			12 (1.3%)
Mental	74			74 (8.2%)
Glossopharyngeal	4			4 (0.4%)
Total	802			906

As the majority of these patients have been treated with some form of radiotherapy when it becomes necessary to block the cervical nerves, this may represent a difficult task owing to the intense fibrosis in the neck area when the cervical chain has been irradiated.

We feel that the posterior approach to the cervical nerves is not precisely an accurate technique and can be very painful for the patient. We prefer to carry out an extradural cervical block with phenol (3). In our hands this technique has proven to be safe and well tolerated by the patient.

REFERENCES

1. Bonica, J. J. (1953): *The Management of Pain.* Lea & Febiger, Philadelphia.
2. Bonica, J. J. (1959): *Clinical Applications of Diagnostic and Therapeutic Nerve Blocks.* Charles C Thomas, Springfield, Ill.
3. Madrid, J. L. (1975): Experience de 363 cas d'analgesie par alcool et phenol. *Cah. Anesthesiol.,* Fr., 23, no. 7, 825–827.
4. Pender, J. W., and Pugh, D. G. (1951): Diagnostic and therapeutic nerve blocks: Necessity for roetgenograms. JAMA, 146:789–801.

Celiac (Splanchnic) Plexus Block with Alcohol for Cancer Pain of the Upper Intra-Abdominal Viscera

Daniel C. Moore

The Mason Clinic, Seattle, Washington 98101

Celiac plexus block is the most effective, least hazardous means of palliative therapy for cancer of the upper intra-abdominal viscera (9,10,14). The celiac plexus can be blocked with 50 ml of 50% alcohol without the alteration of motor, sensory, or visceral function which occurs when most other nerves or plexuses are chemically sectioned. Block of this plexus is definitive treatment for intractable pain from cancer that is limited to one or more of the following upper intra-abdominal organs: (a) stomach and/or duodenum, (b) liver, (c) gallbladder, (d) pancreas, and (e) adrenal glands. Its most frequent use is to alleviate pain from cancer of the pancreas.

RESULTS

In the past 30 years, 168 patients with the established diagnosis of cancer of one or more of the previously noted organs have received 186 alcohol celiac plexus block (18 were reblocked) (Table 1). In these 168 patients, the effectiveness of the alcohol block ranged from 5 days to approximately 1 year. Death from the cancer occurred in 2 days to 14 months following the block. Of the 168 patients, 157 (94%) had good to excellent relief of pain. In addition to pain-relief, other side benefits included: (a) less nausea and vomiting; (b) increased food intake and even occasionally a gain in weight; (c) improved bowel motility, with passing of flatus and stool; and (d) elimination or marked reduction of the need for narcotics. From the time of the block until their death, many patients used only tranquilizers, aspirin with or without codeine, or only small doses of narcotics [first 41 cases document this in a previously published article (3)]. Similar results have been reported by others (2,8,17).

In the patients who had little or no relief, the cancer had metastasized beyond the organs innervated by the celiac plexus. Even though the alcohol blocked the celiac plexus, the patients continued to have pain of a different nature, often in a different area, which was as incapacitating. Therefore, it is advisable to perform a diagnostic block with a long-acting local anesthetic

TABLE 1. *Primary site of cancer of patients treated with alcohol celiac plexus block (1947–1977)*

Site	No.
Pancreas	121
Stomach	11
Liver and bile ducts	7
Gallbladder	2
Liver metastases from:	
Retroperitoneal	2
Rectum	1
Uterus and ovary	5
Lung	11
Kidney	2
Esophagus	6
Total	168

drug—namely, 50 ml of 0.25% bupivacaine (Marcaine®) with 1:200,000 epinephrine—prior to employing alcohol.

TECHNICAL CONSIDERATIONS

Celiac plexus block is not too difficult to master, and complications are minimal provided that the physician performing the procedure: (a) knows the anatomy of the plexus; (b) carries out the technique of the block meticulously; (c) injects the stated amount of alcohol; and (e) employs roentgenography, especially while learning the technique, to determine correct placement of the needles. Because of its high efficacy, it should be used more frequently than it is being used at present. The following detailed discussion of the anatomy and technique of the procedure is included with the hope that it will induce more physicians to learn and use the procedure.

Anatomic Bases

The celiac plexus is situated in the prevertebral region at the level of the body of the first lumbar vertebra. It is composed of right and left celiac superior mesenteric and arteriorenal ganglia and a dense network of nerve fibers that connects them. It surrounds the celiac artery and the base of the superior mesenteric artery. It lies in areolar tissue behind the peritoneum, the stomach, and the omental bursa; in front of the crura of the diaphragm and the commencement of the abdominal aorta; and between the suprarenal glands (Fig. 1).

The celiac plexus contains: (a) the endings of the greater splanchnic nerves, which are made up of branches contributed by the fifth to the ninth or tenth thoracic sympathetic ganglia; (b) the endings of the lesser splanchnic

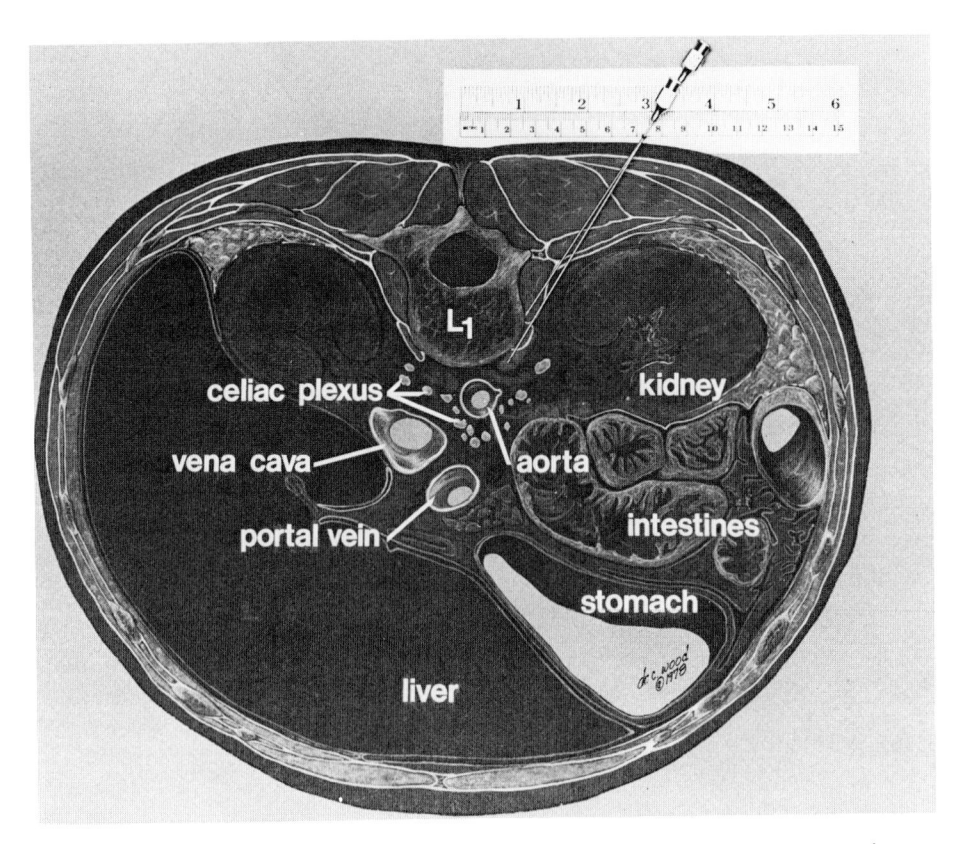

FIG. 1. Schematic cross-section at the level of first lumbar vertebra of a cadaver whose circumference is 36 inches. Size of vertebra, nerves, and organs is scaled accurately. The short-beveled security needles are 20-gauge and 10 cm (4 inches) long.

nerves, composed of branches derived from the ninth, tenth, and sometimes the eleventh thoracic sympathetic ganglia; (c) the endings of the lowest splanchnic nerves, composed of branches contributed by the last thoracic ganglion; and (d) some filaments from the right vagus. The plexus gives off secondary plexuses to the diaphragm, liver, spleen, stomach, adrenal glands, pancreas, ovary and fundus of the uterus, spermatic cord, abdominal aorta, mesentery, small intestine, and colon. While sympathetic and parasympathetic motor fibers themselves do not transmit pain, afferent (sensory) nerve fibers that course with them transmit nociceptive impulses from the viscera.

Technique of Alcohol Block

The posterior approach described by Kappis in 1918, and since advocated in all articles and books describing this block, which were reviewed, is employed (1–17). Prior to performing the block, the anesthetist must explain to the patient its effectiveness in relieving pain, as well as the discomfort experienced during the injection of the alcohol and possible complications. The patient's chart should contain documented evidence of acceptance of the block. As previously mentioned, it is essential to carry out a prognostic block with a local anesthetic before considering alcohol injection. This is done to ascertain that the alcohol block will produce adequate pain relief. For the reasons mentioned below, it is best to carry out the prognostic block at least 12 hr before the alcohol injection is done.

Premedication and/or the Injection of a Local Anesthetic Drug Prior to Injecting Alcohol

The patient is not premedicated or given anesthesia prior to injection of the neurolytic drug, because accurate description of the pain while the alcohol is being injected confirms placement of the needles. Injection of local anesthetic drugs prior to administration of the alcohol is not advised for the same reason, but also because the local anesthetic solution will further dilute the alcohol, resulting in an inadequate block or one of short duration. This does not preclude the use of 3 ml or less of local anesthetic solution while attempts are being made to locate the body of the first lumbar vertebrae.

Position

The patient is placed in the prone position with a pillow between the iliac crests and the rib cage so as to reduce the lumbar curve of the vertebral column to a minimum (Figs. 2 and 3). Any other position increases significantly the likelihood of misplacing the needles.

Landmarks

The landmarks are located by palpation and marked on the skin with a line or an X, using a felt marking pen whose ink when dry will not be washed off by an antiseptic solution (Figs. 2 and 3). The required landmarks are: (a) the spinous processes of the first and second lumbar vertebrae; (b) the cephalad edge of the spinous process of the first lumbar vertebra—the celiac plexus lies at the level of the upper part of the first lumbar vertebra; and (c) a point on the lower borders of the twelfth ribs 5 cm to a *maximum* of 7.5 cm (2 to 3 inches) from the midpoint of the spinous process of either of the marked vertebrae. These distances vary, depending on the size of the patient, and must be measured by a ruler—not estimated (Fig. 1).

The X's marking the cephalad edge of the spinous process of the first lumbar vertebra and those on the twelfth ribs are connected by straight lines. This forms a flat triangle whose apex is seldom more than 2.5 cm (1 inch)

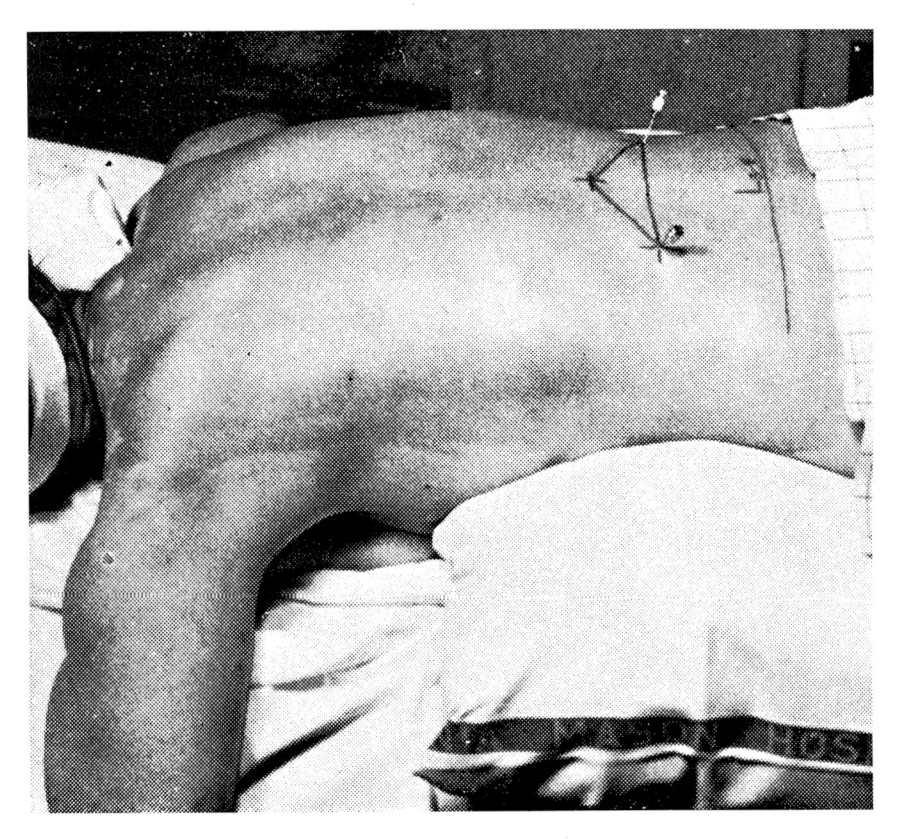

FIG. 2. Lateral view showing the flat triangle formed by joining the three X's which are the landmarks for the celiac plexus block. The straight line between the iliac crests passes through the interspace between the spinous processes of the third and fourth lumbar vertebrae.

above the base (Fig. 2). If the apex of the triangle greatly exceeds 2.5 cm, then either the cephalad edge of the wrong spinous process was marked or the distance from the midline of the spinous process to the 12th rib exceeds 7.5 cm, or both have occurred.

These markings are critical, particularly the maximum of 7.5 cm from the midline to avoid puncture of the kidney or the uteropelvic junction. It is important to remember that the kidneys lie adjacent to the vertebral column and behind the peritoneum, surrounded by loose areolar tissue and a mass of fat (Fig. 4). They are in the same compartment with the celiac plexus, the aorta, and the vena cava (Fig. 1). Moreover, the medial surfaces of the upper and lower poles of the kidney lie approximately 5 cm (2 inches) and 7 cm (3 inches), respectively, from the midline with the right kidney 1 cm lower than the left. Also, the upper poles are at the level of the twelfth thoracic vertebra and the lower poles at the upper border of the body of the

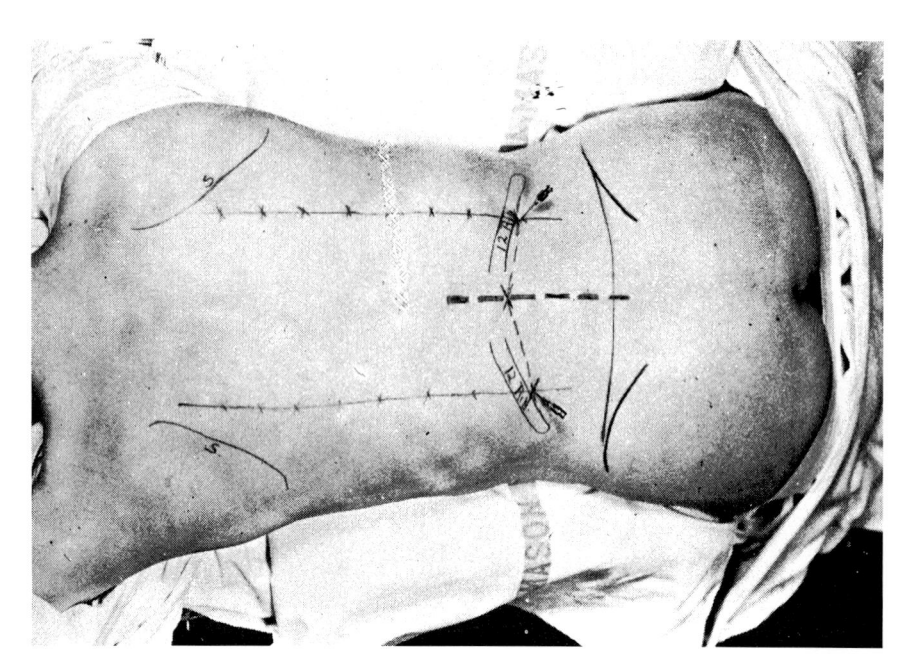

FIG. 3. Posterior view of 4-inch (10.2-cm) needles in place for the execution of the celiac plexus block. Note the direction of the needles as they course along the line from the twelfth rib to the superior edge of the spinous process of the first lumbar vertebra. Also the 55-degree angle formed by the shaft of the needles and the skin.

third lumbar vertebra. Finally, the twelfth ribs lie over the kidneys (Fig. 5).

Therefore, if puncture of the kidneys is to be avoided, the needles must pass medial to them in the 2 to 3 cm (¾ to 1¼ inches) of tissue which lies between the kidneys and the lumbar vertebrae (Figs. 1 and 6). The needle's point may be placed intravascularly or subarachnoidally and withdrawn prior to injecting alcohol with little chance of a complication resulting. Contrarily, if the kidney or the ureteropelvic junction is traumatized when the needle is inserted [and this will occur consistently when the distance for inserting the needle is greater than 7.5 cm (3 inches) from the midline] and if alcohol is injected into or in close proximity to the kidney or the ureteropelvic junction, a serious inflammation may result (17). Sequelae of this may be degeneration of the kidney, extravasation of urine from the ureter, and so forth, requiring nephrectomy.

Neurolytic Solution

A solution of 50 ml of 50% alcohol is preferred. This concentration is prepared immediately prior to its injection by opening ampules of absolute alcohol and mixing their contents with normal saline. Mixing alcohol with a

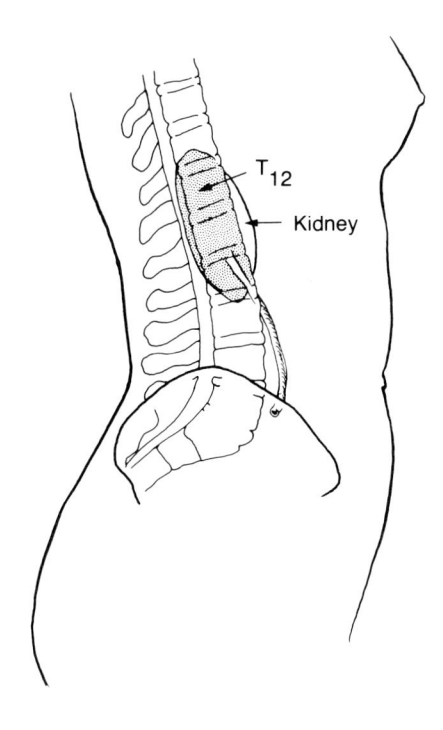

FIG. 4. Schematic drawing showing position of kidneys lateral and opposite to the vertebral column.

local anesthetic solution rather than normal saline will somewhat decrease but not abolish the severe pain from the alcohol, which lasts for 5 to 10 sec. Since the pain from the alcohol is still excruciating and since such a mixture may result in the test dose's giving signs which are difficult to evaluate, I use only normal saline for dilution. Following the injection of the alcohol, the

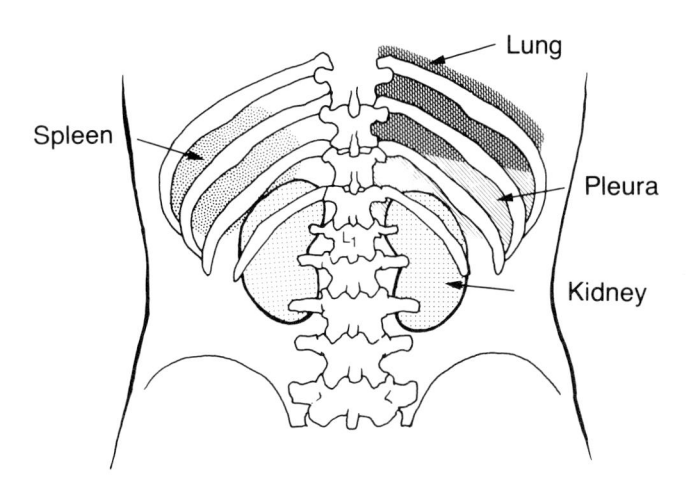

FIG. 5. Schematic drawing of back of the lumbar region, showing position of kidneys in relationship to vertebrae, twelfth rib, pleura, lungs, and spleen.

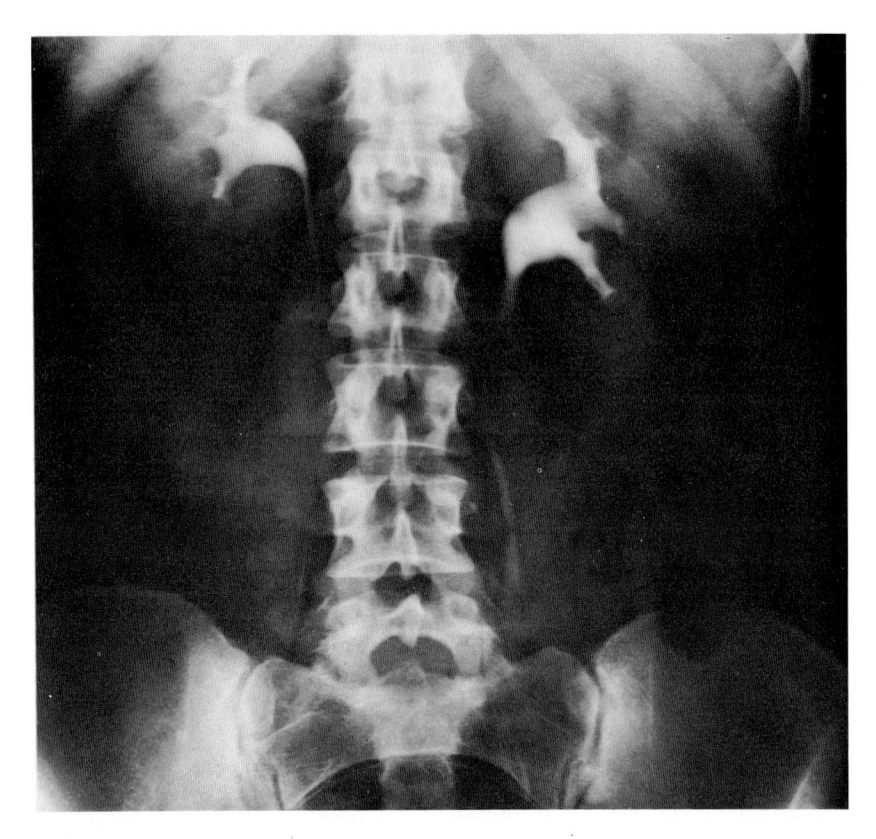

FIG. 6. Intravenous pyelogram showing relationship of kidneys and ureteropelvic junction to vertebrae.

cancer pain is usually markedly reduced or completely abolished in 2 to 10 min, but on occasion 24 hr may be required for maximum effect. The effects of alcohol last 3 weeks to 6 months and on occasion longer. If the block dissipates prior to the patient's death, it is repeated.

Using a smaller amount and stronger concentrations of alcohol is not advocated. The described technique depends on the fact that the solution is injected safely away from the vital organs and diffuses so as to bathe the entire celiac plexus. Pinpoint accuracy of needle placement at the celiac plexus is not necessary. Furthermore, when smaller amounts of absolute alcohol are used, the incidence of unsatisfactory results is higher and the destructive effects greater than required for neurolysis. This increases the possibility of damage to other organs adjacent to the celiac plexus.

Although 50 ml of 6 to 7% aqueous phenol may be used in the same way as alcohol, alcohol is preferred. The onset of analgesia with phenol is somewhat slower, the incidence of satisfactory block less, and the duration shorter. For these reasons, I do not use it.

Placement of the Needles

Although a small-gauge needle may be less painful, two 20-gauge needles are employed, for when they are correctly placed there is no resistance to the injection of the anesthetic solution, and the anesthetist has the feeling that he is injecting intravenously. This feeling indicates correct placement of the needle. If a smaller-gauge needle—for example, a 22-gauge—is used instead, this feeling is decreased, and the physician cannot tell whether the resistance is due to the needle's gauge or whether the needle's point is misplaced under the periosteum of the vertebrae, in an organ's wall, or in other tissue. In the average patient, a 10-cm (4-inch) needle will be sufficient, but on occasion, a 12.5- or 15-cm (5- or 6-inch) needle will be required if the patient is large and/or obese. If in the average-sized patient a needle longer than 10 cm (4 inches) is needed to contact the body of the first lumbar vertebra, the X at the lower border of the twelfth rib is incorrectly placed more than 7.5 cm (3 inches) from the midline of the back.

The following steps are used in blocking the celiac plexus:

The physician stands by the patient at the side into which the needle is to be inserted. A skin wheal is made at the X's on the lower borders of the twelfth ribs using a 26-gauge or smaller needle—if a 30-gauge needle is available, it is used. One of the 20-gauge needles is introduced through the skin wheal at the X at the lower edge of the twelfth rib at a 45-degree angle to the skin. Using the line of the side of the marked triangle as a guide, the needle is slowly advanced as 3 ml or less of local anesthetic solution is injected so as to make its advancement less painful. When the needle contacts the cephalad part of the body of the first lumbar vertebra, the depth of the needle is noted (Fig. 1). The needle should have contacted the lateral side of the body of the vertebra just below the body's midpoint.

To be in the correct position for the celiac plexus block, the needle must be inserted 2 to 2.5 cm (¾ to 1 inch) deeper than the lateral side of the midpoint of the body of the first lumbar vertebra. The needle is then withdrawn 2.5 cm (1 inch), and the angle between its shaft and the skin lateral to the needle is increased by 5 to 10 degrees—that is, from 45 degrees to 50 or 55 degrees—and then the needle is again advanced. This maneuver is repeated, increasing the angle slightly each time, until the needle is felt to slip off the body of the vertebra. At this point, it is advanced another 2 to 2.5 cm (¾ to 1 inch). Now its point should lie in prevertebral areolar tissue which contains the celiac plexus (Figs. 1, 6, and 7). In the average patient, the distance from the skin to the celiac plexus is usually 8.8 to 10 cm (3½ to 4 inches).

So the needle is "walked" slowly anteriorly on the lateral surface of the vertebra; not infrequently contact with the bone is lost, but the needle point is felt to enter into a dense fibrous tissue, which is the periosteum of the vertebra. The periosteum is a valuable landmark because with the next withdrawal of the needle and another slight increase of the angle of the shaft with the skin, the needle will slide anterior to the body of the vertebra. Also, when the needle is inserted *very* slowly on the left side past the body of the vertebra, frequently the pulsation of the aorta may be felt or seen if the needle hub is released. This indicates that the needle is correctly placed. For this reason, placement of the needle first on the left side and then on the right side may be preferable, as the needle's depth on the left side may then be used as a guide for the right side. When the needle's bevel inadvertently is placed in either the aorta or the vena cava, as evidenced by blood appearing at the hub, the needle is withdrawn slowly until blood no longer appears at the hub. Then it is withdrawn another 0.2 to 0.3 cm (⅛ inch) to be certain that it is not in the vessel wall. Puncture of either the aorta or the vena cava is no indication to discontinue the block.

After placing the needle on one side, a second is placed in the opposite side in the same fashion. When the technique is being mastered or in the event of abnormal pathology, posteroanterior and lateral roentgenograms

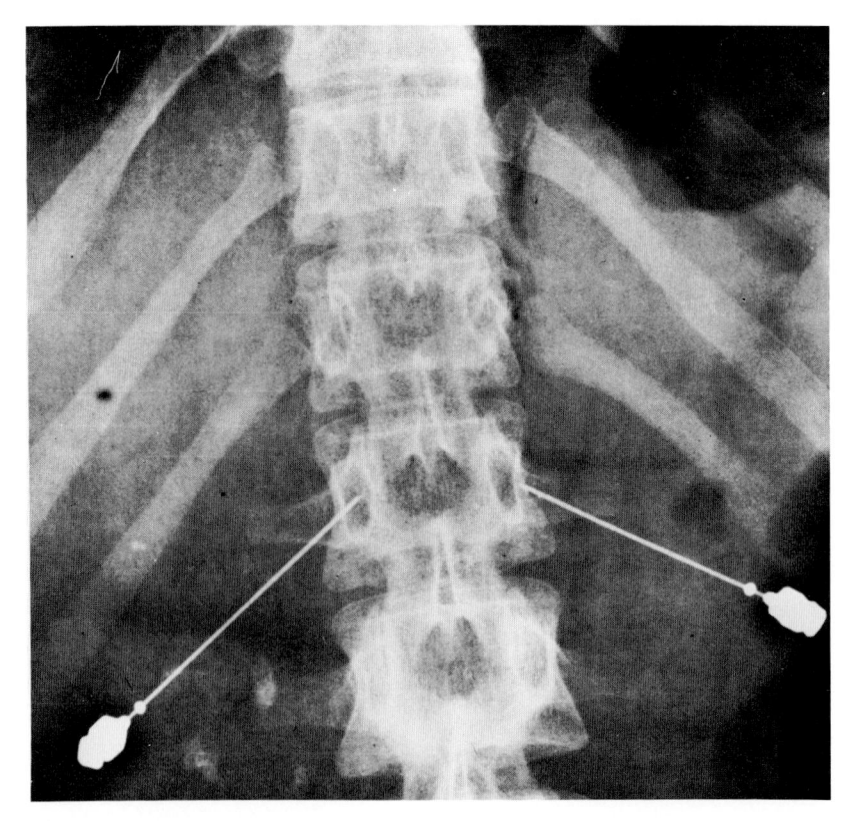

FIG. 7. Posterior-anterior view of needles correctly placed anterior to the body of the first lumbar vertebra.

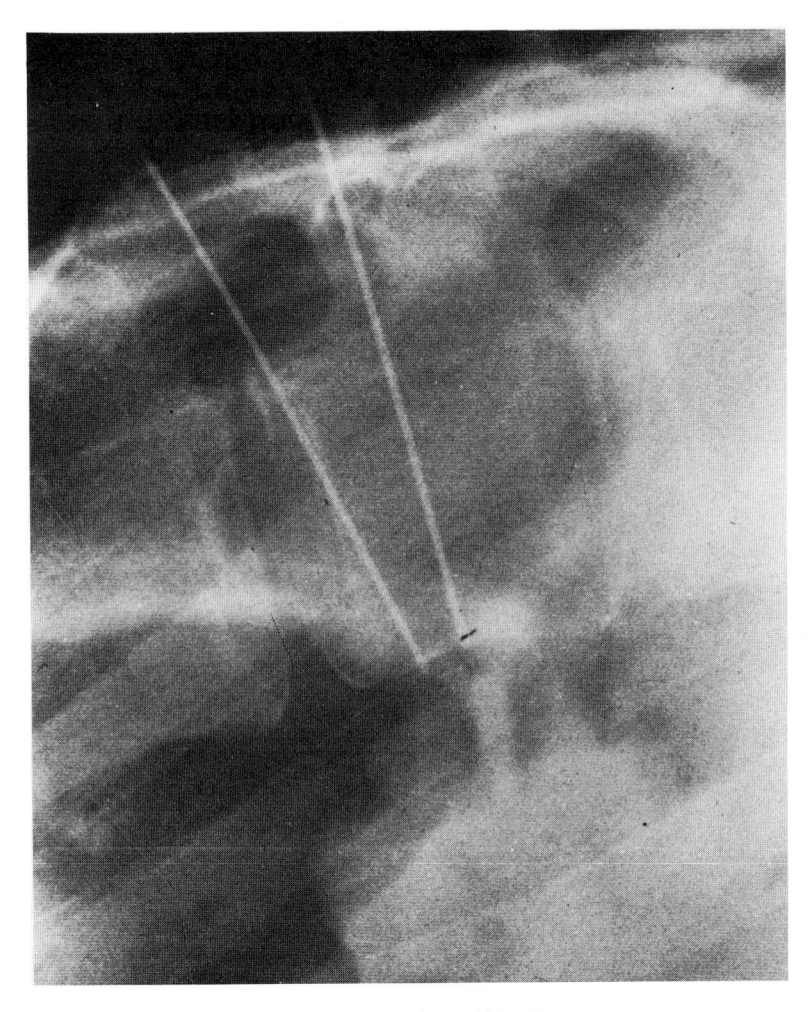

FIG. 8. Lateral view of Fig. 7.

should be taken at this point. These help to rule out epidural or subarachnoid placement of the needle point and confirm its placement anterior to the midpoint of the body of the first lumbar vertebra (Figs. 7 and 8). However, roentgenograms do not rule out intravascular placement. Ideally the needle point should be in this position, but if roentgenograms show the point of the needle to be anterior to the caudad part of the vertebra (rather than at its midpart), nothing further needs to be done because the solution will spread to involve the entire plexus.

After both needles are in place, 2 ml of air is injected through each needle to clear any plugs of tissue which may have entered the needle during its insertion. Then an attempt is made to aspirate for blood or spinal fluid.

When both needles are considered to be properly placed, the syringe filled with dilute alcohol is adapted to the needle and the patient is again warned of the type of pain the alcohol will cause. Aspiration is repeated and if nothing is obtained, 20 to 25 ml of the alcohol are injected at the rate of 2 to 3 ml per sec. As the neurolytic drug is injected, the patient will usually cry out: (a) "It burns like fire," (b) "It is difficult to breathe," or (c) "I cannot stand the pain." Such pain is diagnostic of correct placement of the alcohol, and it subsides in a period of 5 to 10 sec.

Immediately following the injection of one side and even if the patient is still having pain, disconnect the syringe from the needle, *leaving the needle in place,* and refill the syringe. Warn the patient that the pain may increase, and inject another 20 to 25 ml of the alcohol through the second needle. After injection of the first side, the needle is not withdrawn because when the bevels of both needles are correctly placed inside the fascial compartment containing the celiac plexus, injection through the second needle will often force solution to reflux from the first needle. This is another valuable sign that the needles are correctly placed. Subsequently, 2 ml of air are injected through each needle to avoid spilling onto the first lumbar nerve as the needle is withdrawn. Both needles are then removed.

COMPLICATIONS

With the exception of the low blood pressure from block of the celiac plexus and pain in the back from the destructive effects of the neurolytic drug, the complications of celiac plexus block are a result of incorrect landmarks, inaccurately placed needles, or both. If there is any doubt regarding needle placement, posteroanterior and lateral roentgenograms should be taken.

Arterial Hypotension

Following completion of the block, the majority of patients experience hypotension from interruption of the vasoconstrictor fibers to a wide area and the "pooling" of blood in the viscera, particularly in the omentum, the small bowel, and the colon. In the young patient, who can compensate by vasoconstriction in the unaffected vessels, it causes no problem. However, older, arteriosclerotic patients frequently feel faint when they sit up or are ambulated. In 3 days or less, they usually compensate for this splanchnic vascular dilatation.

Oral administration of ephedrine is effective to combat this type of hypotension, but we do not use it. Rather, the patient is warned about fainting or feeling faint when in an upright position or ambulating, and the following orders are written on the patient's chart: (a) wrap both legs to midthigh with a 6-inch elastic bandage or apply elastic stockings; (b) apply a tight abdominal binder before ambulation; (c) when the patient is sitting up for the first time, a nurse should be present and ambulation should be allowed only with an assistant on each side; (d) check blood pressure and pulse every 15 min for 2 hr; and (e) if systolic pressure falls below one-third of the patient's normal, notify Dr. _____, telephone number _____.

Pain

While the cancer pain may be relieved immediately or within a few hours, the patient may experience dull, aching back pain for 24 to 48 hr following the block. Presumably, the tissue irritation from the alcohol causes the pain in the back at the site of the injection. For control, this pain may require small amounts of an analgesic compound—for example, Empirin® #3 which contains phenacetin, 150 mg; acetylsalicylic acid, 200 mg; caffeine, 30 mg; and codeine, 30 mg.

Subarachnoid Injection

When the needles for celiac plexus block are introduced into the skin more than 7.5 cm (3 inches) from the midline and/or at an angle with the skin of less than 45 degrees, the needle may enter the subarachnoid space through an intervertebral foramen or between the lamina of the vertebra.

In more than 3,000 celiac plexus blocks performed with either a local anesthetic solution or alcohol, this has occurred 18 times (0.006%). In all but one case (0.0003%), the spinal fluid dripped from the 20-gauge needle and the needle was withdrawn and placed correctly in the prevertebral space. In the one patient who did receive a subarachnoid injection, the resident physician had not done the prescribed tests prior to injecting the agent. Fortunately, the ensuing total block resulted from a local anesthetic solution and its effects disappeared in a few hours.

Epidural or Lumbar Somatic Nerve Block

Either of these complications may occur if the needle rests in the epidural space, lateral rather than anterior to the body of the vertebra, or in the psoas muscle. In one instance, in an obese, terminally ill woman who had massive ascites, a block was attempted with the patient in a lateral position—a position not used by the author. This compromise in technique coupled with the anatomic distortions of obesity resulted in spread of the alcohol solution to the nerves of the lumbar plexus, and she developed a partial unilateral leg paralysis. Chemical neuropathy with neuralgia (pain) of the first lumbar nerve from slight spillage of the neurolytic drug has been reported, but none of our patients developed such complications.

Puncture of the Lung, Kidney, Blood Vessels, and Other Viscera

Unless a complication occurs, it is difficult to evaluate whether the needles used in celiac plexus block puncture these organs and, if so, how often. Irrespective of the anesthetist's ability, at times they must. However, when a local anesthetic solution is used, complications resulting from this kind of puncture must be minimal and usually go unrecognized. Contrarily, when a neurolytic drug is injected, serious complications (particularly from puncture of the kidney) may result, requiring surgical intervention.

Puncture of the viscera, with peritonitis and hemoperitoneum following a celiac plexus block has not been seen by the author, and none has been noted in the literature. However, grossly bloody urine has been observed once in a patient who also had a pneumothorax from the same block and on whom the landmark for the insertion of the needle was misplaced 12.5 cm (5 inches) from the midline rather than the stated maximum of 7.5 cm (3 inches). Such complications—particularly puncture of the kidney—as previously noted, are more likely to occur when: (a) the needle is inserted more than 3 inches (7.5 cm) from the midline of the spinous process of the first or second lumbar vertebra; (b) the body of the first lumbar vertebra is not contacted by the needle's point prior to advancing it anterior to this vertebra; (c) the needle's point does not lie immediately in front of the body of the lumbar vertebrae but lies 2 cm (¾ inch) or more lateral and/or anterior to the body; and (d) attempts are made to place the needle's point higher than the body of the first lumbar vertebra—that is, at the body of the eleventh thoracic vertebra, as in the supradiaphragmatic technique, which is not advocated by the author.

The following must be emphasized. The major portion of the celiac plexus lies in front of the aorta, but the anesthetist should not attempt to put the needles there because puncture of vital organs is more likely. If the advice of a roentgenologist is sought regarding placement of the needles and if the needles are *correctly* placed 1 cm (⅜ inch) anterior to the body of the vertebra, the roentgenologist may state that the needles are not correctly placed because they are behind rather than in front of the projected location of the aorta (Figs. 7 and 8). *The anesthetist should not move the needles.* The 50 ml of solution will diffuse sufficiently to compensate for the placement of the needle behind rather than in front of the aorta.

Deposit of the neurolytic solution in dilute concentrations in either the aorta or the vena cava can result, but this has not occurred in our series of celiac plexus blocks. Carefully performed aspiration tests and the use of a 20-gauge needle evidently have avoided this complication. Even if 50 ml of 50% alcohol were injected intravascularly, it is doubtful that any untoward effects would result because alcohol infusions are often used for control of pain and other therapy. Whether absolute alcohol or phenol would be equally innocuous is questionable.

Necrosis of Contents in Close Proximity to Celiac Plexus

While necrosis of tissue in the retroperitoneal space from 50 ml to 50% alcohol might be anticipated, repeat autopsy observations have shown no grossly discernable changes.

Blood Levels of Alcohol

Alcohol is readily absorbed following the block as shown by the rapid rise of the drug over the first 20 min. The maximum level measured was 0.021 g/100 ml which is about one-fifth of the common legal standard for intoxication (16).

CONCLUSION

To reiterate, celiac plexus block using a bilateral approach and 50 ml of 50% alcohol relieved safely intractable pain of cancer of the upper intra-abdominal viscera in 94% of patients. Therefore, every physician who treats cancer pain should learn this block.

REFERENCES

1. Adriani, J. (1954): *Nerve Block*. Charles C Thomas, Springfield, Ill.
2. Bonica, J. J. (1953): *The Management of Pain*. Lea & Febiger, Philadelphia.
3. Bridenbaugh, L. D., Moore, D. C., and Campbell, D. D. (1964): Management of upper abdominal cancer pain. *JAMA*, 190:877.
4. Brown, E. M., and Kunjappan, V. (1975): Single-needle lateral approach for lumbar sympathetic block. *Anesth. Analg.*, 54:567.
5. Collins, V. J. (1976): *Principles of Anesthesiology*, 2nd ed. Lea & Febiger, Philadelphia.
6. Dale, W. A. (1952): Splanchnic block in treatment of acute pancreatitis. *Surgery*, 32:605.
7. Hale, D. E. (1963): *Anesthesiology*, 2nd ed. F. A. Davis, Philadelphia.
8. Jones, J. J., and Gough, D. (1977): Coeliac plexus block with alcohol for relief of upper intra-abdominal pain due to cancer. *Ann. R. Coll. Surg. Engl.*, 59:46.
9. Kappis, M. (1919): Sensibilität und lokale anästhesia im chirurgischen gebiet der bauchhöhle mit besonderer berücksichtigung der splanchnicus-anästhesie. *Bruns' Beiträge Zur Klin. Cher.*, 15:161.
10. Labat, G. (1922): *Regional Anesthesia*, 1st ed. Saunders, Philadelphia.
11. Lundy, J. (1945): *Clinical Anesthesia*. Saunders, Philadelphia.
12. Macintosh, R. R., and Bryce-Smith, R. (1953): *Local Anesthesia: Abdominal Surgery*. E. & S. Livingstone, Edinburgh.
13. Moore, D. C. (1965): *Regional Block*, 4th ed. Charles C Thomas, Springfield, Ill.
14. Pauchet, V., Sourdat, P., Labat, G., and D'ormont, R. D. B. (1927): *L'Anesthesie Regionale*. Gaston Dion et Cie, Paris.
15. Southworth, J. L., and Hingson, R. A. (1946): *Conduction Anesthesia*. Lippincott, Philadelphia.
16. Thompson, G. E., Moore, D. C., Bridenbaugh, L. D., et al. (1977): Abdominal pain and alcohol celiac plexus nerve block. *Anesth. Analg.*, 56:1.
17. Walton, F. A. (1952): Coeliac ganglion block. *Can. Med. Assoc. J.*, 67:342.

Chemical Hypophysectomy

John Miles

Centre for Pain Relief, Department of Neurosurgery, Walton Hospital, Liverpool, England

For the last 5 years, in the Centre for Pain Relief in Liverpool, we have been using Moricca's technique of alcohol injection into the pituitary gland for the relief of pain in patients with advanced cancer (1,2). We prefer to call it just that, *alcohol injection into the pituitary gland,* rather than "chemical hypophysectomy" or Moricca's term of "neuroadenolysis" because we would rather *not* imply that the undoubted pain-relieving effect that results, is due necessarily to destruction of the pituitary gland. As you will note, many other exciting explanations are possible.

The technique has been used only when the pain syndrome seemed unlikely to respond to conventional methods such as regional nerve blocks or cordotomy. It has been used particularly for widespread bilateral pain, pain in the head and neck, or midline body pain.

We originally considered that it could be used as an alternative to cordotomy in patients with cancer so advanced as to render the patient unfit for cordotomy. This we no longer believe. Patients being considered for pituitary alcohol injection require as much or more biologic resilience if they are to benefit from it, than do those undergoing cordotomy.

TECHNICAL ASPECTS

To date we have performed 179 injections in 122 patients (Table 1). In 75 instances a single injection was made, but frequently more than one needle was introduced to obtain more complete injection into the gland. Regardless of whether one or more needles were used, a maximum of 1.25 ml of absolute alcohol was injected in increments of 0.1 to 0.2 ml. In all cases 0.5 ml of contrast medium, either water- or oil-soluble, was injected prior to the alcohol. Only one injection was made if a good result had been obtained, or when the patient did not survive long enough to require subsequent injection. Occasionally, although no relief was obtained by the first injection, some other form of treatment was considered more appropriate than repeating it. Otherwise multiple injections were expected.

Thirty-seven patients had a second injection when the pain returned, or if the relief was not sufficient, or when dealing with carcinoma from the breast

TABLE 1. *Pituitary alcohol injection (total experience, 1973–1978)*

Total:	179 Injections in 122 patients
	75 Single
	37 Twice
	10 Three times

when it was considered ethically advisable to achieve pituitary destruction as well as pain-relief. Ten patients underwent a third injection. One to two weeks was the usual interval for elective repeating of the injections.

RESULTS

The quality of pain-relief has been classified as: *excellent* in patients who after the procedure required no analgesics except for perhaps an occasional dose of a nonnarcotic drug; *some relief* was considered to have been achieved when the patient obtained partial relief and would still require nonnarcotic analgesics (but not narcotics) on a regular basis; and *no relief* was considered to occur if the patient still required narcotic analgesics (Table 2).

Seventy-six injections were followed by excellent relief of pain; 59 patients derived some relief of pain, and 26 derived no relief. Eight patients died within the first week and before an assessment was possible. The data on 10 patients are too incomplete to allow accurate assessment.

The duration of pain-relief varied greatly, and so far we have not been able to correlate it with the type of cancer, the sex of the patient, the radiologic evidence of diffusion of contrast within or outside the gland, or even the particular physician who carried out the technique. There have been more than six different doctors administering the procedure.

In the majority of patients the pain-relief has lasted weeks or months (Table 3). The more complete it was, the longer it lasted. The longest relief was most impressive, there being two patients with total suppression of pain for more than 1 year. We cannot guarantee that other medical therapy has not contributed to this relief, but they have certainly had excellent and immediate response without recurrence.

TABLE 2. *Pain-relief after pituitary alcohol injection*

Excellent	76 (42.5%)
Some	59 (33.0%)
None	26 (14.5%)
Died before assessment	8
Untraceable	10
Total	179

TABLE 3. *Duration of pain-relief after pituitary alcohol injection*

Quality	1/52	1/12	3/12	>3/12	Total	Longest
Excellent	17	17	26	16	76	14 months
Some	24	30	5	0	59	6 weeks

TABLE 4. *Types of cancer pain treated by pituitary alcohol injection*

Carcinoma breast	41%
Carcinoma prostate	15%
Carcinoma lung/bronchus	13%
Uterus	10%
Gut (rectum especially)	10%

Pain from almost all forms of cancer has been treated (Table 4). The commonest has been associated with metastases from carcinoma of the breast. The next most frequent has been from carcinoma of the prostate. Usually this has been a picture of slowly progressive infiltration in the pelvic bones or plexus or from distant bony metastases. Usually the sufferer was in good general physical condition. Patients with more fulminating carcinomatoses rarely survive long enough to require surgical treatment specifically for their pain.

SIDE EFFECTS AND COMPLICATIONS

There is a definite morbidity associated with the injection of alcohol into the pituitary gland. There is what one might term an obligatory hormonal morbidity, and this most commonly takes the form of diabetes insipidus. This is common, occurring in over 60% of the patients when their fluid intake and output charts are compared. However, this side effect required treatment in only 20 to 30%. Pitressin® nasal spray is usually sufficient, though Pitressin® injection has been used occasionally. In only 2 cases has the diabetes insipidus continued beyond 6 weeks. Because many of our patients already had had courses of steroids and to prevent corticosteroid deficiency, a dose of 2 mg prednisolone 3 times a day was usually prescribed. It is well to remember that long-surviving patients may require thyroxin.

Morbidity as a result of technical problems occurred, with the most common being cerebrospinal fluid (CSF) rhinorrhea. This occurred to some extent in between 10 and 20% of the patients but usually stopped within a day or so. We have had only 1 patient who took more than 6 weeks to stop leaking. Meningitis must always remain a threat, particularly in the presence of CSF rhinorrhea, and it is our practice to give prophylactive sulfonamide.

Among our patients there have been 2 cases of presumed meningitis successfully treated by antibiotics.

Neurologic complications are of major concern. The most commonly seen complication involves the second and third cranial nerves and is presumably due to the alcohol's diffusing up from the pituitary gland to these structures. In an attempt to minimize this risk, a close observation is kept on the pupils and their ability to react in response to light during the alcohol injection. Five patients have apparently had some deficiency in function of either the second or third cranial nerve following injection. Two of these developed optic nerve impairment with visual-field defects which were marked in the first few days and gradually diminished over succeeding weeks. It is probable that in each of these incidents some permanent deficiency resulted.

Two patients have appeared to show definite evidence of hypothalamic injury. In each there was impairment of conscious level that progressively developed in the days following injection, and in one this was associated with hemiparesis. In each case autopsy confirmed extensive infarction of the pituitary stalk and suggested infarction of the hypothalamus with separation of the ependyma.

We have had 8 deaths within the first week following injections. Two appeared to result from technical failures associated with the transphenoidal puncture. In one of these patients the needle passed through an unsuspected empyema of the sphenoidal sinus which resulted in fatal meningitis. The other patient had a bleeding diathesis associated with her cancer and had a fatal hemorrhage following the puncture. Prior to the injection, the majority of patients were in very poor physical condition due to the advanced state of their cancer. It is this fairly recent experience with some serious complications that has caused us to call into question our previous attitude regarding the fitness of the patient to undertake this procedure. We now feel that the patient must be at least as fit as we consider necessary before undertaking cordotomy.

MECHANISM OF PAIN-RELIEF

As there is usually no alteration in the patient's neurologic and psychologic functions when he is relieved from his pain by this method, we have been very interested to discover an explanation for the analgesic effects. As previously mentioned, in our clinical practice we routinely inject a contrast medium, prior to the injection of alcohol. Consequent, we have observed spread of the contrast out of the gland up the stalk into the hypothalamus and even into the ventricular system in some 20% of patients (Fig. 1). This spread is easily observed during the monitoring of the injection and occurs without excessive pressure. After the route has been opened up, either immediately or late in the injection, all subsequent increments are seen to follow briskly the same track, unless the needle is moved.

We performed a study on cadavers using the same technique but injecting

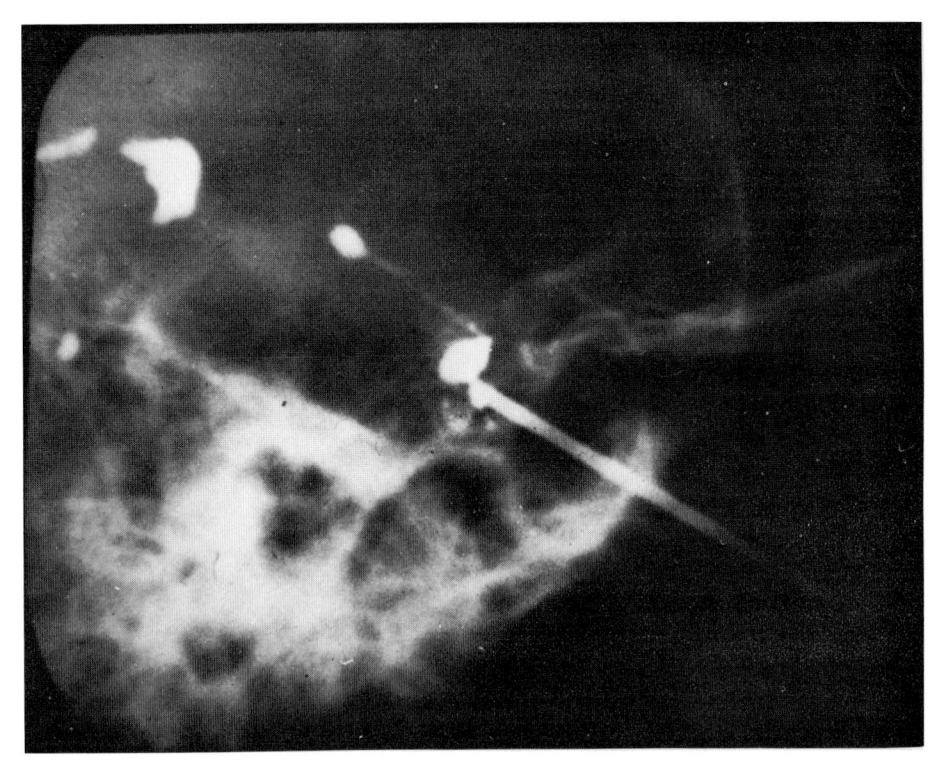

FIG. 1. Lateral radiography of skull, showing spread of iophendylate from the pituitary gland, up the stalk, into the hypothalamus, and into the third ventricle.

a mixture of contrast medium and India ink and observed the same radiologic spread upward to the hypothalamus. However, we also noticed a free movement out of the pituitary gland via the hypophyseal veins to the systemic blood circulation (Fig. 2).

Serial sections of the pituitary, its stalk, and the hypothalamus showed the India ink particles in the portal venous system of the stalk and hypothalamus (Fig. 3). Rupture of the upper ends of the system appeared to have occurred with India ink in the parenchyma of the hypothalamus and within the ependyma of the ventricles.

This suggested the possibility of injury to the hypothalamus, to the hypothalamic-thalamic pathways, and perhaps even the forebrain bundle. Autopsy evidence supported this hypothesis and perhaps explains the very rapid (within minutes or hours) pain-relief that occurs in 10 to 15% of patients. However, since the majority of patients achieve their pain-relief gradually and progressively over the second, third and fourth days, we wondered about the possibility of a chemical explanation.

With the help of Professor H. W. Kosterlitz of Aberdeen University, we

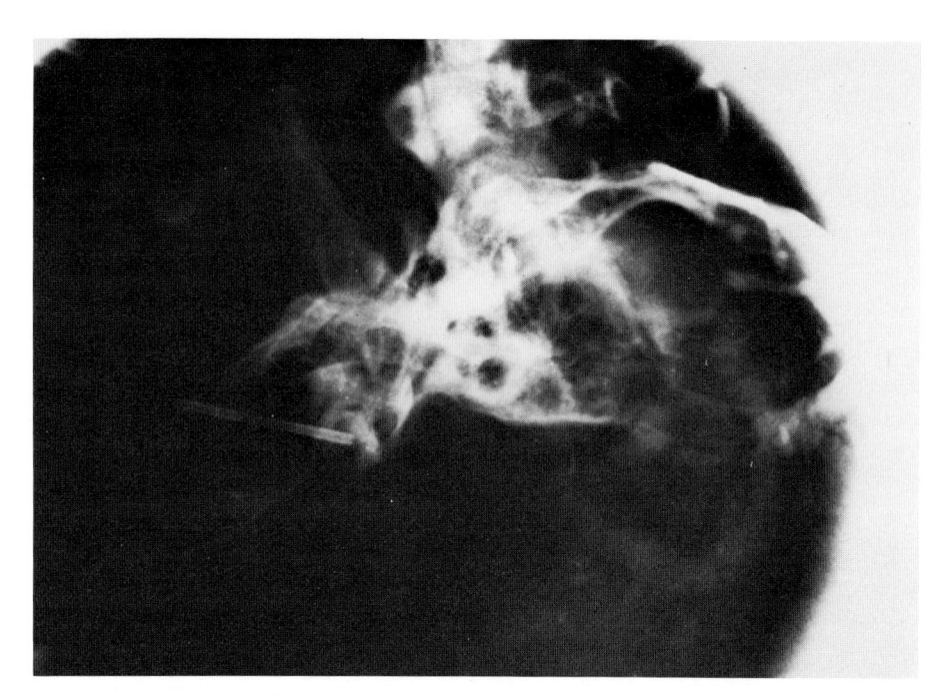

FIG. 2. Lateral radiograph of skull of cadaver during injection of Meglumine Iocarmate showing spread of the contrast medium out into the intracranial veins and sinuses.

sampled lumbar CSF, before, immediately after, and 5 hr after pituitary injection but have failed to show an elevation in either metencephalin or beta endorphin. Nevertheless, we are still wondering about the possibility of this effect's being associated with the currently exciting pituitary/hypothalamic peptide system. Dr. David Bowsher of the Neurobiology Unit at Liverpool University has been challenging patients, whose pain has been relieved by pituitary alcohol injection, with an injection of naloxone. In his initial series of 12 patients, 4 have experienced definite evidence of return of their original pain. This return occurs slowly after 15 to 20 min and lasts for 1 hr and then resolves. Several patients have developed forms of narcotic-withdrawal syndrome that might be associated with their previous medication.

With the help of Dr. Derek Smyth of the Medical Institute for Research, Mill Hill, London, we have just begun to search for the presence and possible elevation of beta endorphin in the blood of patients undergoing pituitary injection. The cadaver study suggests the possibility that there might be a flushing out from the pituitary via the hypophyseal veins of some analgesic peptide, and we await these results.

Naturally we have been interested to know how much pituitary or hypothalamic hormonal suppression results from alcohol injection. It is extremely difficult to subject these patients who are suffering severely from

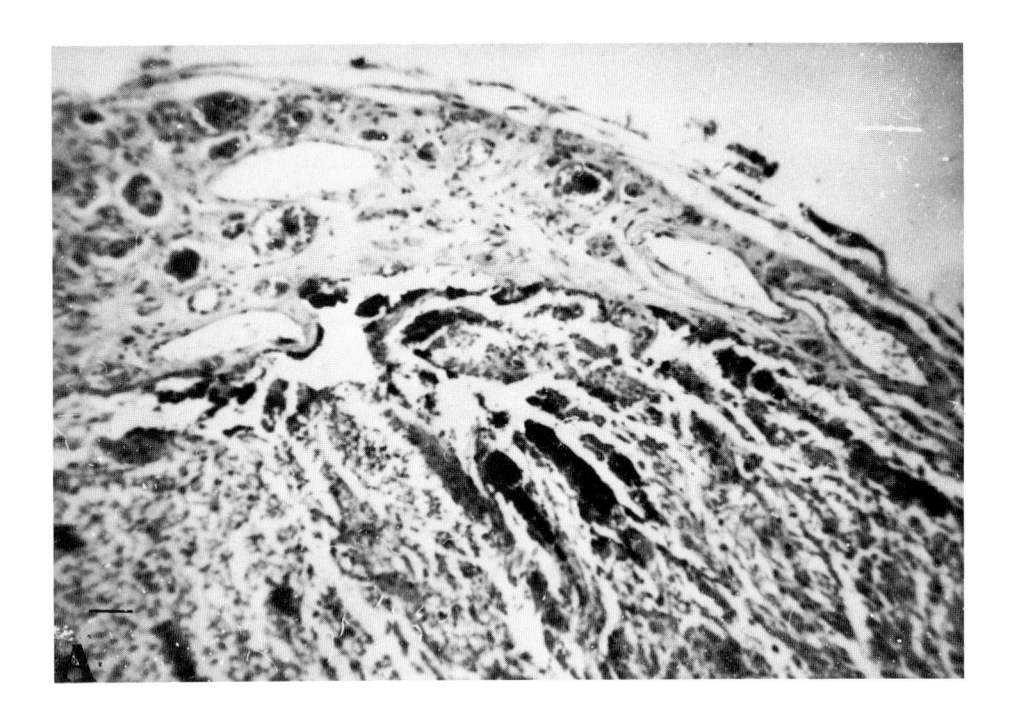

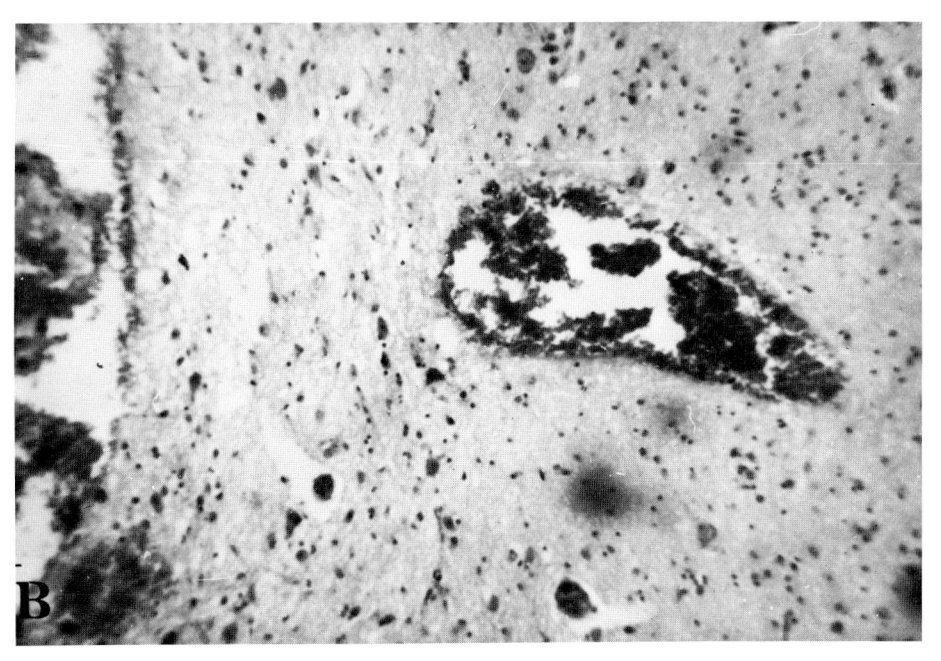

FIG. 3. Photomicrographs showing India ink particles in **(A)** the portal veins of the pituitary stalk; and **(B)** in the upper terminations of the portal veins in the hypothalamus.

very advanced cancer to sophisticated and tedious studies, especially when repetition is necessary. However, we have now developed an endocrinologic protocol condensed into a 4-hr period by which the main pituitary and hypothalamic functions can be assessed, before and 1 month after injection. Dr. Norton Williams, another member of our group, has found that the effects of injection are rather surprising. There is a massive suppression of the growth hormone and prolactin secretion in response to a glucose load; there is a regular and major depression of gonadotrophin activity; there is a rather variable depression of thyroxin output; and there is little or no suppression of ACTH release or of the adrenocortical hormones. Further studies should help in the interpretation of these results.

We obviously do not have a complete explanation for the relief of pain by pituitary alcohol injection and further research needs to be done. The elucidation of the therapeutic effects might result in a considerable advance in our basic knowledge of methods of pain relief and indeed of pain itself.

Despite our lack of understanding of the mechanism of pain-relief, injection of alcohol into the pituitary gland is a simple and very effective procedure for many patients with widespread pain of advanced cancer.

REFERENCES

1. Lipton, S., Miles, J. B., Williams, N., and Bark-Jones, N. (1978): Pituitary alcohol injection for the relief of pain. *Pain,* 5:73–82.
2. Moricca, G. (1974): Chemical hypophysectomy for cancer pain. In: *Advances in Neurology, Vol. 4, International Symposium on Pain,* edited by J. J. Bonica, pp. 707–714. Raven Press, New York.

Chemical Hypophysectomy

Jose L. Madrid

*Department of Anesthesiology and Pain Clinic, Ciudad Sanitaria "10 de Octubre,"
Madrid, Spain*

The endocrine ablation for cancer of the breast was advocated more than 80 years ago, and the role played by the different hormones in breast cancer and its dissemination has been extensively documented. However, it was not until 1953 that Luft and Olivecrona (4) published the results of the first surgical hypophysectomies by way of a frontal craniotomy. This method became a standard procedure for the treatment of advanced cancer of the breast. Since then, the inactivation of the pituitary gland through surgical or nonsurgical methods has been accepted as a therapeutic procedure in the management of cancer of the breast with bone metastases. It has also been observed (10) when total pituitary ablation was accomplished in patients with hormone-dependent tumors, regression of the carcinoma was possible as evidenced by radiologic examination by post-necropsy studies. Moreover, an effective and lasting pain-relief in the majority of these patients was observed which could not be accounted for by tumor regression, because pain-relief developed promptly after the procedure was done.

Surgical ablation of the pituitary gland represents an extensive and risky procedure in many patients. In an effort to develop safer and simpler techniques, extracranial approaches for hypophysectomy have been carried out via the transsphenoidal approach. These include coagulation by radiofrequency, cryohypophysectomy, and implantation of radioactive elements, ^{90}Y, ^{198}Au or ^{32}P (1,2,3,6,11). All these methods have some limitations, as they are associated with severe and important complications or require very expensive apparatus.

In 1963, chemical hypophysectomy was introduced by Moricca (7) at the Regina Elena Cancer Institute in Rome. Essentially, this technique consists of introducing a special needle via transnasal and transphenoidal route into the sella turcica and subsequently injecting absolute alcohol into the pituitary gland (9). In 1976, Moricca (8) reported 2,775 neuroadenolyses, as he came to call the procedure, in a total of 1,139 patients with very impressive results: 86.5% of the patients had excellent pain-relief. Besides, he reported evidence of improvement in the neoplastic disease after neuroadenolysis in the case of hormone-dependent tumors.

Our experience with this technique is related to those patients with diffuse metastatic cancer in whom it was not possible to perform the usual neurosurgical procedures or any appropriate neurolytic nerve block owing to the multiple location of pain. It is important to emphasize that the purpose of the chemical injection of the pituitary was mainly as an analgesic measure rather than as a therapy for the tumor.

MATERIAL AND METHODS

Up to January 1978, we have treated 329 patients with this technique. All patients but one were suffering of intractable pain due to diffuse bone and/or visceral metastases from malignant tumors. The only exception in these series was a case of diabetic retinopathy.

TABLE 1. Age of 329 patients subjected to chemical hypophysectomy

Age group (yrs)	Patients No.	% of total
11–20	1	0.3
31–40	47	14.2
41–50	110	33.4
51–60	86	26.2
61–70	70	21.3
71–80	15	4.6
Total	329	100.0

Our cases consisted of 189 patients with breast carcinoma; 67 patients had prostate carcinoma; 32 patients had some forms of carcinoma of the endometrium; in 24 cases the patients were suffering from lung carcinoma; 11 patients had carcinoma of the pancreas; and 5 cases underwent a chemical hypophysectomy for hypernephroma.

The ages of our patients are represented in Table 1. Our youngest patient was an 11-year-old boy with primary lung carcinoma with diffuse bone metastases, and the oldest patient was an 80-year-old man with carcinoma of the prostate. The largest group of patients treated with chemical hypophysectomy fell into the 41 to 50-years-old group.

A single procedure was performed in 233 patients; 84 patients underwent a second injection 15 days to 4 months after the first one; and 12 patients had a third injection 6 months to 1 year after the second injection, bringing the total number of neuroadenolyses performed to 437.

Technique

The technique we use at the Ciudad Sanitaria "1° de Octubre" General Hospital in Madrid is as follows. Under light, general anesthesia we insert

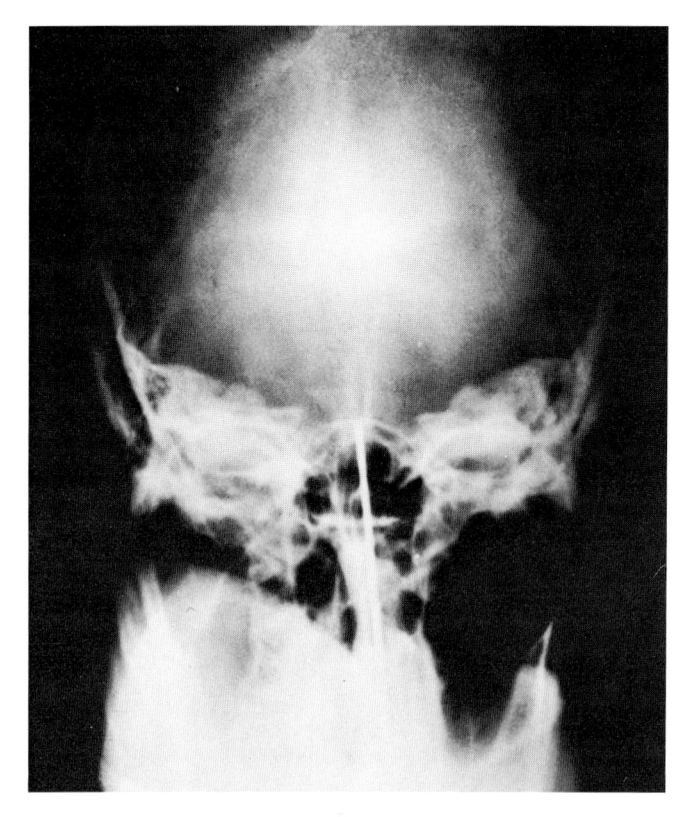

FIG. 1. An anteroposterior roentgenogram taken with Towne's projection permits accurate identification of the sella turcica and the clinoid process, confirming the midline position of the needle.

the Moricca's needle via the right nostril under constant monitoring with an image-intensifier until its tip is just past the floor of the sella turcica. An A-P film taken with Towne's projection enables us to confirm the midline position of the needle into the pituitary fossa (Fig. 1).

Once the correct position of the needle has been achieved, we introduce through the first-placed needle a 20-gauge needle (with stilet) which is 1 inch longer than the first-inserted needle. This second needle has a rubber marker to control the depth into the sella turcica. We feel that with this modification of the original technique the risk of contamination is reduced, and most of the time we are able to feel when the gland has been pierced and the tip of the needle is inside the gland.

After the needle has been properly positioned, we carry out a Queckenstedt test, and if this is negative we confirm the intraglandular position of the needle point by injecting 0.2 ml of Myodil® through the 20-gauge needle. We have observed the spread of the contrast medium moving up the pituitary stalk (Fig. 2A). Once these preliminary steps have been completed, we begin to inject absolute alcohol very slowly, while at the same time we check for

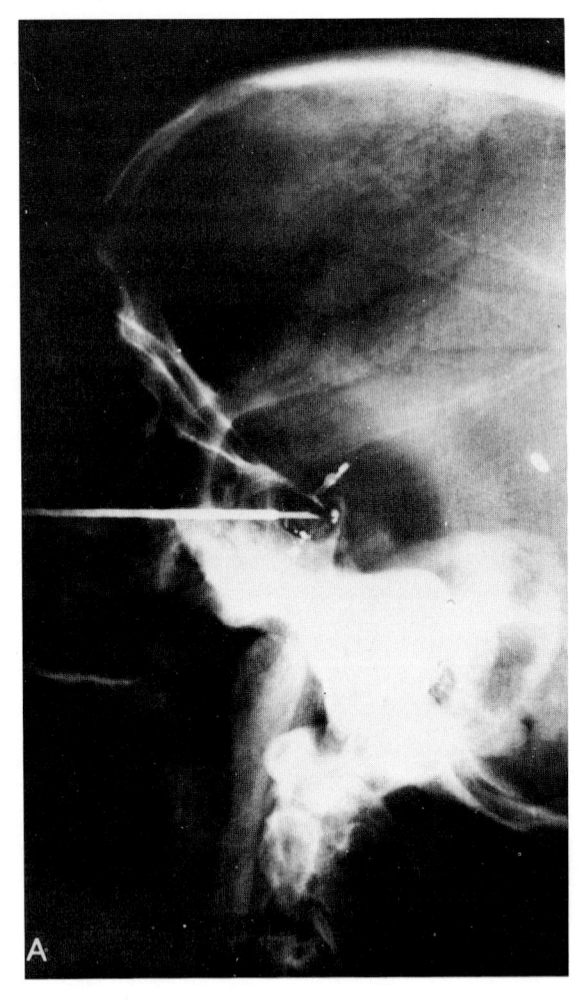

FIG. 2. Lateral roentgenogram showing the position of the needles and diffusion of the Myodil. **A:** After injection of 0.2 ml of Myodil the contrast medium is moving up the pituitary stalk. **B:** After injection of 0.4 ml of alcohol the Myodil® has diffused upward into the third ventricle.

any abnormalities of the pupil or dysfunction of other cranial nerves. After injection of 0.4 to 0.6 ml of alcohol, we are able to observe diffusion of the dye into the third ventricle. Our experiences confirm previous reports by Miles and Lipton (5) about the possibility of the alcohol's using this path (Fig. 2B).

Provided that there are no abnormalities in pupil size, we continue to inject alcohol up to a total of 2 ml. Should dilatation of the pupil appear during injection, we stop the procedure and proceed to inject into the cisterna magna 40 mg of methylprednisolone with the patient still under general anesthesia.

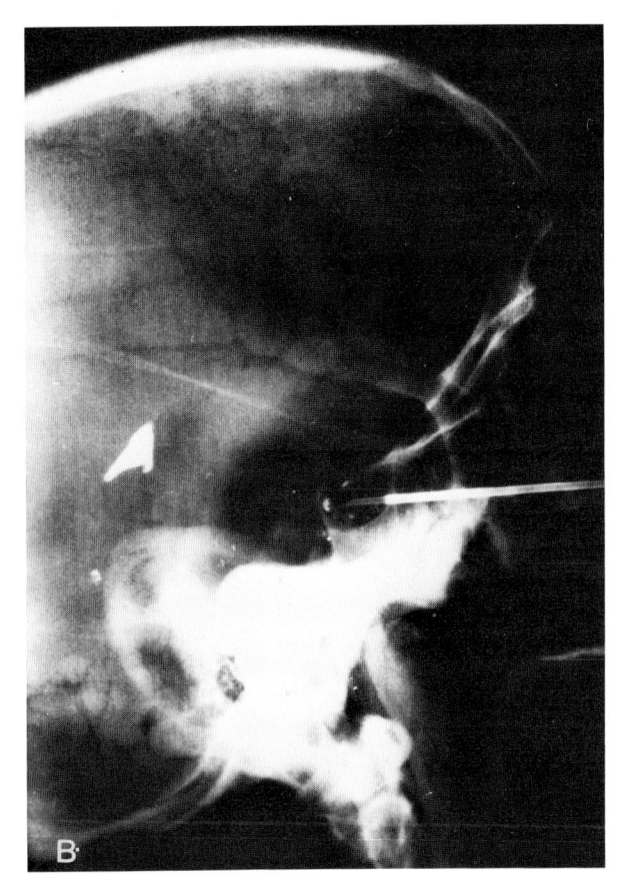

With this procedure the mydriasis has subsided by the time the patient is transferred to the recovery room.

Once the injection has been completed, we insert a nasal tube with two cuffs instead of packing the nostril with gauze as practiced by Moricca. This modification permits a posterior and anterior packing and allows the patient to breathe freely through that nostril.

RESULTS

The immediate results are listed in Table 2. There were no deaths during the procedure, and in general it was well tolerated by the patients in spite of their poor physical condition.

Pain-Relief

Complete pain-relief has been obtained in 221 patients, which represents 67% of the total. We were unable to follow up many of the patients after

TABLE 2. *Immediate results from chemical hypophysectory in 329 patients*

	Patients	
Results	No.	% of total
A. *Pain Relief*		
Complete	221	67.2
Partial	88	26.8
None	20	6.0
B. *Side Effects*		
Anisocoria during injection	32	9.7
Cephalalgia 24–48 hr duration	311	94.5
Cephalalgia 48–72 hr duration	64	19.4
Hyperthermia	28	8.5
Normal diuresis	49	15.0
Diuresis of 3 to 6 L/24 hr	210	63.8
Diuresis of 6 to 8 L/24 hr	62	18.8
Diuresis of more than 8 L/24 hr	8	2.4

leaving the hospital, so we cannot present data on the duration of the pain-relief and correlate it to patient survival. However, we were able to follow some of the patients at regular intervals, and virtually all of them were taking only nonnarcotic analgesics and tranquilizers. Apparently, the combination of hypophysectomy and minor drug therapy provided good relief of pain until the patient's death.

Our longest survival following this procedure was a woman with carcinoma of the breast and multiple bone metastases who died 4 years after she underwent the first treatment. At the time of the first chemical hypophysectomy, this patient was in such agonizing pain that it was necessary to move her on a sheet to the operating table because she would not permit anyone to touch her. On the second day after the hypophysectomy she was able to move around, and after her discharge from the hospital she went to work. She continued to do well for almost a year, when she came back to the hospital complaining of the same type of pain as she did on her first admission. A second chemical hypophysectomy was carried out which made her free of pain for almost another year. A third injection of alcohol into the pituitary gland (assuming there was some left) was performed, giving her partial relief. This together with administration of nonnarcotic analgesics kept her comfortable until her death.

Side Effects and Complications

The most common complication by far in our cases is diabetes insipidus which is transient and usually subsides spontaneously, probably because there is an incomplete destruction of the hypothalamic nuclei by the neurolytic

TABLE 3. Complications of chemical hypophysectomy in 329 patients

	Patients	
Complications	No.	% of total
Rhinorrhea	8	2.4
Diplopia	7	2.2
Hemianopsia	2	0.6
CSF leak	2	0.6
Meningitis	1	0.3
Myxedema	1	0.3
Total	21	6.4

agent. These cases of diabetes insipidus were transitory, and the patients were able to compensate by drinking fluids. Eight patients had diabetes insipidus with production of more than 8 liters of urine in 24 hr. They were treated with Pitressin.® (Table 2, B.)

Eight patients in whom the nasal cavity was packed with a gauze soaked with povidone-iodine developed rhinorrhea. We have not seen rhinorrhea in patients with pneumatic packing of the nasal cavity (Table 3).

Diplopia occurred in 7 patients, 5 of whom recovered and 2 had the complications permanently. Two patients developed right hemianopsia, which persisted during the time we were able to follow them.

Two patients had leak of cerebrospinal fluid (CSF), which persisted for several days and cleared up with bedrest in supine position avoiding any maneuvering tending to increase CSF pressure. One patient developed pneumococcic meningitis, which was treated with high doses of penicillin, and the patient recovered completely. Another patient had a myxedema 30 days after the chemical hypophysectomy and required supportive treatment.

We were able to perform postmortem studies in 5 patients who died after chemical hypophysectomy. All of them presented a complete necrosis of the anterior pituitary lobe, while the posterior lobe was apparently intact (Figs. 3 and 4). None of these cases had evidence of pathologic damage of the hypothalamic nuclei. However, in one case we found leptomeningeal edema and some hemorrhagic changes in the lower part of the infundibulum which could be attributable to the effect of alcohol (Fig. 5).

DISCUSSION

Although not exempt from controversy, the important feature of this technique is its simplicity and efficacy, which permit it to be used in those hospitals lacking the facilities to carry out more complicated and expensive techniques to relieve intractable painful syndromes due to neoplastic diseases. The dramatic pain-relief obtained in the majority of these patients *cannot* be

A

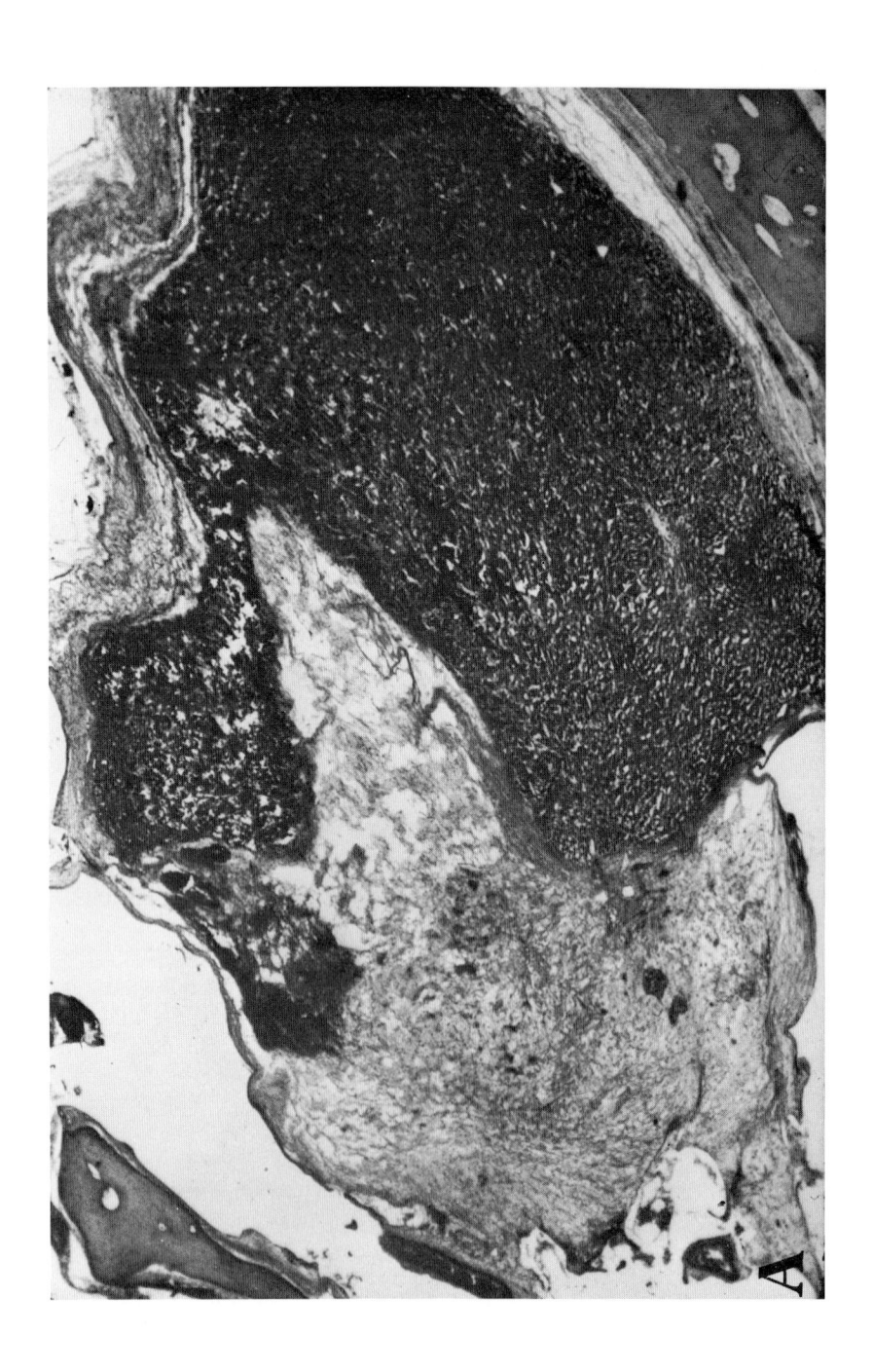

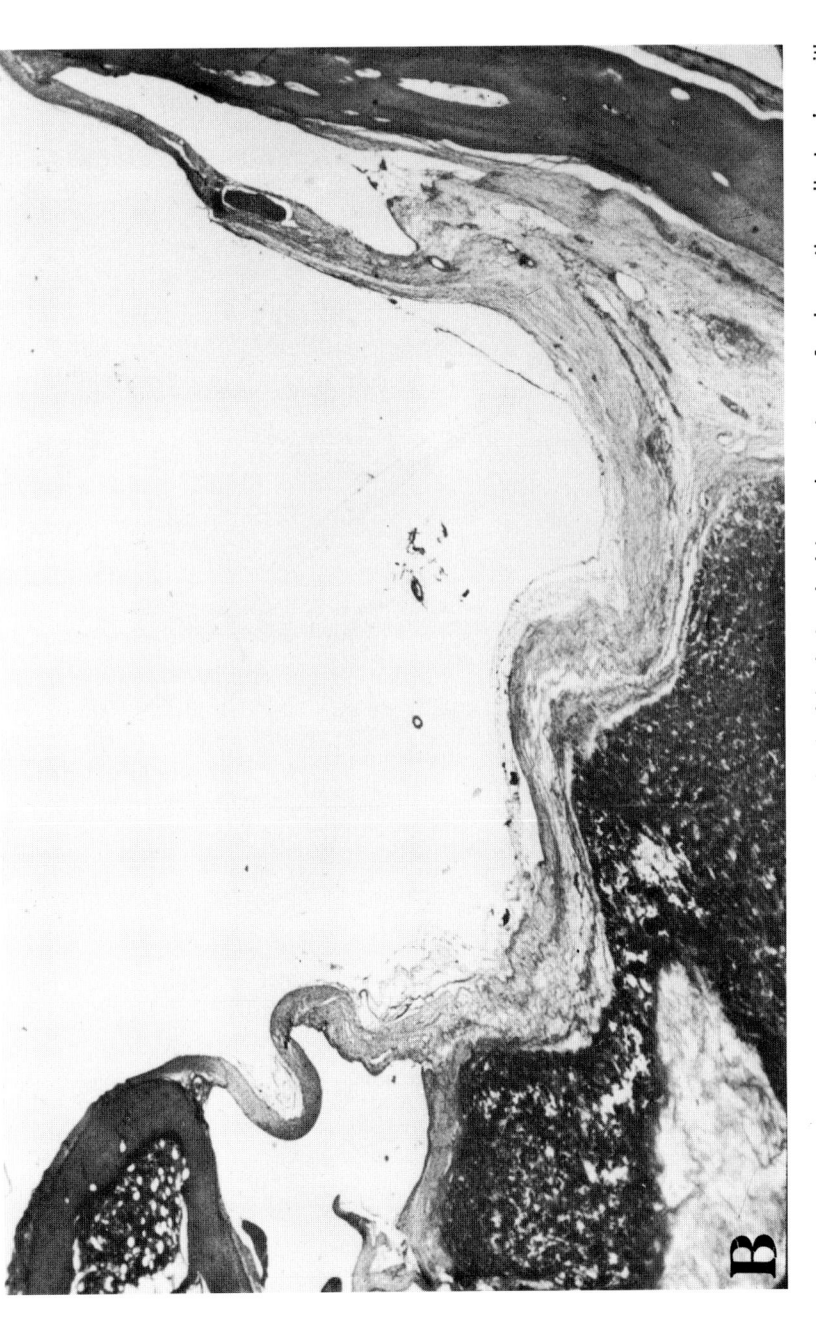

FIG. 3. Autopsy specimens taken from a patient who had had chemical hypophysectomy. **A:** shows the sella turcica with the pituitary gland *in situ*. On the left upper corner the anterior clinoid process can be seen. The anterior part of the pituitary gland shows a total necrosis, whereas the posterior part seems to be intact. **B:** View of the superior aspect of the pituitary gland. Note that the otherwise intact tentorium remains attached to the bone, but its surface is sunken due to a volume decrease of the sella turcica content.

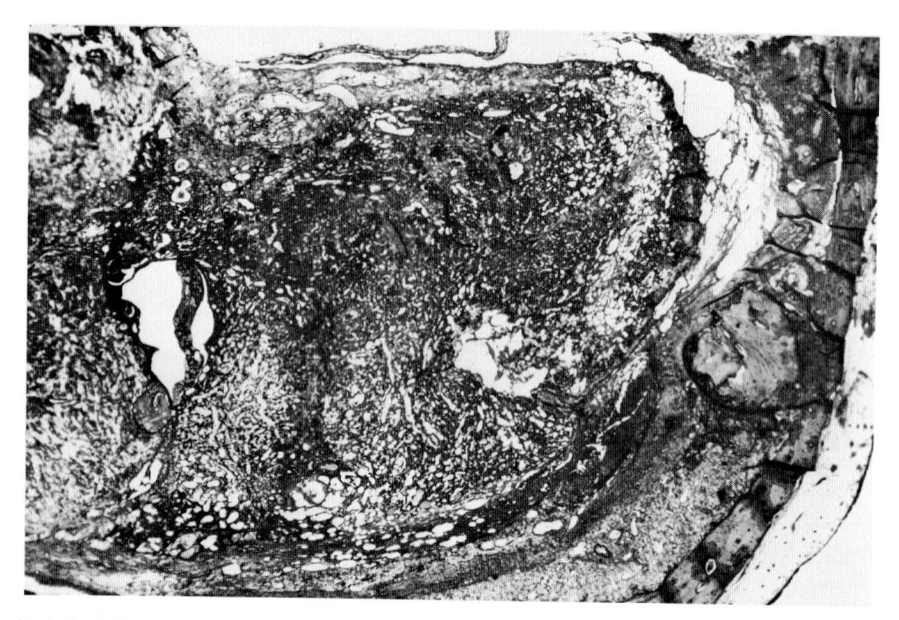

FIG. 4. Autopsy specimen of another patient showing the changes following an injection of alcohol in the anterior pituitary gland. The pituitary lobe has been replaced by necrotic material and extensive fibrosis.

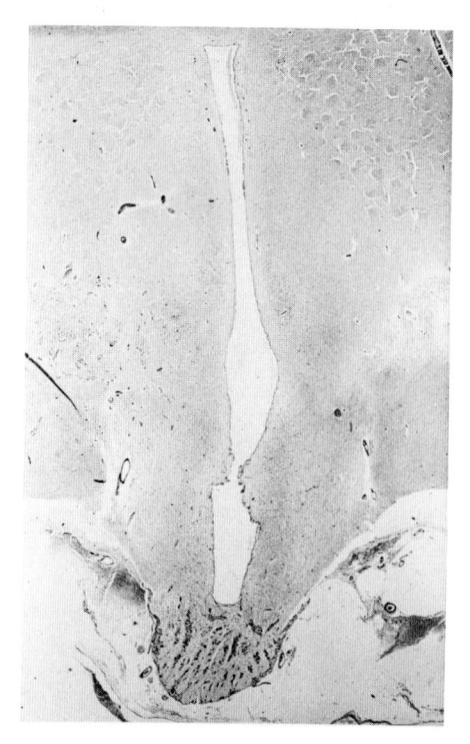

FIG. 5. Coronal section of the hypothalamus and third ventricle. In the upper part of the interthalamic commissure, while in the lower part of the infundibulum can be seen a leptomeningeal edema and some hemorrhagic changes in the neurovascular zone attributable to the effects of alcohol.

attributed solely to removal of some hormones, because similar results can also be seen in patients with non-hormone-dependent tumors.

Moricca's hypothesis regarding progressive involvement of the hypothalamohypophysis connections by direct action of the alcohol is a plausible explanation of the mechanism of action of chemical hypophysectomy. However, there are probably other mechanisms operative with this procedure. These are discussed by Miles (*this volume*).

While there are still many questions that need to be answered to explain the exact mechanisms of pain-relief with this technique, there is no doubt that it is an extremely useful procedure in patients with widespread pain of advanced cancer. Our favorable experience is especially impressive in view of the fact that most of the patients sent to us could not be relieved of pain with any other method and were in poor physical condition. As a result of our experience, our staff considers chemical hypophysectomy as a unique method to relieve advanced cancer pain.

REFERENCES

1. Adams, J. E., Seymour, R. J., Earll, J. M., Tuck, M., Sparks, L. L., and Forsham, P. H. (1968): Transsphenoidal cryohypophysectomy in acromegaly. Clinical and endocrinological investigation. *J. Neurosurg.*, 28:100–104.
2. Hartog, M., Doyle, F., Fraser, R., and Joplin, G. F. (1965): Partial pituitary ablation with implants of gold-198 and yttrium-90 for acromegaly. *Br. Med. J.*, 2:396–398.
3. Joplin, G. F., Fraser, R., Steiner, R., Laws, J., and Jones, E. (1961): Partial pituitary ablation by needle implantation of gold-198 seeds for acromegaly and Cushing's disease. *Lancet*, 2:1277–1280.
4. Luft, R., and Olivecrona, H. (1953): Experiences with hypophysectomy in man. *J. Neurosurg.*, 10:301–316.
5. Miles, J., and Lipton, S. (1976): Mode of action by which pituitary alcohol injection relieves pain. In: *Advances in Pain Research and Therapy, Vol. 1: Proceedings of the First World Congress on Pain,* edited by J. J. Bonica and D. Albe-Fessard, pp. 867–869. Raven Press, New York.
6. Molinatti, G. M., Camanni, F., Massara, F., Olivetti, M., Pizzini, A., and Giuliani, G. (1962): Implantation of yttrium 90 in the sella turcica in 16 cases of acromegaly. *J. Clin. Endocrinol. Metab.*, 22:599–611.
7. Moricca, G. (1974): Chemical hypophysectomy for cancer pain. In: *Advances in Neurology, Vol. 4: International Symposium on Pain,* edited by J. J. Bonica, pp. 707–714. Raven Press, New York.
8. Moricca, G. (1977): Neuroadenolysis (alcoholization of the pituitary) for intractable cancer pain. In: *Anaesthesiology. Proceedings of the VI World Congress on Anaesthesiology.* Excerpta Medica, Amsterdam.
9. Moricca, G. (1968): The management of cancer pain. In: *Progress in Anaesthesiology. Proceedings of the IV World Congress of Anaesthesiology,* pp. 266–270. Excerpta Medica, Amsterdam.
10. Pearson, O. H., Ray, B. S., Harrold, C. C., West, D. C., Li, M. C., Maclean, J. P., and Lipsett, M. B. (1956): Hypophysectomy in treatment of advanced cancer. *JAMA*, 161:17–21.
11. Rand, R. W. (1966): Cryosurgery of the pituitary in acromegaly: Reduced growth hormone levels following hypophysectomy in 13 cases. *Ann. Surg.*, 164:587–592.

Hypophysectomy for Relief of Pain of Disseminated Carcinoma of the Prostate

Charles R. West, Anthony M. Avellanosa, Alfonso M. Bremer, and Kazuo Yamada

Roswell Park Memorial Institute, Buffalo, New York 14263

The first hypophysectomy for disseminated prostatic carcinoma was performed some 30 years ago (17). At that time, craniotomy was the only practical technique available for carrying out the hypophysectomy. Since this intracranial procedure was usually considered when orchiectomy and estrogen therapy had failed, and since the medical condition of these patients was frequently somewhat deteriorated after relapse, the risks of craniotomy were often regarded as unacceptable. Thus, a number of techniques of less extensive surgery for accomplishing hypophysectomy were eventually worked out (2,14). One of these was the transsphenoidal stereotaxic cryohypophysectomy, a technique considered safe and one which did not require general anesthesia and the usual preparation for major surgery (1,8,10,11,14,20). After the transsphenoidal stereotaxic cryohypophysectomy was performed in a number of patients, it was found that the procedure did not effect a complete ablation of the adenohypophysis. In fact, Norrell et al. (11) found total cryodestruction of the anterior lobe in only 4 of 18 cases. It is of interest that they found little correlation between the quality and duration of response and the anatomical completeness of the adenohypophysectomy in patients with disseminated prostatic carcinoma.

The present report provides data on the direct correlation between functional ablation of the growth hormone (GH) response to insulin-induced hypoglycemia following hypophysectomy and overall remission in patients with disseminated prostatic carcinoma. Our findings support previous findings that total functional adenohypophyseal destruction is not necessary to achieve satisfactory remission of signs and symptoms of widespread carcinoma of the prostate.

RATIONALE FOR HYPOPHYSECTOMY

The underlying theoretic basis for the palliation of symptoms and signs achieved by hypophysectomy in patients with disseminated carcinoma of the prostate is that it removes the source of trophic hormones which support the metabolic activity of the tumor. Huggins and Hodges (6) proposed that androgens under influence of gonadotropins stimulate growth of prostatic carcinoma and concluded that by removing the testes as the main source or by inhibiting its effects with estrogen therapy, growth of the cancer would often be retarded. Extragonadal androgens may be effectively eliminated from circulation by hypophysectomy and or adrenalectomy, and thus these procedures may be regarded as a rational extension of the orchiectomy.

The mechanism by which pain of osseous metastases is relieved following hypophysectomy, especially when tumor regression cannot be demonstrated, is not clear. However, elucidation of this may be provided soon by the accumulation of information on the highly specific opiate receptors and opioid peptides (α-endorphins, β-endorphins, and enkephalins) recently described in the pituitary and in the hypothalamus (4,7,12,19) and implicated in the regulation of pain (5,7). Indeed, Moricca (9) has presented clinical data which indicate that relief of pain of cancer following hypophysectomy is not limited to patients with endocrine-sensitive tumors (breast and prostate). Thus, since radioimmunoassay techniques have already been developed (15), it would be of great interest to determine the role of endorphins and enkephalins in modulating pain, especially that associated with cancer. Furthermore, it would also be useful to determine whether the hypophysectomy procedure is in some way related to release of endogenous, opioid-like compounds into the general circulation.

INDICATIONS FOR CRYOHYPOPHYSECTOMY

In the sequence of the hormonal regimen for treatment of disseminated carcinoma of the prostate, hypophysectomy may be considered after orchiectomy and estrogen therapy have been proved ineffective. Under these conditions, the main indication for cryohypophysectomy is pain of widespread metastases, usually in the bones of the spinal column, of the pelvis, and of the lower extremities. Metastases in the liver or in other viscera are not contraindications to cryohypophysectomy, nor is advanced age (1,2). Many of these patients will obtain gratifying relief of subjective and objective signs and symptoms in what are often the final weeks or months of their lives (2,10,11,14,17).

PATIENTS AND METHODS

All of these patients treated at Roswell Park Memorial Institute had histologically proved prostatic carcinoma and demonstrated dissemination of disease, despite previously beneficial orchiectomy and estrogen hormonal therapy. They also had substantial bone pain as the main indication for cryohypophysectomy. Adenohypophysectomy was achieved either under direct vision following open craniotomy (8 patients) or following stereotaxic cryoablation (19 patients) under topical anesthesia and sedation. Retrospective review of the records of these patients revealed that those who had general medical conditions judged to be extremely poor were usually treated by cryohypophysectomy. Furthermore, only those patients who underwent GH assay during insulin-induced hypoglycemia once during the preoperative (control) and twice during the postoperative (experimental) period were included for analysis in this report.

Initial workup included detailed history and general physical examination. Laboratory studies included: roentgenological skeletal survey, determination of body weight, concentrations of serum acid and alkaline phosphatase, blood glucose (fasting), urea nitrogen, electrolytes, urinalysis, and peripheral vein hematocrit. All these studies were repeated postoperatively. None of the patients suffered from preexisting diabetes mellitus.

Growth Hormone Assay

In the present study, the GH assay was used to determine an index of adenohypophyseal ablation. Plasma levels were determined in all patients during insulin-induced hypoglycemia following overnight fast as described by Garcia et al. (3). Human GH assay so performed was an accurate measure of adenohypophyseal function (16) and thus was a means of comparing indices of subjective and objective remission. All patients included here underwent GH assay once within 10 days prior to surgery and twice during the postoperative period. The initial postoperative GH assay was performed 2 weeks to 1 month following surgery and repeated between the third and ninth month. The period of hypoglycemia was always carried out with continuous monitoring of blood pressure, pulse, and level of consciousness and a physician in constant attendance. There were no untoward occurrences during the GH assay procedure.

Clinical Criterions for Response

These were as previously described by Scott and his associates (17). Subjective responses were: (a) pain-relief, (b) sense of well-being and (c) improved appetite. Objective responses were: (a) decreases in serum acid phosphatase level, (b) sustained decreases in serum alkaline phosphatase levels (c) weight gain (d) improved radiological appearance of osseous metastases, and (e) improvement in anemia designated by increase in relative hematocrit or stability of hematocrit values at 30% or greater. A persistent deterioration of any of these criterions, when evaluated at monthly intervals, indicated progression of the disease.

Surgical Technique

The techniques used to perform adenohypophysectomy following craniotomy were as previously described by Poppen (13). Those for the stereo-

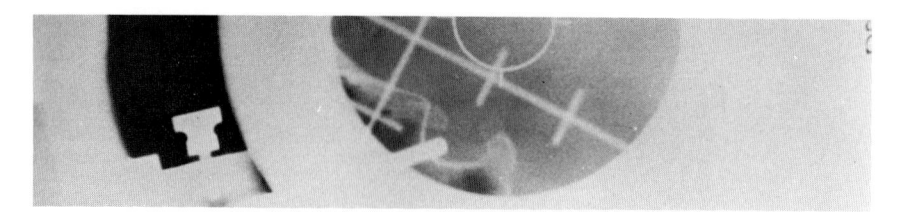

FIG. 1. Transsphenoidal insertion of cryoprobe into the antero-inferior quadrant of the sella turcica.

taxic transsphenoidal cryoablations were as described by Rand et al. (14) with modifications of Norrell et al. (11). Biplane fluoroscopy facilitated placement of a 2.7 mm cryoprobe through the sphenoid sinus and through the floor of the sella turcica. With the cryoprobe properly placed at the target point as shown in Fig. 1, a single midline lesion was created with the probe temperature at $-180°$ to $-190°$ C for 20 min. Routine operative and postoperative hormonal management is described elsewhere (10).

Calculations and Expressions of Data

It has already been shown that insulin-induced hypoglycemia is associated with hypophyseal release of GH (16). Data which we obtained from hormonal assay were plotted as a response curve (Fig. 2). As presented here,

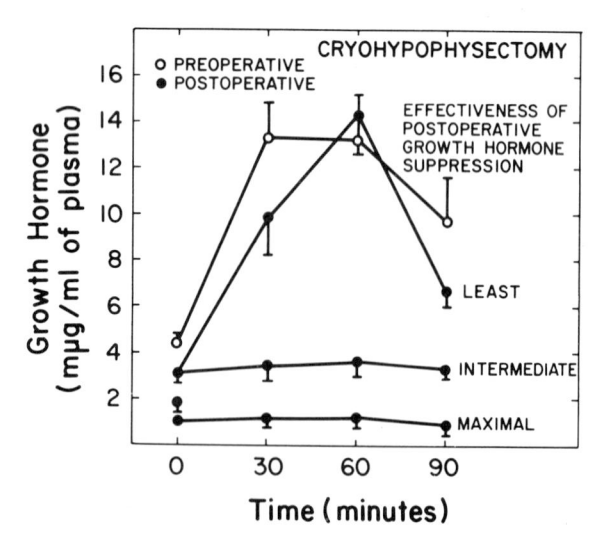

FIG 2. Concentrations of plasma growth hormone and of blood glucose plotted as functions of time following start of intravenous infusion of insulin. Each plotted point represents mean values with standard error of mean (vertical half bars) for 8 to 16 determinations from 8 patients.

numerical integration (18) of data points that describe the curve over the 90-min assay period yielded a single value that reflected the data determined for the entire assay period and permitted direct statistical comparison of groups of data. The survival period of patients was calculated from the time of hypophysectomy to the time of death.

RESULTS

When the plasma levels of glucose fell to less than 50% of the corresponding fasting level after start of intravenous infusion of insulin (0.1 units/kg, regular insulin), the absence of a characteristic increase in plasma GH (Fig. 2) was an indication of suppression of adenohypophyseal function (15). It should be emphasized that valid assessment of anterior pituitary function by GH provocation during the postoperative period is best delayed for at least 2 to 4 weeks, since transient injury by surgical insult might yield an erroneous index of anterior pituitary functional integrity if considered as permanent (10). Thus, in order to avoid this possible error in our study, GH response to insulin-induced hypoglycemia was repeated twice in all cases.

Profound suppression of plasma GH levels secondary to insulin provocation was detected after the pituitary gland was removed under direct vision (Fig. 3). However, the responses following cryohypophysectomy were variable, reflecting varying degrees of adenohypophyseal destruction (Table 1). In fact, as shown in Table 1, three patterns of suppression indicated average

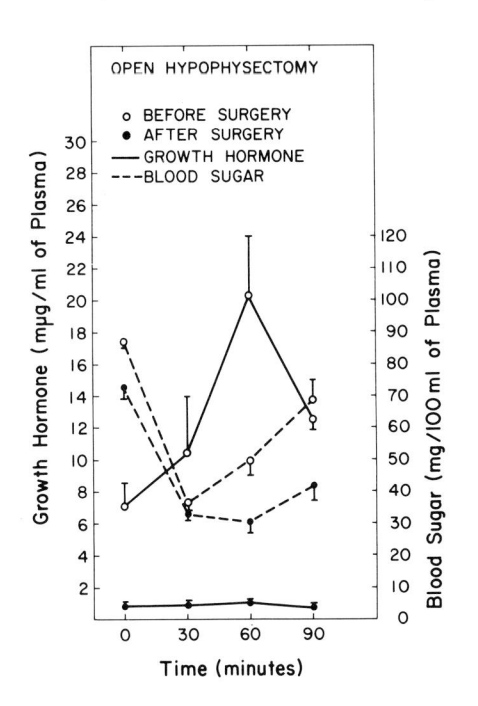

FIG. 3. Concentration of plasma growth hormone plotted as a function of time after start of insulin infusion. Each plotted point represents mean values with standard error of mean (vertical half bars) for 10 or more determinations from 5 or more patients in each group designated.

TABLE 1. *Human growth hormone (GH) responses to insulin-induced hypoglycemia[a]*

Procedure	Integrated average GH level, over 90-min period (mμg/ml of plasma)		Index of adenohypophyseal ablation[b] (%)
	Preoperative	Postoperative	
Craniotomy with hypophysectomy	**8/8** 15.6(±0.9)	**8/16** 0.94(±0.03)	93.9
Stereotaxic cryohypophysectomy	**19/19** 13.5(±1.8)	Maximal reduction **7/14** 1.3(±0.12)[c]	90.3
		Intermediate reduction **5/10** 3.6(±0.6)[c]	73.3
		Least reduction **7/14** 10.5(±0.8)[c]	22.2

[a] Data tabulated represent mean values (±SEM) for the number of determinations indicated in boldface (no. of patients/no. determinations). All patients underwent GH assay once preoperatively and twice in the postoperative period.

[b] Based on GH suppression; mean differences between respective preoperative and postoperative values are significant at the level of $p < .001$ and are expressed as percent decrease from preoperative values.

[c] Significance of mean difference between adjacent postoperative values at the level of $p < .001$.

reductions of insulin-induced GH levels of 22.2% (least), 73.3% (intermediate) and 90.3% (maximal).

Correlation of the test results with corresponding criterions for clinical remission in the respective groups indicated that the operative procedure was either clinically effective or not effective (Table 2). When adenohypophyseal function was reduced by 73% (intermediate, Tables 1 and 2), it was as effective in extending the postsurgical time of survival and duration of clinical remission as the more totally ablative cryosurgical procedure (maximal, Tables 1 and 2). Furthermore, distinction between the clinical efficacy of open hypophysectomy versus cryohypophysectomy in prolongation of re-

TABLE 2. *Remission and survival periods[a] for two operative procedures*

	Stereotaxic cryosurgical adenohypophysectomy			Craniotomy with adenohypophysectomy
	Least[b]	Intermediate[b]	Maximal[b]	
No. of patients	7	5	7	8
Age, year	70.40, (+1.76)	65.0, (+1.78)	67.14, (+2.40)	58.09, (+1.30)
Duration of remission, mo.				
Subjective	0.87, (±0.52)	10.25, (±3.84)	7.54, (±2.22)	5.11, (±1.48)
Objective	0.12, (+0.05)	7.60, (±3.04)	6.25, (±2.55)	6.78, (+2.62)
Survival following adenohypophysectomy, mo.	4.80, (+1.3)	13.58 (+3.0)	13.57, (+2.83)	10.88, (+2.36)

[a] Following adenohypophysectomy for disseminated prostatic carcinoma; values tabulated represent means (±SEM).

[b] Categories of least, intermediate, and maximal effectiveness of GH suppression refer to similar categories designated in Table 1 and Fig. 2; GH indicates growth hormone.

mission and survival times disappeared when at least 73% of anterior pituitary function was destroyed by the cryogenic lesion. Although effective hypophysectomy achieved by either direct or indirect techniques was associated with some improvement of survival time and of subjective and objective remission ($p < 0.05$), dramatic relief of pain was often the most gratifying. In all of the patients reported here who had 73% or more suppression of GH, pain-relief occurred within 4 days or less of the surgical procedure.

COMMENT

More than 50% of the patients with disseminated carcinoma of the prostate who have relapses following previous castration and estrogen therapy will benefit from hypophysectomy (2,8,10,11,17). We found that cryohypophysectomy was the better choice of the two procedures used when the medical condition of the patients precluded extensive surgery. It was clear that total anterior pituitary ablation was not necessary to achieve effective remissions from prostatic carcinoma (11). Furthermore, a specific laboratory criterion which permits a determination of the technical adequacy of the hypophysectomy procedure has been provided by the data presented in this report.

REFERENCES

1. Conway, L. W., and Collins, W. F. (1969): Results of transsphenoidal cryohypophysectomy for carcinoma of the breast. *N. Engl. J. Med.*, 281:1–7.
2. Fergusson, J. D., and Phillips, D. E. H. (1962): A clinical evaluation of radioactive pituitary implantation in the treatment of advanced carcinoma of the prostate. *Br. J. Urol.*, 34:485–492.
3. Garcia, J. F., Linfoot, J. A., Manougian, E., Born, J. L. and Lawrence, J. H. (1967): Plasma growth hormone studies in normal individuals and acromegalic patients. *J. Clin. Endocrinol. Metab.*, 27:1395–1402.
4. Goldstein, A., Lowney, L. T. and Pal, B. K. (1971): Stereospecific and nonspecific interactions of the morphine congener levorphanol in subcellular fractions of the mouse brain. *Proc. Natl. Acad. Sci. USA*, 68:1742–1747.
5. Guillemin, R., Ling, N., and Burgus, R. (1976): Endorphines, peptides, d'origine hypothalamique et neurohypophysaire à activité morphinomimétique. Isolement et structure moléculaire de l'alpha-endorphine. *C.R. Acad. Sci. (Paris)*, 282:783–785.
6. Huggins, C., and Hodges, C. V. (1941): Studies on prostatic cancer: I. Effects of castration, of estrogen and of androgen on serum phosphatase in metastatic carcinoma of prostate. *Cancer Res.*, 1:293–297.
7. Hughes, J. T. (1975): Isolation of an endogenous compound from the brain with and pharmacological properties similar to morphine. *Brain Res.*, 88:295–298.
8. Maddy, J. A., Winternitz, W. W., and Norrell, H. (1971): Cryohypophysectomy in management of advanced prostatic cancer. *Cancer*, 28:322–328.
9. Moricca, G. (1974): Chemical hypophysectomy for cancer pain. In: *Advances in Neurology, Vol. 4: International Symposium on Pain*, edited by J. J. Bonica, pp. 707–714. Raven Press, New York.
10. Murphy, G. P., Reynoso, G., Schoonees, R., Gailani, S., Bourke, R., Kenny, G. M., Mirand, E. A. and Schlach, D. S. (1971): Hypophysectomy and adrenalectomy for disseminated prostatic carcinoma. *J. Urol.*, 105:817–825.

11. Norrell, H., Alves, A. M., Winternitz, W. W. and Maddy, J. (1970): A clinicopathological analysis of cryohypophysectomy in patients with advanced cancer. *Cancer,* 25:1050–1060.
12. Pert, C. B., and Snyder, S. H. (1973): Opiate receptor: Demonstration in nervous tissue. *Science,* 179:1011–1014.
13. Poppen, J. L. (1960): *An Atlas of Neurosurgical Techniques.* W. B. Saunders Co., Philadelphia.
14. Rand, R. W., Dashe, A. M., Paglia, D. E., Conway, L. W. and Solomon, D. E. (1964): Stereotactic cryohypophysectomy. *JAMA,* 189:255–259.
15. Rossier, J., Bayon, A., Vargo, T. M., Ling, N., Guillemin, R., and Bloom, F. (1977): Radioimmunoassay of brain peptides: Evaluation of a methodology for the assay of β-endorphin and enkephalin. *Life Sci.,* 21:847–852.
16. Roth, J., Glick, S. M., Yalow, R. S. and Berson, S. A. (1963): Hypoglycemia: A potent stimulus to secretion of growth hormone. *Science,* 140:987–988.
17. Scott, W. W. and Schirmer, H. K. A. (1962): Hypophysectomy for disseminated prostatic cancer. In: *On Cancer and Hormones: Essays in Experimental Biology,* pp. 175–204. University of Chicago Press, Chicago.
18. Sokolnikoff, I. S. and Redheffer, R. M. (1958): *Mathematics of Physics and Modern Engineering,* p. 717. McGraw-Hill, New York.
19. Terenius, L. (1973): Characteristics of the "receptor" for narcotic analgesics in synaptic plasma membrane fractions from rat brain. *Acta Pharmacol. Toxicol.,* 33:377–384.
20. Tytus, J. S., and Ries, L. (1961): Further observation on rapid freezing and its possible applications to neurosurgical techniques. *Bull. Mason Clin.,* 15:51–61.

Discussion

Part II. Management of Pain of Advanced Cancer: Nerve Blocks

D. C. Moore and G. Moricca (Moderators)

Moricca (Rome): I listened with great satisfaction and interest to the discussions of Madrid, Miles, and Lipton.

But I would like to underline the fact that their results on pain treatment must and can be even better. Our results are better. In Italy also, Acampora in Napoli, Casini in Cagliari, Francesconi in Merano, and Pasqualucci in Perugia often obtain better results. Why? Because I have always been aggressive against pain and my friends feel the same way.

Well, in this case, to repeat the treatment with two or more needles and with greater quantities of neurolytic permits one to obtain far better results. Results that are not obtainable, it must be underlined, with any other medical, surgical method or with any other kind of method.

And this is due not only to the more or less total destruction of hypophyseal tissue but also and mainly to the hypothalamic effect obtainable with the neuroadenolytic treatment in a totally atraumatic way. Neuroadenolysis, a delicate technique but very sure in expert hands, permits one to dominate pain considered intractable generally with only one block. Being atraumatic, it can be done on poor-risk patients.

Why remove the ovaries and testicles when you can strike at a higher level with better results? Why use chemotherapy for pain treatment? Why not recur to neuroadenolysis in hormone-conditioned tumors; neuroadenolysis not only cures the pain but also fights the evolution of the neoplasia; later one can recur to polychemotherapy.

Bond (Glasgow): Dr. Miles, how often are changes in mental functions observed after hypophysectomy? What form do these changes take? How long do they last?

Miles (Liverpool): In our series we have seen recognizable mental changes in fewer than 10 patients. In the patients in whom I suspected hypothalamic injury this took the form of obtunded behaviour. The patient was withdrawn, and in one of them she also had a hemiparesis. One of these two died and we saw evidence of specific hypothalamic injury. In the rest of the cases, euphoria and some degree of lack of insight has been the usual; and in these instances it has lasted only a few weeks.

Meissner (Stuttgart): Dr. Bonica, what kind of written consent of the patient do you have that the patient is informed about the method to be used and about possible complications?

Bonica (Seattle): As I indicated, an essential requisite for carrying out nerve block procedures and for carrying out any management of pain in patients with chronic pain, including cancer pain, is to thoroughly inform the patient of exactly what is going to be done, why it is being done, what is to be expected, and what are the possible complications. Now, in discussing complications, one has to be very sensitive and supportive, indicating that one has had much experience and most patients do not get complications. It is important for them to realize that complications may occur, that failure may occur. And it is up to the patient and to the family to decide whether or not they wish to undertake the risk. In the U.S.A. we must obtain written consent and the patients must be informed in ordinary language so that they understand what they are undergoing.

Swerdlow (Manchester): How is it possible to avoid complications with intrathecal block?

Bonica: You can predict that with a block in the thoracic dermatomes there is almost no chance whatsoever of paralyzing the bladder or the rectum. Muscular paresis is going to occur when a chemical is applied to the cervicothoracic region or in the lumbosacral region and when you are injecting in the middle and lower thoracic dermatomes. You also avoid complications by keeping the dose down. One should not normally inject more than 1 ml of solution, possibly with the exception of the thoracic region, which we are going to be talking about tomorrow. By injecting 2 and 3 cc as I have seen and heard done, you are inviting complications.

In other words, you really have to have great skill and experience, and this must be obtained during a period of training in a setting where individuals who have wide experience can teach you how to do it. You said that it can't happen that injection in the trunk will produce complications in the low limbs, but I know it has been produced. It was very obviously a serious technical error that can be avoided by proper technique.

Questioner: Dr. Gerbershagen, will you comment on the use of intrathecal-water publication by King and Jewett for treatment of intractable cancer pain?

Gerbershagen (Mainz): It has been tried for several years now to inject either water or hypertonic cold or warm saline into the subarachnoid space. We have done it only 3 times with water and about 5 or 6 times with hypertonic saline. It was very painful to the patient in spite of premedication with meperidine, and the effect lasted about 3 days. It is a damaging procedure, because there are histopathological changes that are quite widespread in comparison to the change you see with phenol or alcohol. Regarding intrathecal phenol, we recommend to do a diagnostic block first for practice, and you can get one nerve with 0.5 ml of tetracaine.

Houde (New York): Dr. Miles, regarding the challenge of naloxone to patients whose pain had been relieved by pituitary alcohol injection; were they on narcotics?

Miles: No, they had not been on narcotics for at least 2 weeks.

Schulkes (Amsterdam): Dr. Swerdlow, what were the types of complications encountered in your series?

Swerdlow: Headache, paresthesia, numbness, hyperesthesia, and the two major complications—muscular paresis, weakness of an arm or of a leg, and bladder and bowel weakness.

Questioner: Dr. Swerdlow, how did you define good and fair pain-relief?

Swerdlow: Good relief after the block means that the patient doesn't require any analgesics at all or nothing more than the mild ones. Fair relief means that he has a lot less pain than he used to have, but he still requires a certain amount of medication and maybe some limitation in his activities. As far as I am concerned, poor relief is no relief.

I was very interested in Moore's presentation and would like to make one point. I firmly believe that it is not necessary to inject 25 cc on each side. I think that it is too much. I think that 15 cc on each side is quite enough, and I have made this point to several colleagues in this business; having tried 15 cc, they absolutely agree.

Moore (Seattle): I disagree. Our failures have been with less than 50 ml.

Hildebrandt (Göttingen): Dr. Miles, is thermocoagulation of the pituitary gland an alternative to alcohol injection?

Miles: I don't know that anyone has tried pituitary ablative surgery for the range of cancers that are being treated by alcohol injection. Certainly hypophysectomy by any route has been known to be associated with an amazingly rapid relief of pain in some patients. And the implication, as I see it, is that surgery by whatever means might damage the area of the hypothalamus, as Madrid showed.

Bonica: Regarding nerve blocks and narcotics, and this applies also to neurosurgery, I must assume that people who do these procedures have the skill and experience that we stressed this morning. First of all, it is best to refer the patients early. Often people will prescribe narcotics for months before they think about sending the patient for nerve block. I think that this does several disservices to the patient. First, the degree of analgesia with successful blocks is greater than with narcotics, without some of the side effects. Second, it is important to remember that the pain of the cancer stimulates respiration and counteracts the depressive effects of the narcotics. If the patient has had large doses of narcotics and we then produce either a block or a neurosurgical relief of pain, there is a danger that the patient will have trouble with respiratory depression. I have seen patients develop apnea following a nerve block. Thirdly, the fact that the patient requires narcotics after the block or after hypophysectomy or neurosurgery does not really mean that the procedure has failed to produce analgesia. It may well be that the patient has developed physiologic and psychologic dependence; and although his nociceptive input has been eliminated, either partially or totally, his body still requires narcotics in order to feel well. Finally, I want to dispel the misconception that the continuous use of narcotics is contraindicated in patients with block. One of the serious mistakes one can make is when a patient has been on narcotics for a long period of time and one gets a very good block or successful neurosurgery procedure; if one suddenly stops the narcotics, the patient is likely to develop a withdrawal syndrome and will feel very uncomfortable from the absence of the narcotic drugs. It is a misconception that narcotics are bad to give to patients with chronic pain, including patients with cancer. I think we should forget about the problem of addiction in patients with cancer.

General Comments on Ablative Neurosurgical Procedures

Carlo A. Pagni

2nd Chair of Neurosurgery, University of Torino, Torino, Italy

In the past, ablative neurosurgical procedures for pain-relief have been based on the hypothesis that pain is due to activation of specific fibers, tracts, and centers whose destruction would block nociceptive impulses. However, if pain were simply a sensory modality conducted along such specific systems, we should be able to permanently relieve patients by appropriate destruction of these pathways somewhere in their course. As is now well known, such is not the case. What is worse, activity in sensory relays does not disappear following interruption of afferent systems. On the contrary, following such procedures activity can be triggered by nonnoxious stimulation and exaggerated by deafferentation (70).

In the last decade or so, evidence has been adduced that pain is *not* simply due to activation of specific fibers in peripheral nerves or tracts in the central nervous system consisting of long, ascending fibers with the same origin, function, and termination and collected in discrete regions of the neuraxis; or centers located in specific thalamic nuclei or cortical areas where sensory impulses are brought to consciousness to produce pain (1,27, 30,63,70). Sensory mechanisms for localization of the source of painful excitations are only part of the many systems which subserve pain and its affective components. Nociceptive transmission involves not only the long afferents but also short neurons which extend from the spinal cord to the hypothalamus and terminate not only in pain "centers" but also activate a large number of subcortical and cortical structures. Moreover, neuronal systems subserving pain are open to many excitatory and inhibitory influences coming from many sources (nociceptive and other neural systems) which can enhance or block nociceptive impulses at every level of the central nervous system (1). Thus, it seems that pain is due to the activation of many diffuse paths and of many gating mechanisms which allow patterns of activity to develop in widespread subcortical and cortical structures (8).

In less than 70 years about 15 different neurosurgical operations have been devised to treat intractable pain. Certain procedures have been temporarily abandoned in favor of a new one, and then resumed to avoid the drawbacks of the latest procedure (100,101). Moreover, the good results reported with a new operation often keep eluding surgeons who try to duplicate them. The obvious conclusion is that surgical procedures for pain do not produce as satisfactory relief as claimed by their proponents. In this report, I will attempt to give a brief overview and evaluation of the most widely employed ablative procedures for cancer pain based both on personal experience and data found in the literature.

SYMPATHECTOMY

Sympathectomy is of limited usefulness for cancer pain. As White and Sweet (102) state, "pain from carcinoma generally does not arise as long as the disease is confined to a viscus." Nevertheless, pain due to visceral infection, distention, ulceration, or other pathophysiology can be relieved by sympathectomy which interrupts not only the sympathetic motor fibers, but also the afferent (sensory) fibers which supply the viscus. An example of this is the surgical (or chemical) splanchnicectomy to relieve the pain of carcinoma of the pancreas. However, the pain caused by cancer of the abdominal or thoracic viscera usually becomes severe and intractable when the tumor involves somatic spinal nerves or nerve trunks. At this point, only extensive denervation by rhizotomy or interruption of central pain pathways will produce adequate relief.

SPINAL DORSAL RHIZOTOMY

Dorsal rhizotomy of spinal nerves was the first operation successfully employed in the surgery of pain (Fig. 1). However, accurate analyses of long-term results was not attempted until recently. These have shown that the results are not as good as might be expected after complete denervation of a painful area produced by cutting an adequate number of nerve roots. Usually, the operation has been an immediate, complete success, but in a few months patients start anew to complain of pain (46).

In analysis of the results in a group of patients, Loeser (46) found no technical factors accounting for the lack of long-term success of rhizotomy: therefore, he suggested that abnormal physiologic phenomena are at work. Coggeshall et al. (12) suggests that some unmyelinated nociceptive fibers arising from cells of the dorsal ganglion but running in the anterior roots might be responsible for the recurrence of pain. Consequently, Osgood et al. (65) introduced the technique of posterior root "ganglionectomy," which should interrupt even these sensory fibers which pass through the anterior root. However, evidence to support this hypothesis is still lacking. Failures from dorsal rhizotomy are also accounted for by the fact that cancer is a progressive disease which spreads and involves adjacent nerves which have not been surgically interrupted. Although this is undoubtedly true in certain

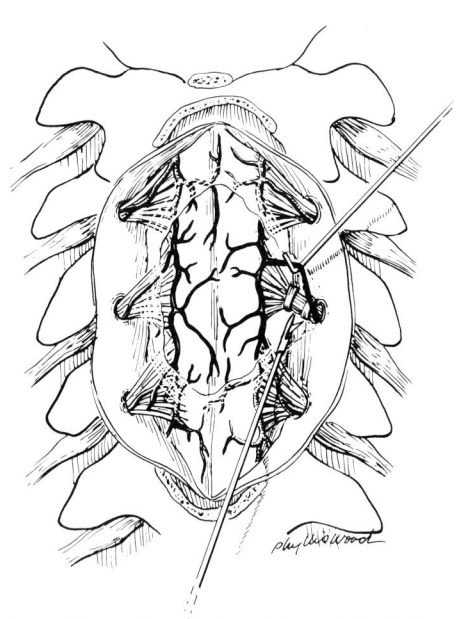

Nerve clipped; Artery deflected; Nerve divided between clips;

FIG. 1. Spinal dorsal rhizotomy. (Courtesy of Loeser, J. D., in: Bonica, J. J.: *The Management of Pain,* 2nd edition, *in preparation*).

cases, failures have been observed even if the denervation was adequate: Pain "recurs" even in permanently denervated and analgesic areas. In such cases, there is not recurrence of the original pain; an entirely new, strange, annoying, burning or aching, unbearable sensation develops which patients never had before. The abnormal sensation is referred to the anesthetic area or deep under the anesthetic skin: Sometimes denervated limbs feel like a painful phantom (70). In other words, recurrence of "pain" really represents the development of "anesthesia dolorosa": the source of pain does not lie in the peripheral nerves or roots, but in the central nervous system. Initially, deafferentation is followed by decrease of activity in the deafferented central sensory pathways but later spontaneous, persistent, abnormal firing patterns develop which give rise to the sensations patients call pain (see literature in ref. 70). Furthermore, cancer may damage nerve trunks with consequent loss of large, myelinated axons followed by disinhibition of small fibers, resulting in excessive neuronal firing in central pain pathways which contributes to the pain. Further deafferentation by rhizotomy could exaggerate the abnormal firing.

In contrast, nearly four decades ago, Ray (75) and recently Barrash and Leavens (2) reported good results following extensive dorsal rhizotomy. However, Ray (75) did not mention long-term results. The opinions of Barrash and Leavens (2) are based on 72 cases of cancer pain: 40 patients were completely relieved and 10 were satisfactorily relieved. They believe that rhizotomy is a safe and effective procedure for severe intractable pain including that due to cancer.

I obtained favorable results with extensive rhizotomy used to relieve cancer pain in the trunk, upper limb, and shoulder but only in patients who survived less than 4 months. If survival was longer, there was either recurrence or painful anesthesia. In patients with cancer pain in the face, head, and neck, rhizotomy of cranial nerves and cervical spinal roots sometimes gives longer relief (Fig. 2). Moreover, denervation of the neck is well tolerated and suppression of shooting pains is sufficient to make patients more comfortable (71,72). Rhizotomy can successfully be employed even in pain limited to the perineum and sacrococcygeal region due to rectal and anal carcinoma in patients submitted to colostomy (7,20,37). Bilateral rhizotomy from S_5 to S_2 (some of which are to be spared on one side if there are no bladder disturbances) can afford complete relief: The area of perineal and perianal anesthesia is small and well tolerated without anesthesia dolorosa (7,20,37). Unfortunately, if carcinoma spreads to invade lumbar spinal nerves or roots, the operation proves inadequate.

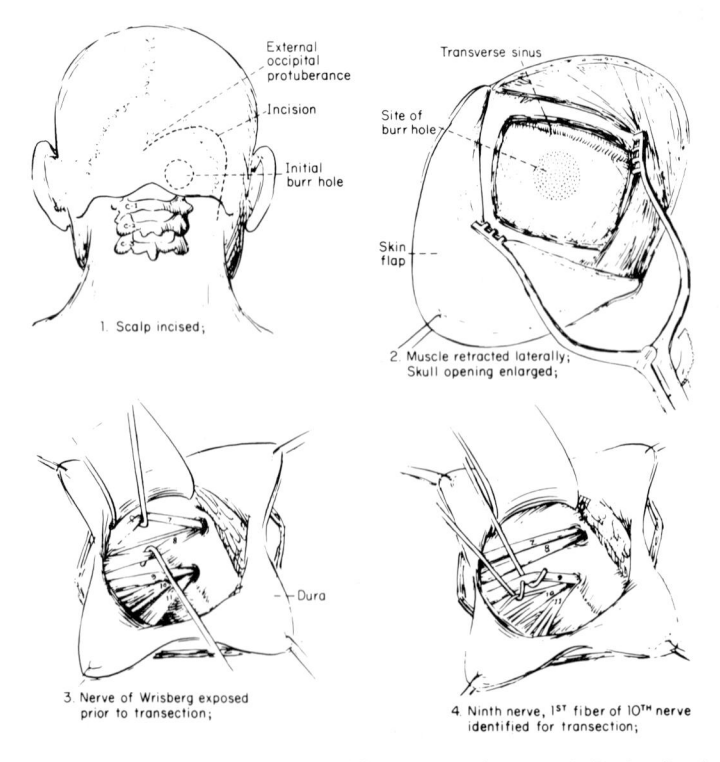

FIG. 2. Section of the VII and IX nerves. (Courtesy of Loeser, J. D., in: Bonica, J. J.: *The Management of Pain,* 2nd edition, *in preparation*).

A significant disadvantage of dorsal rhizotomy is massive denervation of an arm or leg which makes the limb virtually useless. To avoid this, Sindou et al. (87) introduced the "selective spinal posterior rhizotomy" or "radicletomy" or "rhizidiotomy." With the aid of the operative microscope only small-caliber fibers which, as the rootlets enter the cord are collected in a small lateral bundle, are cut; the large, myelinated fibers bound for the posterior funiculi, collected medially, are spared. Only pain sensation should be abolished, leaving intact other sensory modalities. The purposes of the operation are: (a) to spare inhibitory input on nociceptive afferents thus preventing failures due to deafferentation; and (6) to avoid functional impairment of limbs due to massive denervation. Sindou et al. (87,88) reported that among the 20 patients subjected to this procedure, 13 obtained complete relief and 3 partial relief of pain and that, "the best indication would seem to be painful disease of upper limb . . . and cervical roots (mainly Pancoast-Tobias syndrome) where high cervical cordotomy is often inefficient and extensive posterior rhizotomy too severe." (88) Vlahovitch and Fuentes (97) share this opinion, although in their patients they combined "radicletomy" and total rhizotomy. Experience with the procedure is, however, limited.

Percutaneous thermocoagulation of cranial and spinal nerves is a new technique with less risk and is thus worthwhile in patients in very poor condition (38). However, the experience with this procedure is limited.

ANTEROLATERAL CORDOTOMY

Anterolateral cordotomy or spinothalamic tractotomy aims at sectioning the spinothalamic tract in the anterolateral quadrant of the cord, wherein are located the ascending pathways which primarily transmit nociceptive information coming from the opposite side of the body. I will *not* discuss the indications, technique, and complications of the procedure but will limit my comments to the efficacy of open cordotomy and percutaneous cordotomy in relieving pain in the lower half of the body. This will include comments on the problem of recurrence on long-term followup.

Open Cordotomy

Complete unilateral transection of the anterolateral quadrant (Fig. 3) at upper thoracic or cervical levels produces, in nearly every patient, analgesia in the contralateral half of the body, and bilateral section produces bilateral analgesia. Immediate relief of pain is achieved in nearly 60 to 80% of patients (74,102). However, the number of failures rises at long-term followup: Broadly speaking, the incidence of recurrence of pain is about 30 to 50%. Unfortunately, details are often lacking in the published reports. Criteria for evaluation of the results and the length of survival are quite different in the various published series, thus precluding comparison of different series found

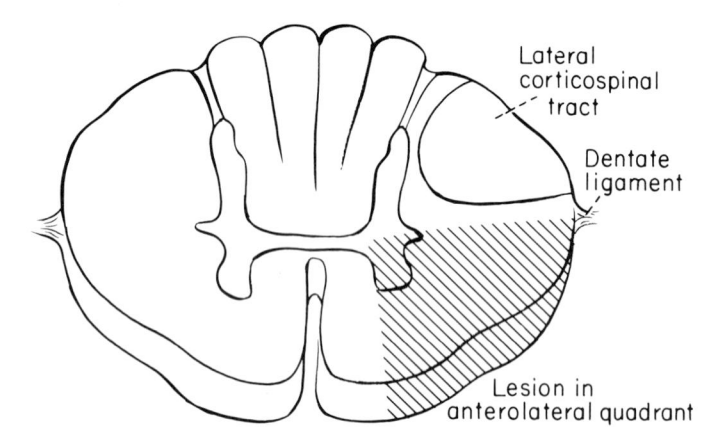

FIG. 3. Cordotomy lesion. (Courtesy of Loeser, J. D., in: Bonica, J. J.: *The Management of Pain*, 2nd edition, *in preparation*).

in the literature. My own personal experience is based on 24 patients I have been able to personally follow up. Among this group, more than 75% of the patients had recurrence of pain 3 months after the procedure was done. This figure is higher than currently estimated in the literature. However, it compares quite well with Bohm's report (6) which, oddly enough, is never quoted even in the most complete reviews on the subject. He reported that out of 29 patients who had bilateral thoracic cordotomy, 20 had recurrence of pain at 3½-months follow-up and only 9 patients who survived only 2 months died free from pain. In other words, there was a recurrence of pain in all surviving patients at 3½ months. No better were the results noted by Siegfried and Krayenbühl (86), who reported that after a few weeks 50% of the patients had recurrence of pain.

The obvious question is, "why the disappearance of analgesia?" Incomplete section of the spinothalamic tract with only temporary damage to ascending fibers has been blamed for the recurrence. Although this may be true in some cases, neuroanatomic studies have shown that fading of analgesia occurs even with complete bilateral sections of the anterolateral quadrant (11,28,63,70,102). Moreover, usually there is not simple recurrence of the pain for which the patient was operated on; patients complain of a new kind of pain, of disagreeable, unbearable sensations (dysesthesia). Peripheral stimuli can give rise to hyperpathia. These symptoms are identical to those of "central pain" and are often more annoying and sometimes more excruciating to the patients than the original cancer pain (11,68,70). Recovery of sensibility and the related symptomatology are not simply due to recovery of function of injured long ascending fibers, but in part due to transmission of impulses by other multisynaptic or alternative spinal pathways which can and often do display abnormal spontaneous activity (11,34,

63,70). These pathways are diffuse and intermingled with other cord tracts. Total interruption of them will never be possible without severe impairment of other functions.

Reliable information is scanty about the effectiveness of cordotomy at C_1-C_2 for the relief of pain in the shoulder and upper arm. The number of patients reported is usually small (6,9,24,25,48,64,66,100), or the problem is not thoroughly discussed (53,57). White and Sweet (102) state that "cervical cordotomy has a very poor chance of producing lasting analgesia of the arm," and Schürmann (82) states that, "with cervical cordotomy at level of C_1-C_2 permanent analgesia very rarely extends higher than C_8-D_1," being ineffective for relief of pain in the shoulder and upper limb. None of the 6 patients I was able to personally follow up for more than 3 months obtained permanent analgesia of, and good relief of pain in the shoulder and arm. In the opinion of White (100) shoulder and upper limb pain is better treated by some form of leucotomy or thalamotomy; others prefer selective posterior rhizotomy (44,88,97) or mesencephalic tractotomy (53). The mechanisms of fading of analgesia, recurrence of pain, and occurrence of central pain are probably the same as in thoracic cordotomy.

Percutaneous Cordotomy

In 1963, Mullan et al. (59) introduced the technique of percutaneous cordotomy. The procedure, refined by others (15,26,41,45,79) entails the interruption of the anterolateral quadrant of the cord by percutaneous insertion of a coagulating probe in the spinal cord at upper or lower cervical level. It is a relatively minor surgical procedure: Operative mortality seems very low (1 to 3%) even following bilateral procedures, and complications are less than those occurring with open cordotomy (78). Percutaneous cordotomy seems to offer the patients the same pain-relief as open cordotomy (26,78) with a rate of immediate success up to 96% (94). However, long-term follow-up studies do not always detail precise results.

Impressively large series of cases are only of moderate interest, because pain-relief seems to have been assessed only at discharge (26,56,60,94) and correlations between survival and pain-relief are sometimes lacking (26,41, 56,60,94). Only Rosomoff (78) made an accurate study of 100 cases of bilateral cordotomy at long-term follow-up. Cancer pain and noncancer pain were grouped together, with results not given separately for pain in the upper or lower half of the body. Rosomoff (78) obtained "complete relief" postoperatively in 80 out of 100 cases (80%); at 6-weeks follow-up, 42 out of 63 (67%) patients were still free from pain; at 3 months the rate was 31 out of 49 (63%); at 6 months, 18 out of 36 (50%) of the patients remained pain-free; at 1 year 9 out of 30 (less than 27%) were still relieved. It seems, therefore, that results of percutaneous cordotomy are neither better nor worse than those of open cordotomy. There is no report in the literature containing a detailed analysis of long-term results and failures in patients with pain of the upper limb and shoulder (56). Lorenz et al. (47) state ". . . failures and bad results were mainly due to difficulties in achieving complete abolition of pain arising from the brachial plexus and not sufficient level of anaesthesia."

Perhaps the most relevant point in Rosomoff's report (78) is that percutaneous cordotomy was given to 34 patients who died in 6 weeks, and to another 13 who died between 6 weeks and 3 months, i.e., high-risk patients in very poor condition, "the majority (of which) had died pain-free." It seems to me the best definition of the role of percutaneous cordotomy in surgery for pain was given by Mullan (58): "Percutaneous cordotomy . . . extends the indication for cordotomy to those patients who are too ill for the open surgical procedure. It does not, however, extend it to types of pain that do not respond to the classical surgical method." Another important advantage is that the procedure may be repeated if necessary. This led to the extension of indications to many patients with advanced cancer who had only a few days or weeks of life-expectancy. That could explain why percutaneous cordotomy "seems" to afford higher success rate than open cordotomy even in upper-half body pain. Clearly, an operation which abolishes pain for 2 to 3 weeks in a patient who will survive for such a short time may not be as successful in relieving pain and suffering if the patient had lived 4 to 6 weeks or longer.

In summary, success of cordotomy—by open or percutaneous method—is strictly tied to the duration of survival of the patient. As to when either open or percutaneous cordotomy is indicated, if the patient is in fair condition with several months of life-expectancy, the open technique done with the aid of the operative microscope which allows better visualization of anatomic landmarks and more complete transection of anterolateral quadrant is to be preferred. In patients with very short life-expectancy, when limited damage to the anterolateral quadrant is sufficient to relieve pain during the last few days or weeks of life, percutaneous cordotomy is to be preferred.

MEDULLARY TRACTOTOMY

Spinothalamic tractotomy at medullary level was undertaken with the hope of attaining better results in pain of upper limb than those given by spinal cordotomy (Fig. 4). No more than 68 cases have been reported, many of which involved pain caused by nonmalignant disease (5,102). It appears that no fewer than 43 out of 56 cases were permanently relieved of upper limb pain at some years follow-up. Maybe the good results are due to the fact that lesions impinged on the extralemniscal pain pathways at bulbar level.

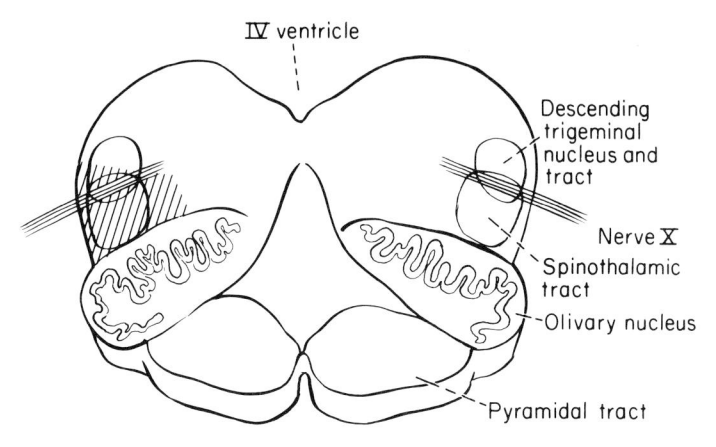

FIG. 4. Medullary tractotomy. (Courtesy of Loeser, J. D., in: Bonica, J. J.: *The Management of Pain,* 2nd edition, *in preparation*).

MESENCEPHALIC TRACTOTOMY

Spinothalamic tractotomy at mesencephalic level was introduced by Dogliotti (17) and Walker (98). The operation entails high operative mortality, complications, and frequent occurrence of central pain and dysesthesia (70,72). Thus, it was given up in spite of the fact that it seemed indicated for pain in face, neck, and upper limb.

The introduction of stereotactic technique by Speigel and Wycis et al. (91) renewed interest in mesencephalotomy. In fact, stereotactic midbrain tractotomy is an operation with low mortality and rare complications (70,72). Furthermore, the stereotactic lesion can be extended beyond the spinothalamic tract to impinge on the reticular formation where polysynaptic pain pathways are supposed to exist (62,77,103). The hope was it would be possible to obtain longer relief of pain and to avoid risk of central pain. The method was employed only in small series of patients with cancer pain (27,31,61,95,103). Opinions about the efficacy of the operation differ: Some writers reported only poor results (103); others believe mesencephalotomy is the technique of choice for the treatment of pain in the head, neck, and arm (61); still others believe that for relief of pain due to cancer it is necessary to combine mesencephalotomy with bilateral cingulotomy (96).

In 1976, Mazars et al. (53) reported they performed 224 stereotactic mesencephalotomies of which 8 were done bilaterally. Of this group, 152 patients had cancer pain. They state the, ". . . effect on pain was immediate and excellent." This is worth noting for patients with cervical and cephalic pain, ". . . which is not relieved by other less valuable procedures." Relief was permanent and complete even in the upper thoracic region and the incidence of complications was very low, but statistical analysis of the results was not reported. Mazars et al. believe that for pain in the lower half of the body cordotomy is still more effective than mesencephalotomy (53). The results reported by Mazars and his colleagues are impressive and suggest further trial of the method.

COMMISSURAL MYELOTOMY

Commissural myelotomy consists of section of the pain fibers at the midline of the cord where they cross to ascend in the contralateral anterior quadrant. It was intended to give large bands of bilateral analgesia in the torso and/or limbs, depending on the cord-splitting level. It would then seem possible to obtain bilateral pain-relief with a single operation, without damage to other spinal tracts and major complications. Successes of the procedure have been rather elusive. Only Wertheimer and Lecuire (99) reported satisfactory results in a large series of cases submitted to lumbar myelotomy for bilateral pain of the legs, pelvis, and perineum. The incidence of complications consisting in operative death, radicular pain, leg dysesthesia, paresis, and/or bladder and/or bowel dysfunction were high. Of 80 patients followed up, 27 (33%) were completely relieved, 25 (32%) were improved, and in 28 (35%) the procedure failed. In 1963, Dargent et al. (16) reviewed the same series and reached the conclusion that commissural myelotomy is effective only for vaginal and visceral pain, and that for rectal and leg pain, cordotomy is preferred.

This operation seemed a matter of only historical interest rather than of practical value, when in 1964, Lembcke (40) reported impressive results in 12 patients submitted to cervical myelotomy. All the patients were relieved and analgesia persisted up to 10 years in 6 long-term survivors; no serious complication occurred. This prompted new interest in the procedure which was employed both for pain in the lower half of the body (10,13,36,44,53, 89,90) and for cervical, upper limb, and thoracic pain (32,73,83). Wertheimer and Lecuire's standard incision was 2 to 3 cm long and a few mm deep (99). Currently most surgeons try to produce a deeper incision with complete splitting of the cord in two halves for several centimeters (10,13, 36,73,90).

As is always the case in surgery for pain, some are happy with the results while others are not. The former group includes Lembcke (40) and Broager (10), who state they gave up bilateral cordotomy in favor of commissural myelotomy. In contrast, Papo and Luongo (73) reported that while pain was completely relieved in all patients, it remained absent for only several weeks: Severe pain recurred within 2 months.

Everyone who has performed commissural myelotomy agrees that, in spite of extensive splitting of the cord, defects in pain and temperature appreciation are relatively mild, that no permanent extensive analgesia ensues and that hypalgesia, when present, fades away in a few weeks. On the contrary, disturbances due to dorsal column injury (loss of positional sense, tactile hypoesthesia, dysesthesia, tingling, ataxia) are frequent and may be marked (44,73). The mechanism by which myelotomy abolishes pain, even if temporarily, is far from clear. Schwarcz (83) suggested pain-relief was due to interruption of extralemniscal polysynaptic pathways close to the central gray matter of the spinal cord: Myelotomy acts like an intralaminar thalamotomy. Sourek (89) and Papo and Luongo (73) report that a close correlation exists between signs of posterior column damage and pain-relief: When these fade away, pain usually recurs, suggesting a role of injury or irritation of dorsal column system responsible for the relief of pain. It seems to me myelotomy is a rather mysterious operation whose mechanisms, indications, and results are far from clear.

STEREOTACTIC THALAMOTOMY

Stereotactic thalamotomy aroused the hope that combined destruction of both the spinothalamic system (VPL-VPM nuclei) and the polysynaptic pathways (CM, Pf, intralaminar, limitans nuclei) might afford longer analgesia and pain-relief than other operations, without occurrence of central pain. Regrettably, experience has shown that it is nearly impossible to achieve persistent analgesia and pain-relief by this technique: In about 70 to 80% of cases pain recurs in a few weeks or months (69). Moreover, destruction of the VPL-VPM nuclei frequently gives rise to central pain (11,51,52,67,69).

Mark et al. (49,50) suggested that the suppression of pain by thalamotomy is not due to lesion of the VPL-VPM nuclei, but to involvement of nonspecific pathways in the CM-Pf-intralaminar complex whose destruction might afford relief of pain without sensory loss and risk of central pain. In my experience unilateral lesions limited to the CM-Pf-intralaminar complex yield only transient results (67,69). Furthermore, clinical-anatomic studies of both personal and published case reports of patients relieved of pain (49,50,93) demonstrate that the lesion actually destroys a variable part of the dorsomedial nucleus with a leucotomic effect which might play a critical role in securing relief of pain in absence of any sensory loss.

An attempt to improve the results was made with bilateral lesions of the basal thalamus including VPL-VPM, CM-Pf-intralaminar complexes: Sometimes results reached the expectation (4,14,35,92). Pulvinarectomy, introduced by Richardson (76) affords no better results for some (22,69), while others are satisfied with this procedure (104).

Stereotactic thalamotomy seems a method of limited practical value. Because of its very low mortality and complication rate, it can be employed in patients in very poor condition with pain of the head, face, neck, and upper limb when other procedures are not indicated or might not be tolerated (72). Therefore, I have read with interest the reports by Fairman (18) and Sano (80) that unilateral or bilateral lesions of the internal medullary lamina including the CM, Pf, and limitans ("thalamolaminotomy") and of the posteromedial hypothalamus ("posteromedial hypothalamotomy") give excellent and persistent relief even in diffuse cancer pain. These data suggest the method merits further trial.

Tractotomy of the descending root of the trigeminal nerve, known as Sjöqvist's operation, is employed for head and face cancer pain. This topic is discussed elsewhere in this volume.

PSYCHOSURGERY

Since the Freeman and Watts statement, "The results of lobotomy . . . have been so gratifying that further efforts in the earlier control of intractable pain are unwarranted" (23), the procedure has been considered for patients with intractable cancer pain. Lobotomy seems to work in that it changes the attitude of the patient toward his pain (23), removes the anticipation and memory of the pain (85), and alters affective and emotional response to it (55); but it does not alter the perception of pain.

Unfortunately, bilateral lobotomy invariably produces apathy and severe psychologic deterioration. Because of this serious complication, less destructive procedures were introduced: unilateral lobotomy (81), undercutting of the frontal cortex (54,84), progressive radiofrequency frontal lobotomy (29), bilateral frontal topectomy (39), and dorsomedial stereotactic thalamotomy (92) (Fig. 5). However, even with those procedures, pain-relief invariably seems to be associated with, and depend on, severe emotional and mental defects. Pain is relieved only so long as changes of personality persist; should they subside, there is recurrence of complaints.

To avoid psychic disturbances, White and Sweet (102) introduced graduated bilateral coagulation of medial frontal white matter. With this procedure small areas of frontothalamic projection fibers are destroyed in successive steps, at intervals of several days. In this way it seems possible to

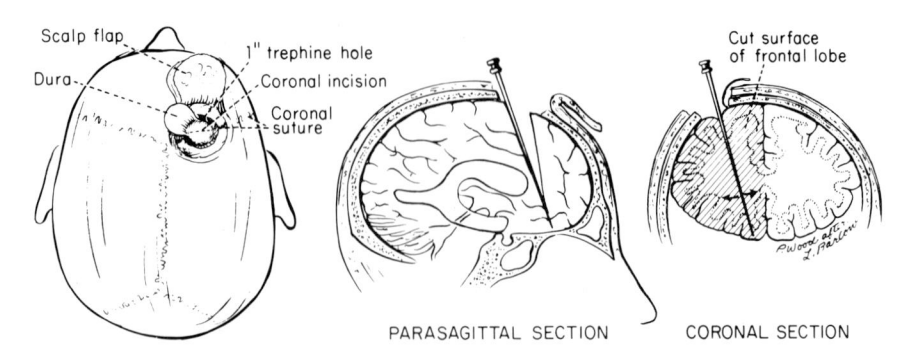

FIG. 5. Prefrontal lobotomy. (Courtesy of Loeser, J. D., in: Bonica, J. J.: *The Management of Pain,* 2nd edition, *in preparation*).

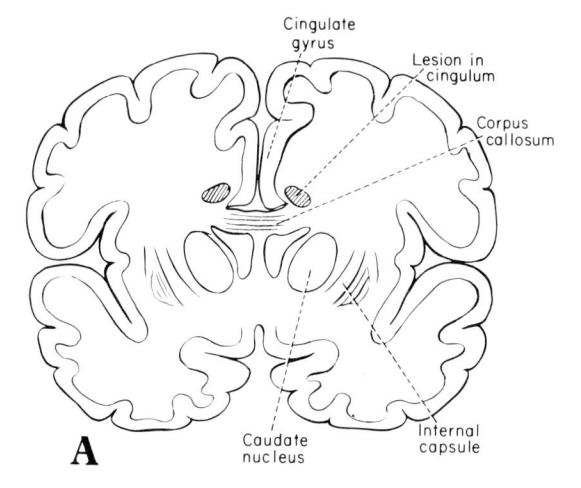

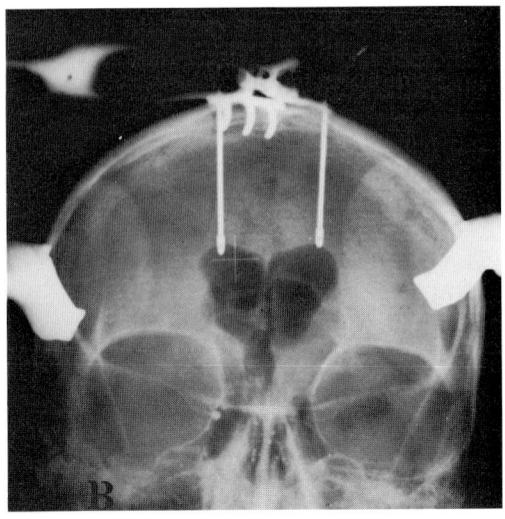

FIG. 6. A and B: Cingulotomy. (Courtesy of Loeser, J. D., in: Bonica, J. J.: *The Management of Pain*, 2nd edition, *in preparation*).

afford pain-relief without severe mental deterioration. Bertrand et al. (3) attempted to obtain the same result by means of stereotactic section of the frontothalamic pathways. Lindstrom et al. (42,43) performed frontal lobotomy by means of ultrasonic beam; "considerable relief from pain" was obtained in 45 of 48 patients thus treated without the mental defects of frontal lobe surgery.

In 1962, Folz and White introduced "cingulotomy" (21). In the cingulum run pathways mediating activities of the limbic system to the entire forebrain; these pathways play a major role in emotional behavior. The hope was to succeed in modifying emotional reaction to pain, relieving suffering with minimal psychic impairment. Foltz and White (21) reported excellent relief at 6 months to 1 year follow-up in a group of patients who showed marked emotional reaction to pain. Recently, Hurt and Ballantine (33) in reporting the results of bilateral cingulotomy in 32 patients with cancer pain, stated they "were unable to document unwanted changes in intellect, memory, personality or other psychological functions in these patients." Marked to complete relief was achieved in 37% of patients, slight to moderate in 28%: but there was "a tendency to progressive decrease in the initial degree of pain relief" (33). It seems, therefore, that cingulotomy has, at least partially, fulfilled expectations (Figs. 6A and B). Duration of relief, however, is briefer than following more-mutilating frontal operations with the attendant persistent mental impairment.

My experience is limited to 4 cases of frontothalamic section (3), 4 cases of cingulotomy (21), 4 of graduated frontal coagulation, and 2 of dorsomedial thalamotomy (92). As far as I can judge by this limited experience, relief of suffering was achieved only with concomitant personality changes and mental deterioration. Thus, I am rather inclined to agree with Falconer (19), who considers frontal surgery a procedure of therapeutic desperation. The less-mutilating procedures in more experienced hands might afford satisfactory relief with only minor personality changes.

CONCLUSIONS

It seems to me that neurosurgical ablative procedures are not always the final answer for relief of pain in cancer. Experience has taught us that if persistent and massive noxious stimuli, as those provoked by cancer, impinge on the central nervous system, not even the largest interruption of the so-called 'pain pathways' might permanently abolish pain and suffering. Owing to vicarious pathways, at least a part of those impulses surface consciousness as pain. Furthermore, sensory deprivation, due both to peripheral or central nervous system lesions, triggers spontaneous discharges in central pain which contribute to the patient's suffering.

However, in cancer pain, surgery has still a definite place. Owing to the fact that patients with malignant disease have a short period of survival, appropriate peripheral or central pain pathways interruption can afford dramatic relief for some months. I think we cannot obtain complete relief for much more than 3–4 months.

Somebody could ask himself whether such a formidable procedure as a surgical operation is reasonable in patients with very short life expectancy. We must recall that in very advanced cancer, for patients who will not survive more than a few weeks, less destructive procedures have been introduced, such as percutaneous cordotomy and stereotactic surgery. They can be employed without major complications. The appropriate procedure must be chosen on the basis of localization of pain, general conditions, and life expectancy. Appropriate selection of operation in selected cases will give the most gratifying results.

REFERENCES

1. Albe-Fessard, D. (1972): Central pathways for noxious stimuli. In: *Cervical Pain*, edited by C. Hirsch and Y. Zotterman, pp. 179–193. Pergamon Press, Oxford.
2. Barrash, J. M., and Leavens, M. E. (1973): Dorsal rhizotomy for the relief of intractable pain of malignant tumor origin. *J. Neurosurg.*, 38:755–757.
3. Bertrand, C., Martinez, N., and Hardy, J. (1966): Frontothalamic section for intractable pain. In: *Pain*, edited by R. S. Knighton and P. R. Dumke, pp. 531–535. Little, Brown, Boston.
4. Bettag, W. (1966): Results of treatment of pain by interruption of the medial pain tract of the brain stem. *Excerpta Medica Int. Cong. Series*, 110:771–775.
5. Birkenfeld, R., and Fisher, R. G. (1963): Successful treatment of causalgia of upper extremity with medullary spinothalamic tractotomy. *J. Neurosurg.*, 20:303–311.
6. Bohm, E. (1960): Chordotomy for intractable pain due to malignant disease. *Acta Psychiatr. Scand.*, 35:145–155.
7. Bohm, E., and Franksson, C. (1958–1959): Coccigodynia and sacral rhizotomy. *Acta Chir. Scand.*, 116:268–274.
8. Bowsher, D. (1974): Thalamic convergence and divergence of information generated by noxious stimulation. In: *Advances in Neurology, Vol. 4: International Symposium on Pain*, edited by J. J. Bonica, pp. 223–232. Raven Press, New York.
9. Brihaye, J., and Rétif, J. (1961): Comparison des résultats obtenuse par la cordotomie anterolaterale au niveau dorsal et auniveau cervical. (À propos de 109 observations personnelles). *Neurochirurgie*, 7:258–277.
10. Broager, B. (1974): Commissural myeolotomy. *Surg. Neurol.*, 2:71–74.
11. Cassinari, V., and Pagni, C. A. (1969): *Central Pain. A Neurosurgical Survey*. Harvard University Press, Cambridge.
12. Coggeshall, R. E., Appelbaum, M. L., Facem, M., Stubbs, T. B., III, and Sykes, M. T. (1975): Unmyelinated axons in human ventral roots, a possible explanation for the failure of dorsal rhizotomy to relieve pain. *Brain*, 98:157–166.
13. Cook, A. W., and Kawakamy, Y. (1977): Commissural myeolotomy. *J. Neurosurg.*, 47:1–6.
14. Cooper, I. S. (1965): Clinical and physiologic implications of thalamic surgery for disorders of sensory communication. Part 1. Thalamic surgery for intractable pain. *J. Neurol. Sci.*, 2:493–519.
15. Crue, B. L., Todd, E. M., Carregal, E. J. A., Wright, W. H., and Maline, D. B. (1970): Posterior approach for high cervical percutaneous radiofrequency stereotaxic cordotomy. In: *Pain and Suffering. Selected Aspects*, edited by B. L. Crue, pp. 35–41. Charles C Thomas, Springfield, Ill.
16. Dargent, M., Mansuy, L., Colon, J., and De Rougemont, J. (1963): Les problèmes posé par la douleur dans l'evolution des cancer gynécologiques. *Lyon Chir.*, 59:62–83.
17. Dogliotti, A. M. (1938): First surgical sections in man, of the lemniscus lateralis (pain-temperature paths) at the brainstem, for the treatment of diffused rebellious pain. *Anesth. Analg.*, 17:143–145.
18. Fairman, D. (1976): Neurophysiological basis for the hypothalamic lesion and stimulation by chronic implanted electrodes for the relief of intractable pain in cancer. In: *Advances in Pain Research and Therapy, Vol. 1: Proceedings of the First World Congress on Pain*, edited by J. J. Bonica and D. Albe-Fessard, pp. 843–847. Raven Press, New York.
19. Falconer, M. A. (1948): Relief of intractable pain of organic origin by frontal lobotomy. *Res. Publ. Assoc. Nerv. Ment. Dis.*, 27:707–714.
20. Felsöőry, A., and Crue, B. L. (1976): Results of 19 years experience with sacral rhizotomy for perineal and perianal cancer pain. *Pain*, 2:431–433.

21. Foltz, E. L., and White, L. E. (1966): Rostral cingulotomy and pain "relief." In: *Pain,* edited by R. S. Knighton and P. R. Dumke, pp. 469–491. Little, Brown, Boston.
22. Farioli, B., and Guidetti, B. (1975): Effects of stereotactic lesions of the pulvinar and lateralis posterior nucleus on intractable pain and dyskinetic syndromes in man. *Appl. Neurophysiol.,* 38:23–70.
23. Freeman, W., and Watts, J. W. (1950): *Psychosurgery in the Treatment of Mental Disorders and Intractable Pain.* Charles C Thomas, Springfield, Ill.
24. French, L. A. (1974): High cervical tractotomy: Technique and results. *Clin. Neurosurg.,* 21:239–245.
25. French, L. A., Chou, S. N., and Story, J. L. (1966): Cervical tractotomy: Technique and clinical usefulness. In: *Pain,* edited by R. S. Knighton and P. R. Dumke, pp. 311–320. Little, Brown, Boston.
26. Gildenberg, P. L. (1974): Percutaneous cordotomy cervical. *Clin. Neurosurg.,* 21:246–256.
27. Glees, P. (1953): The central pain tract. *Acta Neuroveg.,* 7:160–174.
28. Graf, C. I. (1960): Consideration in loss of sensory level after bilateral cervical cordotomy. *Arch. Neurol.,* 3:410–415.
29. Grantham, E. G. (1951): Prefrontal lobotomy for relief of pain, with a report of a new operative technique. *J. Neurosurg.,* 8:405–410.
30. Hassler, R. (1960): Die zentrale Systeme des Schmerzes. *Acta Neurochir.,* 8:423–535.
31. Helfant, M. H., Leksell, L., and Strang, R. R. (1965): Experiences with intractable pain treated by stereotaxic mesencephalotomy. *Acta Chir. Scand.,* 129:573–580.
32. Hitchcock, E. (1974): Stereotactic myelotomy. *Proc. R. Soc. Med.,* 67:771–772.
33. Hurt, R. W., and Ballantine, H. T. (1974): Stereotactic anterior cingulate lesions for persistent pain: A report on 68 cases. *Clin. Neurosurg.,* 21:334–351.
34. Kerr, F. W. L. (1975): Neuroanatomical substrates of nociception in the spinal cord. *Pain,* 1:325–356.
35. Kim, Y. K., and Umbach, W. (1972): Comparative evaluation of different psychosurgical methods. In: *Present Limits of Neurosurgery,* edited by I. Fusek and Z. Kunc, pp. 465–469. Avicenum, Praha.
36. King, R. B. (1977): Anterior commissurotomy for intractable pain. *J. Neurosurg.,* 47:7–11.
37. Kühner, A. (1976): La valeur des interventions sur les racines sacrées dans le traitement des syndromes douloureux du bassin. *Neurochirurgie,* 22:429–436.
38. Lazorthes, Y., Verdie, J. C., and Lagarrigue, J. (1976): Thermocoagulation percutanée des nerfs rachidiens à visée analgésique. *Neurochirurgie,* 22:445–453.
39. Le Beau, J., Bouvet, M., and Rosier, M. (1950): Traitement des douleurs irréductibles par la topectomie. *Sem. Hop.,* 24:1946–1952.
40. Lembcke, W. (1964): Über die mediolongitudinale Chordotomie im Halsmarkbereich. *Zentrabl. Chir.,* 89:439–443.
41. Lin, P. M., Gildenberg, P. L., and Polakoff, P. P. (1966): An anterior approach to percutaneous lower cervical cordotomy. *J. Neurosurg.,* 25:553–560.
42. Lindstrom, P. A. (1972): Prefrontal sonic treatment—sixteen years' experience. In: *Psychosurgery, Proc. 2nd Int. Congr. Psychosurg.,* edited by L. Laitinen and K. Vaernet, pp. 357–376. Charles C Thomas, Springfield, Ill.
43. Lindstrom, P. A., Moench, L. G., and Rovnanek, A. (1964): Prefrontal sonic treatment. *Curr. Psychiat. Ther.,* 4:143–149.
44. Lippert, R. G., Hosobuchi, Y., and Nielsen, S. L. (1974): Spinal commissurotomy. *Surg. Neurol.,* 2:373–377.
45. Lipton, S., Dervin, E., and Heywood, O. B. (1974): A stereotactic approach to the anterior percutaneous electrical cordotomy. In: *Advances in Neurology, Vol. 4: International Symposium on Pain,* edited by J. J. Bonica, pp. 689–694. Raven Press, New York.
46. Loeser, J. D. (1972): Dorsal rhizotomy for the relief of chronic pain. *J. Neurosurg.,* 36:745–750.
47. Lorenz, R., Grumme, T., Herrmann, D., Palleske, H., Kühner, A., Stende, U., and

Zierski, J. (1975): Percutaneous cordotomy. In: *Advances in Neurosurgery Vol. 3*, edited by H. Penzholz, M. Brock, J. Hamer, M. Klinger, and O. Spoerri, pp. 178–185. Springer, Berlin.
48. Mansuy, L., Sindou, M., Fischer, G., and Brunon, J. (1976): La cordotomie spinothalamique dans les douleurs cancéreuses. *Neurochirurgie,* 22:437–444.
49. Mark, V. H., Ervin, F. R., and Hackett, T. P. (1960): Clinical aspects of stereotactic thalamotomy in the human. I. The treatment of chronic severe pain. *Arch. Neurol.,* 3:351–367.
50. Mark, V. H., Ervin, F. R., and Yakovlev, P. I. (1963): Stereotactic thalamotomy III. Verification of anatomical lesion site in the human thalamus. *Arch. Neurol.,* 8:528–538.
51. Maspes, P. E., and Pagni, C. A. (1965): Studio critico degli interventi stereotassici eseguiti a livello talamico per il trattamento dei dolori incoercibili. *Riv. Pat. Nerv. Ment.* Atti Congr. Naz. Soc. Ital. Neurol., pp. 1–154.
52. Maspes, P. E., and Pagni, C. A. (1974): A critical appraisal of pain surgery and suggestions for improving treatment. In: *Recent Advances on Pain: Pathophysiology and Clinical Aspects,* edited by J. J. Bonica, P. Procacci, and C. A. Pagni, pp. 201–255. Charles C Thomas, Springfield, Ill.
53. Mazars, G., Merienne, L., and Cioloca, C. (1976): État actuel de la chirurgie de la douleur. *Neurochirurgie [Suppl.],* 1:1–164.
54. McKissock, W. (1951): Rostral leucotomy. *Lancet,* 2:91–94.
55. Merskey, H., and Spear, F. G. (1967): *Pain: Psychological and Psychiatric Aspects.* Baillière, Tindall and Cassell, London.
56. Müke, R., and Correia, A. (1975): Potentials and limits of percutaneous cervical cordotomy. In: *Advances in Neurosurgery, Vol. 3,* edited by H. Penzholz, M. Brock, J. Hamer, M. Klinger, and O. Spoerri, pp. 195–198. Springer, Berlin.
57. Mullan, S. (1971): The surgical relief of pain. *Clin. Neurosurg.,* 18:208–224.
58. Mullan, S. (1974): Percutaneous cordotomy. In: *Advances in Neurology, Vol. 4: International Symposium on Pain,* edited by J. J. Bonica, pp. 677–682. Raven Press, New York.
59. Mullan, S., Harper, P., Hekmatpanah, J., Torres, H., and Dobbin, G. (1963): Percutaneous interruption of spinal pain tracts by means of a strontium 90 needle. *J. Neurosurg.,* 20:931–939.
60. Mullan, S., Hekmatpanah, J., Dobbin, G., and Beckman, F. (1965): Percutaneous intramedullary cordotomy utilizing the unipolar anodal electrolytic lesion. *J. Neurosurg.,* 22:548–553.
61. Nashold, B. S. (1972): Extensive cephalic and oral pain relieved by midbrain tractotomy. *Confin. Neurol.,* 34:382.
62. Nashold, B. S., Wilson, W. P., and Slaughter, D. G. (1969): Stereotactic midbrain lesions for central dysaesthesia and phantom pain. *J. Neurosurg.,* 30:116–126.
63. Noordenbos, W. (1959): *Pain: Problems Pertaining to the Transmission of Nerve Impulses Which Give Rise to Pain.* Elsevier, Amsterdam.
64. Ogle, W. S., French, L. A., and Peyton, W. T. (1956): Experiences with high cervical cordotomy. *J. Neurosurg.,* 13:81–87.
65. Osgood, C. P., Dujovni, M., and Faille, R. (1976): Microsurgical lumbosacral ganglionectomy technique, anatomic rationale, and surgical results. In: *Advances In Pain Research and Therapy, Vol. 1: Proceedings of the First World Congress on Pain,* edited by J. J. Bonica and D. Albe-Fessard, pp. 855–862. Raven Press, New York.
66. Owens, G. (1966): Panel discussion. Unsolved problems. In: *Pain,* edited by R. S. Knighton and P. R. Dumke, pp. 540–545. Little, Brown, Boston.
67. Pagni, C. A. (1966): Discussion by Erwin, F. R., Brown, C. E., and Mark, V. H., Striatal influences on facial pain. *Confin. Neurol.,* 27:88–89.
68. Pagni, C. A. (1969): Fisiopatologia del dolore. *Atti. VI Congr. Naz. Soc. Ital. Med. Fis. Riabil.,* pp. 77–116. Mattioli, Fidenza.
69. Pagni, C. A. (1974): Place of stereotactic technique in surgery for pain. In: *Advances in Neurology, Vol. 4: International Symposium on Pain,* edited by J. J. Bonica, pp. 699–706. Raven Press, New York.

70. Pagni, C. A. (1977): Central pain and painful anesthesia. In: *Pain—Its Neurosurgical Management. Part II: Central Procedures*, edited by H. Krayenbühl, P. E. Maspes, and W. H. Sweet, pp. 132–257. Karger, Basel.
71. Pagni, C. A. (1979): Therapy of cancer pain in the head and neck. Role of neurosurgery. In: *Advances in Pain Research and Therapy, Vol. 2*, International Symposium on Pain of Advanced Cancer, edited by J. J. Bonica and V. Ventafridda. Raven Press, New York.
72. Pagni, C. A., and Maspes, P. E. (1970): Problems in the surgical treatment of pain in malignancies of the head and neck. In: *Current Research in Neurosciences, Vol. 10*, edited by H. T. Wycis, pp. 138–153. Karger, Basel.
73. Papo, I., and Luongo, A. (1976): High cervical commissural myelotomy in the treatment of pain. *J. Neurol. Neurosurg. Psychiatry*, 39:705–710.
74. Piscol, K. (1975): Open spinal surgery for intractable pain. In: *Advances in Neurosurgery, Vol. 3*, edited by H. Penzholz, M. Brock, J. Hamer, M. Klinger, and O. Spoerri, pp. 157–169. Springer, Berlin.
75. Ray, B. S. (1943): The management of intractable pain by posterior rhizotomy. *Res. Publ. Ass. Res. Nerv. Ment. Dis.*, 23:391–407.
76. Richardson, D. E. (1967): Thalamotomy for intractable pain. *Confin. Neurol.*, 29:139–145.
77. Roeder, F., and Orthner, H. (1961): Erfahrungen mit stereotaktischen Eingriffen. III Mitteilung. Über zerebrale Schmerzoperationen, insbesondere mediale Mesencephalotomie bei thalamischer Hyperpatie und bei Anaesthesia dolorosa. *Confin. Neurol.*, 21:51–97.
78. Rosomoff, H. L. (1969): Bilateral percutaneous cervical radiofrequency cordotomy. *J. Neurosurg.*, 31:41–46.
79. Rosomoff, H. L., Carroll, F., Brown, J., and Sheptak, P. (1965): Percutaneous radiofrequency cervical cordotomy: Technique. *J. Neurosurg.*, 23:639–644.
80. Sano, K. (1977): Intralaminar thalamotomy (thalamolaminotomy) and posteromedial hypothalamotomy in the treatment of intractable pain. In: *Pain—Its Neurosurgical Management. Part II: Central Procedures*, edited by H. Krayenbühl, P. E. Maspes, and W. H. Sweet, pp. 50–103. Karger, Basel.
81. Scarff, J. E. (1950): Unilateral prefrontal lobotomy for the relief of intractable pain. Report of 58 cases with special consideration of failures. *J. Neurosurg.*, 7:330–336.
82. Schürmann, K. (1972): Fundamental principles of the surgical treatment of pain. In: *Pain—Basic Principles—Pharmacology—Therapy*, edited by R. Janzen, W. D. Keidel, A. Herz, and C. Steichele, pp. 181–193. Thieme, Stuttgart.
83. Schvarcz, J. R. (1976): Stereotactic extralemniscal myelotomy. *J. Neurol. Neurosurg. Psychiat.*, 39:53–57.
84. Scoville, W. B. (1949): Selective cortical undercutting as a means of modifying and studying frontal lobe function in man. *J. Neurosurg.*, 6:65–73.
85. Scoville, W. B. (1972): Psychosurgery and other lesions of the brain affecting human behavior. In: *Psychosurgery, Proceedings of the 2nd International Congress on Psychosurgery*, edited by E. Hitchcock, L. Laitinen, and K. Vaernet, pp. 5–21. Charles C Thomas, Springfield, Ill.
86. Siegfried, J., and Krayenbühl, H. (1972): Clinical experience in the treatment of intractable pain. In: *Pain—Basic Principles—Pharmacology—Therapy*, edited by R. Janzen, W. D. Keidel, A. Herz, and C. Steichele, pp. 202–204. Thieme, Stuttgart.
87. Sindou, M., Fischer, G., Goutelle, A., and Mansuy, L. (1974): La radicellotomie postérieure sélective. Premiers résultats dans la chirurgie de la douleur. *Neurochirurgie*, 20:391–408.
88. Sindou, M., Fischer, G., and Mansuy, L. (1976): Posterior spinal rhizotomy and selective posterior rhizidiotomy. In: *Pain—Its Neurosurgical Management. Part I: Procedures on Primary Afferent Neurons*, edited by H. Krayenbühl, P. E. Maspes, and W. H. Sweet, pp. 201–250. Karger, Basel.
89. Sourek, K. (1969): Commissural myelotomy. *J. Neurosurg.*, 31:524–527.
90. Sourek, K. (1977): Mediolongitudinal myelotomy. In: *Pain—Its Neurosurgical*

Management. Part II: Central Procedures, edited by H. Krayenbühl, P. E. Maspes, W. H. Sweet, pp. 15–34. Karger, Basel.
91. Spiegel, E. A., Wycis, H. T., Marks, M., and Lee, A. J. (1947): Stereotaxic apparatus for operations on the human brain. *Science*, 106:349–350.
92. Spiegel, E. A., Wycis, H. T., Szekely, E. G., and Gildenberg, P. L. (1966): Medial and basal thalamotomy in so-called intractable pain. In: *Pain*, edited by R. S. Knighton and P. R. Dumke, pp. 503–517. Little, Brown, Boston.
93. Sugita, K., Mutsuga, N., Takaoka, Y., and Doi, T. (1972): Results of stereotactic thalamotomy for pain. *Confin. Neurol.*, 34:265–274.
94. Tasker, R. R. (1977): Open cordotomy. In: *Pain—Its Neurosurgical Management. Part II: Central Procedures*, edited by H. Krayenbühl, P. E. Maspes and W. H. Sweet, pp. 1–14. Karger, Basel.
95. Torvik, A. (1959): Sensory motor and reflex changes in two cases of intractable pain after stereotactic mesencephalic tractotomy. *J. Neurol. Neurosurg. Psychiatry*, 22:299–305.
96. Turnbull, I. M. (1972): Bilateral cingulotomy combined with thalamotomy or mesencephalic tractotomy for pain. *Surg. Gynecol. Obstet.*, 134:958–962.
97. Vlahovitch, B., and Fuentes, J. M. (1975): Résultats de la radicellotomie sélective postérieure à l'étage lombaire et cervical. *Neurochirurgie*, 21:29–42.
98. Walker, E. A. (1942): Mesencephalic tractotomy. A method for the relief of unilateral intractable pain. *Arch. Surg.*, 44:953–962.
99. Wertheimer, P., and Lecuire, J. (1953): La myélotomie commissurale postèrieure. À propos de 107 observations. *Acta Chir. Belg.*, 52:568–574.
100. White, J. C. (1966): Cordotomy: Assessment of its effectiveness and suggestions for its improvement. *Clin. Neurosurg.*, 13:1–19.
101. White, J. C., and Kjellberg, R. N. (1973): Posterior spinal rhizotomy. A substitute for cordotomy in the relief of localized pain in patients with normal life expectancy. *Neurochirurgia*, 16:141–170.
102. White, J. C., and Sweet, W. H. (1969): *Pain and the Neurosurgeon. A Forty Years Experience*. Charles C Thomas, Springfield, Ill.
103. Wycis, H. T., and Spiegel, E. A. (1962): Long-range results in the treatment of intractable pain by stereotaxic midbrain surgery. *J. Neurosurg.*, 19:101–107.
104. Yoshimasu, N. (1972): Functional anatomy of the internal medullary lamina based on the results of stereotaxic surgery. *Brain and Nerve*, 24:1277–1292. (In Japanese.)

Percutaneous Cervical Cordotomy

Sampson Lipton

Associated Department of Neurological Sciences, Liverpool University, Walton Hospital, Liverpool L9 1AE England

In 1905, Spiller (16) showed that pain and temperature sensation are transmitted through the anterolateral spinal tract. Seven years later, Spiller and Martin (17) reported a patient in whom section of the anterior quadrant of the spinal cord abolished intractable pain. Since then, sectioning of the anterolateral quadrant (ALQ), commonly known as cordotomy, or anterolateral tractotomy, has been used widely to relieve severe, intractable pain located below the cervical spinal segments. Until 15 years ago, the procedure was carried out through a laminectomy and a subsequent section of the tracts at the upper thoracic levels.

In 1963, Mullan (11) first described the technique of percutaneous cordotomy at C_{1-2}. Destruction of the ALQ was achieved through a needle inserted via a posterolateral approach and a radioactive strontium–tipped probe placed in ALQ. Subsequently, techniques entailing lateral, anterior, and posterior approaches were developed (1,6).

Because the percutaneous technique is a minor surgical procedure, it has been largely used for the relief of severe pain of advanced cancer. In this presentation, I will discuss: (a) the anatomic bases of cervical percutaneous cordotomy; (b) techniques of lateral, anterior, posterior, and bilateral percutaneous cervical cordotomy; and (c) the results obtained by our group for patients with cancer.

ANATOMIC CONSIDERATIONS

The anterolateral quadrant of the spinal cord contains crossed sensory fibers which transmit sensations interpreted as pain, heat, and cold. Also in this region are the spinocerebellar tracts, and ataxia may result when these are destroyed. Moreover, in the C_1-C_2 region of the spinal cord are located the respiratory reticular fibers lying close to the anterior horn cells, and these may be destroyed by cordotomy at this level.

The posterior quadrant of the spinal cord contains the cerebrospinal or motor tract, and this is contiguous anterolaterally with the sensory tracts. The dentate ligament at the C_1-C_2 level tends to separate the anterior sen-

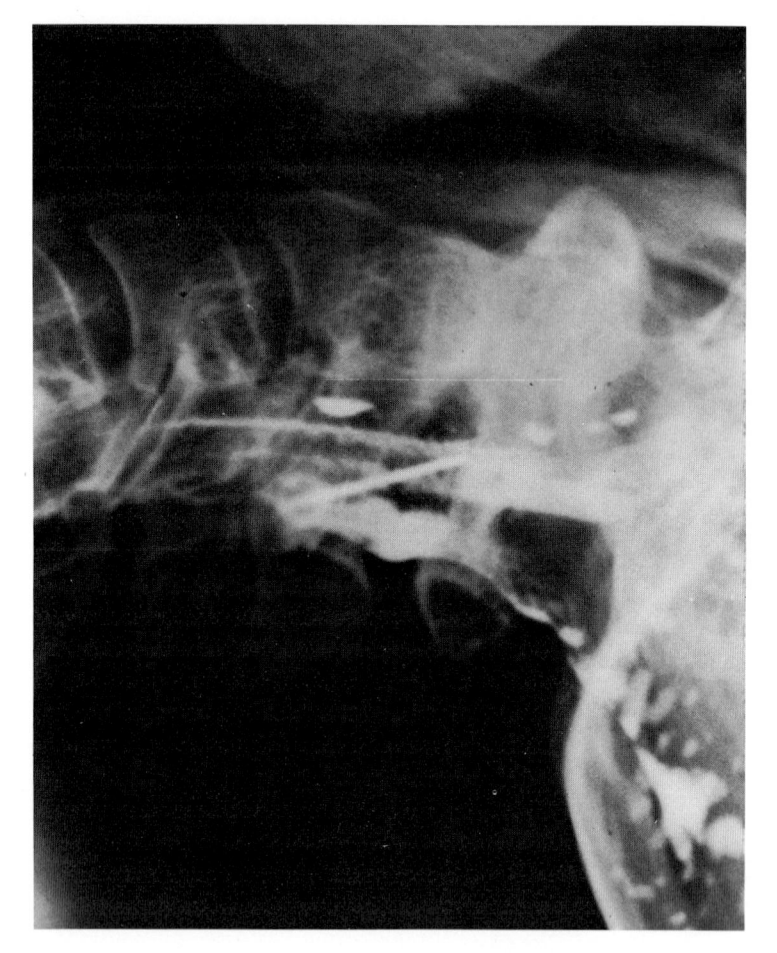

FIG. 1. Lateral roentgenograms of the cervical spine taken in the course of a lateral percutaneous cervical cordotomy. The needle is in place after being inserted through the interspace between C_1 and C_2 vertebra. Injection of the radio-opaque emulsion outlines the anterior border of the spinal cord, the dentate ligament, and the posterior dura. Note that the point of the spinal needle is anterior to the dentate ligament.

sory quadrant from the posterior motor nerve fibers. The position of the ALQ is between the anterior border of the spinal cord anteriorly and the dentate ligament posteriorly.

The cervicomedullary junction is a portion of the spinal cord where rapid rearrangements of nerve fibers are made. Above this level the motor fibers are anteriorly situated while below, the sensory fibers are anterior. Thus, over a short distance, motor fibers move posteriorly, while sensory fibers move anteriorly. This takes place over a definite section of the spinal cord, whose length varies in different patients. Occasionally at the C_1-C_2 level, the motor decussation has not been completed and the motor fibers have not moved completely posteriorly, while the sensory fibers remain partially posteriorly (18).

Another important anatomic fact is that when pain fibers enter the posterior root of the spinal cord, they ascend for a few segments and then cross to the opposite ALQ. However, this crossover is not 100%, and occasionally little, if any, crossover takes place. There are authenticated cases where sectioning of one ALQ has produced analgesia on the same side of the body instead of the contralateral side (20).

The pain fibers in the anterolateral quadrant are segmented in that the sacral fibers are close to the dentate ligament, and those from lumbar, dorsal, and cervical regions lie successively anteriorly The upper cervical pain fibers lie close to the anterior horn cells and the respiratory fibers. A cordotomy, which produces a high level of analgesia by destruction of the cervical fibers, tends to destroy the respiratory fibers also (5,13).

Nerve fibers which control micturition lie close to the lateral horn and may be destroyed in any cordotomy. Bilateral cordotomies at any level of the spinal cord may interfere with micturition. Bilateral cordotomies at the C_1-C_2 level may also interfere with respiration. Loss of reticular respiratory fibers bilaterally produces a peculiar form of apnea in which the patient can breathe voluntarily but does not breathe automatically (4). These patients, therefore, tend to develop a form of sleep apnea ("Ondine's Curse"). This respiratory problem can be avoided by carrying out cordotomy on one side, using the lateral approach, and on the other side, using the anterior approach at the C_5-C_6 level; i.e., below the respiratory reticular fibers and below the outflow of the phrenic nerve. Alternatively, a bilateral C_1-C_2 cordotomy can avoid respiratory problems if the level of analgesia is kept below C_7 on one side. If a patient has reduced lung-function, then a unilateral cordotomy will increase the disability by reducing ventilatory power (8).

TECHNICAL CONSIDERATIONS

The anterior approach can be used at any cervical level but usually is done at C_5-C_6. The lateral approach can be carried out only at the C_1-C_2 space, as the anatomic configuration of the cervical facet joints (zygoapophyseal joints) closes the other spaces. The posterior approach can be made at the C_1-C_2 space or between the base of skull and C_1 if a cervicomedullary lesion is to be made. The technique of the lateral approach will be discussed first.

As previously mentioned, the first technique of percutaneous cervical cordotomy described by Mullan in 1963 (11) entailed the use of ionizing radiation to destroy the ALQ. A spinal needle was inserted from a posterolateral approach, and the tip of the spinal needle was placed against the vertebral body anteriorly. Through this needle was inserted a probe tipped with radioactive strontium which was forced against the bone. The spinal needle was then withdrawn to uncover the radioactive-tipped probe, and a mathematical calculation was used to estimate the irradiation time. This technique led to pain-relief in the lower limb in 1 to 2 weeks. Relief of pain in the arm required a higher dose of radioactivity and took longer to develop. Further, the radiation destruction of nerve fibers was progressive. If the patient lived long enough, damage spread to the contralateral side of the spinal cord and even posteriorly; paresis and even paraparesis could develop.

In 1965, Mullan (12) described a modification entailing the use of a direct electrical current to achieve destruction of the ALQ. This worked well, but a period of at least 20 min was required for adequate analgesia to develop. In the same year, Rosomoff and his co-workers (14) used a radiofrequency current which produced thermocoagulation of the nerve fibers in the ALQ. This method produces a very rapid destruction of the nerve tissues; much more care had to be taken to position the needle correctly. Our center has employed a technique for percutaneous cordotomy based upon the work of Mullan and Rosomoff.

LATERAL PERCUTANEOUS CERVICAL CORDOTOMY

Instrumentation. For the lateral percutaneous cervical cordotomy, the patient lies supine with the head fixed in a special head-holder. A spinal needle of sufficient size to allow the electrode to pass through it is used. The electrode has a stop on it so that only 4 mm of its tip protrudes through the spinal needle. Moreover, the terminal 2 mm of the electrode is free of insulation, and the tip is sharpened. A lesion generator is used to produce the radiofrequency current; and the complete apparatus, which includes the head-holder, micromanipulator to raise or lower the spinal needle, the electrode kit and lesion generator, is sold commercially.[1] Commercial lesion generators usually contain facilities for impedance measurements and a range of stimulation frequencies from 2 to 100 Hz.

Technique of puncture. Under local anesthesia, the spinal needle is inserted approximately 1 cm below and behind the mastoid process and advanced into the subarachnoid space anterior to the dentate ligament. Ten ml of air or 1 to 2 ml of myodil emulsion[2] is injected. Air outlines the anterior border of the spinal cord, whereas myodil outlines the dentate ligament (3,4,10,14) (Figs. 1 and 2). Which of these is used depends upon the patient's life-expectancy; if the patient has a long life-expectancy, air is used, because this avoids the risk of arachnoiditis in those patients sensitive to myodil. The majority of my patients have a short life-expectancy due to inoperable cancer; usually, I employ myodil.

---

[1] The apparatus the author uses is that of Owl Instruments Limited, 61 Alness Street, Downs View, Ontario, Canada, M3J 2H2.
[2] The myodil emulsion is made up by shaking 3 ml of iophendylate with 6 ml of saline or CSF in a 20-ml syringe with air.

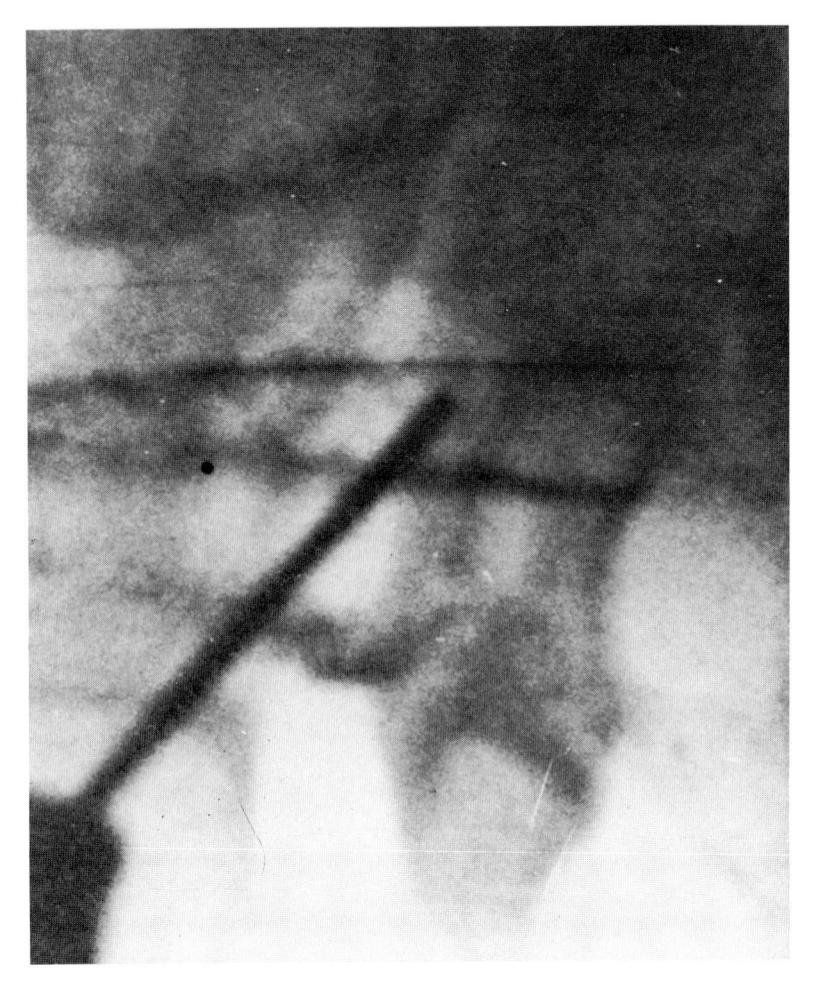

FIG. 2. Close-up of normal appearance after injection of radio-opaque emulsion.

After the injection of air or myodil, the position of the spinal needle is checked by lateral and anteroposterior X-rays using an image-intensifier. The lateral film helps to place the tip of the needle in relation to the dentate ligament or anterior border of the spinal cord (Fig. 3). The anteroposterior film taken through the open mouth allows visualization of the tip of the spinal needle in relation to the pedicles laterally and the odontoid process medially. If penetration is deeper than the lateral border of the odontoid process, the spinal needle has been inserted too deeply (8,10,14,15) (Fig. 4).

The spinal needle is then aimed 1 to 2 mm anterior to the dentate ligament or 3 mm posterior to the anterior border of the spinal cord. Impedance measurements are then used to insert the electrode. When the tip of the electrode is in the cerebrospinal fluid, resistance is about 200 ohms. When the electrode tip is half in the spinal cord and half in the cerebrospinal fluid, the

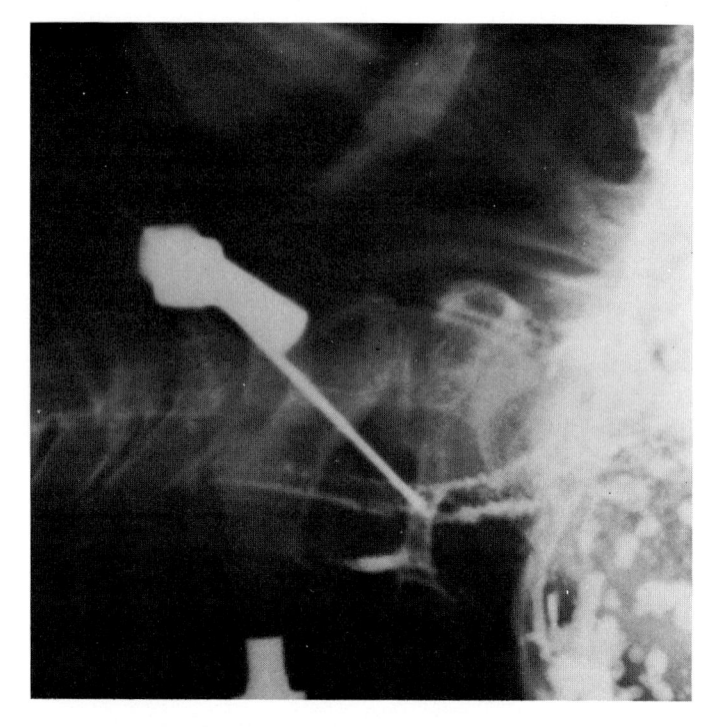

FIG. 3. The hub of the spinal needle is elevated and its tip depressed. Also note that the dentate ligament is depressed.

resistance is slightly higher, approximately 300 ohms. When the tip is entirely in the spinal cord, the resistance rises rapidly to 800 ohms or more.

Stimulation technique. Initial stimulation is at 2 Hz; and at 2 V, stimulation of motor fibers and anterior horn cells may occur. This is shown by rhythmic contractions of the small muscles of the ipsilateral neck causing a turning movement of the head and of the ipsilateral trapezius as well, causing elevation of the shoulder. At this voltage, there should be no activation of arm, body, or leg muscles. If there is, the electrode is too close to the corticospinal tract, and its position must be altered. If the voltage is increased to 4 or 5 V, contractions of the ipsilateral limb or trunk muscles may occur.

Stimulation is then carried out at 100 Hz and 0.2 V; the patient may describe sensation on the contralateral side. These sensory hallucinations may take any form, such as pain, tingling, pins and needles, or sensations of hot or cold wind on the skin. Occasionally, these sensations are ipsilateral, and occasionally bilateral. If consistent ipsilateral sensory hallucinations are produced, the only method of determining whether the patient has an uncrossed sensory tract is by carrying out a small coagulation and observing the development of analgesia. In the author's experience, this has invariably been on the contralateral side; but it must be recognized that sooner or later

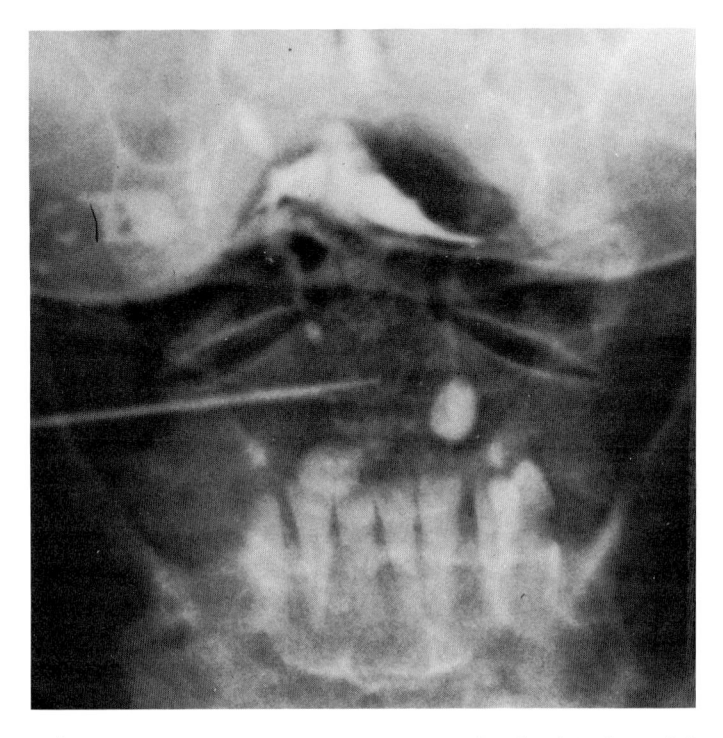

FIG. 4. Anteroposterior view through the open mouth showing the relationship of the tip of the spinal needle and the electrode protruding through it to the odontoid process.

a patient with one of the rare uncrossed sensory tracts will appear, so care must be taken (8,12,19).

Coagulation. Before carrying out coagulation, sensation to pinprick on both sides of the body should be checked; the mere presence of the electrode can produce alterations of sensation in the contralateral side. On rare occasions, the insulated portion of the electrode or even the spinal needle could have been inserted into cord tissue, and this may show itself by a Brown-Sequard syndrome. If penetration of the cord in this fashion occurs, the needle should be withdrawn, the cordotomy postponed and the patient observed for 24 hr. Recovery of normal sensation and power begins in about 15 min and improves rapidly. The following day, the percutaneous cordotomy can be carried out in the usual fashion.

There are two methods of coagulating the ALQ. One is by using a current of about 50 milliamperes (mA) for short periods of time, beginning with 2½ sec and rising to 30 sec in small increments. Testing of analgesia is always carried out between each increment. The second method is to use a time of 30 sec and vary the current beginning with 20 mA, rising to 50 mA and again testing contralateral sensation between each increment. The actual current and time used will depend on the lesion generator; if a commercial instrument is used, these parameters will be indicated by the manufacturer. It is best to err on the cautious side, as a larger lesion can always be made; but damage cannot be eradicated once it has occurred. The series of coagulations continues until analgesia covers the painful area with a few segments to spare. The final coagulation used is repeated 3 times to make sure all fibers in the coagulated region are destroyed.

During coagulation, the ipsilateral arm and leg are carefully observed for the development of weakness: a sign of spread of the lesion to the corticospinal tract. This is quite easily carried out by asking the patient to flex the ipsilateral knee or hold the ipsilateral arm in the air while coagulating. After each coagulation, the grip can be tested as can dorsiflexion of the foot (7).

RESULTS

Analgesia. It is difficult to obtain an accurate figure for this, as many authorities have not published full details (3,8,10). In the author's series, 75% of patients with intractable cancer pain were free of pain until they died. A further 8% had exceedingly good relief of pain, which was not complete but was controlled by simple analgesics, such as aspirin or paracetamol. A further 8% had partial relief of pain which wore off in a variable period, while 9% obtained ineffectual relief of pain or were failures. Of the last two groups, totaling 17%, more than one-third (7%) had successful repeat cordotomies. This brings the total success rate to 90% (8).

Mortality. Mortality depends primarily on selection of patients. In our institution, if the patient is expected to live at least 2 weeks, a cordotomy will be carried out. Over the years, increasingly ill patients have been accepted for the lateral percutaneous cervical cordotomy, and the mortality has increased also. It is now 6.2% in the first postoperative week. The majority of these deaths occurred in patients who had respiratory problems before the cordotomy. The number of percutaneous cervical cordotomies carried out at the Centre for Pain Relief, Walton Hospital, Liverpool, is approaching 700. Fewer than 50 cordotomies have been carried out on patients with long life-expectancies. It is these patients who, in the main, develop dysesthesiae beginning some 6 months postoperatively.

Side effects and complications. Horner's syndrome after a lateral C_1-C_2 percutaneous cervical cordotomy is invariably present in successful cordotomies. It is usually marked in the first few weeks and gradually decreases over a period of months. No cardiovascular disturbances have developed in any of our patients subjected to percutaneous cervical cordotomy. Ataxia is rare but may be masked by weakness and therefore not noted. A few cases have been seen to involve the lower limb and usually improve within 3 weeks. Hemiparesis was present to some extent in 90% of the patients postoperatively. However, 40% of the patients did not have any practical disability; 40% recognized that they had weakness; and 20% were unsteady when they turned around or went up or down stairs due to a weak lower limb. About 10% of the patients had enough weakness to require a walking aid, but the majority of these did not require this walking aid after 1 month. Two percent of patients had a permanent hemiparesis sufficient to prevent them from walking without help. Normally, the leg is affected to a greater degree than the arm; this probably being a reflection of the closeness of the motor fibers to the leg of the ALQ.

Abnormalities of micturition are rare after unilateral cordotomy (1.5%). However, after bilateral cordotomy, urinary problems are much more frequent.

Significant respiratory complications occurred in 8.7%, and approximately half these (4.6%) were fatal. They are very rare after unilateral cordotomy, but more common after a bilateral lesion. These figures are higher than those of most other authorities.

Bilateral Percutaneous Cervical Cordotomy

The two possible complications of bilateral percutaneous cervical cordotomy at the upper cervical level have already been mentioned (14). These are sleep apnea, which has a 50% mortality rate, and problems with micturition, which occur in almost all cases. It is wise, therefore, to consider procedures which can avoid a high bilateral percutaneous cervical cordotomy. Often, a high cordotomy can be combined with an intrathecal phenol block for the pain on the other side. As both these lesions will be made on the same side of the spinal cord, both respiratory and bladder problems can be avoided. Alternatively, a high lateral percutaneous cervical cordotomy can be combined with an anterior percutaneous cervical cordotomy at the C_5-C_6 level.

If a bilateral cordotomy has to be carried out, it is best to have an interval of a week between the two sides, and to aim the electrode on one side cephalad, and on the second side, caudad to try to ensure that the two lesions are not made at exactly the same spinal level. If the analgesic level of one of these lesions can be kept below C_7, there should be no respiratory problems. Great care must be taken when a cordotomy is performed on a patient with pulmonary deficiencies contralateral to the cordotomy (3).

Anterior Percutaneous Cervical Cordotomy

In 1966, Lin (6) reported an anterior approach to the anterolateral quadrant using a lower disk space. The technique consists of inserting the spinal needle through the disk space between C_5 and C_6, entering the subarachnoid space and placing an electrode into the anterolateral tract from

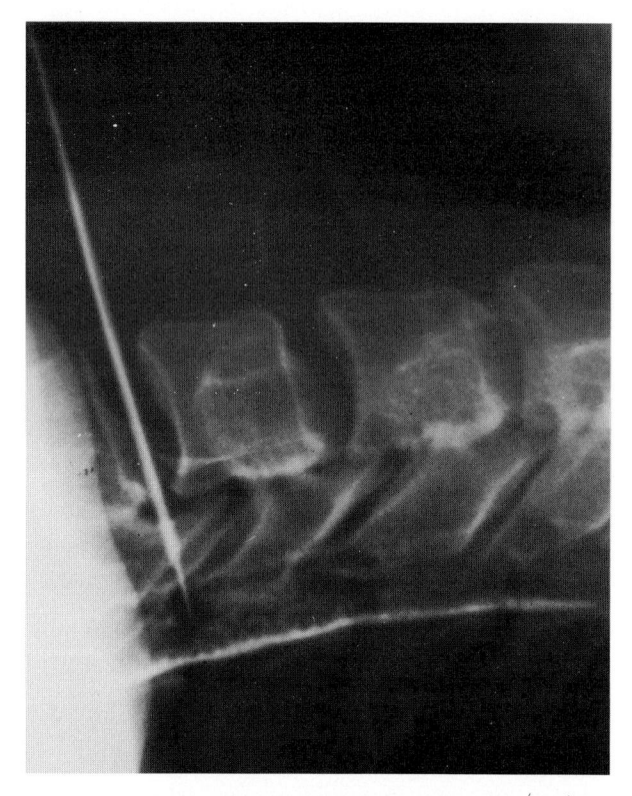

FIG. 5. Anterior-approach percutaneous cordotomy. Note that the spinal needle is in position through the disk space with the electrode protruding. An injection of radio-opaque emulsion has outlined the subarachnoid space with the posterior dura showing up well.

an anterior position. The target is exactly the same as that in the lateral approach, namely 2 mm anterior to the dentate ligament. A series of calculations have to be made from X-ray films to ensure that the direction of the spinal needle is correct. If cervical or thoracic sensory fibers are to be destroyed, the target is 3 to 4 mm from the midline on the contralateral side, whereas for sacral or lumbar pain, the target is 8 mm from the midline. In the anteroposterior direction, the target is 8 mm behind the posterior edge of the vertebral body (Fig. 5).

This technique is difficult because the spinal needle is gripped by the disk material and, once the tip of the needle has entered the disk, its direction cannot be altered. Therefore, this needle must be aimed directly at the target from the very beginning.

The technique is much safer than C_1-C_2 lateral cordotomy because respiratory abnormalities do not occur, as the lesion is made below the outflow of the phrenic nerve. The patient's normal diaphragmatic activity is preserved on the side of the lesion. However, the electrode approaches the sensory fibers by passing through the anterior horn cells, and there is a high risk of damage to the motoneurons. Depending on the level used, there may be weakness of muscles in the upper or lower arm; and, if a lower cervical space is used, in the hand itself. This weakness recovers usually within a week.

Because of the difficulty of approach, a number of stereotactic methods have been designed to help in placing the spinal needle on the correct line (2,9).

Posterior Percutaneous Cervical Cordotomy

Crue et al. (1) reported the technique of using the posterior approach to the anterolateral quadrant of the spinal cord. A bipolar needle is used for recordings, and then the same electrode is used as a monopolar lesion electrode. With the patient lying prone, the electrode is inserted through the skin and muscles of the posterior part of the neck through the C_1-C_2 interspace and thence through the epidural and subarachnoid spaces and into the substance of the spinal cord. A stereotactic frame is used to line up the spinal needle and electrode on the target. The target, of course, is exactly the same as that used in the lateral or anterior approach cordotomy. At the C_1-C_2 level, the target is 3 to 4 mm lateral from the midline; it is assumed that the midline of the odontoid process corresponds to the midline of the spinal cord. The electrode is inserted until it is 1 to 2 mm from the anterior border of the spinal cord.

Stimulation studies are carried out as in the previous techniques with both 2-Hz and 100-Hz stimulation. The position is also checked by X-ray films or through an image-intensifier, and a lesion is made in similar fashion to that previously described for the lateral percutaneous cordotomy. The lesion begins close to the anterior horn and cervical fibers so the initial analgesia tends to develop in the upper part of the body and spreads downward. Lesions closer to the dentate ligament tend to cause analgesia in the lower limb, which spread upward. Posterior percutaneous cervical cordotomy is, therefore, of more value when a high level of analgesia is required.

This technique is more complicated than the other two; and, as the electrode traverses the corticospinal tract, there is more danger of hemiparesis. It requires sophisticated apparatus and highly skilled operators.

CONCLUSION

It is obvious that the techniques of percutaneous cervical cordotomy described in this presentation offer a range of procedures which provide analgesia in the spinal dermatomes. We have found the lateral percutaneous cervical cordotomy the simplest to carry out, although the correct technique must be meticulously followed to prevent complications. Anterior percutaneous cervical cordotomy is technically difficult because the needle is gripped by the intervertebral disk. It does, however, provide a method of avoiding sleep apnea.

The posterior approach has limited application because of its technical difficulty. It has advantages when a very high level of analgesia is required and will produce a higher level of analgesia than the lateral approach. A very small number of patients who have had this procedure have been reported.

The lateral percutaneous cervical cordotomy and the surgical (open) cordotomy provide the most satisfactory and the most profound relief of pain for the intractable pain of inoperable cancer that can be obtained at the present time. The mortality depends on selection of patients; but, because surgical trauma is avoided with the percutaneous technique, its mortality in very ill patients is much lower than that of open (surgical) cordotomy. The lateral percutaneous cervical cordotomy is best for unilateral pain below the C_5 dermatome; but because it has to be performed at the C_1-C_2 space, analgesia may well arise unexpectedly up to the C_5 dermatome; and there is the remote possibility of paresis of the upper limb. For these reasons, when pain is present bilaterally at lumbar and sacral levels, a surgical bilateral, upper-dorsal cordotomy may have advantages in controlling the level of analgesia in patients able to withstand a major operation.

REFERENCES

1. Crue, B. L., Todd, E. M., Carregal, E. J. A., Wright, W. H., and Maline, D. B. (1970): Posterior approach for high cervical percutaneous radiofrequency stereotactic cordotomy. In: *Pain and Suffering—Selected Aspects,* edited by B. L. Crue, Ch. 5. Charles C Thomas, Springfield, Ill.
2. Fox, J. L., and Green, R. C. (1968): Percutaneous stereotaxic cordotomy. II. A guidance technique for the anterior approach. *Acta Neurochir. (Wien),* 18:318–326.
3. Ganz, E., and Mullan, S. (1977): Chapter 2. In: *Persistent Pain—Modern Methods of Treatment,* edited by S. Lipton, pp. 21–33. Academic Press, London and New York.
4. Hitchcock, E., and Leece, B. (1967): Somatotopic representation of the respiratory pathways in the cervical cord of man. *J. Neurosurg.* 27:320–329.
5. Krieger, A. J., and Rosomoff, H. L. (1974): Sleep-induced apnoes. I. A respiratory and autonomic dysfunction syndrome following bilateral percutaneous cervical cordotomy. *J. Neurosurg.,* 39:168–180.
6. Lin, P. M., Gildenberg, P. L., and Polakoff, P. P. (1966): An anterior approach to percutaneous lower cervical cordotomy. *J. Neurosurg.,* 25:535–560.
7. Lipton, S. (1968): Percutaneous electrical cordotomy in relief of intractable pain. *Br. Med. J.,* 2:210.
8. Lipton, S. (1973): Percutaneous cervical cordotomy. *Proc. R. Soc. Med.,* 66:607–609.
9. Lipton, S., Dervin, E., and Heywood, C. B. (1974): A stereotactic approach to the anterior percutaneous electrical cordotomy. In: *Advances in Neurology, Vol. 4: International Symposium on Pain,* edited by J. J. Bonica, pp. 689–694. Raven Press, New York.
10. Mullan, S. (1971): Percutaneous cordotomy. *J. Neurosurg.,* 35:360–366.
11. Mullan, S., Harper, P. V., Hekmatapanah, J., Torres, H., and Dobbin, G. (1963):

Percutaneous interruption of spinal pain tracts by means of a strontium 90 needle. *J. Neurosurg.,* 20:931.
12. Mullan, S., Mallis, M., Karasick, J., Vailati, G., and Beckman, F. (1965): A reappraisal of the unipolar anodal electrolytic lesion. *J. Neurosurg.,* 22:531.
13. Nathan, P. (1963): The descending respiratory pathway in man. *J. Neurol. Neurosurg. Psychiatry,* 26:487–499.
14. Rosomoff, H. L. (1969): Bilateral percutaneous cervical radio-frequency cordotomy. *J. Neurosurg.,* 31:41–46.
15. Rosomoff, H. L., Carroll, F., Brown, J., and Sheptak, P. (1965): Percutaneous radiofrequency cervical cordotomy technique. *J. Neurosurg.,* 23:639.
16. Spiller, W. G. (1905): The occasional clinical resemblance between caries of the vertebra and lumbothoracic syringomyelia, and the location within the spinal cord of the fibers of the sensation of pain and temperature. *Univ. Pa. Med. Bull.,* 18:147–154.
17. Spiller, W. G., and Martin, E. (1912): The treatment of persistent pain of organic origin in the lower part of the body by division of the anterolateral column of the spinal cord. *JAMA,* 58:1489–1490.
18. Taren, J. A., Davis, R., and Crosby, E. C. (1969): Target physiologic corroboration in stereotaxic cervical cordotomy. *J. Neurosurg.,* 30:569–584.
19. Tasker, R. R., and Organ, L. W. (1973): Percutaneous cordotomy. Physiological identification of target site. *Confin. Neurol. (Basel),* 35:110–117.
20. Voris, H. C. (1951): Ipsilateral sensory loss following cordotomy. Report of a case *Arch. Neurol. (Chicago),* 65:95.

Spinal Posterior Rhizotomy and Commissural Myelotomy in the Treatment of Cancer Pain

I. Papo

Neurosurgery Division, Regional General Hospital, 60100 Ancona, Italy

Unlike open cordotomy, which has been widely used for the treatment of cancer pain, spinal rhizotomy and commissural myelotomy have been erratically used and the subjects of controversies. It is beyond the scope of this brief report to deal exhaustively with pathophysiologic and practical aspects concerning these two procedures. Therefore, I shall confine my remarks to data that will help ascertain the proper role of rhizotomy and myelotomy in the treatment of cancer pain.

SPINAL RHIZOTOMY

Spinal posterior rhizotomy has been infrequently used in the treatment of cancer pain for two reasons. First, cancer is a progressive disease which tends to spread and involve the adjacent areas innervated by nerve roots not severed by the rhizotomy. Consequently, the area denervated surgically often becomes too limited to ensure permanent or at least long-lasting relief. Second, the overlap in spinal dermatomes requires that a significant number of nerve roots must be sectioned to produce a band of analgesia broad enough to secure permanent analgesia in the entire area to which pain is referred. This requires an extensive laminectomy which may not be tolerated by debilitated patients with advanced cancer. Moreover, despite the large laminectomy and extensive rhizotomy, there is no guarantee of good results both in terms of quality and duration of pain-relief. In addition, extensive sensory denervation of limbs gives rise to severe disability. For these reasons, even in the past when ablative surgery was much more popular and used more frequently than at present, spinal rhizotomy was used infrequently for the treatment of cancer pain.

Spinal rhizotomy still may be of practical value in two circumstances: When pain is limited to only a few spinal segments, and when the tumor is localized with no tendency to spread into the surrounding regions.

The largest series of patients subjected to dorsal rhizotomy for cancer pain was reported by Barrash and Leavens (2), who operated on 72 patients. In this group the rhizotomy was done in the following regions: cervical, 17; cervicothoracic, 8; thoracic, 25; thoracolumbar, 2; lumbar, 3; lumbosacral, 3; sacral, 13; and thoracolumbosacral, 1. Altogether, 18 additional operations were needed. The results were as follows: complete relief in 40 patients (57%); good relief in 10 (14%); moderate relief in 8 (12%); minimal relief in 5 (7%); and no relief in 5 (7%). In 2 (3%) patients the results could not be evaluated. According to Barrash and Leavens, dorsal rhizotomy is a valuable procedure in the management of cancer pain.

These very favorable results, however, are not borne out by other reports in the literature in which the percentage of early and, more importantly, late failure is significantly higher. White and Sweet (34) treated a total of 34 patients: Early relief was achieved in 19, but pain recurred subsequently due to extension of disease in 4 patients. In 12 patients rhizotomy was ineffective, and finally 2 patients with advanced cancer died. In Loeser's series (18) only 43% of 13 patients operated for cancer pain benefited permanently from rhizotomy. This procedure was effective in only 5 out of 18 patients treated by Onofrio and Campa (20). Loeser and Onofrio and Campa state that preoperative regional anesthetic blocks are not reliable in predicting the later therapeutic efficacy of posterior rhizotomy. However, to make a more precise assessment of the practical value of this operation, the site, type, and extent of pain must be taken into account.

Cervical Rhizotomy

Painful syndromes in the neck are often successfully managed, as White and Sweet (34) pointed out, by sectioning 3 to 6 roots. I have also satisfactorily treated 3 patients by sectioning 3 or 4 roots. In most of these patients, good results are achieved without residual neurologic disorders. However, pain strictly limited to the neck is rather uncommon.

Cervicobrachial Rhizotomy

Posterior rhizotomy has also been used for the treatment of pain in the apex of the chest and/or in the upper arm due to breast (10,20,34) and lung cancer (23). In such cases, often as many as 8 or 9 roots must be divided to relieve pain in the entire area. Such extensive denervation requires a very large laminectomy which cannot be withstood by patients in poor physical condition.

Except for Ray's favorable report (23), in which no details are given, the results reported in the literature are, on the whole, not very gratifying (10,20,34). Even with extensive denervations, failures and early recurrences occur not infrequently. Moreover, as was previously emphasized, extensive rhizotomies lead to severe disability of the upper limb.

In spite of these considerations, Sindou et al. (27) believe that because other procedures attempted for the relief of cervicobrachial pain are often dangerous or ineffective or both, spinal rhizotomy has a definite role in cancer patients with this type of pain. It is especially indicated in patients with not very advanced Pancoast-Tobias tumors and in patients in whom the function of the upper limb is already lost.

Thoracic Rhizotomy

Dorsal rhizotomy of several thoracic segments may be indicated in patients in good physical condition who have severe segmental neuralgic pain caused by metastasis or collapse of a thoracic vertebra. It is also indicated in patients with thoracic segmental pain caused by a localized tumor which is not likely to spread extensively. On the other hand, in patients with thoracic pain caused by advanced cancer and who are predicted to have a short life-expectancy, chemical rhizotomy is preferable.

Sacral Rhizotomy

For the management of sacrococcygeal and perineal pain from pelvic malignancies (rectal or cervix carcinoma), sacral rhizotomy has also been reported by several writers (3,6,7,9,11,20). Guillaume and Sigwald (11) recommend rhizotomy only in cases of pudendal neuralgia and for pain strictly located in the anal and coccygeal region. They believe this operation should not be done for patients with deep pain. Bohm and Franksson (3) reported on 7 patients complaining of superficial coccygeal pain treated by bilateral rhizotomy of the lowermost 2 or 3 sacral roots. In 3 patients, one of whom lived more than 3 years, relief was complete until death, while the remainder developed subsequent pain caused by recurrence of abdominopelvic tumor. Onofrio and Campa (20) reported long-term relief of perineal pain caused by rectal cancer in only 2 of 7 patients subjected to this procedure.

Kuhner (15) treated 4 patients suffering from rectal cancer pain and 1 from prostatic carcinoma pain. In one patient the S_4 and S_5 roots were sectioned, in the remainder, the rhizotomy included S_3 as well. Coccygodinia was permanently abolished in all the patients. Of 4 patients who also had associated pain, complete relief was obtained in 2 and significant relief in the other two.

Crue et al. (6,7,9) advocate the complete section of the dural sheath together with all spinal roots below S_1 using a simplified technique. The whole dural sheath is divided between two ligatures through a small opening in the bone. In patients having good bladder control, S_2 is spared at least on the less painful side. Crue and his associates believe sacral rhizotomy is effective for treatment of perineal, sacral, and coccygeal pain either superficial or deep. The operation should be performed only in patients with pain of at least 3 months' duration, life-expectancy should be at least 3 months, and all the patients should have a previous colostomy. They reported on 29 patients treated with this technique. Of these, 1 died and the results could not be assessed, while the results obtained in the other 28 patients were as follows: satisfactory in 20; fair in 5; poor in 2; and total failure in 1. Sciatic pain associated with perineal pain caused the poor results, both observed in patients with carcinoma of the cervix.

Personally, I have used Crue's technique in 4 patients suffering from superficial and deep perineal and sacrococcygeal pain from rectal carcinoma. All of them had previous colostomies. In 3 patients, phenol rhizotomy had failed to relieve the pain, and in 1 pain recurred 3 months after an effective subarachnoid neurolysis but subsequent neurolytic injections proved ineffective. In all patients but one who had severe drug addiction, pain was satisfactorily relieved. They remained pain-free until death 3 to 8 months after sacral rhizotomy. I should add, however, that despite sparing of S_2 roots bilaterally, vesical function which was already impaired, was permanently lost.

Sacral rhizotomy is of value in the treatment of pain strictly limited to sacrococcygeal and perineal region whether it is deep or superficial. Because of the very limited denervation produced by this procedure, recurrence of pain due to the spread of pelvic cancer beyond the boundaries of the analgesic area is relatively frequent. The procedure fails to relieve sciatic pain even if S_1 is divided and also fails to relieve abdominopelvic visceral pain. Since phenol rhizotomy produces excellent results in most patients with saddle pain, surgical rhizotomy should be reserved only for patients in whom phenol rhizotomy has failed.

POSTERIOR RHIZIDIOTOMY

In recent years, Sindou and his associates (26,27) have suggested a modified technique to achieve selective section of those rootlets considered primarily responsible for nociceptive transmission. They call this procedure *selective posterior rhizidiotomy*. This is achieved by making an incision 1 mm deep into the spinal cord to interrupt the ventrolateral portion of each rootlet supplying the painful area. In this way the pain-conducting fibers are interrupted in Lissauer's tract. Theoretically, rhizidiotomy should obviate the most disabling complication of total posterior rhizotomy. For the treatment of cancer pain Sindou et al. (26,27) performed rhizidiotomy at the cervical and lumbosacral levels, with results which can be considered very worthwhile. Of 16 patients with different pain syndromes subjected to this procedure, 13

(81%) were relieved satisfactorily. Valuable results were also reported by Vlahovitch and Fuentes (31).

Of course rhizidiotomy should be considered only for the treatment of pain involving roots whose section would entail functional disability (e.g., roots subserving the upper and lower limbs). I have done rhizidiotomy on 2 patients with Pancoast's tumors with pain in the upper chest and the upper limb limited to C_8 and T_1 spinal segments. Total rhizotomy of T_2-T_5 was combined with rhizidiotomy of C_8 and T_1. Pain was abolished with no major disability, but the interval for follow-up is still too brief to make a reliable assessment of the results achieved.

Although rhizidiotomy is certainly a more selective and less dangerous technique than total posterior rhizotomy, it is nonetheless a major surgical operation which requires extensive laminectomy. Therefore, its indications are limited and not substantially different from those of conventional dorsal rhizotomy.

COMMISSURAL MYELOTOMY

Commissural myelotomy at different levels and with different techniques is a recurrent topic in neurosurgery. Since this operation was devised for the management of pain by Armour (1) over a half a century ago, its popularity has waxed and waned. Its very attractive theoretical basis may account for such an undulating history. It would seem quite logical that neurosurgeons should aim at producing bilateral pain-relief with a single harmless procedure, which does not damage the corticospinal, respiratory, micturitory, or other main spinal tracts. Unfortunately, the results produced by commissural myelotomy have been far from what one would have expected. Consequently, neurosurgeons have become disenchanted and myelotomy has been abandoned for a period of time. In a paper published in 1976, Lungo and I (21) reviewed the literature, and since then several other reports have been published (5,14,25,29,30).

To begin with, we must distinguish between two kinds of commissurotomies, according to the technique used to divide the anterior commissure: open commissurotomy, which can be done at different levels required by the location of the painful area; and stereotactic myelotomy, as suggested by Hitchcock (12,13), which is performed in the upper cervical spinal cord.

Conventional Myelotomy

Conventional myelotomy aims at dividing the spinal commissures through a perfectly midline incision. Review of the literature reveals that the depth and the extent of the incision have become increasingly greater. In fact, the French authors who first performed myelotomy on a large scale (19,32,33) during the 'forties and early 'fifties, used to make a small incision 3 mm deep and 2.5 to 3 cm long into the spinal cord. Later, Sourek (28) advocated a complete division of the spinal cord in two halves over the length of 2.5 to 4 cm. More recently, Cook and Kawakami (5) and King (14) carried out complete myelotomies of up to 100- to 110-mm long in an attempt to interrupt all the decussating fibers subserving the painful area.

Despite these very long commissurotomies, clear-cut bands and levels of well-defined thermoanalgesia are very seldom observed. In some patients no analgesia at all can be demonstrated. Moreover, the published results achieved by myelotomy are somewhat contradictory. Mansuy and associates (19) and Wertheimer and his associates (32,33) of Lyon in the initial report stated that myelotomy provided satisfactory results in most patients with bilateral pain. However, subsequently they reanalyzed the same material (8) and concluded that myelotomy was effective only for the treatment of vaginal and visceral pain, whereas rectal and lower limb pain were not significantly influenced. Cordotomy, therefore, should be preferred in most patients.

Sourek (29) believes myelotomy is an effective technique for the management of pain located in lower half of the body, whereas pain located in the apex of the chest and in the upper limbs would recur in most cases after cervical commissurotomy. In contrast, Lembcke (16) reported favorable results in all the 12 patients treated with cervical myelotomy. Still different, were the results reported by Cook and Kawakami (5), who succeeded in relieving pain in the upper part of the body with myelotomy but the procedure was unsatisfactory for lower limb pain due to pelvic cancer. Lippert, Hosobuchi and Nielsen (17) pointed out that the results after myelotomy are gratifying in patients with pain located in the midline or in bilaterally innervated structures, but they are much less favorable in patients with spinal or lower limb pain. In Sunder, Plassmann and Grunert's (30) series of 56 patients, 50 of them with cancer pain, permanent relief was obtained in about one-third of the cases.

Stereotactic Myelotomy

Our results (21) with stereotactic myelotomy have been much less favorable than those reported by Hitchcock (12,13) and Schvarcz (24,25). Although immediate relief is obtained in nearly all patients, it very seldom lasts long enough to keep patients pain-free until death among those who survive for more than 2 or 3 months.

General Evaluation

An overall assessment of commissural myelotomy is very difficult for many reasons. First of all, the surgical technique is not yet standardized: There are no reliable, widely accepted criteria for how long the incision should be in order to interrupt all the fibers subserving a given painful area, though it is generally agreed that the depth of the incision should extend to the anterior sulcus of the spinal cord. Secondly, the sensory changes are too unreliable to allow any physiologic appraisal of the effects of myelotomy. Moreover, the mechanism of therapeutic action of commissurotomy is still hypothetical: none of the explanations suggested is substantiated by definite anatomic or physiologic evidence. Although ascending systems are likely to be involved, the reduced transmission of nociceptive impulses brought about by myelotomy is often insufficient to ensure permanent or even long-lasting relief. In a significant percentage of patients when the effects of the surgical trauma wear off and some fibers not divided anatomically recover their previous function, pain recurs.

In establishing criteria for the use of myelotomy in the treatment of cancer pain, the practical drawbacks of this operation must also be borne in mind. Myelotomy is a major surgical procedure that should be considered with great caution and reservation in the treatment of patients in poor condition and with short life-expectancy. Moreover, even with the largest myelotomies there is no reasonable guarantee of long-lasting results. Therefore, this operation should not be considered as a routine procedure in patients with long life-expectancy. Complications must also be considered. Postoperative dysesthesia may be very distressing and sometimes last several weeks. Temporary disorders of propioception or somatic motor disturbances occur in a significant percentage (4).

Considering the location of pain, we have concluded that commissurotomy for upper chest and upper limb cancer pain may be of some value in selected patients, although there are differences of opinion regarding its efficacy for these conditions. As I have already stressed in the discussion of posterior rhizotomy, virtually all techniques suggested for the treatment of cancer pain in these sites fail to produce adequate relief in a substantial percentage of patients. Since there is no standard effective treatment for these unfortunate patients, myelotomy may be indicated in patients with lung cancer in whom respiratory function is already impaired and life-expectancy rather short. In contrast, commissurotomy will not be very effective for the treatment of bilateral lower limb pain from pelvic or spinal cancer. Moreover, abdominal and saddle pain, which may be relieved by myelotomy, is also satisfactorily controlled in most patients with the much less traumatic phenol rhizotomy.

Survey of the literature does not provide useful criteria for selecting patients for commissural myelotomy. Consequently the indications for this procedure still remain a matter of controversy and personal opinions of various writers. Piscol (22) in assessing open spinal operations for cancer pain, recommends myelotomy only for lower trunk pain, but even in these cases bilateral open cordotomy is a much more reliable and no more traumatic operation.

To conclude, I believe that one should be very cautious about recommending commissural myelotomy as the initial therapeutic modality for the relief of pain of advanced cancer. Less traumatic and better-established procedures should be considered before myelotomy. I believe that on the whole, specific indications for myelotomy seem to be exceedingly rare.

REFERENCES

1. Armour, D. (1927): Lettsorian lecture on the surgery of the spinal cord and its membranes. *Lancet*, 1:691–697.
2. Barrash, J. M., and Leavens, M. E. (1973): Dorsal rhizotomy for the relief of intractable pain of malignant tumor origin. *J. Neurosurg.*, 38:755–757.
3. Bohm, E., and Franksson, C. (1959): Coccygodinia and sacral rhizotomy. *Acta Chir. Scand.*, 116:278–284.
4. Broager, B. (1974): Commissural myelotomy. *Surg. Neurol.*, 2:71–74.
5. Cook, A. W., and Kawakami, Y. (1977): Commissural myelotomy. *J. Neurosurg.*, 47:1–6.
6. Crue, B. L., and Todd, E. M. (1964): A simplified technique of sacral rhizotomy for pelvic pain. *J. Neurosurg.*, 21:835–837.
7. Crue, B. L., Todd, E. M., Wright, W. H., and Maline, D. B. (1970): Sacral rhizotomy for pelvic pain. In: *Pain and Suffering*, edited by B. L. Crue, pp. 24–30. Charles C Thomas, Springfield, Ill.
8. Dargent, M., Mansuy, L., Colon, J., and De Rougemont, J. (1963): Les problèmes posés par la douleur dans l'évolution des cancer gynécologiques. *Lyon Chirurgical*, 59:62–83.
9. Felsoory, A., and Crue, B. L. (1976): Results of 19 year experience with sacral rhizotomy for perineal and perianal cancer pain. *Pain*, 2:431–433.
10. Grant, F. C. (1941): Surgical methods for relief of pain. *JAMA*, 116:567–571.
11. Guillaume, J. Sigwald (1947): Coccygodinie rebelle traitée par radicotomie bilatérale de S5. *Guérison. Rev. Neurol.*, 54:60.
12. Hitchcock, E. (1970): Stereotactic cervical myelotomy. *J. Neurol. Neurosurg. Psychiatry*, 33:224–230.
13. Hitchcock, E. (1974): Stereotactic myelotomy. *Proc. R. Soc. Med.*, 67:771–772.
14. King, R. B. (1977): Anterior commissurotomy for intractable pain. *J. Neurosurg.*, 47:7–11.
15. Kuhner, A. (1976): La valeur des interventions sur les racines sacrées dans le traitement des syndromes douloureux du bassin. *Neurochirurgie*, 22:429–436.
16. Lembcke, W. (1964): Ueber die mediolongitudinale Chordotomie im Halsmarkbereich, *Zbl. Chir.*, 89:439–443.
17. Lippert, R. G., Hosobuchi, Y., and Nielsen, S. L. (1974): Spinal comissurotomy. *Surg. Neurol.*, 2:373–377.
18. Loeser, J. D. (1972): Dorsal rhizotomy for the relief of chronic pain. *J. Neurosurg.*, 36:745–750.
19. Mansuy, L., Lecuire, J., and Acassat, L. (1944): Technique de la myelotomie commissural posterieure. *J. Chirurgie*, 60:206–213.
20. Onofrio, B. M., and Campa, H. K. (1972): Evaluation of rhizotomy: Review of 12 year experience. *J. Neurosurg.*, 36:751–755.
21. Papo, I., and Luongo, A. (1976): High cervical commissural myelotomy in the treatment of pain. *J. Neurol. Neurosurg. Psychiatry*, 39:705–710.
22. Piscol, K. (1975): Open spinal surgery for (intractable) pain. In: *Advances in Neurosurgery, Vol. 3*, edited by H. Penzholz, M. Brock, J. Hamer, M. Klinger, and O. Spoerri, pp. 157–169. Springer, Berlin.
23. Ray, B. S. (1943): The management of intractable pain by posterior rhizotomy. *Res. Publ. Ass. Res. Nerv. Ment. Dis.*, 23:391–407.
24. Schvarcz, J. R. (1974): Spinal stereotactic surgery. In: *Recent Progress in Neuro-*

logical Surgery, edited by K. Sano and S. Ishii, pp. 234–245. Excerpta Medica, Amsterdam.
25. Schvarcz, J. R. (1976): Stereotactic extralemniscal myelotomy. *J. Neurol. Neurosurg. Psychiatry*, 39:53–57.
26. Sindou, M., Fischer, G., Goutelle, A., and Mansuy, L. (1974): La radiacellectomie sélective postérieure. Premiers résultats dans la chirurgie de la douleur. *Neuro-Chirurgie*, 20:391–408.
27. Sindou, M., Fischer, G., and Mansuy, L. (1976): Posterior spinal rhizotomy and selective posterior rhizidiotomy. *Prog. Neurol. Surg.*, 7:201–250. Karger, Basel.
28. Šourek, K. (1969): Commissural myelotomy. *J. Neurosurg.*, 31:524–527.
29. Šourek, K. (1977): Commissural myelotomy. *Prog. Neurol. Surg.*, 8:15. Karger, Basel.
30. Sunder-Plassmann, M., and Grunert, V. (1976): Commissural myelotomy for drug-resistant pain. In: *Clinical Microneurosurgery*, edited by W. Th. Koos, F. W. Boeck, and R. F. Spetzler, pp. 165–170. Thieme, Stuttgart.
31. Vlahovitch, B., and Fuentes, J. M. (1975): Résultats de la radicellectomie sélective postérieure à l'étage lombaire et cervical. *Neuro-Chirurgie*, 21:29–42.
32. Wertheimer, P., and Lecuire, J. (1953): La myélotomie commissurale postérieure. À propos de 107 observations. *Acta Chir. Belg.*, 52:568–574.
33. Wertheimer, P., and Sautot, J. (1949): Les résultats de la myélotomie commissurale postérieure (à propos de 69 observations). *Con. Méd.*, 74:413–414.
34. White, J. C., and Sweet, W. H. (1969): *Pain and the Neurosurgeon: A Forty-year Experience*. Charles C Thomas, Springfield, Ill.

Open Cordotomy in the Treatment of Cancer Pain

I. Papo

Neurosurgery Division, Regional General Hospital, 60100 Ancona, Italy

Open cordotomy, either at the cervical or thoracic level, has been one of the most debated topics in neurosurgery for more than 50 years. All technical, pathophysiologic and clinical problems concerning this operation have been exhaustively dealt with in innumerable reports, monographs, and meetings, so that a further appraisal of them appears to be unnecessary. Since the introduction of percutaneous cervical cordotomy 15 years ago and its subsequent widespread use, open cordotomy has been rather neglected and has been the subject of only a few reports. Hence, at present the question arises as to whether it is still rational to perform open cordotomy for the treatment of cancer pain.

Differences of opinion exist regarding the usefulness and indication for open cordotomy for this purpose. Tasker (6), who performs percutaneous cordotomies routinely, believes this procedure can be applied in nearly all patients, even if they are suffering from terminal cancer and in very poor condition. According to him, open cordotomy should be carried out only in the following instances: (a) in uncooperative patients in whom motor and sensory tracts cannot be localized safely by electrical stimulation; (b) in patients with craniospinal malformations in whom no reliable anatomic landmarks are available; and (c) in the unusual cases in which the neurosurgeon is unable to localize sensory and motor pathways. According to Tasker the mandatory indications for open cordotomy would be exceedingly rare.

These opinions, however, are not shared by everyone. For instance, Kuhner (1), who also has ample experience with percutaneous cordotomy, is of the opinion that open and percutaneous cordotomies have the same indications. Percutaneous tractotomy is of course a much less traumatic procedure. However, it has some drawbacks, particularly when a bilateral operation is required. Piscol (5) suggests that open thoracic cordotomy is preferred for the treatment of unilateral or bilateral pain located in the lower half of the body.

In comparing the two procedures, we acknowledge that percutaneous cordotomy is a simple, safe, and effective technique with minimal discomfort for the patients, provided that it is done by experienced surgeons who perform this operation routinely in a large number of patients. If percutaneous cordotomy is done only occasionally, it is likely to take longer to perform and may also be distressing to the patient. On the other hand, open cordotomy done with an operative microscope for magnification is also a safe operation which produces excellent results. Magnification makes anatomic landmarks perfectly clear, and the section of the anterolateral column can be achieved precisely without impinging upon the corticospinal tract. The complication rate of microsurgical cordotomy is negligible, and the level of analgesia is usually satisfactory and long-lasting. Finally, the whole procedure can be completed in 25 to 30 min under general anesthesia.

RESULTS

Analgesia

In the past 2 years I have performed open thoracic cordotomy on 24 patients. In 3 of them a two-stage operation was done at 3- to 6-month intervals. All patients operated on were complaining of excruciating pain in one lower limb mostly from rectal and cervix carcinoma. In all of the patients except 2, extensive analgesia and excellent pain-relief was achieved and persisted until death, which occurred 4 to 12 months later. In 2 patients, despite a very broad section of the anterolateral column, the level of analgesia dropped from T_6 to L_4 in a few weeks, leaving a band of hypalgesia from T_{11} to L_4. Fortunately, both patients had previously been complaining of sciatic pain which was completely eliminated and did not recur.

Complications

No permanent complications were observed with the unilateral operation. However, in the patients in whom pain developed in the contralateral side after the first operation, a second cordotomy on the opposite side resulted in mild weakness of one lower limb and transient urinary retention.

DISCUSSION

On the basis of personal experience, I emphasize that magnification has significantly improved the results of open cordotomy both in terms of quality and safety. In the past, a certain rate of unpredictable short-term failures were observed even with massive open sections of the anterolateral columns (7). Many explanations have been suggested, but none of them is entirely satisfactory. The degree of drop of the level of analgesia remains unpredictable.

In order to establish guidelines for the use of open cordotomy, especially in view of the favorable results produced by percutaneous cordotomy during the past decade, it is necessary to consider the different circumstances in which both techniques are done. If a neurosurgeon performs open cordotomy extensively, the results will be good and the procedure can be used. However, since the vast majority of neurosurgeons do only a few cordotomies a year, the results are likely to be less favorable.

If a percutaneous cordotomy is the routine procedure, I would share Tasker's point of view but on different grounds. First of all, even though open cordotomy under magnification is a safe and effective procedure, it still entails significant surgical trauma and, consequently, there is much more postoperative pain and morbidity, which require a longer hospital stay. Secondly, psychologic factors must also be taken into account: most patients with severe pain of advanced cancer have already been subjected to previous therapy which includes surgical operations with long hospital stays. Consequently, they dislike hospitals and are reluctant to undergo further operations. In contrast, most physicians do not consider percutaneous cordotomy as a major operation and, therefore, this procedure is accepted more readily. Thirdly, percutaneous cordotomy can be carried out in patients in poor physical condition who do not tolerate major surgical operations. Finally, there is no definite evidence that open cordotomy produces better or more lasting analgesia than percutaneous cordotomy (1,2,4).

Some indications for open cordotomy still exist. I believe that for the treatment of bilateral lower limb pain, open thoracic cordotomy should be preferred unless anterior percutaneous tractotomy is performed at a lower cervical level. Moreover, open and percutaneous cordotomies can be properly combined for the treatment of bilateral pain. Open cordotomy is also indicated when neurosurgeons do not perform percutaneous cordotomy. Apart from its specific indications for bilateral lower limb pain, unilateral pain in the lower limb in patients in relatively good condition seems to be the most valuable indication for open thoracic cordotomy. A two-stage procedure is done when pain develops in the contralateral side weeks and months after the first operation.

High or low open cervical cordotomy, as suggested by Mansuy et al. (3), does not seem to provide substantial advantages to warrant its routine use. Finally, for some types of cancer pain, the rationale for open cordotomy, whether unilateral or bilateral, is doubtful when other simpler therapeutic modalities to relieve the pain are available.

REFERENCES

1. Kuhner, A. (1976): La cordotomie cervicale percutanée. *Neuro-Chirurgie,* 22:261–280.
2. Lorenz, R., Grumme, Th., Hermann, H. D., Palleske, H., Khuner, A., Steude, U., and Zierski, J. (1975): Percutaneous cordotomy. In: *Advances in Neurosurgery, Vol. 3,* edited by H. Penzholz, M. Brock, J. Hamer, M. Klinger, and O. Spoerri, pp. 178–185. Springer, Berlin.
3. Mansuy, L., Sindou, M., Fischer, G., and Brunon, J. (1976): La cordotomie spino-

thalamique dans les douleurs cancéreuses. Résultats d'une série de 124 malades opérés par abord direct postérieur. *Neuro-Chirurgie,* 22:437–444.
4. Muke, R., and Correia, A. (1975): Potentials and limits of percutaneous cervical cordotomy. In: *Advances in Neurosurgery, Vol. 3,* edited by H. Penzholz, M. Brock, J. Hamer, M. Klinger, and O. Spoerri, pp. 195–198. Springer, Berlin.
5. Piscol, K. (1975): Open spinal surgery for (intractable) pain. In: *Advances in Neurosurgery, Vol. 3,* edited by H. Penzholz, M. Brock, J. Hamer, M. Klinger, and O. Spoerri, pp. 157–169. Springer, Berlin.
6. Tasker, R. R. (1976): Open cordotomy. *Prog. Neurol. Surg.,* 7:14. Karger Basel.
7. White, J. C., and Sweet, W. H. (1969): *Pain and the Neurosurgeon: A Forty-year Experience.* Charles C Thomas, Springfield, Ill.

Medullary Tractotomy for Cephalic Pain of Malignant Disease

Albino Bricolo

Department of Neurosurgery, Ospedale Civile, 37100 Verona, Italy

In spite of varying reports of its efficacy, it is time to reconsider Sjöqvist's (26) brilliant idea of medullary tractotomy as a neurosurgical procedure for the relief of cancer pain in the face and head. However, we still do not have a method which is always applicable and effective in relieving serious cancer pain in this region. This is due to the fact that nociceptive (pain) impulses from these areas are transmitted by several sensory cranial nerves and possibly by the upper cervical dorsal roots. In addition to the major nerve supply to the face by the trigeminal nerve, some somatic sensory fibers of the facial, glossopharyngeal, and vagal nerves transmit pain from the auricle, external auditory meatus, tympanic membrane, posterior third of the tongue, tonsils, tonsillar pillars, uvula, part of the soft palate, and pharynx (1,2,4,7,9, 13,25,27,29). The relief of severe cancer pain in this region remains a challenging problem (3).

Operations including mesencephalic spinothalamic tractotomy, trigeminal tractotomy, multiple rhizotomy, stereotactic mesencephalotomy, and thalamotomy have been proposed for the treatment of this type of pain (20,22,32). The most widely used operation is the section of multiple sensory roots done through a posterior fossa craniectomy and cervical laminectomy and section of the trigeminal nerve, the nervus intermedius, the glossopharyngeal nerve, the upper vagal rootlets, and the upper dorsal roots of the cervical nerves. Apart from the not infrequent failure to produce complete and persistent denervation of the painful area, this procedure subjects the patient to a significant risk of paralytic keratitis, dyspnea, dysphagia, facial and recurrent laryngeal nerve palsy (23,24,30,32).

An alternative operation could be bulbar tractotomy, which is derived from Sjöqvist's (26) trigeminal tractotomy. This technique is based upon the fact that the pain and temperature fibers of the seventh, ninth, and tenth cranial nerves are located in the medulla and upper cervical cord in close proximity to the descending trigeminal tract (13). This procedure, which Kunc (13,14,15,16) has continued to improve, theoretically is the most physiologic one: A small incision relieves pain in the face and anterior two-thirds of the head with preservation of touch sensation and the corneal reflex. Nevertheless, it has never achieved widespread use and has been abandoned by many neurosurgeons because of unpredictable results. Moreover, there has been a high incidence of complications including ipsilateral ataxia and loss of proprioception, paralysis of recurrent laryngeal nerve, lateropulsion, and contralateral analgesia (4,6,17,31). The failures and complications have been due primarily to errors of identification of the descending trigeminal tract in the medulla.

We believe that many of these problems can be obviated as described by Hosobuchi and Rutkin by localizing the anatomic structures with the aid of a surgical microscope, by using a physiologic means of identifying the descending trigeminal tract (8), and producing a precise lesion of the tract with radiofrequency. Recently, we have introduced two new technical aids which should and have improved the results: monitoring of evoked potentials from peripheral stimulation and using a more refined apparatus for producing the radiofrequency lesion. This is a preliminary report of our experience.

OPERATIVE TECHNIQUE

The operation is done under general anesthesia, with the patient in the prone position and head flexed. We prefer this to the sitting position because it prevents loss of large amounts of cerebral spinal fluid and allows the use of controlled respiration with a negative pressure phase, which serves to decrease the risk of air embolism.

After endotracheal anesthesia is established and before the operation is started, a pin electrode is inserted respectively into the supraorbital, infraorbital and mental foramina, coupled with a second pin electrode inserted into the overlying skin to provide intraoperative stimulation of each branch of the trigeminal nerve. Two other electrodes are applied percutaneously for stimulation of the median nerve at the wrist and the peroneal nerve at the neck of the fibula.

A midline incision is made beginning at the inion and extending caudad to the spinous process of C_5. This provides very ample exposure of the suboccipital region and the posterior arch of the atlas and facilitates the performance of tractotomy and, if necessary, rhizotomy of C_2. If section of the lower cervical sensory roots is also required, this incision can be extended caudad so that the laminectomy can be enlarged. The posterior arch of the atlas is first removed, and then 1 cm or more of the posterior rim of the foramen magnum is removed by approaching it from the bottom with a Cloward-Harper laminectomy rongeur.

Once this is accomplished, a longitudinal dural incision is made starting about 5 mm lateral to the midline, ipsilateral to the patient's pain at the level of C_2 and extending the incision cephalad. As the incision approaches the marginal sinus, it is carried slightly more lateral and any bleeding is promptly controlled. Initially, the dura is incised without opening the arachnoid and is then reflected laterally. Only after achieving effective hemostasis is the arachnoid opened to expose the medulla and the upper cervical cord. A Zeiss surgical microscope is used for the remainder of the procedure to facilitate precise identification of nervous structures. Only minimal traction with a spatula inserted below and slightly medial to the cerebellar tonsils is required to identify the obex.

Anatomic Considerations

A clear understanding of the anatomy of the dorsal surface of the medulla and upper cervical cord is essential for optimum results. Lateral to the important anatomic landmark of the obex, the clava and cuneate tubercle are seen; more laterally and ventrally are the bulbar and spinal rootlets of the accessory nerve as they leave the lateral surface of the medulla. Between the point from which the accessory nerve rootlets emerge and the dorsolateral sulcus that limits laterally the fasciculus cuneatus, lies the tuberculum cinereum, which is the bulge made by the fibers of the descending spinal tract of V overlying the caudal nucleus of the trigeminal nuclear complex. These fibers, which conduct pain and temperature, are the proximal branches of neurons whose cell bodies are in the gasserian ganglion. They enter the pons and then turn caudally at the trigeminal spinal tract terminating below the obex. These fibers become most accessible in the lower medulla near the surface within the tuberculum cinereum.

These descending fibers are arranged in a segmental fashion with the ophthalmic fibers lying ventrally and laterally, the mandibular fibers dorsomedially, and the maxillary fibers between them (4,5,15,21,26,27). Tactile fibers, for the most part, turn cephalad after entering the pons. The sensory fibers of the seventh, eighth, and tenth cranial nerves which transmit pain cross the trigeminal spinal tract at their respective levels and descend with it into the cervical spinal cord (1,4,5,17,27). Kunc's contributions (15) are fundamental to the accurate definition of the topographic relationship between the two tracts. The extratrigeminal facial pain fibers, named by Kunc (15) "tractus spinalis, nervi facialis, glossopharyngii and vagi communis," form a narrow bundle that descends between the fasciculus cuneatus and the adjacent trigeminal spinal tract.

Neurophysiologic Consideration

Since the boundaries of the tuberculum cinereum as well as the posterior sulci of the spinal cord are frequently not easily distinguishable, there has always been a need to localize the descending trigeminal tract by means other than anatomic landmarks (4,11,12). In Kunc's (15) procedure, a more precise position of the tract is determined by a delicate local stimulation with a thin needle with the patient under local anesthesia. This direct mechanical stimulation produces a subjective painful response referred to the area of the face supplied by those fibers being stimulated. This technique, especially when carried out by Kunc himself, permits the operator to perform precise and successful tractotomies (16). Furthermore, with the patient awake it is possible to check immediately the results of the section done and to extend it as necessary. To obtain optimal results, it is necessary to use local anesthesia and to have an awake and intelligent patient who responds promptly and correctly to the stimulation. However, because the fibers of the trigeminal tract are primary neurons (33) and their stimulation is often very painful, the stimulation may impair the patient's cooperation (17) and his responses can be misleading (15–32). Moreover, many patients are so stressed by the operation that they are unable to indicate precisely the area in which they feel the stimulation-induced pain.

In view of this, the recording of evoked potentials from the dorsal surfaces of the medulla and upper cervical cord produced by the stimulation of the peripheral trigeminal, median, and popliteal nerves, as suggested by Mullan (19) and carried out by Hosobuchi and Rutkin (8), seems to be a more practical and accurate neurophysiologic method to delineate the descending trigeminal tract and the adjacent funiculi and to preclude the dis-

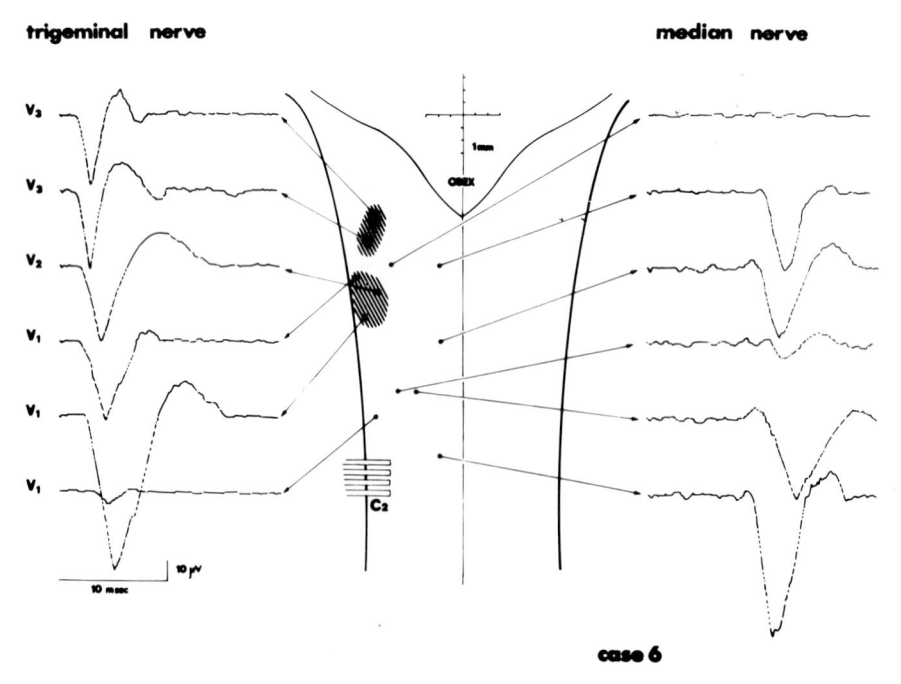

FIG. 1. Case 6 (O.P., 47 yrs). Evoked potentials from the dorsal surface of the medulla and upper cervical cord elicited by ipsilateral trigeminal and median nerve stimulation (monophasic square-wave, 3 Hz, 10 mA, 0.1 msec). Hatching areas indicate radio-frequency lesions.

comfort often experienced with local anesthesia. We have adopted the technique of Hosobuchi and Rutkin (8) which proved very satisfactory, using the O.T.E. Biomedica Neuroaverage 1239 for stimulation and for recording the data.

By monitoring the evoked potentials recorded from the dorsolateral surface of the medulla and upper cervical cord through bipolar concentric electrodes (0.45-mm diameter, 0.07-sq-mm recording area; DISA 9013 K, 0512) it is easy to make a neurophysiologic map that outlines exactly the position of the tract (Fig. 1). The ipsilateral median and/or popliteal nerve is first stimulated, and the dorsal surface of the medulla is systematically explored from the midline in a lateral and caudad-cephalad directions at the emergence of the C_2 posterior rootlets. In this way, we can outline precisely the lateral boundary of the fasciculus cuneatus, which consists of a line beyond which no evoked responses are elicited. After this important boundary is determined, each of the three peripheral branches of the trigeminal nerve is separately stimulated and evoked response recorded from the space between the lateral boundary of the fasciculus cuneatus and the origin of bulbar and spinal accessory rootlets. In this way, it is possible to trace the limits of the descending trigeminal tract and the position within it of the three trigeminal divisions.

Producing the Lesion

Formerly, we made the incision with a scalpel blade prepared so that 5 mm of the cutting edge was exposed. However, now we prefer to produce the lesion with radiofrequency by inserting a stainless-steel electrode insulated with Teflon® which is 0.7 mm in diameter with a 3-mm uninsulated tip into the descending tract to a depth of 1 to 2 mm. Using the Owl Cordotomy System (Model OCS1) and placing the ground electrode subcutaneously in the shoulder region, we make a lesion with a current of 30 mA at 22 to 30 V for 30 sec. This technique permits us to make a precise lesion in the trigeminal tract. If superficial blood vessels are in the way, they are carefully displaced before the electrode is inserted into the medulla.

The majority of authors consider the obex as the most important anatomic landmark in determining the level of tractotomy. However, since the position of the obex is not constant in relation to the inner bulbar structures (17, 32), others prefer to measure the distance from above the uppermost C_2 rootlet rather than below the obex (15). But even these landmarks are far from being reliable, because the distance between them is not constant, varying from 16 to 20 mm.

For these anatomic reasons and other considerations the sites of the incisions used by neurosurgeons have not been uniform. The original incision employed by Sjöqvist (26) in his first procedure in 1938 was much higher, at a level between the middle and the lower third of inferior olive. However, because of certain disadvantages, the level of incision was lowered progressively as far as 5, 6 or 8 mm or more below the obex and extended from the accessory rootlets to the emergence of the C_2 posterior root (5,10,18,28).

The electrophysiologic mapping obtained by evoked responses, which indicates the somatotopic localization of the trigeminal spinal tract, permits us to make the radiofrequency lesions more precisely than do the anatomic landmarks. The point from which the widest potential is evoked by stimulation of the peripheral trigeminal branch is the target zone to be destroyed. Thus, with one or more well-placed lesions, a complete analgesia is achieved of all three divisions of the trigeminal nerve. Moreover, since the pain tracts of the seventh, ninth, and tenth cranial nerves lie between the trigeminal spinal tract and the fasciculus cuneatus, these are also interrupted by extending the lesion dorsomedially to reach the neurophysiologic boundary of fasciculus cuneatus. In addition, the posterior rootlets of the upper two or three cervical nerves can be divided if necessary.

Our previous failures in eliminating pain deep in the ear and posterior oral cavity were probably due to the fact that the incision did not extend dorsally as far as it should have been because of our fear of endangering the fasciculus cuneatus and thereby producing an ipsilateral ataxia.

RESULTS

Ten patients have been treated with the technique described above. These included 7 males and 3 females whose ages ranged from 44 to 71 years. The data are summarized in Table 1. We have had no deaths due to this operation. Despite the poor physical status of some patients due to pain and malnutrition, we were able to discharge all of them from our services. Of these, 8 returned home and 2 were returned to the referral hospital. None had postoperative complications, and those who were able to be out of bed before the operation resumed activities and were able to swallow again. A mild and transitory ataxia in the ipsilateral upper extremity appeared in 2 patients, but none complained of unpleasant dysesthesias or hyperpathia, and those who had no eye neoplastic involvement retained the corneal reflex.

All of the patients experienced immediate complete relief of cancer pain. At their discharge, 1 to 2 weeks later, the results on pain were still very good; 8 patients were pain-free, and 2 developed pain which was less than the original pain. One of the latter, the first operated in this series, developed a pain in the jaw which had been spared by analgesia, and this was due to the fact that the C_2 posterior root had not been sectioned. The second patient (Case 8) in whom pain in the neck persisted, probably would have had complete relief if the C_3 posterior root had been sectioned.

A careful postoperative examination revealed that 9 patients had complete ipsilateral analgesia in all of the three divisions of the trigeminal, as well as analgesia in the distribution of the seventh, ninth and tenth cranial

TABLE 1. *Etiology, site of pain, and results of medullary tractotomy (MT) in 10 patients.*

Case		Age	Sex	Site of pain	Cause	Operation	Pain-relief
1	B.F.	44	M	R. face, ear, throat, jaw	Pharyngeal cancer	MT	Partial
2	C.T.	57	F	L. face, ear, throat	Pharyngeal cancer	MT	Complete
3	C.A.	42	M	R. face, fronto-temp. scalp	Ethmoidal cancer	MT C_1-C_2	Complete
4	B.F.	68	M	L. face, jaw, tongue, throat	Tongue cancer	MT	Complete
5	P.L.	71	M	L. face, tongue, jaw	Lip cancer	MT	Complete
6	O.P.	47	F	L. face, ear, jaw, neck	Pharyngeal ca. cervical metastasis	MT C_2-C_3	Complete
7	B.A.	56	M	L. face, ear, throat	Laryngeal cancer	MT	Complete
8	P.A.	62	F	L. face, ear, neck	Osteogenic sarcoma	MT C_2	Partial
9	M.L.	70	M	R. face, ear, tongue	Maxillary cancer	MT	Complete
10	S.U.	46	M	R. face, neck	Laryngeal cancer	MT C_2-C_3	Complete

nerves (Fig. 2). Tactile sensation was generally spared, even in those patients who had hypoalgesia and analgesia on the face prior to operation as a result of cobalt or surgical therapy. As expected, the neck was also anesthetic in patients who had section of the posterior root of C_3. Our longest follow-up examination has been 6 months, at which time the results were the same as at discharge.

CONCLUSIONS

Our case material is not large enough and the follow-up periods not sufficiently long to allow definite conclusions. However, we feel the following comments are warranted.

The procedure is essentially an extracranial operation. Therefore, it is simpler and less traumatic than any of the other procedures that have been proposed and used for the surgical treatment of pain of cancer of the face and neck. The results of the procedures are quite satisfactory: Pain-relief is achieved while touch sensation and the corneal reflex are preserved, and there are minimal operative risks and complications. In view of this, we wonder why most neurosurgeons prefer a more radical procedure, e.g., multiple rhizotomy, which sacrifices all of the facial sensations in order to relieve

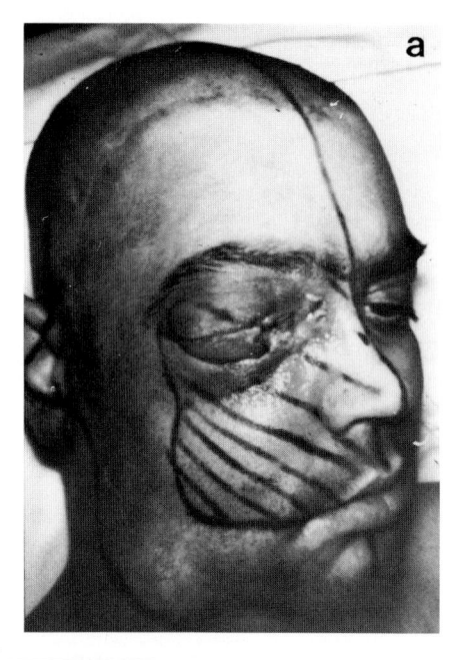

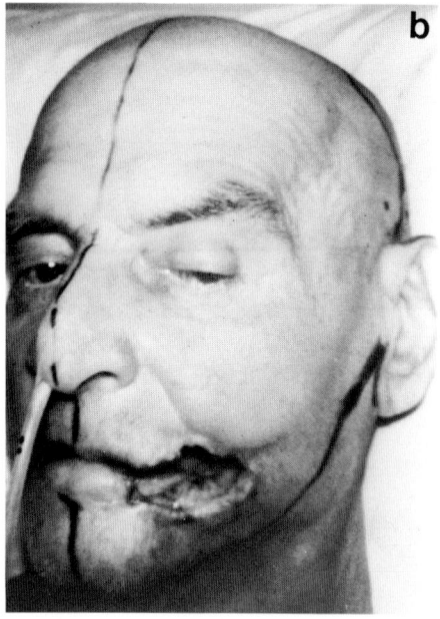

FIG. 2. **A:** Case 3 (C.A., 42 yrs). Complete relief of pain following right-sided medullary tractotomy and section of C_1 and C_2 posterior roots. **B:** Case 5 (P.L., 71 yrs). Complete relief of pain following left-sided medullary tractotomy. Black line delineates area of complete analgesia; hatching that of anesthesia.

pain and why they consider this more physiologic bulbar tractotomy as only of mere historical interest. These attitudes are probably due to inconsistent results obtained because of the difficulty in localizing precisely the trigeminal tract. We believe that now the neurophysiologic monitoring and precise localization of the tract can be achieved, descending trigeminal tractotomy will become the procedure of choice.

ACKNOWLEDGMENTS

The collaboration of Dr. Galeazzo Sciarretta, of the Bioengineering Research Group of Verona, is gratefully acknowledged for arrangement of electrophysiological instrumentation.

I am also indebted to Mrs. Francesca Pistorelli for her help in translation and typing of the manuscript.

The work is supported in part by the N. H. Marastoni Foundation of Verona.

REFERENCES

1. Brodal, A. (1969): *Neurological Anatomy in Relation to Clinical Medicine.* Oxford University Press, Oxford.
2. Crosby, E. C., Humphrey, I., and Lauer, E. W. (1962): *Correlative Anatomy of the Nervous System.* Macmillan, New York.
3. D'Errico, A. (1973): Mesencephalic and medullary tractotomies. In: *Neurological Surgery,* edited by R. Youmans, pp. 1758–1763. Saunders, Philadelphia.
4. Falconer, M. A. (1949): Intramedullary trigeminal tractotomy and its place in the treatment of facial pain. *J. Neurol. Neurosurg. Psychiatry,* 12:297–311.
5. Grant, F., and Weinberger, L. (1941): Experiences with intramedullary tractotomy. *Surg. Gynecol. Obstet.,* 72:747–751.
6. Guidetti, B. (1950): Tractotomy for the relief of trigeminal neuralgia. *J. Neurosurg.,* 7:499–502.
7. Hamby, W., Shinners, B., and Marsh, I. (1948): Trigeminal tractotomy: Observations on forty-eight cases. *Arch. Surg.,* 57:171–174.
8. Hosobuchi, Y., and Rutkin, B. (1971): Descending trigeminal tractotomy. Neurophysiological approach. *Arch. Neurol.,* 25:115–125.
9. Humphrey, T. (1955): Pattern formed at upper cervical spinal cord levels by sensory fibers of spinal and cranial nerves. *Arch. Neurol. Psychiatry,* 73:36–49.
10. Kempe, L. G. (1970): *Operative Neurosurgery, Vol. 2.* Springer, Berlin.
11. Kerr, F. W. L. (1963): The divisional organization of afferent fibres of the trigeminal nerve. *Brain,* 86:721–732.
12. King, R. B., and Meagher, J. N. (1955): Studies of trigeminal nerve potentials. *J. Neurosurg.,* 12:393–402.
13. Kunc, Z. (1960): La localisation des trajets de la douleur des nerfs IX, X et VII dans la moelle allongée et la possibilité de leur tractotomie séléctive. *Acta Neurochir.,* 8:327–334.
14. Kunc, Z. (1965): Treatment of essential neuralgia of the 9th nerve by selective tractotomy. *J. Neurosurg.,* 23:494–500.
15. Kunc, Z. (1966): Significance of fresh anatomic data on spinal trigeminal tract for possibility of selective tractotomies. In: *Pain,* edited by R. Knighton and P. Dumke, pp. 351–363. Churchill Ltd., London.
16. Kunc, Z. (1977): Data obtained by means of trigeminal tractotomy. *J. Neurosurg. Sci.,* 21:115–120.

17. McKenzie, K. G. (1955): Trigeminal tractotomy. *Clin. Neurosurg.,* 2:50–69.
18. Mracek, Z. (1977): Surgical management of intractable pain due to malignant tumours in the face and neck. *J. Neurosurg. Sci.,* 21:123–125.
19. Mullan, J. F. (1971): Personal communication.
20. Nashold, B. S., Jr., Slaughter, D. G., Wilson, W. P., and Zorub, D. (1977): Stereotactic mesencephalotomy. *Prog. Neurol. Surg.,* 8:35–49.
21. Olivecrona, H. (1942): Tractotomy for relief of trigeminal neuralgia. *Arch. Neurol. Psychiatry,* 47:544–552.
22. Pagni, C. A., and Maspes, P. E. (1970): Problems in the surgical treatment of pain in malignancies of the head and neck. *Topical Probl. Psychiat. Neurol.,* 10:138–153.
23. Pagni, C. A., and Maspes, P. E. (1972): The relief of intractable pain in malignant disease of the head and neck by stereotactic thalamotomy or sensory root section. In: *Pain,* edited by J. P. Payne and R. A. P. Burt, pp. 204–207. Livingstone, London.
24. Pagni, C. A., Maspes, P. E., Visca, A., and Bollati, A. (1969): Riflessioni sul problema del trattamento chirurgico delle algie cranio-cervico-facciali da neoplasia maligna. *Min. Neurochir.,* 13:29–33.
25. Reney, R., Reney, A., and Hunter, C. (1950): Treatment of major trigeminal neuralgia through section of the trigemino-spinal tract in the medulla. *Am. J. Surg.,* 80:11–30.
26. Sjöqvist, O. (1938): Studies on pain conduction in the trigeminal nerve. A contribution to surgical treatment of facial pain. *Acta Psychiat. Neurol.,* Suppl. 17.
27. Taren, J. A. (1964): The position of the cutaneous components of facial, glossopharyngeal and vagal nerves in the spinal tract of V. *J. Comp. Neurol.,* 122:389–398.
28. Taren, J. A., Kahn, E., and Humphrey, T. (1969): The surgery of pain. In: *Correlative Neurosurgery,* edited by E. Kahn et al., pp. 464–508. Charles C Thomas, Springfield, Ill.
29. Walker, A. E. (1966): Neuralgias of the glossopharyngeal, vagus, and intermedius nerves. In: *Pain,* edited by R. Knighton and P. Dumke, pp. 421–429. Churchill Ltd., London.
30. Wetzel, N. (1966): The relief of pain of malignant disease in the head and neck by sensory root section. In: *Pain,* edited by R. Knighton and P. Dumke, pp. 431–437. Churchill Ltd., London.
31. White, J. C. (1962): Evaluation of operations for relief of pain. *Neurol. Méd-chir.,* 4:1–28.
32. White, J. C., and Sweet, W. H. (1969): *Pain and the Neurosurgeon.* Charles C Thomas, Springfield, Ill.
33. Zverina, E. (1977): Location of trigeminal neuralgia development. Preoperative stimulation of descending trigeminal tract. *J. Neurosurg. Sci.,* 21:109–110.

Percutaneous Thermocoagulation of the Gasserian Ganglion in the Treatment of Pain in Advanced Cancer

*Jean Siegfried and **Giovanni Broggi

*Neurochirurgische Klinik, Universitätsspital Zürich, CH-8091 Zürich, Switzerland; and
**Division of Neurosurgery, Istituto Neurologico "C. Besta," via Celoria, 11, 20133 Milano, Italy

Percutaneous controlled thermocoagulation of the gasserian ganglion permits a clinically complete or partial selective destruction of pain fibers with preservation of some touch sensitivity, carries little stress or danger, has a low complication rate, and can be performed on old patients and/or those in poor general condition with the patient practically ambulatory throughout. After being established as one of the operations of choice in the neurosurgical treatment of classic idiopathic trigeminal neuralgia, its use in symptomatic facial pain appears promising. In our first 6 patients with metastatic or direct invasion of the middle fossa and/or of the face by carcinoma, we obtained good relief of pain (11). Now we have had more experience in patients with pain in one or more trigeminal divisions caused by advanced cancer and managed in two different hospital centers. This report contains a summary of our results.

METHODS AND MATERIALS

In the 6-year period extending from February 1972, to February 1978, 1,106 patients have been operated on in Zürich (742) and Milan (364) for trigeminal pain. In these rather large series, only 20 patients (12 in Zürich, 8 in Milan) were suffering from symptomatic trigeminal pain of advanced cancer. The youngest patient was 37 years old and the oldest 80 years old. The age distribution shows that the majority of patients were between 60 and 70 years old.

The sites of the cancer producing pain in one or more trigeminal divisions are listed in Table 1, and the diagnosis of cancer is listed in Table 2. The general condition of all patients was poor to very poor. They were suffering

TABLE 1. *Site of the cancer producing pain in one or more trigeminal divisions*

Site	No. of pts.
Mandible	5
Epipharynx-mandible	4
Tongue	3
Base of the skull	3
Cerebellar angle	2
Middle fossa	2
Ear-mandible	1

from intractable pain, and most of them were taking narcotics. Carbamazepine was tried in all cases without success. Preoperatively, a diminution of sensitivity (hypesthesia and hypalgesia) was found in 9 patients and hyperpathia noted in 5 patients.

In each patient the technique of percutaneous controlled thermocoagulation of the gasserian ganglion described by Sweet (15) and subsequently by us (12) was used. The anterior approach of Härtel (6) to the foramen ovale with local anesthesia or in some cases with a short-lasting intravenous general anesthetic was used. The needle is introduced into the skin usually 3.0 cm lateral to the labial commissure. The visual landmarks for direction of the electrode are derived from the intersection of a plane 3 cm in front of the ear canal with that passing through the middle of the pupil. Lateral and submento-vertex X-ray views confirm the position of the electrode in the gasserian ganglion through the foramen ovale. For localization of the electrode within the ganglion, low-voltage stimulation (100 to 300 mV, 60-cycle square-wave pulse of 1-msec duration) was performed; nonpainful sensation of itching or tingling in the field of projection of one, two, or sometimes three divisions of the trigeminal nerve permits correct adjustment of the position of the electrode tip. Under an ultra-short-acting barbiturate, one or more radiofrequency coagulations with a temperature of 60°C to 70°C for 1 min are carried out until a dense hypalgesia or analgesia to pinprick in the division mediating the pain is obtained.

TABLE 2

Diagnosis	No. of pts.
Carcinoma	9
Metastasis	5
Fibrosarcoma	4
Cylindroma	2

RESULTS

In patients with cancer pain, a long follow-up is not possible. Moreover, 5 patients could not be evaluated for more than a few weeks after the operation and did not answer the questionnaire we sent them after discharge. Dramatic pain-relief was observed immediately after the operation in all patients, but this relief lasted only a few days in 5 patients. In 6 patients the pain recurred slowly after 1 month, when it was still much less intense than before the operation; but subsequently it gradually became worse and eventually was as intense as before the operation.

Table 3 summarizes the follow-up and shows that about one-half of the patients operated on got very good benefit from the operation with long-

TABLE 3. *Follow-up time and results*

Follow-up	No. of pts.	Pain-free	Less pain	No effect
1 month	20	9	6	5
3 months	15 (2)[a]	9	0	6
12 months	10 (3)[a]	7	0	3
18 months	5 (1)[a]	2	0	3
24 months	2	1	0	1

[a] In bracket: up to death.

lasting effect. The diagnosis of the cancer pain does not play any role, but the site of the cancer producing pain is decisive. As long as the pain is localized in one or more trigeminal divisions, one can expect a favorable result. In two cases, further improvement was obtained with an additional thermorhizotomy of glossopharyngeal nerve. Three cases with bone destruction and deep, burning pain were not improved.

Analgesia with hypesthesia was noted in all the patients, and total anesthesia developed in 3 patients. No complications occurred, except itching which was reported by 5 patients.

DISCUSSION

Face and throat pain in advanced cancer pain are common, and the incidence of severe and intractable pain is higher than with malignancy at other sites. Rather surprisingly, the number of patients operated on by us is very small in view of our large experience with the surgical management of facial pain. Cancer pain in the trigeminal region represents only 1.8% of our operations for trigeminal pain. The diagnosis of the cause of pain usually is seen as manifestly clear in patients with demonstrated tissue damage due to the neoplastic disease, and complaints have often a major emotional component.

However, the patients generally state or imply that the emotional effects are necessarily secondary to the pain rather than a primary cause of pain (16). We are thus involved with a chain of morbid processes in which a primary disorder (cancer pain) leads to a second component (emotional pain), which in turn aggravates the first one. In this vicious circle, neurosurgery has a role to play, and pain produced by cancer is certainly one of the best indications for pain surgery.

Combined multiple rhizotomies of cranial nerves and upper cervical nerves are old methods (2,3) and are still indicated in control of pain from malignant tumors involving the face, head, and neck (8,9). A review of several important series made by Sindou et al. (13), included a total of 254 patients of deep and/or extensive cervical and cervicofacial cancers treated by different cranial nerve operations often combined with upper cervical rhizotomy. Of the total, 53% of the patients derived good results (generally short survival), and there was an 18% mortality. The high mortality rate could be explained by the almost invariably precarious state of the patient operated on and the extensive trauma produced by the surgery. The same interpretation can be given for other techniques. Gros et al. (4) reported 24 cases of cervicofacial pain due to cancer, for which they combined an upper cervical rhizotomy and a medullary trigeminal tractotomy complemented by section of the ninth cranial nerve in all the cases and by section of the tenth nerve in 5 cases. They obtained good initial results in 70% of the patients; but this decreased 44% until death, which occurred, on an average, around the sixth month after the operation. Their mortality rate was about 20% (4).

Destruction of only one or two cranial nerves for face and throat pain are rarely mentioned. In his personal experience of 1,433 patients with facial pain treated with alcohol injection of trigeminal nerve, Harris (5) had very few patients with symptomatic pain caused by disseminated sclerosis, antral abscess, sinusitis, etc., but none had advanced cancer. In a series of 637 patients subjected to extradural preganglionic neurotomy (Spiller-Frazier operation), Ruge (10) mentions only one case of carcinoma.

The introduction of the percutaneous coagulation technique by Sweet has led to a resurgence of interest in the neurosurgical treatment of trigeminal pain and its use in cases of advanced cancer. Sweet (14) himself reported on a series of 20 patients of whom 4 were completely relieved until death from 3 weeks to 3 months later. The remainder, after varying short periods of partial or total relief, had recurrence of pain on the same or the opposite side as the lesion spread. Single cases have been reported with success by others (1,7,11).

Our personal experience with this technique in patients with cancer pain suggests the following indications and guidelines:

1. The pain caused by cancer must be localized and tissues supplied by one or more trigeminal branches.

2. If the glossopharyngeus nerve is involved in the pain process, percutaneous thermocoagulation of this nerve can be combined with that of the gasserian ganglion.
3. The preexistence of anesthesia and/or analgesia in the pain area due to destruction of trigeminal roots by the cancer itself is a contraindication to the operation, because the goal of the procedure (analgesia) is already present. An anesthesia or analgesia dolorosa cannot be cured by surgical interruption of pain pathways.
4. Patients with deep, burning pain involving nerve fibers other than those in the trigeminal nerve will derive little or no relief from thermocoagulation of the gasserian ganglion.

SUMMARY

Under strict indications, good to very-good relief of facial cancer pain can be achieved by the percutaneous, controlled thermocoagulation of the gasserian ganglion. This is a procedure devoid of stress, suitable for old patients as well as patients in poor general condition, and has a low complication rate. A series of 20 cases is reported and the indications discussed.

REFERENCES

1. Broggi, G. (1975): Thermorhizotomy in trigeminal neuralgia: Preliminary considerations in 46 cases. *Adv. Neurosurg.,* 3:297–300.
2. Dandy, W. E. (1929): Operative relief from pain in lesions of the mouth, tongue and throat. *Arch. Surg. (Chicago),* 19:143–148.
3. Fay, T. (1926): Intracranial division of glossopharyngeal nerve combined with cervical rhizotomy for pain in inoperable carcinoma of the throat. *Ann. Surg.,* 84:456–459.
4. Gros, C., Cordier, M., Vlahovitch, B. and Roilgen, A. (1963): Neurotomie combinée et traitement des algies cervico-cranio-faciales d'origine néoplasique. *Ann. Chir.,* 17:533–539.
5. Harris, W. (1940): An analysis of 1433 cases of paroxysmal trigeminal neuralgia (trigeminal-tic) and the end-results of Gasserian alcohol injection. *Brain,* 63:209–224.
6. Härtel, F. (1914): Die Behandlung der Trigeminusneuralgie mit intrakraniellen Alkoholeinspritzungen. *Deutsch. Z. Chir.,* 126:429–552.
7. Onofrio, B. M. (1975): Radiofrequency percutaneous Gasserian ganglion lesions. Results in 140 patients with trigeminal pain. *J. Neurosurg.,* 42:132–139.
8. Pagni, C. A., and Maspes, P. E. (1970): Problems in the surgical treatment of pain in malignancies of the head and neck. *Topical Prob. Psychiat. Neurol.,* 10:138–153.
9. Pagni, C. A., and Maspes, P. E. (1972): The relief of intractable pain in malignant disease of the head and neck by stereotactic thalamotomy or sensory root section. In: *Pain,* edited by R. Janzen, W. D. Keidel, A. Herz, and C. Steichele. Georg Thieme Verlag, Stuttgart.
10. Ruge, D., Brochner, R., and Davis, L. (1958): A study of the treatment of 637 patients with trigeminal neuralgia. *J. Neurosurg.,* 15:528–536.
11. Siegfried, J. (1977): 500 percutaneous thermocoagulations of the Gasserian ganglion for trigeminal pain. *Surg. Neurol.,* 8:126–131.
12. Siegfried, J., and Vosmansky, M. (1975): Technique of the controlled thermoco-

agulation of trigeminal ganglion and spinal roots. *Adv. Tech. Standards Neurosurg.,* 2:199–209.
13. Sindou, M., Fischer, G., and Mansuy, L. (1976): Posterior spinal rhizotomy and selective posterior rhizidiotomy. *Prog. Neurol. Surg.,* 7:201–250.
14. Sweet, W. H. (1976): Controlled thermocoagulation of trigeminal ganglion and rootlets for differential destruction of pain fibers: Facial pain other than trigeminal neuralgia. *Clin. Neurosurg.,* 23:96–102.
15. Sweet, W. H., and Wepsic, J. G. (1974): Controlled thermocoagulation of trigeminal ganglion and rootlets for differential destruction of pain fibers. Part 1: Trigeminal neuralgia. *J. Neurosurg.,* 40:143–156.
16. Woodforde, J., and Fielding, J. R. (1975): Pain and cancer. In: *Pain,* edited by M. Weisenberg, pp. 326–331. C. V. Mosby Co., St. Louis.

Percutaneous Differential Radiofrequency Rhizotomy of Glossopharyngeal Nerve in Facial Pain Due to Cancer

*Giovanni Broggi and **Jean Siegfried

*Division of Neurosurgery, Istituto Neurologico "C. Besta," via Celoria 11, 20133 Milan, Italy; and **Neurochirurgische Universitätklinik, Kantonsspital Zurich, 100 Ramistrasse, Zürich, 8022, Switzerland

Pain sensitivity of the face and the anterior part of the tongue depends on the trigeminal nerve, while the external ear, oropharynx, larynx, epipharynx, and posterior part of the tongue are innervated by the glossopharyngeal and vagal nerves. The surgical treatment of pain in all these regions may include the partial or total section of these three nerves (7).

After the introduction of percutaneous radiofrequency (RF) differential trigeminal rhizotomy (5) for treatment of trigeminal neuralgia, pain due to cancer in the territory of the trigeminal nerve innervation also has been successfully treated by this technique (Siegfried and Broggi, *this volume*). However, facial pain due to cancer is seldom confined to the trigeminal territory, especially when the base of the skull has been invaded by metastases or there is diffusion of the primary tumor.

Until recently, the surgical treatment of 9th and 10th nerve neuralgia entailed opening of the posterior fossa or extracranial section of the nerve at the posterior foramen lacerum. However, this second surgical approach is not easy in the presence of a tumor or when tissues are modified by previous radiation therapy.

Moreover, the approach to the 9th and 10th nerves through the posterior fossa is not free of operative risk, even when a microsurgical technique is used (4). This operative risk is increased in the cancer patient, who is usually debilitated by the disease and by chemotherapy. Selective bulbar tractotomy (3), indicated when both trigeminal and glossopharyngeal neuralgia are present, poses a similar surgical risk.

Recently (1,6) a percutaneous approach like the one successfully used for trigeminal neuralgia has been proposed for treatment of glossopharyngeal neuralgia. We now suggest the use of this technique for treatment of facial and rhinopharyngeal pain due to cancer.

METHODS AND MATERIAL

In our departments during the past year we have treated 4 patients with glossopharyngeal neuralgic pain with percutaneous RF differential rhizotomy of the 9th nerve at the extracranial side of the posterior foramen lacerum. Two of these patients had cancer of the face.

Case 1 (INM). Male, 50 years old; had a carcinoma of the larynx treated by direct surgery and by two courses of radiation therapy. The pain was located in the right face, in the territory of the 2nd and 3rd trigeminal root, in the ear, in the external auditory canal, and in the tonsillar pillar. The trigeminal pain was continuous, unbearable, burning. The 9th nerve pain was paroxysmal and of the lightning type, triggered by swallowing.

On April 4, 1977, percutaneous RF differential rhizotomy of the trigeminal nerve was done, and 10 days later this same technique was used to produce a rhizotomy of the glossopharyngeal nerve. The pain in the face completely disappeared with analgesia in the territory of the trigeminal nerve. The glossopharyngeal neuralgia also disappeared, but 6 months later the patient had a recurrence of this pain, and on October 3, 1977, a second percutaneous RF rhizotomy of the glossopharyngeal nerve was performed. To date, the patient has remained pain-free. No neurological deficit followed the surgery except for the sensory deficit in the territory of the 5th and 9th nerves. No cardiac problems were present either during or after the surgery.

Case 2 (KSZ). A 68-year-old female had carcinoma of the epipharynx with

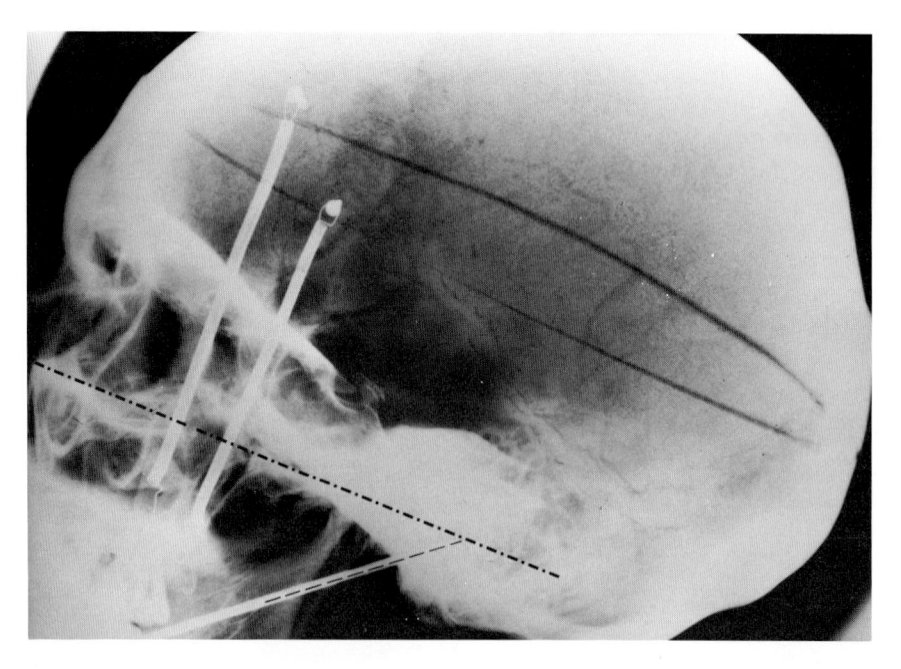

FIG. 1. Lateral X-ray of the dry skull, with the needle inserted in the pars nervosa of the posterior foramen lacerum. Note the angle to the plane passing through the internal auditory meatus and the inferior margin of the orbit.

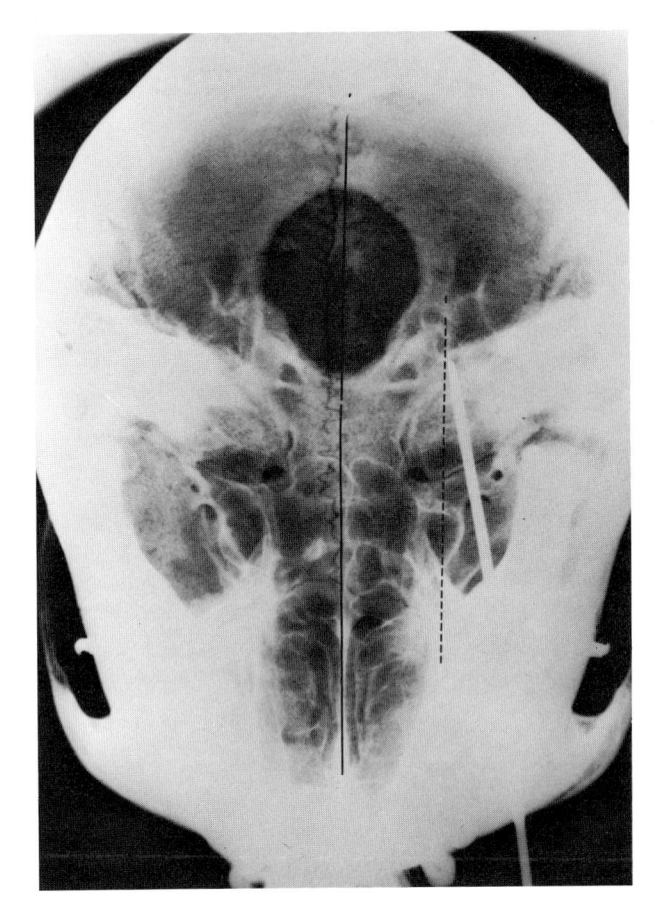

FIG. 2. A-P view of the X-ray of the dry skull. The needle is inserted in the pars nervosa of the posterior foramen lacerum. Note the angle to the plane parallel to the midsagittal plane.

pain referred to the mandibular region accompanied by typical glossopharyngeal neuralgia on the left. On January 31, 1978, she underwent in a single session trigeminal and glossopharyngeal percutaneous RF differential rhizotomies. Promptly after the procedure, she had pain-relief associated with analgesia in the mandibular and lower lip regions. She also had difficulty in swallowing, which lasted for 3 weeks and a permanent deficit of the left 12th cranial nerve. No other neurologic deficits followed this percutaneous surgery. She has remained pain-free to the present time.

TECHNIQUE

The technique of 9th nerve percutaneous rhizotomy is similar to the percutaneous approach to the trigeminal ganglion (1). The needle is inserted into the skin of the cheek 2.5 mm lateral to the labial commissure, and is directed under fluoroscopic control along two planes: one of a 12° angle to

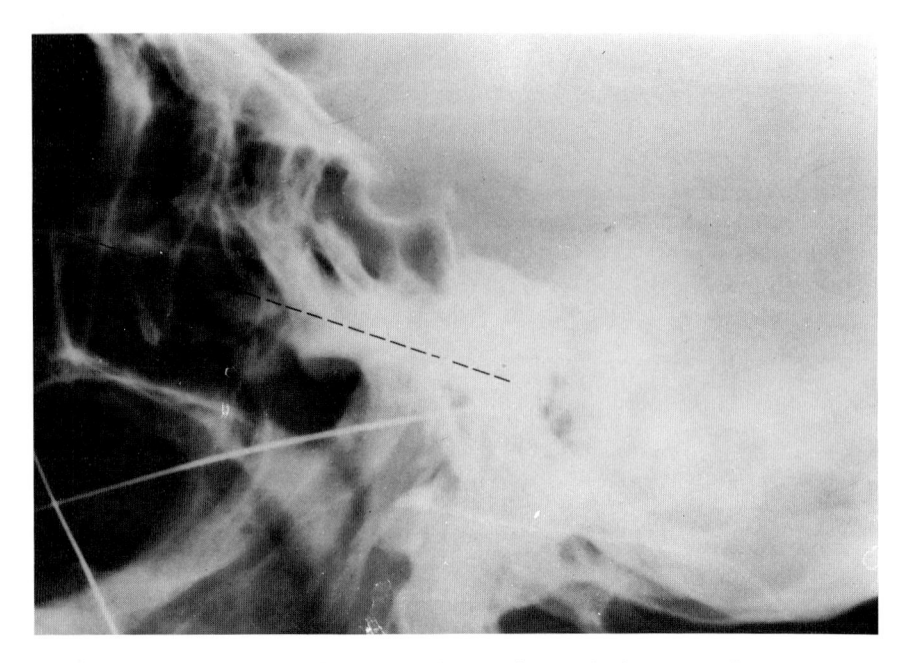

FIG. 3. Case no. 1: Lateral view of the X-ray taken with the image fluoroscopic intensifier. Note that the needle inserted in the position where RF coagulation was performed after electrophysiological control makes an angle to the plane passing through the internal auditory meatus and the inferior margin of the orbit equal to that in the model in Fig. 1.

the vertical plane passing through the pupil of the eye, the second at a 40° angle to the plane passing through the internal auditory meatus and the inferior margin of the orbit.

The needle is advanced to a point lateral to the internal carotid artery where its tip should be at the medial portion of the posterior lacerum. This position is checked with X-ray, then electrophysiologic control is carried out by checking the impedance and evoking 9th, 10th, and 12th nerve responses to confirm the exact position of the needle. EKG monitoring is also recommended. Thiopental sodium (Pentothal®) is administered as a single bolus before the RF coagulation in order to produce amnesia and partial analgesia. The temperature of the probe should be kept between 65°C and 75°C. The lesion is repeated if intraoperative evaluation indicates this is necessary.

Despite the necessity to pass through the tumor or through a tissue hardened by radiation therapy, no difficulties greater than those encountered in noncancer patients have been experienced.

DISCUSSION

A tumor that causes glossopharyngeal neuralgia is rare, but Dandy (2) has also reported a similar case in 1927. In our series, glossopharyngeal nerve involvement in facial pain due to cancer is not infrequent. On the basis of our very limited experience with these 2 patients, we speculate that graded RF percutaneous rhizotomy is a safe and successful technique for the treatment of glossopharyngeal pain due to cancer. It produces minimal trauma, and it can be easily applied to debilitated patients. Since facial pain due to cancer often is not limited to single cranial-nerve involvement, the surgeon can perform the two rhizotomies within a few days or even in the same session as in our second case. Moreover, the hospitalization period is very short, and there is no postoperative pain or morbidity which often follows general anesthesia in the sitting position. Also, the procedure is more readily accepted by patients who believe that it entails no more than a needle puncture. Finally, the operative risk is almost nil, with no mortality and a very selective morbidity.

REFERENCES

1. Broggi, G. (submitted): Percutaneous differential radiofrequency rhizotomy of the glossopharyngeal nerve. *Surg. Neurol.*
2. Dandy, W. E. (1927): Glossopharyngeal neuralgia (tic douloureux): Its diagnosis and treatment. *Arch. Surg.,* 15:198–214.
3. Kunc, Z. (1965): Treatment of essential neuralgia of the ninth nerve by selective tractotomy. *J. Neurosurg.,* 23:494–500.
4. Laha, R. K., and Jannetta, P. J. (1977): Glossopharyngeal neuralgia. *J. Neurosurg.,* 47:313–320.
5. Sweet, H. W. (1976): Treatment of facial pain by percutaneous differential thermal trigeminal rhizotomy. *Prog. Neurol. Surg.,* 7:153–179.
6. Tew, J., Jr. (1977): Percutaneous rhizotomy in the treatment of intractable facial pain (trigeminal, glossopharyngeal and vagal nerves). In: *Current Techniques in Operative Neurosurgery,* edited by H. H. Schimedek and W. H. Sweet, pp. 409–426. Grune & Stratton, New York.
7. White, J. C., and Sweet, W. H. (1970): *Pain and the Neurosurgeon: A Forty Year Experience,* pp. 265–302. Charles C Thomas, Springfield, Ill.

Stereotaxic Thalamolaminotomy and Posteromedial Hypothalamotomy for the Relief of Intractable Pain

Keiji Sano

Department of Neurosurgery, University of Tokyo, Tokyo, Japan

The word *pain* has two meanings, one is the pain sensation and the other the suffering. Or one can say that the pain has two aspects, the sensory-discriminative and the emotional-motivational. This is also true with *il dolore, la douleur,* or *der Schmerz.* Moreover, pain sensation can be classified into the truly discriminative "epicritic" pain and the diffuse, or poorly localized "protopathic" pain.

Intractable pain is mainly concerned with this protopathic pain and the associated suffering. The ideal treatment of pain is to cure or minimize the protopathic pain and the suffering without impairing epicritic, discriminative pain sensation. With thalamolaminotomy and posteromedial hypothalamotomy, we are able to achieve such desired results.

THALAMOLAMINOTOMY (INTRALAMINAR THALAMOTOMY)

Since stereotaxic procedures were introduced, but especially during the last three decades, most of our surgical efforts to relieve pain have been concentrated in various parts of the thalamus. In our clinic, one operative procedure on the internal medullary lamina for the relief of intractable pain, which we call intralaminar thalamotomy, or thalamolaminotomy, has been carried out since 1963 (12). The internal medullary lamina comprises the intralaminar nuclei [n. centralis lateralis (CL), centre médian (CM), n. limitans (Lim), etc.] and their adjacent fibers. Standard stereotaxic techniques were used for stimulation and recording at the time of thalamotomy. The technique of the procedure has been reported in detail elsewhere (9,10, 12,13) and is illustrated in Fig. 1.

Clinical Investigations

Neuronal Unit Discharge

In recent cases, before inserting stimulating or lesion-making needles, we have inserted tungsten microelectrodes, 5–10 Megohms, with the tip 1 to 2

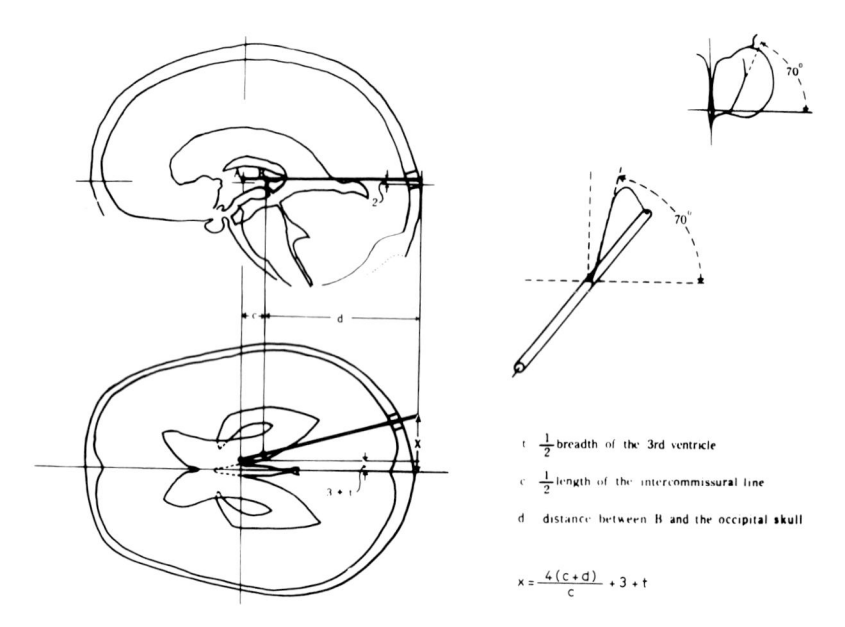

FIG. 1. Technique of thalamolaminotomy. A = point 2–4 mm above the midpoint of the intercommissural line and 3 mm lateral to the wall of the third ventricle. B = point 2–4 mm above the posterior commissure and 7 mm lateral to the wall of the third ventricle. (Courtesy of Sano, K. (1977): In: *Progress in Neurological Surgery*, edited by H. Krayenbühl et al. 8:50–103. Karger Basel.)

μm in diameter, into the brain, in order to investigate spontaneous and evoked neuronal unit discharges from various areas near the target area. With pin pricks of the skin over the wide areas of the body and extremities, both contra- and ipsilateral increase of unit discharge was observed in the nucleus parafascicularis and the center median. Some units also responded to the application of heat to the skin, but did not respond to tactile stimulation.

We have found two types of units, fast-responding and slow-responding. The former units responded with a latency of about 30 to 40 msec and showed a shorter duration of discharge. The latter units responded with a long latency (several hundred msec) and had a longer duration.

In addition, electrical stimulation (1,3,6 Hz and 60,100 Hz, 5–20v̄) of the internal medullary lamina and the adjacent structures was carried out in every 2 mm of the needle (0.8 mm in diameter) track with the parameters mentioned above in order to obtain an accurate localization of the target. Figure 2 (left figure) summarizes the results of high-frequency (60,100 Hz) stimulation in patients under local anesthesia. The stimulated points are projected on the horizontal (+4) plane of the Schaltenbrand and Bailey Atlas (14). Black circles mean that the points showed sensory effects induced by stimulation, whereas white circles mean that the stimulation of the points did not elicit somatic sensation, but produced "unpleasant" sensation which

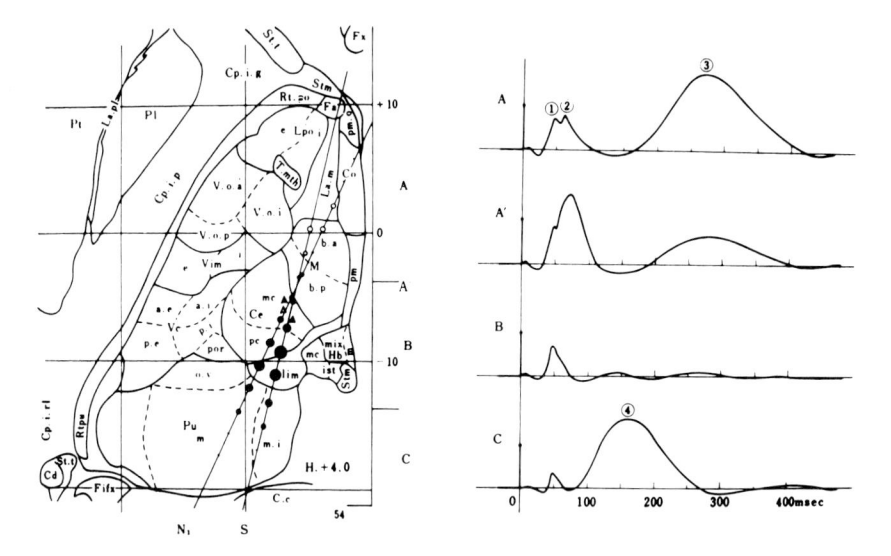

FIG. 2. Left = needle tracks. Right = evoked potentials. *Black circles* = pain effect, the size of the circle being proportional to the effect. *White circles* = unpleasant sensation. *Triangles* = motor effect. (Courtesy of Sano, K. (1977): In *Progress in Neurological Surgery*, edited by H. Krayenbühl et al. 8:50–103. Karger Basel.)

was poorly localized anywhere in the body. The sizes of the circles are proportional to the sensitivity to the stimulation.

As seen in Fig. 2, the white circles are seen in the medial and anterior part of the thalamus (A, left). The black circles are distributed in a wide area of the posterior half of the internal medullary lamina (B, left) which ranges from about 4 mm to 14 mm posterior to the midpoint of the intercommissural line in the anteroposterior direction. The nucleus parafascicularis, the parvocellular portion of the centre médian and the n. limitans are especially sensitive to stimulation. The more forward or upward the stimulating point moves, the weaker the response.

The general character of the sensory responses to the high-frequency stimulation of this area was a diffuse, burning pain in the contralateral half of the body or the whole body. Not infrequently, the spontaneous pain of the patient was exaggerated at a lower intensity than the threshold to produce diffuse, burning pain, irrespective of the side of stimulation.

Among the intralaminar nuclei, the centre médian (CM) occupies the largest area. Although it certainly plays an important role in the perception of pain, it is unlikely that all its parts are related to pain. Only the posterior part which corresponds to the parvocellular portion of the nucleus, is closely related to pain. Several writers have reported the effects of stimulation of the centre médian, but these have differed from author to author. This variety of effects might be partly due to the difference of stimulating points and partly to the difference of parameters. In our experience, the parvocellular portion of the centre médian, the n. parafascicularis (pf) and the n. limitans (Lim) form a most essential area for pain.

High-frequency stimulation of the middle portion of the internal medullary lamina, from the midpoint of the intercommissural line to the point 8 mm behind the midpoint (i.e., the part medial to the Vop and Vim nuclei of Hassler (14) and probably corresponding to the magnocellular portion of the CM), produced, in some patients, tremor and rigidity and in other patients, trembling in the contralateral extremities. These points are represented by triangles in Fig. 2 (A', left). In cases with extrapyramidal disorders, stimulation of this portion markedly increased tremor and rigidity. Cortical evoked potentials produced by low-frequency (1,3,6 Hz) stimulation showed a good correlation with the sensory-motor effects and were characteristic of each zone (Fig. 2, right).

Conclusions

These data and experimental studies on cats (5,10) led to the following conclusions: (a) The faster-conducting fibers of the spinothalamic tract (fast A-delta) course in the lateral side of the medulla and then turn inside, joining in the lemniscal system, and terminate finally in the specific sensory nucleus of the thalamus contralateral to the side of stimulation. A part of them may terminate in the PO (6,7). (b) The slower-conducting fibers (slow A-delta) course in the more medial part of the medulla; some of them terminate in the lateral part of the central gray, others to the ventral part of the internal medullary lamina of the thalamus, and finally, the rest of the fibers reach the posterior hypothalamus. Some of the slower fibers project also to the side ipsilateral to the side of stimulation. (c) The role of the hypothalamus in pain perception should be emphasized not only because of its effects upon the autonomic and emotional responses to stress, but also because the slow A-delta fibers end here. (d) Unitary discharges could be recorded from various parts in the thalamus which reacted to selective C-fiber stimulation. The results obtained indicate that unitary elements reactive to the C-fiber impulses are widely scattered in the medial structures in the thalamus. But at the same time, they show that the C-fibers terminate most densely in the intralaminar nuclei such as the CM and the CL. We could not find cells in the n. ventralis posterolateralis (VPL) which were activated by the C-fiber stimulation. However, this does not exclude the existence of C-fiber terminals in this nucleus, because the number of cells tested were relatively few.

The latencies of reactions varied very much, ranging from 400 msec to, in most cases, several hundred msec. The longest one was about 2,000 msec, but, in this case, evaluation of the response was very difficult. These results are compatible with those of Albe-Fessard and Kruger (1), as well as those of Collins and Randt (2) who described that the mean latency of the midbrain responses to C-fiber stimulation was 560 msec. The cells in the ventral part of the CM probably receive both slow A-delta and C-fibers. Experimental studies suggest that the intralaminar nuclei exert facilitatory effects upon the specific sensory system and the latter exerts inhibitory effects on the former.

Thus, the specific sensory system and the intralaminar structures constitute a "diencephalic control system" of sensation.

Therapeutic Application

For the relief of intractable pain, the B zone of the lamina where stimulation produces increase of spontaneous pain and burning sensation, namely the zone including the intralaminar nuclei, the parvocellular portion of the centre médian, the n. parafascicularis, the n. limitans with the adjacent fibers, was sterotaxically destroyed.

Patients with thalamic pain; pain due to malignancy; atypical facial pain due to trauma, herpes zoster, carotid basilar anastomosis, etc., causalgia, tabes dorsalis, and other types of central pain in which long-term medication had not been effective, have been subjected to this standard procedure. In some cases stereotaxic destruction of the centre médian–parafascicular complex (usually from the frontal burr hole) was performed.

Results

Table 1 summarizes the results of operations on 41 patients at the time of discharge and 3 months later. Although not shown in the table, the results at 1-year follow-up were the same as those at 3-months follow-up. The numbers in parentheses are cases of stereotaxic destruction of the centre médian–parafascicular complex, while all of the others are cases of thalamolaminotomy. As expected, some patients had less pain-relief at 3 months than at the time of discharge.

The data in Table 1 make it obvious that standard thalamolaminotomy is more effective than the centre médian–parafasciculotomy. The longest follow-up is more than 10 years in a patient with thalamic syndrome who still is pain-free. Except in four instances, the procedure was done bilaterally with an interval of 7 to 10 days. The thalamolaminotomy was especially effective for thalamic pain and other types of central pain. However, pain due to cancer recurred several months later, although when it recurred the pain was still of a tolerable degree as compared with the preoperative state.

No severe complications were observed. Very slight disturbance of consciousness, confusion, or hallucinations were seen in several patients on the second or third postoperative day mostly after the second-stage operation, but they recovered within a week.

In all patients, normal sensations remained intact after the operations.

TABLE 1. Results with thalamolaminotomy (in 41 patients)

Cause or type of pain	No. of patients	At discharge				3 Months			
		Complete	Good	Fair	Little or none	Complete	Good	Fair	Little or none
Thalamic pain	9	3	4(1)[a]	—	(1)	3	3(1)	1	(1)
Cancer pain	13	3(1)	(1)	5(3)	—	4(1)	—	4(4)	—
Trigeminal neuralgia	4	1	3	—	—	1	2	1	—
Causalgia	4	3	—	—	1	3	—	—	1
Tabes dorsalis	1	—	—	—	1	—	—	—	1
Other central pain	10	2	2(3)	1	2	2	1(2)	1	3
Total	41	13	14	9	5	14	9	11	6
% of Total		33%	34%	22%	11%	34%	22%	27%	17%

[a] Numbers in parentheses indicate results with the stereotaxic destruction of the centrum medianum–n. parafascicularis complex.

Sensory testing for touch, pressure, temperature and even pain (by pin prick) revealed that these sensations were not impaired compared with the preoperative state.

Autopsy was obtained in 4 cases, 3 of patients with cancer and 1 with thalamic pain. In these cases, the sites of stereotaxic lesions were examined, and with the aid of Nauta Gygax method, the degenerated fibers from the lesion sites were tracked (16). The terminal degeneration was found in the n. ventrocaudalis parvocellularis (Vcpc) and in the second somatosensory cortex on the ipsilateral side. No degenerated axons were found in the medial thalamic nuclei. From these findings, it may be concluded that the posterior portion of the internal medullary lamina has definite connections at least with Vcpc and the second somatosensory cortex, but no connection with the dorsomedial nucleus.

POSTEROMEDIAL HYPOTHALAMOTOMY

This procedure entails making a small stereotaxic lesion in the posterior (ergotropic) hypothalamus which is actually the continuation of the periaqueductal gray. I introduced the procedure in 1962 (8,11), in order to normalize the ergotropic and trophotropic balance for the treatment of violent, very aggressive, and restless behaviors mostly in cases with epilepsy and mental retardation.

Based on the experimental data in animals and on the fact that painful stimuli always cause signs of sympathetic discharges, we started to perform the posteromedial hypothalamotomy for intractable pain in 1971. In the same year, Fairman (4) reported the effects of the posteromedial hypothalamotomy in 12 patients with intractable pain due to metastatic malignant tumor.

Studies of neuronal unit discharges at the time of operation showed the existence of neurons responding to C fiber impulses and A delta fiber impulses in the postero-medial hypothalamus. Electrical stimulation of the area elicited signs of sympathetic discharge (11) and EEG changes similar to those produced by intravenous injection of epinephrine as reported by Venes et al. (15).

There was no operative mortality. As indicated, this procedure was more effective in the treatment of intractable pain due to malignant tumors than that due to other causes (Table 2).

The operation was done bilaterally in 6 patients and unilaterally in 14. It seems that for pain due to lesions below the neck, the operation on the contralateral side was most effective, whereas for pain due to lesions in the face and the head, the operation on the ipsilateral side was more effective.

There was no impairment of sensation noticed after the operation. In our series, regression of metastases of malignant tumors has rarely been ob-

TABLE 2. Results with posteromedial hypothalamotomy for pain-relief (in 20 patients)

Cause or type of pain	No. of patients	At discharge				3 Months			
		Complete	Good	Fair	Little or none	Complete	Good	Fair	Little or none
Cancer pain	13	9	3	1	—	9	—	2	2
Causalgia	2	1	1	—	—	—	—	1	1
Neuralgia	4	—	2	2	—	—	—	2	2
Thalamic pain	1	—	—	1	—	—	—	—	1
Total	20	10	6	4	—	9	—	5	6
% of Total		50%	30%	20%	—	45%	—	25%	30%

served, although patients' lives may have been prolonged because of increased appetite and discontinuance of narcotic analgesics.

Five patients with intractable pain due to malignant tumors who lived pain-free for 1 to 3 months following the procedure, after death were submitted to autopsy. The degenerated axons from the lesion site were searched for with the aid of the Nauta-Gygax method. Degenerated fibers were found in the ipsilateral nucleus ventrocaudalis parvocellularis (Vcpc), the second somatosensory cortex, the rolandic sensory cortex, the n. parafascicularis (pf), the pallidum, and downward in the reticular formation. Many of the axons probably terminated in the Vcpc. Moreover, it is noteworthy that no degenerated axons were found in the medial nuclei. It may be concluded that the posteromedial portion of the hypothalamus has connections at least with the Vcpc and probably with the n. parafascicularis and the somatosensory cortices, but no connection with the dorsomedial nucleus.

DISCUSSION

The data suggest that neurons throughout the length of the brain stem, particularly those of the nuclei of the medial two-thirds of the reticular formation, contribute axons to the ascending reticular pathway. This pathway divides at the mesencephalo-diencephalic junction, one portion running a ventral

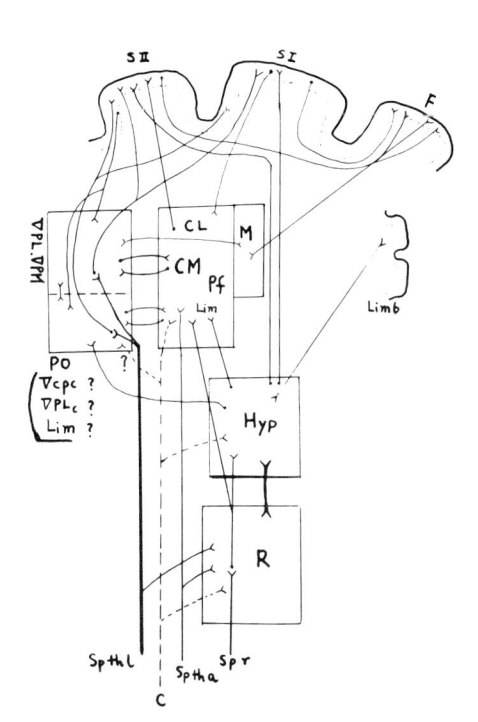

FIG. 3. Diagram of pathways related to pain. C = C fibers; CL = n. centralis lateralis; CM = centrum medianum; F = frontal lobe; Hyp = hypothalamus; Lim = n. limitans; Limb = limbic cortex; M = medial nuclei; Pf = n. parafascicularis; PO = posterior nuclear group; R = brain stem reticular formation; SI = rolandic sensory cortex; SII = second sensory cortex; Spr = spino-reticulo-thalamic pathways; Sptha = anterior spinothalamic tract; Spthl = lateral spinothalamic tract; Vcpc = n. ventro-caudalis parvocellularis; VPL = n. ventralis postero-lateralis; VPM = n. ventralis postero-medialis; VPLc = VPL caudalis. (Courtesy of Sano, K. (1977): In: *Progress in Neurological Surgery*, edited by H. Krayenbühl et al. 8:50–103. Karger Basel.)

course to the hypothalamus, the other ascending and terminating within the intralaminar nuclei of the thalamus (Fig. 3).

According to Dafny and his associates (3), in the posterior hypothalamus of cats there are neurons which respond to somatosensory, visual, and acoustic stimuli respectively; that is to say, there is convergence of impulses of various modalities at the single-cell level. Our data suggest that the posterior hypothalamus in man as well as in the cat contains neurons responding to A-delta as well as C-fiber impulses.

Thus, it is apparent that the hypothalamus is playing a role in sensory functions. Stimulation of the posteromedial hypothalamus in man, however, does not produce any definite sensation but a very unpleasant feeling or great fear. Probably the hypothalamus is important in coloring the emotional aspect of sensations and in provoking autonomic-endocrine responses. This suggests that the posterior hypothalamus is related to unpleasant, fearful, or horrible feelings and sympathetic discharges and endocrine changes which often accompany pain.

SUMMARY

The internal medullary lamina of the thalamus with its nuclei is a composite structure with functional topographic differences: Namely, the anterior, middle, and posterior portions are concerned with emotional, motor, and sensory activities respectively.

The posterior portion of the internal medullary lamina, including the center median (parvocellular portion), n. parafascicularis, n. centralis lateralis, n. limitans, has neurons which respond to slower A-delta-fiber impulses and C-fiber impulses. This portion of the medullary lamina exerts facilitatory influences on the specific sensory system and the latter, in turn, exerts inhibitory influences upon the former, thus both constituting the diencephalic control system of sensation. This posterior portion of the internal medullary lamina has connections, proved by means of the Nauta-Gygax method, with the n. ventrocaudalis parvocellularis and the second sensory cortex. Stereotaxic lesion of the posterior portion of the internal medullary lamina—the intralaminar thalamotomy or the thalamolaminotomy—produces effective relief of intractable pain, especially of central pain, somehow producing no sensory deficits.

The posteromedial hypothalamus has neurons which respond to slower A-delta fiber and C-fiber impulses. Stimulation of this area produces signs of sympathetic discharge (such as rise in blood pressure, tachycardia, pupillary dilation), neck movement, ocular movements, endocrine changes and EEG changes (desynchronization or slow waves of high voltage in the cortical leads) and an unpleasant feeling or fear or horror, but no pain. The posteromedial hypothalamus has connections, proved by means of Nauta-Gygax method, with the n. ventrocaudalis parvocellularis and the n. parafascicularis and probably with the somatosensory cortices.

Stereotaxic lesions of the posteromedial hypothalamus, called posteromedial hypothalamotomy, produce relief of intractable pain due to malignancy, but are not so effective for central pain. No sensory deficits are noted after the operation.

The rationale of the thalamolaminotomy and the posteromedial hypothalamotomy may be that both procedures make lesions not only in one of the main end-stations of the C-fibers and the slow A-delta fibers, but also in the portions that exert influences on the specific sensory system, and thus decrease the intensity of volleys of impulses and change the pattern of impulses which can be interpreted as pain.

REFERENCES

1. Albe-Fessard, D., and Kruger, L. (1962): Duality of unit discharge from cat centrum medianum in response to natural and electrical stimulation. *J. Neurophysiol.*, 25: 1–20.
2. Collins, W. F., and Randt, C. T. (1960): Midbrain evoked responses relating to peripheral unmyelinated or "C" fibers in cat. *J. Neurophysiol.*, 23:47–53.
3. Dafny, N., Bental, E., and Feldman, S. (1965): Effect of sensory stimuli on single unit activity in the posterior hypothalamus. *Electroenceph. Clin. Neurophysiol.*, 19:256–263.
4. Fairman, D. (1972): Hypothalamotomy as a new perspective for alleviation of intractable pain and regression of metastatic malignant tumors. In: *Present Limits of Neurosurgery*, edited by I. Fusek and Z. Kunc, pp. 525–528. Avicenum, Prague.
5. Ishijima, B., and Sano, K. (1971): Responses of specific and non-specific thalamic nuclei to the selective A-δ and C-fiber stimulation, and their interactions in cat's brain. *Neurol. Med. Chir. (Tokyo)*, 11:84–100.
6. Mountcastle, V. B., and Henneman, E. (1952): The representation of tactile sensibility in the thalamus of the monkey. *J. Comp. Neurol.*, 97:409–439.
7. Poggio, G. F., and Mountcastle, V. B. (1960): A study of the functional contributions of the lemniscal and spinothalamic systems to somatic sensibility. *Johns Hopkins Hosp. Bull.*, 106:266–316.
8. Sano, K. (1962): Sedative neurosurgery with special reference to posteromedial hypothalamotomy. *Neurol. Med. Chir. (Tokyo)*, 4:112–142.
9. Sano, K. (1967): The role of the internal medullary lamina in pain. *Anales del XII Congreso Latinoamericano de Neurocirugia*, pp. 937–952.
10. Sano, K. (1977): Intralaminar thalamotomy (thalamolaminotomy) and posteromedial hypothalamotomy in the treatment of intractable pain. In: *Prog. Neurol. Surg. Vol. 8*, edited by H. Krayenbühl et al. pp. 50–103. Karger, Basel.
11. Sano, K., Mayanagi, Y., Sekino, H., Ogashiwa, M., and Ishijima, B. (1970): Results of stimulation and destruction of the posterior hypothalamus in man. *J. Neurosurg.*, 33:689–707.
12. Sano, K., Yoshioka, M., Ogashiwa, M., Ishijima, B., and Ohye, C. (1966): Thalamolaminotomy. A new operation of relief of intractable pain. *Confin. Neurol.*, 27:63–66.
13. Sano, K., Yoshioka, M., Sekino, H., Mayanagi, Y., Yoshimasu, N., and Tsukamoto, Y. (1970): Functional organization of the internal medullary lamina in man. *Confin. Neurol.*, 32:374–380.
14. Schaltenbrand, G., and Bailey, P. (1959): Einfürung in die Stereotaktischen Operationen mit einem Atlas des menschlichen Gehirns. Thieme, Stuttgart.
15. Venes, J. L., Collins, W. F., and Taub, A. (1972): Evoked cerebral cortical activity from small peripheral nerve fibers in cat. *Electroenceph. Clin. Neurophysiol.*, 33: 207–214.
16. Yoshimasu, N. (1972): Functional anatomy of the internal medullary lamina based on the results of stereotaxic surgery. *Brain & Nerve*, 24:1277–1292 (in Japanese).

Central Gray Stimulation for Control of Cancer Pain

Donald E. Richardson

Department of Neurological Surgery, Louisiana State University School of Medicine, and Hotel Dieu Hospital Pain Rehabilitation Unit, New Orleans, Louisiana 70119

This presentation includes a discussion of a new technique for pain-relief that has been applied to only a few patients suffering from cancer pain. A detailed analysis of indications, contraindications, complications, successes, and failures is not available. However, experience to date suggests that this technique has advantages over many others for the control of cancer pain. The potential for control of bilateral pain involving any area of the body from the scalp to the perineum with one operative procedure that can be done under local anesthesia seems to make the procedure ideal for many cancer patients.

Brain stimulation for pain-relief was first done by Heath in 1960 (5). Stimulation of the medial septal area in a woman with carcinoma of the cervix with pelvic pain resulted in pain-relief that was associated with euphoria and a feeling of being intoxicated. Gol (4) did stimulation of this area in several patients with mixed results but, in general, poor pain-relief. Adams and Hosobuchi have stimulated the main sensory nucleus of the thalamus, a procedure comparable to dorsal column stimulation with pain-relief in the area of produced paresthesias (6).

Interest in periaqueductal gray stimulation for pain-relief developed after the report published in 1969 by Reynolds that stimulation of small areas of the central gray produced marked behavioral analgesia in animals (8). This lead was vigorously pursued by Mayer, Liebeskind, Akil, and associates (7) who have been able to produce analgesia consistently by stimulating the area of the dorsal raphe nucleus in the rat. Analgesia was sufficient to allow surgical procedures on the animal without apparent pain and was not associated with motor paralysis or impairment of other sensory modalities. Akil has demonstrated that brain-stimulation analgesia is dependent upon an intact serotonin system, is reduced by dopamine depletion, and is inhibited by norepinephrine (1,2).

Dr. Akil and I carried out a series of experiments in cats and found that stimulation produced analgesia and changes in the evoked response in the medial thalamus comparable to those produced by morphine (9). In addition, naloxone, a morphine antagonist, inhibits these changes in animals (8).

Naloxone given to patients prior to stimulation of the periaqueductal gray also blocks the effect of stimulation with reduction of analgesia (11). In addition, we have measured endogenous opiates in the ventricular fluid of patients undergoing stimulation for pain control and have been able to demonstrate a rise in enkephalin-like compounds in the fluid following stimulation (3). These findings would indicate that the endogenous opiate system, as well as the serotonin system, is involved in the effect of stimulation of the periventricular gray for pain control.

A trial of acute stimulation in 5 patients undergoing thalamotomy was then carried out, with demonstration of excellent bilateral analgesia in 1 and hypalgesia in another 3 patients (10). We found that periaqueductal stimulation produced nystagmus and vertigo, whereas stimulation of the periventricular gray matter in the very medial thalamus produced excellent analgesia with minimal side effects. We have now operated on a large number of patients utilizing a chronic depth-electrode system with an induction receiver and external transmitter that allows chronic self-stimulation for pain control (11). In our published series of 30 patients, 4 patients with cancer pain have been operated on (12). These and 2 additional patients are reported here in detail.

TECHNIQUE

Our present approach is to insert a single, 4-contact, pull-down, platinum-electrode (1) in each patient even if the pain is bilateral. Insertion is done through a coronal burr hole on the side opposite the more intense pain.

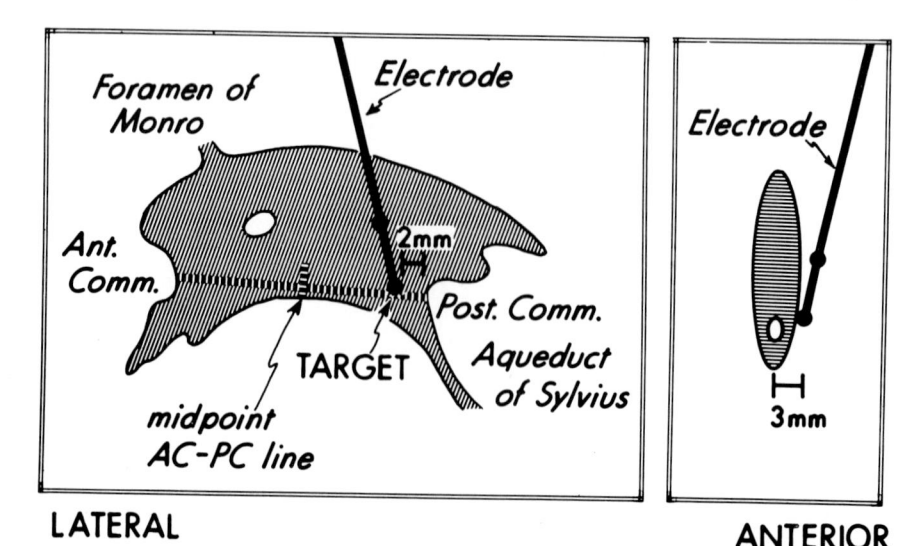

FIG. 1. Placement of electrode for stimulation of periventricular grey.

The procedure is done with a Trent Wells stereotaxic instrument under local anesthesia. Stimulation testing is then carried out for optimum placement based on adequacy of pain-relief and minimal side effects. After the final positioning of the electrode, fine percutaneous leads are brought out through a needle-puncture site some distance from the burr hole, and the electrode is locked in place at the burr hole site by a spherical plug (Fig. 1).

Following surgery, a period of testing of stimulation for effectiveness and side effects is carried out usually lasting approximately 2 weeks. A second procedure for internalization of the system is then done under general anesthesia. The receiver is implanted in the pectoral area and connected to the two most effective electrode contacts through a mating connector in the parietal area, and the percutaneous wiring is removed. A period of parameter-selection, frequency of stimulation, and patient-instruction for proper use of the system is usually necessary. Internal settings on the transmitter allow variations of pulse width, frequency, and maximum voltage which are selected during the period of testing to minimize side effects and maximize pain-relief. The patient is instructed to slowly increase the variable voltage control until side effects are noted and then to reduce the voltage until no side effects are felt, following which a period of stimulation is carried out, typically 10 to 30 min in duration.

RESULTS

The results in 6 cancer patients will be presented in detail with a brief history, since the series is too limited for statistical analysis.

Patient #1. W. S. was a 63-year-old male with recurrent carcinoma of the colon following abdominoperineal resection. His pain was perineal, spreading to the back and legs, increased by lying on his back or standing. Dihydrocodeinone (Percodan®) and morphine 15 mg intramuscularly were insufficient for complete pain-relief prior to surgery, and he was confined in bed lying on his left side most of the time. The electrode was implanted in early September of 1973, on the right side. Following surgery, stimulation at 1 V, 20 Hz, for 20 min every 4 to 5 hr allowed the patient to ambulate and to lie on his back for the first time in months. He described the pain as "floating away." At high current levels, he reported a startled reaction and some dizziness, felt frightened and apprehensive, and demonstrated mild nystagmus. Sensory side effects consisting in a warm sensation down his back were noted at effective pain-relieving levels of stimulation. He remained free of pain on stimulation until he died 2 months following surgery from uremia.

Patient #2. B. M. was a 60-year-old male with a Pancoast tumor of the lung with brachial plexus and spine invasion. He had severe bilateral pain in the neck, shoulders, arm, and chest. Prior to surgery, meperidine (Demerol®), 100 mg every 3 hr, was interspaced with phenothiazines, resulting in partial pain-relief. He was operated on in June of 1974, with implantation in the right periventricular area. Following surgery, he could be maintained almost free of pain with stimulation for 20 min every 2 to 4 hr and amitriptyline (Elavil®), 100 mg daily. Side effects during stimulation consisted of paresthesias of heat in the left face and arm. His disease progressed rapidly, and he expired 2 months following surgery (Fig. 1).

Patient #3. C. G. was a 55-year-old female with carcinoma of the breast with generalized bone metastasis which produced pain in the right shoulder, back, right leg, and both knees. She also had burning in the left leg secondary to previous high thoracic chordotomy. Dihydromorphinone (Dilaudid®), 2 mg every 4 hr, was ineffective in relieving pain, as well as was a previous hypophysectomy. She was implanted April of 1976, on the left side and obtained good relief with stimulation 3 times a day for 30 min. Side effects were heat paresthesias in the left leg and a "locking of her eyes." She did well for 6 months, and then back and right flank pain increased secondary to metastasis to the L_3 vertebra. Increase in stimulation to 10 min every 2 hr controlled pain for 2 more months. She then had a pathologic fracture of the spine which caused severe pain that required resumption of narcotic medication by mouth.

Patient #4. G. S. was a 52-year-old male with carcinoma of the bladder and local recurrence causing low back, pelvic, perineal, and right leg pain. Bed rest and oral codeine, 90 mg every 4 hr, did not relieve his pain, which was markedly increased by ambulation. An electrode was implanted on the left in September, 1976. Following surgery, stimulation for 15 min every 2 to 4 hours and oral amitriptyline, 100 mg daily, gave 80 to 90% relief of his pain while ambulating. Side effects during stimulation were either absent or consisted of slight warmth in the trunk. Pain-relief remained excellent for 5 months until he died from uremia.

Patient #5. J. M. was a 48-year-old female with recurrence of pelvic cancer and consequent perineal and pelvic pain bilaterally. In addition, she had a feeling of pressure described as "sitting on a lump" that was disturbing. In March of 1977, a right periventricular electrode was inserted, and pain-relief was dramatic. However, following surgery, she had persistent complaints of the pressure or lump sensation that disturbed her and had anxiety and depression that was exacerbated by the constant reminder of the pressure of the pelvic mass and perineal drainage. Other physicians placed her on narcotics again, and she discontinued stimulation.

Patient #6. H. L. is a 54-year-old male with generalized peritoneal recurrence of carcinoma of the colon. He developed deep midline and bilateral upper-lumbar and lower-thoracic back pain and upper-abdominal midline pain of constant, aching character. Prior to surgery, he was using meperidine, 100 mg intramuscularly every 2 to 3 hr. A right PVG electrode was inserted in April of 1978, and stimulation every 4 hr produced 80% pain-relief. The addition of amitriptyline, 100 mg at bedtime, gave complete pain-relief with use of the stimulator on a 2-time per day basis. There are no side effects during stimulation, but if stimulation is increased to near maximum for the transmitter, he has blurring of vision.

DISCUSSION

We have demonstrated in this small number of patients that periventricular gray stimulation is effective in relieving severe and widespread pain from recurrent cancer, and that the side effects are mild and easily tolerated. Three obvious problems are demonstrated by these patients. First, on the basis of the fact that 2 patients died only a few months after the electrode implantation, I would advocate not using this procedure unless life-expectancy is predicted to be 4 or more months. Of course it is difficult to predict life-expectancy in these patients, but if the condition of the patient suggests a very short life, I would use percutaneous brain stimulation so as to avoid general anesthesia and the added expense of internalization of the system.

The second problem that has emerged from our experience is that central stimulation may prove insufficient in patients whose disease progresses and whose pain intensity increases. Our experience is not extensive enough to solve this problem, but in the patients with nonmalignant, chronic pain we have operated on, we also have had failures when the pain problem was static or increased. Obviously, the procedure is not perfect and an unknown failure rate will have to be anticipated.

Another limitation of the technique is that associated symptoms, such as pressure or mass effect produced by the tumor growth, are not affected by stimulation. It appears that stimulation affects only pain caused by noxious sensory input. A careful questioning of patients regarding specific type of discomfort and "pain" will help avoid this problem. Anxiety and depression are not controlled by stimulation and should be treated by additional means. The addition of amitriptyline, a tricyclic antidepressant, has improved stimulation results in a number of patients who, prior to surgery, had no effect from the drug. We think this is due to the increased effectiveness of dopamine and serotonin produced by this drug and predicted by Akil's work in animals (2). At present, we routinely place all patients on amitriptyline or a similar tricyclic following surgery. Narcotic addiction also is not controlled by stimulation, nor are withdrawal symptoms modified by stimulation.

Tolerance from excessive stimulation has been observed in rats and also in some patients with chronic, benign pain not included in this report. However, tolerance can be controlled by using the least-effective duration of frequency of stimulation. It can be reversed by discontinuing stimulation for a few days, the addition of tricyclics, norepinephrine (disulfiram), or, more recently, tryptophan.

SUMMARY

The number of patients is too small for a significant analysis of complications and failures. However, our limited experience suggests that brain stimulation in the area of the periventricular gray substance has the promise of being an effective method of relieving severe cancer pain. The procedure can control widespread and bilateral pain with minimal side effects and minimal surgery.

REFERENCES

1. Akil, H., and Liebeskind, J. C. (1975): Monaminergic mechanisms of stimulation-produced analgesia. *Brain Res.,* 94:279–296.
2. Akil, H., and Mayer, D. J. (1972): Antagonism of stimulation produced analgesia by PCPA, a serotonin synthesis inhibitor. *Brain Res.,* 44:692–697.
3. Akil, H., Richardson, D. E., Hughes, J., and Barchas, J. D. (1979): Elevation in levels of enkephalin-like material in the ventricular CSF of pain patients upon analgetic focal stimulation. *Science,* 201 (4354): 463–465.

4. Gol, A. (1967): Relief of pain by electrical stimulation of the septal area. *J. Neurol. Surg.*, 5:115–120.
5. Heath, R. G., and Mickle, W. A. (1960): Evaluation of seven years of experience with depth electrode studies in human patients. In: *Electrical Studies on the Unanesthetized Brain,* edited by E. R. Ramey and D. S. O'Doherty. Haber, New York.
6. Hosobuchi, Y., Adams, J. E., and Rutkin, B. (1973): Chronic thalamic stimulation for the relief of facial anesthesia dolorosa. *Arch. Neurol.,* 29:158–161.
7. Mayer, D. J., Wolfle, T. L., Akil, H., Carder, B., and Liebeskind, J. C. (1971): Analgesia resulting from electrical stimulation in the brain stem of the rat. *Science,* 174:1351–1354.
8. Reynolds, D. V. (1969): Surgery in the rat during electrical analgesia induced by local brain stimulation. *Science,* 164:444–445.
9. Richardson, D. E., and Akil, H. (1975): Comparison of analgesic brain stimulation, peripheral nerve and dorsal column stimulation to morphine sulfate: Effects on evoked responses to noxious input. In: *Abstracts of the First World Congress on Pain (Florence, Italy, 1975),* p. 262. International Association for the Study of Pain, Seattle.
10. Richardson, D. E., and Akil, H. (1977): Pain reduction by electrical brain stimulation in man, Part I: Acute administration in periaqueductal and periventricular sites. *J. Neurosurg.,* 47:178–183.
11. Richardson, D. E., and Akil, H. (1977): Pain reduction by electrical brain stimulation in man, Part II: Chronic self-administration in periventricular gray matter. *J. Neurosurg.,* 47:184–194.
12. Richardson, D. E., and Akil, H. (1977): Long-term results of periventricular gray self-stimulation. *Neurosurgery,* 1:199–202.

Thalamic and Hypothalamic Stimulation

David Fairman

Av. Quintana 49, 8C, Buenos Aires, Argentina

This paper will describe the results of thalamic and hypothalamic stimulation for pain-relief in a series of 750 consecutive patients with intractable pain caused by a malignant neoplasm. My patients can be divided into two groups on the basis of the target selected: intralaminar nucleus of the thalamus (630 patients) or hypothalamic periventricular nucleus (120 patients). The results are contained in Tables 1 and 2.

In 1972, we first performed repetitive stimulation through implanted electrodes in the hypothalamic periventricular nucleus and observed that pain-relief was obtained which outlasted the stimulus for varying periods. We did not need to make a lesion in this region to obtain pain-relief. Effective results were obtained when the stimulation varied between 3 and 4 msec, and total remission of pain was obtained not in stages but instantaneously. These satisfactory results of repetitive stimulation lasted from 1 hr to several days. Repetitive stimulation can be performed as often as necessary (Fig. 1).

Table 2 shows the tabulation corresponding to the hypothalamic procedure for the relief of intractable pain in our series of 120 neoplastic patients in pain.

An essential objective has been to select the optimal target point for electrical stimulation to alleviate pain. Gybels (4) reported interesting studies on electrical stimulation of the thalamic nucleus VPL for the relief of intractable pain. Mazars (7) stated that the integrity of VPL is essential for effective relief of pain by thalamic electrical stimulation. Richardson (8) showed that electrical stimulation of the periaqueductal gray area can be a satisfactory treatment for intractable pain. Most of the reports include patients with various chronic pain syndromes including cancer pain, postherpetic neuralgia, atypical facial neuralgia, phantom limb, and thalamic syndrome. We believe that confusion arises because there is no distinction made between different types of pain. The preoccupation with correct target selection has overlooked the important fact that a prerequisite for success is the proper selection of patients. Target selection should be based upon a careful diagnosis of the type of pain experienced by the patient. In our experience, the essential prerequisite for effective pain-relief by hypothalamic stimulation is the selection of patients based upon the type of pain. This

TABLE 1. Stereotactic thalamic tractotomy

Number of cases	Site of carcinoma	Percent
294	Lung	46
122	Head—Neck	19
99	Uterus	15
81	Breast	12
34	G.I. Tract	5
Total 630		100

selection is easier in patients with benign diseases, but in patients with neoplasms the problem is much more complex. The evaluation of the genesis of pain in patients with cancer must establish whether the intractable pain is due to excessive nociception by nerve-fiber compression or due to reduced nervous impulses or deafferentation.

Although deafferentation has been known to affect the central nervous system, it has only recently been incorporated in interpretations of the mechanisms of pain. Therapeutic implications are, of course, derived from understanding of mechanisms. The concept of deafferentation is supported by experimental studies such as those performed by Eccles and McIntyre (2). These investigators severed the dorsal roots of the seventh and first sacral nerves just distal to the dorsal ganglion; i.e., they interrupted the sensory impulses along the root. They found that in a period of time varying between 21 and 40 days there was reduced synaptic efficacy which could be largely restored by brief bursts of repetitive stimulation. Loeser and Ward (6) demonstrated that experimental chronic deafferentation produced by dorsal rhizotomy or hemicordotomy resulted in alterations in both spontaneous and evoked activity. The pathological process that leads to hyperactivity seems to be secondary to chronic deafferentation. Although proof of this concept will require further studies, it can be stated that reduction of the input to the central neurons may produce an increased output in response to a standard stimulus.

TABLE 2. Hypothalamotomy repetitive stimulation and/or lesion.

Number of cases	Site of carcinoma	Percent
54	Lung	45
21	Head—Neck	18
19	Uterus	16
14	Breast	11
12	G.I. Tract	10
Total 120		100

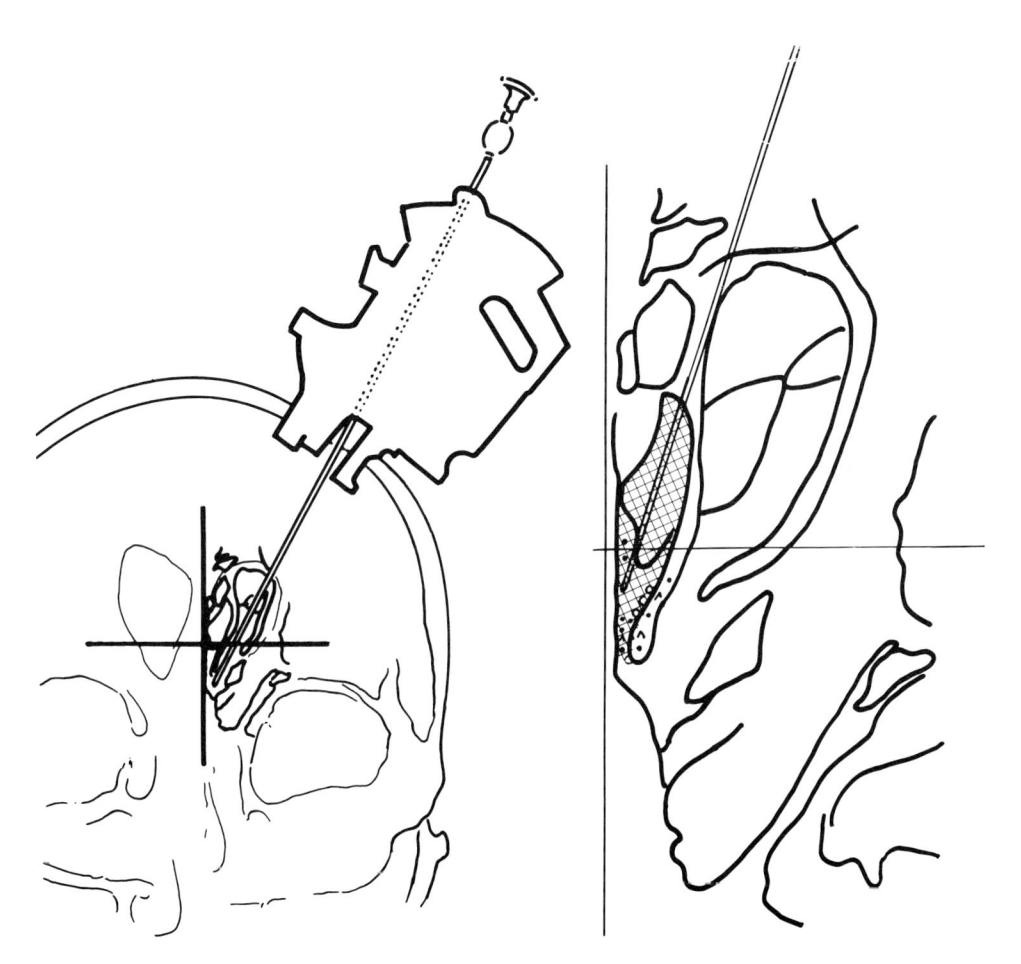

FIG. 1. A. Schema of stereotaxic approach to the hypothalamus. B. Enlargement showing points subjected to stimulation and the different effects mapped on frontal section of the Schaltenbrand-Bailey Atlas.

The concept of deafferentation is pivotal, because it constitutes the indication for repetitive stimulation. The first human experimental studies of deafferentation were performed in 1905 by Head (5) who, after sectioning the superficial radial nerve of his own forearm, described observations made over a 2-year period on the recovery sensation after neurorrhaphy. He observed that the first fibers to regenerate were unmyelinated and of very small diameter. Stimulation of these unmyelinated, free nerve endings produced only unpleasant sensations: a crude, poorly localized sensation of pain. He designated this type of painful sensation "protopathic."

The gradual return of the myelinated, larger fibers was associated with the reappearance of light touch, appreciation of intermediate grades of warmth and cold, and two-point discrimination. He designated this type of sensibility "epicritic." Head postulated that in a normal nerve, these two systems of fibers complemented each other and that the epicritic fibers not only suppressed the unpleasant and diffuse type of protopathic pain but also added the finer modalities of sensation.

We suggest that there is a similarity between these experimental works and the process of deafferentation observed in pain due to neoplastic involvement of peripheral nerves.

As Denny-Brown (1) pointed out, the paraneoplastic neuropathy is a degenerative lesion characterized by demyelinization as well as alterations in the diameter of the nerve fiber. Impulse transmission is probably altered. This process constitutes a process similar to deafferentation. There normally exists an equilibrium between the inhibitory and excitatory impulses transmitted respectively by the myelinated and unmyelinated fibers. Impulses transmitted by the myelinic fibers control the impulses transmitted by the unmyelinated fibers. In the paraneoplastic neuropathy, the process of deafferentation produces a disequilibrium resulting in the protopathic type of severe and diffuse pain due to the lack of inhibition of the epicritic myelinated fibers upon the protopathic unmyelinated ones. In our experience, the optimal procedure for the relief of intractable pain produced by a paraneoplastic neuropathy is electrical stimulation through implanted hypothalamic electrodes and not the surgical interruption of the pain pathways at any level.

In other cases of pain produced by the primary tumor itself or by metastasis, we suggest the presence of a dual mechanism. When compression of the nerve fibers or plexuses is obvious, the excess of nociceptive stimuli is responsible for the production of pain. But, at the same time, there can also be an infiltration process of the neoplastic cells along the perivascular spaces of the nerve fibers. This infiltration can cause a gradual process of demyelinization and partial destruction of the nerves, especially affecting the larger, rapidly conducting fibers which are more susceptible to this. These anatomic changes produce a reduction of nervous impulses so that the pain may be considered to be due to deafferentation. The diminution of the myelinated fibers causes a lack of inhibition of the unmyelinated C pain-conducting fibers. Because of this dual mechanism, we perform repetitive hypothalamic stimulation followed, when necessary, by a lesion at the intralaminar thalamic nucleus.

In 1969 (3), we developed the hypothesis that the hypothalamic periventricular system modulates both inhibitory and excitatory influences of synaptic transmission of pain impulses by blocking the pathways connecting the brainstem reticular formation to the different areas of the paleo- and neocortex which underlie the conscious experience of pain. In Fig. 2, we can see the diagram of the modulating periventricular hypothalamic system (MPHS) that constitutes an area of convergence for the different volleys of sensory, motor, and autonomic fibers which share adjacent neuronal circuits. This hypothesis includes the concept that a dynamic competition for the use

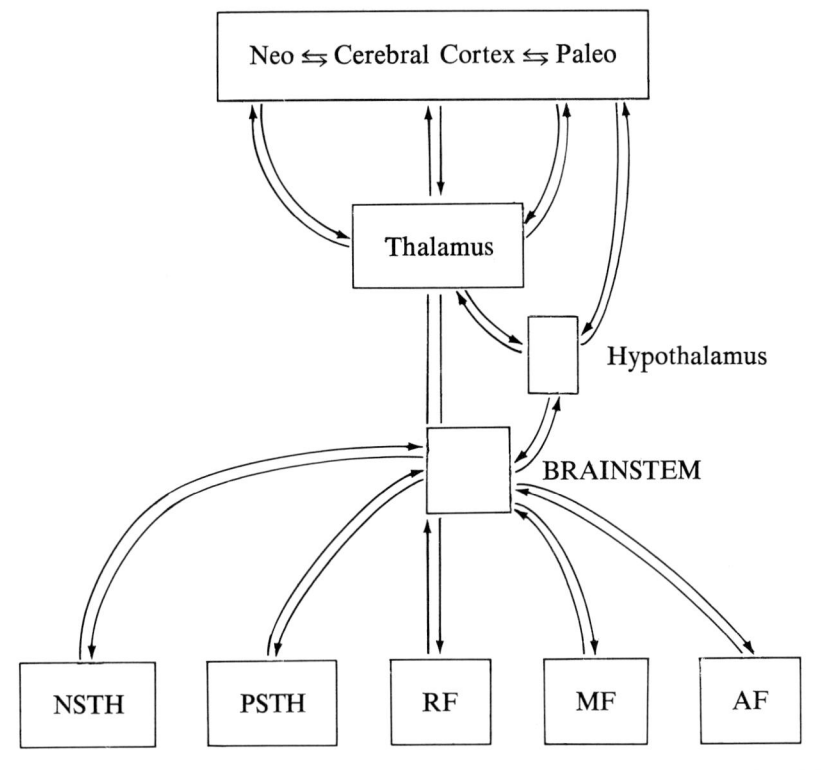

FIG. 2. Theory of the Modulating Periventricular Hypothalamic System (MPHS). NSTH, neospinothalamic; PSTH, paleospinothalamic; RF, reticular formation; MF, motor fibers; and AF, autonomic fibers.

of the same neuronal circuits between the pattern of pain impulses and the pattern of impulses elicited by adequate stimulation results in the effective blocking of the pain impulses.

Our thalamic target is the intralaminar nuclei and our hypothalamic target is the hypothalamic periventricular nuclei whether we perform a surgical lesion or stimulation. We are, therefore, attacking the same neuronal circuits at different levels. We are influencing the phylogenetically old pathways which mediate protopathic pain through the paleospinothalamic tract which relays to the second sensory area.

From the anatomical standpoint, this is the most circumscribed area where repetitive stimulation produces effective and long-lasting results. We are aware, however, that not only at the subcortical level but also at all levels of the nervous system, including the peripheral receptors and the transmission pathways, there exists a process of interrelation. This interaction between the sensory, motor, and autonomic systems is established continuously through the excitatory and inhibitory impulses.

Our theory of the MPHS is based on the fact that the hypothalamus is the highest correlation center of the autonomic nervous system. It integrates at all levels the sensory-motor and motor-sensory systems playing an essential role in the mechanism of pain. Moreover, our model is consistent with the studies suggesting that the hypothalamus could be the coordinating center of the whole brainstem reticular system and, therefore, the primary regulator of cortical activity and consciousness.

At the present stage of our knowledge, many questions can be asked concerning the effects of the mechanism by means of which hypothalamic repetitive stimulation may produce the relief of pain. Therefore, further studies are needed before the exact relationship between electrophysiological alterations of the neural metabolism and repetitive stimulation is established.

REFERENCES

1. Denny-Brown, D. (1948): Primary sensory neuropathy with muscular changes associated with carcinoma. *J. Neurol. Neurosurg. Psychiat.,* 11,1:73–78.
2. Eccles, J. C., and McIntyre, A. K. (1953): The effects of disuse and activity on mammalian spinal reflexes. *J. Physiol.,* 121:492–516.
3. Fairman, D. (1976): Neurophysiological basis for the hypothalamic lesion and stimulation by chronic implanted electrodes for the relief of intractable pain in cancer. In: *Advances in Pain Research and Therapy,* edited by J. J. Bonica and D. Albe-Fessard, pp. 843–847. Raven Press, New York.
4. Gybels, J. (1972): Supraspinal control of experimental pain sensation in man. In: *Pain,* pp. 128–131. Thieme, Stuttgart.
5. Head, H., Rivers, W. H. R., and Sherren, J. (1905): The afferent nervous system from a new aspect. *Brain,* 28:99–115.
6. Loeser, J. D., and Ward, A. A. (1967): Some effects of deafferentation of neurons of the cat spinal cord. *Arch. Neurol.,* 17:629–636.
7. Mazars, G., Merienne, L., and Cioloca, C. (1976): Etat actuel de la chirurgie de la douleur. *Neurochirurgie,* 22,1:1–164. Masson, Paris.
8. Richardson, D. E., and Akil, H. (1973): Pain relief by electrical stimulation of the brain in human patients. *Excerpta Medica,* 219:79.

Dorsal Column and Peripheral Nerve Stimulation for Relief of Cancer Pain

John D. Loeser

Department of Neurological Surgery, University of Washington School of Medicine, Seattle, Washington 98195

Electrical stimulation of the peripheral nerves and spinal cord has not yet received an adequate trial in the management of chronic pain due to cancer. It is difficult at this time to present meaningful data on the results obtained; any predictions which I make for the future are based as much upon hope as knowledge. Neurosurgeons have not reported many of their cases; thorough evaluations are often lacking and data are fragmentary. Impediments to clinical research are myriad; my inability to provide an answer to the questions of the efficacy of peripheral nerve stimulation (PNS) or spinal cord stimulation (DCS or PISCES) is based upon both the paucity of reported cases and the methods of evaluation.

We should be cognizant of some of the factors which have led to this unhappy state of affairs. In the United States, governmental regulations have made clinical research and the development of new technologies far too cumbersome. Manufacturers of equipment cannot control the applications of their inventions by well-intentioned but often misguided surgeons. Patient-selection criteria are frequently ignored for reasons of convenience or financial gain. The victim of all this is, of course, the hapless patient.

Practical implanted electrical stimulators have been available for approximately 10 years. These have been manufactured in the United States by Medtronic, Inc, and Avery Laboratories; I am not aware of other commercial suppliers. Many research groups have designed their own equipment for experimental purposes, but the clinical literature seems to report exclusively on Medtronic and Avery stimulators.

These implanted stimulators are inductance-coupled to an antenna driven by a cigarette-pack-sized, battery-operated transmitter; the electronic components have been highly reliable and are certainly safe. There have been no reports of electrical malfunctions resulting in patient problems such as seizures, myocardial dysrhythmia, or other phenomena unrelated to stimulation of the desired neural structures. Batteries do wear out, antenna lead wires break, patients destroy their transmitters by immersing them in bathtubs or dropping them out of windows; the stimulator systems are, in fact, quite durable. The major difficulties have occurred in the electrode system and its interface with the neural tissues. Lead wires break from metal fatigue, electrodes shift in position and become encased in fibrous tissue and this reduces or eliminates their effectiveness. Of course, there are some surgical complications such as infection, rejection of foreign bodies, CSF leaks, and damage to neural tissues. By far the most common long-term problem is related to electrode migration or loss of stimulation efficacy thought to be due to fibrosis about the sites of stimulation.

MECHANISM OF ACTION

Our abilities to cope with failures to achieve pain-relief with electrical stimulation would be enhanced by some comprehension of why electrical stimulation does relieve pain. Review of the more extensive data on patients with pain due to benign diseases suggests that there are few, if any, predictors of long-term efficacy of PNS, DCS, or PISCES systems. All investigators have commented upon the importance of excluding patients whose emotional states preclude meaningful interpretation of the effects of stimulation, but few other generalities emerge. It does seem to be generally true that stimulation must elicit paresthesias in the region of pain to lead to relief of that pain. There is a much higher incidence of immediate pain-relief than long-term amelioration of symptoms. Some of this is undoubtedly placebo effect, but stimulation may also lose its efficacy over time because of mechanisms less related to psychologic factors and related supratentorial functions and more readily ascribed to synaptic or axonal changes. We should, therefore, be cognizant of the fact that long-term stimulation of the spinal cord or peripheral nerves in man has never been shown to be either safe or hazardous. Patients with pain due to cancer are obviously not a suitable group to study for data on long-term hazards of stimulation, but the short and variable lifespans of patients with pain due to cancer make analyses of the efficacy of this mode of therapy quite complicated. I know of not one carefully planned and well-executed study on the efficacy of peripheral nerve or spinal cord stimulation for the relief of pain secondary to cancer. The situation is scarcely better for chronic pain due to benign diseases.

PERIPHERAL NERVE STIMULATION

Peripheral nerve stimulation (PNS) requires the application of an electrode directly upon the nerve to be stimulated via an open surgical procedure. Electrodes have been placed upon such nerves as the sciatic, femoral, ulnar, or median and about the brachialplexus (Fig. 1). The radio receiver is usually implanted subcutaneously in the thigh, abdomen, or supraclavicular fossa. There are very few patients with pain due to cancer who have had a peripheral nerve stimulator implanted (2,12). This is probably due to the

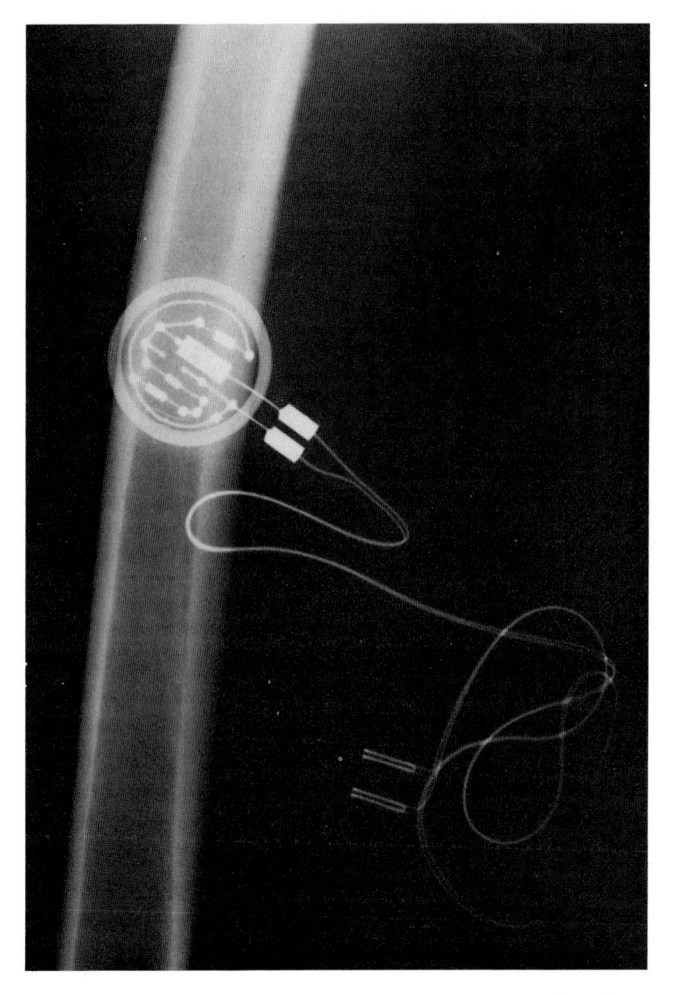

FIG. 1. Lateral X-ray of a sciatic-nerve stimulator and implanted radio receiver in a patient with chronic leg and buttock pain. The receiver is activated by placing an antenna on the skin directly over the receiver.

relative rarity of cancer pain originating from an extremity as well as the limited dissemination of this technique for pain-relief amongst the medical community.

The advantages of peripheral nerve stimulation should not be overlooked; it is a simple, nondestructive procedure for pain-relief. Patients do not have to tolerate a neurologic deficit to be relieved of their pain. The surgery required to insert the electrode and radio receiver can be performed under local anesthesia with minimal surgical risk to the patient. Paresthesias are restricted to the distribution of the nerve being stimulated; one must be certain that all of the noxious sensory inputs are via this nerve. It is desirable to carry out carefully performed local anesthetic block of the nerve before peripheral nerve stimulation is attempted. This procedure should eliminate sensation from the painful region and help predict the effects of PNS.

There is still ambiguity as to whether the locus of noxious sensation must be distal to the site of stimulation for pain-relief to occur. I have one patient whose sciatic-nerve stimulator relieves her pain due to arachnoiditis and epidural adhesions. Peripheral nerve stimulation could relieve pain due to neoplastic invasion of plexuses or epidural space. I believe that the small number of patients with chronic, severe pain in an extremity secondary to cancer can be considered for peripheral nerve stimulation before subjecting them to ablative neurosurgical procedures.

SPINAL CORD STIMULATION

Electrical stimulation of the spinal cord has been utilized since the pioneering work of Shealy approximately 10 years ago (14). The most commonly used commercially available components are manufactured by Avery Laboratories and Medtronic, Inc. In addition, there are parochial experimental devices.

The original concept was that electrical stimulation delivered to the dorsal columns of the spinal cord was responsible for the relief of pain. For this reason, electrodes were designed for implantation via a laminectomy directly upon or within the dura covering the midline dorsum of the spinal cord (Fig. 2). Several varieties of electrode sizes and configurations were evaluated; none were totally satisfactory. Bipolar stimulation proved superior to monopolar; flexible lead wires resistant to fracture by repeated movement were developed.

Surgical complications have been all too common, and morbidity ensued for a significant number of the patients (10,13,16). Among the complications described have been: wound infection, CSF fistula, subdural or epidural hematoma, spinal cord compression, and migration of the radio receiver within its subcutaneous pocket. Some patients have complained of a new pain associated with the implanted equipment. A significant number of patients have described a change in the effects of DCS so that what was a pain-relieving electrical stimulation becomes not only ineffective in alleviating the spontaneous pain but itself becomes unpleasant.

Although the initial concept involved stimulation of the dorsal columns, it became obvious from animal experimentation, human trials, and, later, planned ventral electrode placements, that the actual neural tissues stimulated by the electrodes were uncertain and that stimulation applied to the ventral surface or from dorsal to ventral surfaces could also be effective in relieving pain. The actual current pathways are difficult to determine and the physiologic basis of pain-relief from DCS is uncertain. Whether the effect of electrical stimulation is to activate certain axons which inhibit pain

TABLE 1. *DCS and PNS for cancer pain*

Author	Year	Type[a]	No. of pts.	% Success
Burton (1)	1975	DCS	1	?
Campbell (2)	1976	PNS	3	0
Clark (3)	1975	DCS	3	67
Freidberg (5)	1975	DCS	1	100
Hunt (6)	1975	DCS	1	0
Long (7)	1975	DCS	6	50
Medtronic (4)	1976	PISCES	9	44
Miles (8)	1974	DCS	2	100
Nashold (9)	1972	DCS	1	0
Nielson (10)	1975	DCS	18	61
North (11)	1977	PISCES	2	50
Picaza (12)	1975	PNS[b]	5	60
Pineda (13)	1975	DCS	4	50
Shealy (14)	1969	DCS	2	100
Shelden (15)	1975	DCS	17	47
Sweet (16)	1974	DCS	3	67

[a] PNS = peripheral nerve stimulation; DCS = dorsal column stimulation; PISCES = percutaneously inserted spinal-cord electrode system.
[b] Acute stimulation only.

or to block transmission in axons subserving pain sensations is uncertain. Many patients have reported pain-relief outlasting stimulation by minutes or hours; the neural substrates for such prolonged effects are unknown. Recent studies have suggested that a central neurohumoral system (enkephalins) may be activated by electrical stimulation.

Problems in patient-selection have plagued the assay of the clinical efficacy of dorsal column stimulation. As we might predict, patients whose pain behavior is largely under the control of environmental or emotional factors do not often get relief from DCS. Patients with pain due to cancer do not usually fall into that category and should, therefore, be reasonable candidates for DCS. Table 1 includes all the published cases I can find of DCS for the treatment of cancer pain. Fifty-one patients is not an impressively large group upon which to base an analysis of the efficacy of this treatment modality (1,3,5–10,13–16). Why has not dorsal column stimulation received a wider trial?

The first answer must be that it has, but the patients have not been carefully followed and reported. It is said that over 3,000 DCS units have been employed; roughly 10% of these patients appear in the literature. Data is therefore lost for scientific analysis, although surgeons received fees and manufacturers sold equipment. The development of new technologies cannot be facilitated by this style of slipshod data-collection. Since impressively good results often get reported, my suspicion is that a large proportion of the

1. Electrode sutured to inner surface of dura;

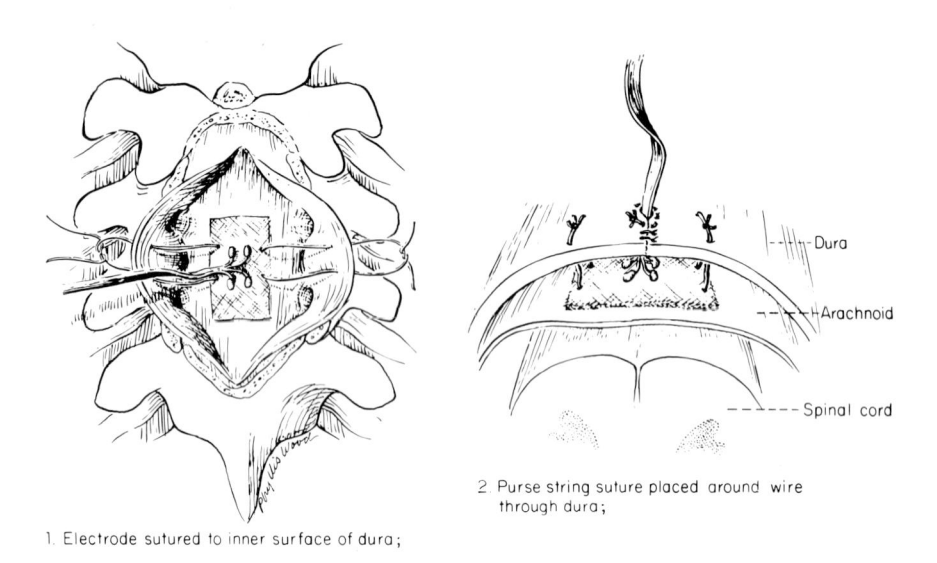

2. Purse string suture placed around wire through dura;

FIG. 2. The insertion of a dorsal column stimulator in the subdural space over the thoracic spinal cord. The lead wires are connected to an implanted radio receiver.

unreported patients did not benefit from DCS. Available case reports suggest that roughly one-half of the patients with pain due to cancer have reported significant relief of their pain when implanted with a dorsal column stimulator (7). Review of the reported cases does not generate any predictors of long-term efficacy. It does seem to be true that paresthesias must be perceived by the patient in the region of the pain if symptomatic relief is to occur.

The insertion of a dorsal column stimulator requires a laminectomy and is usually done with general anesthesia. It is, therefore, a major operation which may not be well tolerated by a terminally ill patient. On the other hand, DCS offers the promise of pain-relief without destruction of any portion of the nervous system and without new neurologic deficits. Almost all of the reported cases have utilized midline dorsal placement of the stimulating electrodes, although some investigators have tried other stimulation sites. Optimal localization of the electrodes has not yet been established (Fig. 2).

The initial enthusiasm for DCS has waned as its modest long-term efficacy and significant complication rate have become apparent. The development of a much simpler electrode system has re-kindled an interest in spinal cord stimulation for pain-relief (4). The PISCES® equipment (Percutaneous Insertion of Spinal Cord Electrode System) eliminates the surgical hazards of DCS but has added new problems with electrode stability. Two flexible electrodes are inserted into the epidural space via standard needles and then threaded into the desired position under fluoroscopic observation. The elec-

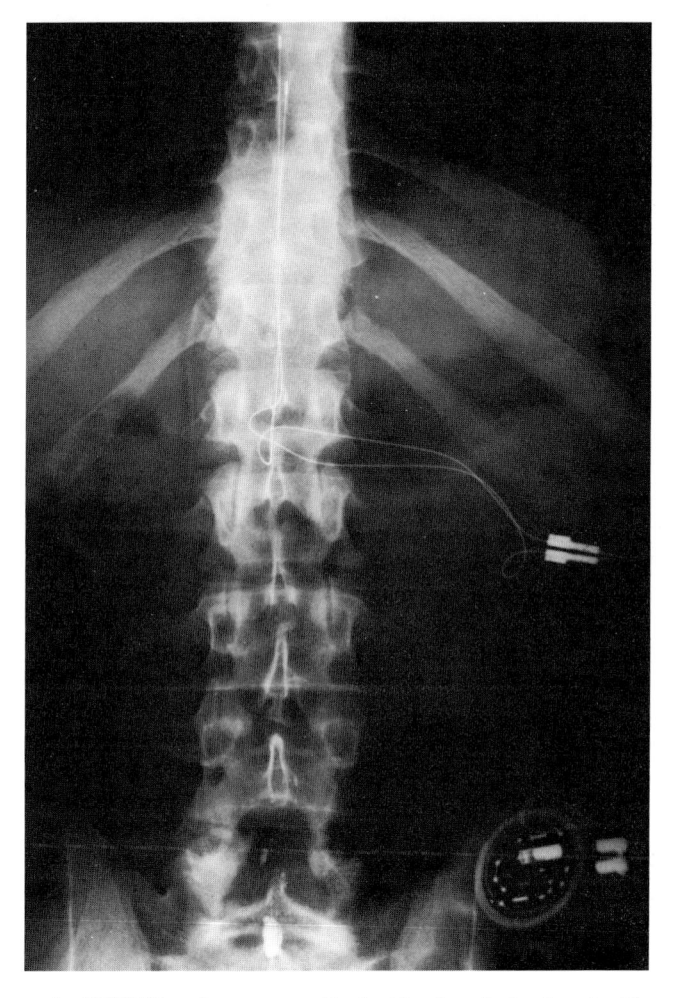

FIG. 3. X-ray of a PISCES system on a patient with chronic back pain. The electrodes were inserted percutaneously at L_1–L_2 and connected to an implanted radio receiver, which can be seen in the left lower quadrant.

trode lead wires are then passed through the skin and connected to an external stimulator (Figs. 3 and 4). The patient then undergoes a trial period; if stimulation is effective, the lead wires are removed and the electrodes connected to an implanted receiver identical to that used for DCS or PNS. This system has eliminated the need for a major surgical procedure and has proven to have a very low rate of complication. The major drawback has been migration of the epidural electrodes hours, days, or months after insertion, with subsequent loss of stimulation efficacy. New electrodes will be required with some type of anchoring devices if this technique is to gain widespread clinical evaluation.

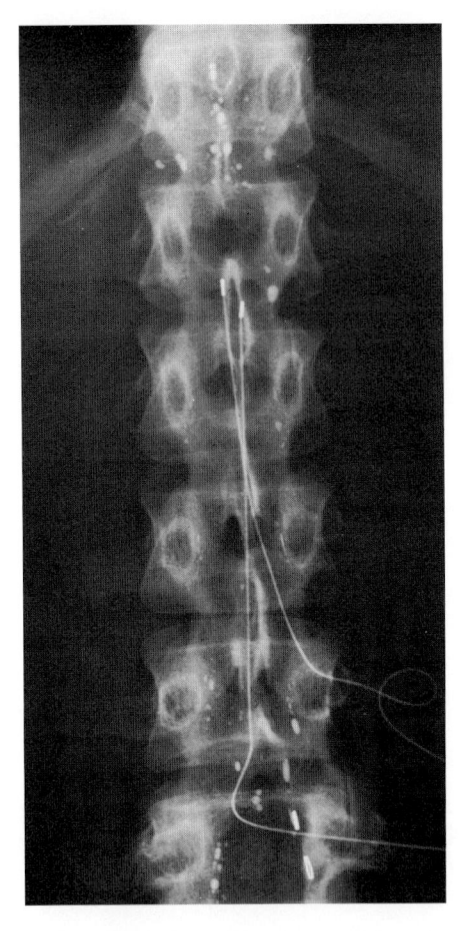

FIG. 4. X-ray of PISCES electrodes in the lumbar epidural space. During the evaluation period, these electrodes are connected to an external stimulator. If stimulation relieves the patient's pain, they are connected to a permanent, implanted radio receiver.

A limited number of patients with pain due to cancer have been reported to have received a PISCES trial; approximately 50% appear to have significant long-term relief (4,11). Experience is too limited to permit a meaningful evaluation.

CONCLUSIONS

In conclusion, I believe that electrical stimulation of the peripheral nerves or spinal cord has the potential for providing pain-relief to patients with cancer. The major problems seem to be related to the perfection of stimulation electrodes and the trial of this technique in a large enough group of patients to generate valid data on the likelihood of pain-relief for other patients with cancer. Clinical efficacy should be demonstrated in well-controlled studies before electrical stimulation of nerve or spinal cord becomes a readily available therapeutic modality.

REFERENCES

1. Burton, C. (1975): Dorsal column stimulation: Optimization of application. *Surg. Neurol.*, 4:171–176.
2. Campbell, J. N., and Long, D. M. (1976): Peripheral nerve stimulation in the treatment of intractable pain. *J. Neurosurg.*, 45:692–699.
3. Clark, K. (1975): Electrical stimulation of the nervous system for control of pain: University of Texas Southwestern Medical School experience. *Surg. Neurol.*, 4:164–166.
4. *Clinical Status Report Medtronic PISCES System Model 3401.* Medtronic, Inc., Minneapolis. 1976.
5. Freidberg, S. R. (1975): Neurosurgical treatment of pain caused by cancer. *Med. Clin. North Am.*, 59:481–485.
6. Hunt, W. E., Goodman, J. H., and Bingham, W. G., Jr. (1975): Stimulation of the dorsal spinal cord for treatment of intractable pain: A preliminary report. *Surg. Neurol.*, 4:153–156.
7. Long, D. M., and Erickson, D. E. (1975): Stimulation of the posterior columns of the spinal cord for relief of intractable pain. *Surg. Neurol.*, 4:134–141.
8. Miles, J., Miles, J., Hayward, M., Bowsher, D., Mumford, J., and Molony, V. (1974): Pain relief by implanted electrical stimulators. *Lancet*, 1:777–779.
9. Nashold, B. S., and Friedman, H. (1972): Dorsal column stimulation for control of pain. Preliminary report on 30 patients. *J. Neurosurg.*, 36:590–597.
10. Nielson, K. D., Adams, J. E., and Hosobuchi, Y. (1975): Experience with dorsal column stimulation for relief of chronic intractable pain. *Surg. Neurol.*, 4:148–152.
11. North, R. B., Fischell, T. A., and Long, D. M. (1977): Chronic stimulation via percutaneously inserted epidural electrodes. *Neurosurg.*, 1:215–218.
12. Picaza, J. A., Cannon, B. W., Hunter, S. E., Boyd, A. S., Guma, J., and Maurer, D. (1975): Pain suppression by peripheral nerve stimulation. *Surg. Neurol.*, 4:105–114.
13. Pineda, A. (1974): Dorsal column stimulation and its prospects. *Surg. Neurol.*, 4:157–163.
14. Shealy, C. N. (1969): Dorsal column electrohypalgesia. *Headache*, 9:99–102.
15. Shelden, C. H., Paul, F., Jacques, D. B., and Pudenz, R. H. (1975): Electrical stimulation of the nervous system. *Surg. Neurol.*, 4:127–132.
16. Sweet, W. H., and Wepsic, J. G. (1974): Stimulation of the posterior columns of the spinal cord for pain control: Indications, technique and results. *Clin. Neurosurg.*, 21:278–310.

Transcutaneous Nerve Stimulation in Cancer Pain

V. Ventafridda, E. P. Sganzerla, C. Fochi, G. Pozzi, and G. Cordini

Department of Pain Therapy and Rehabilitation, National Cancer Institute, Milan, Italy; Department of Anesthesiology, Universita degli Studi, Milan, Italy

In the past 10 years there has been a renewed interest in transcutaneous electrical nerve stimulation (TENS) as a means of controlling pain. This simple method of pain modulation was known to the Romans, who used electric eels as current generators. In the 19th century, electrical stimulation was used widely for the treatment of various pain syndromes, and the first electrostatic portable stimulators known as "magneto-electric machines" were built. Because of variable and unpredictable results, electroanalgesia was eventually abandoned by most workers. Although Martini et al. (5) in 1943 demonstrated the analgesic effect of the application of electrical currents to the cat's spinal cord, it was not until after the publication of the gate control theory of pain by Melzack and Wall in 1965 (6) that interest in this method of analgesia was resumed. Of the various techniques developed, transcutaneous electrical nerve stimulation has been the most widely used because it is simple, can be applied on the skin, and produces no important side effects.

Published clinical data reveal that TENS may be acutely beneficial in a large number of patients treated for various pain syndromes, but its efficacy usually declines over a long-term period (7). Results obtained in the management of cancer pain vary among different authors reporting data. In a previous paper (12) we reported good to excellent results in about 43% of the patients with cancer pain managed with this modality. Best results were obtained in patients with moderate initial pain, especially when the pain was located in the head and neck regions and when evident trigger points or hyperalgesic areas were found. Good results were also achieved in patients with post-herpetic neuralgia and with early phantom-limb pain that followed cancer therapy. Using the time that the stimulator was employed by the patient as a criterion, long-term results were less favorable. In 159 patients who obtained an initial benefit from TENS, only 56 (35%) were still using it after 1 month. After 10 days, 92 (58%) had already returned the device, as they did not feel it could help their pain anymore.

In order to obtain a more careful clinical assessment and to better identify the role of TENS in controlling cancer pain, we studied a group of 37 patients who, according to our past experience, were expected to obtain an effective control of their pain with this method. We used a detailed pain-profile questionnaire to assess the efficacy of the technique.

MATERIAL AND METHODS

We evaluated 37 patients with intractable cancer pain or other painful conditions in which cancer was a primary cause. All of them were evaluated with a simplified pain-profile questionnaire according to the model developed

TABLE 1. *Pain profile scoring matrix*

Grade	Daily duration of pain	Intensity of pain	Activity level	Drugs
0	No pain	None	Normal	None
1	Having pain up to 25% of time	Mild	Slightly restricted activity	Antiinflammatory agents
2	Up to 50% of time	Discomforting	Moderately restricted	Psychotropic drugs
3	Up to 75% of time	Distressing	Severely restricted	Hypnotics pentazocine
4	Up to 100% of time	Horrible or excruciating	Incapacitated	Narcotics

by Piccaza, Ray, and Shealy (10). Four major criteria for assessing pain and pain relief were used: (a) severity of pain; (b) the percentage of time each day the pain was present; (c) the effect of pain on physical activity; and (d) the use of drugs (Table 1). In all of the patients, TENS was achieved with a commercially available stimulator and electrodes.[1] Optimal setting of electrical output for pain-relief was empirically determined on an individual basis, by testing the whole range of tolerable outputs in various combinations of pulse width, intensity, and frequency. In every patient, we tried to induce a tolerable tingling sensation, carefully avoiding painful levels of stimulation. Rubber electrodes were usually applied over pain trigger areas, over nerve trunks supplying the painful areas, or over an area of the painful region which, according to the patients, gave the best analgesia. All the patients continued to use the device as long as they obtained some definite benefit from it.

Before entering the study group, all patients were instructed in the use of the stimulating device and used it for a first trial period of 48 hr. All patients who after this first trial obtained a satisfactory pain-relief from the

---

[1] EPC-Mini—STIM-TECH, Minneapolis, Minnesota.

stimulator were invited to use it as long as they derived benefit from it. At the beginning of the control period and at 10, 20, and 30 days, they were invited to return to the pain clinic where they filled out the pain-profile questionnaire and were clinically evaluated.

For every category of the pain profile and for the total score, the differences observed between the beginning of the treatment and the 10-, 20-, and 30-day evaluations have been calculated. Wilcoxon's t-test has been applied to the differences of total scores.

RESULTS

As in our previous experience, this group of patients' TENS had a very high rate of success in the first days of use which rapidly declined during subsequent evaluations. Although the intensity of pain was markedly reduced in 35 (96%) patients during the first 10 days of treatment, only 4 (11%) of the patients experienced reduction of their pain intensity after 30 days. Physical activity initially increased in 28 (76%) patients. This declined to 19% (7 patients) at 30 days. A similar pattern was noted in the total time each day the pain was present or absent: The presence of pain was reduced in 32 (86%) patients at the time of the first evaluation, and 4 (11%) at the last evaluation. In contrast, drug intake was reduced initially in only 13 (35%) patients; but after 1 month, it was reduced in 20 (54%) patients.

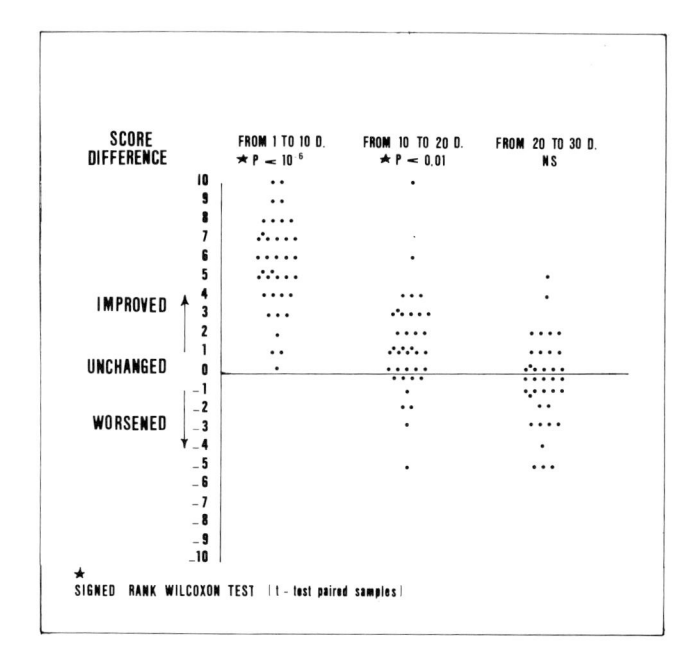

FIG. 1. Total score: differences at 10, 20, and 30 days.

TABLE 2. Results at 30th. day in 37 oncological patients treated with T.E.N.S.

Pain character	Pain site	No. patients	Major +5 +2	Medium +1 −0	Minor −1 −5
Somatic pain	Head and neck	13	3	6	4
with overt	Chest wall	5	—	—	5
trigger points	Abdominal	1	—	1	—
20 patients	Limbs	1	—	—	1
Dysesthesic pain	Phantom (limb)	6	3	1	2
17 patients	Postherpetic neuralgia (chest wall)	8	—	6	2
	Post. surg. neuralgia (chest wall)	3	—	1	2

The differences between the total scores are shown in Fig. 1, which demonstrates that while in the first 10 days, 36 patients (96%) had an overall improvement, follow-up showed significant declines in the effect of the stimulator; and at 30 days, only 27% of the patients still enjoyed an improvement in their pain problem. This was not statistically significant.

Considering the type of pain (Table 2), the best results at 30 days were observed in 3 patients with head and neck pain and in 3 patients with initial phantom-limb pain and to a lesser degree in 6 patients with postherpetic

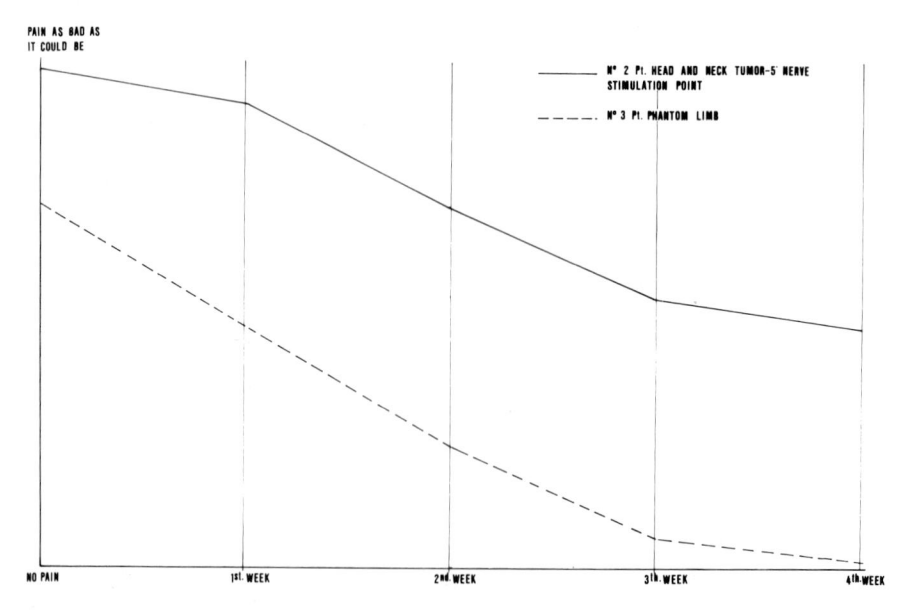

FIG. 2. Worst pain experienced during the week recorded by visual analogue on 5 patients under TENS study.

neuralgia. In the patients who benefited from TENS, there was a constant decrease of pain-appreciation evaluated with the visual analogue technique (2) (Fig. 2).

None of the subjects suffered a complication due to the use of the stimulating device. Skin irritation was avoided by instructing the patients about the frequent cleaning of the electrodes and changing of the conductive paste.

DISCUSSION

Our results with TENS show that in treating patients with chronic pain syndromes of oncologic origin, the long-term usefulness of the stimulating device is quite limited. Even if a high percentage of patients initially respond well to this method of pain modulation, the success rate declines rapidly. After a month or so, it continues to be effective in only a small percentage of patients.

One of the most important factors in the successful use of TENS is the correct positioning of the electrodes and the optimal adjustment of the electrical output. This has to be done with the patient's collaboration, and it is a time-consuming procedure. The patient must be aware of the pain-reducing mechanism of TENS. Pulse width, intensity, and rate combinations have different results for each subject. In order to avoid unpleasant overstimulation and still provide effective levels, these must be carefully determined. Once the analgesic effect is obtained, it is important to test the device for at least 48 hr. Only with such a trial can we determine the correct use and efficacy of the device. Thereafter, the patient must be encouraged to use the stimulator as long as he likes, which may extend from 2 to 3 hr to the entire day.

The presence of a trigger point in an area related to a peripheral nerve fiber is a positive indication for TENS treatment. Richly innervated skin areas are more suitable to pain modulation. Patients suffering from compression by large masses over the cervical nerve trunks or neoplastic involvement on the maxillofacial tissues may get immediate relief. Electrodes must avoid areas of skin erosion or hypesthetic areas. Even if there are no differences between placebo and TENS (11), the placebo effect offered by the use of the stimulating device and its autoregulation by the patient may be useful in diverting the subject's attention from his illness.

Our observations on personality profiles obtained by submitting patients to the MMPI test before treatment indicate that those who had benefit for more than 10 days by the use of TENS revealed significant alterations on their clinical scales compared with the subjects who refused the device at the outset (Fig. 3).

The benefits derived from TENS may be increased by combined therapy with psychotropic drugs and anti-inflammatory agents (13). In fact, antidepressant compounds, such as aminotriptyline with electric stimulation, are

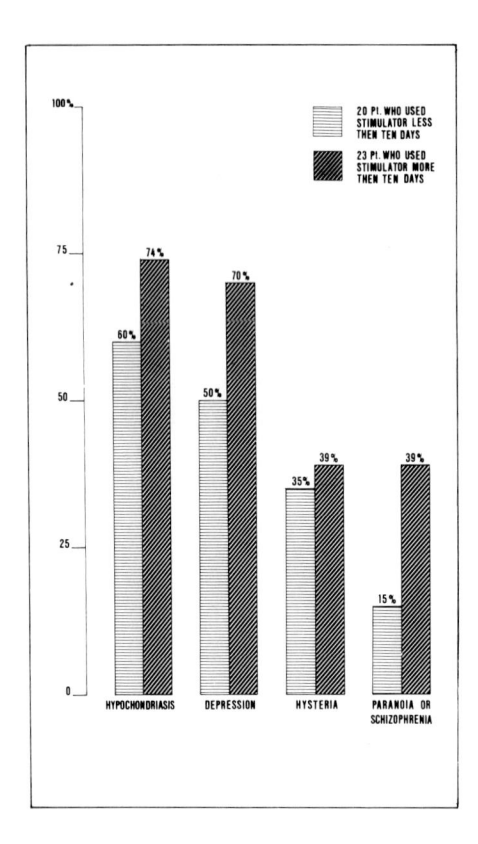

FIG. 3. MMPI significant percent scales with T > 70 on 43 patients who underwent TENS study.

effective in controlling pain from postherpetic neuralgia occurring during chemotherapy for systemic tumors. Electrodes must be placed around the herpetic area until the patient feels a tingling sensation. The tricyclic compound (75 mg daily) not only counteracts the depression, but also restores normal sleep-wakefulness cycling.

Although only a few patients with cancer pain derive long-lasting benefits from TENS, we feel that this simple and innocuous method is worthy of clinical application. Drug-use reduction is a clear index that TENS is worth a trial in oncologic pain control before utilizing more destructive or toxic methods.

REFERENCES

1. Ebersold, M. J., Laws, E. R., Stonnington, H. H., and Stillwell, G. K. (1975): Transcutaneous electrical stimulation for treatment of chronic pain: A preliminary report. *Surg. Neurol.*, 4:96–98.
2. Huskisson, E. C. (1974): Measurement of pain. *Lancet*, 9:1127–1131.
3. Loeser, J. D., Black, R. G., and Christman, A. (1975): Relief of pain by transcutaneous stimulation. *J. Neurosurg.*, 42:308–314.

4. Long, D. M. (1974): External electrical stimulation as a treatment of chronic pain. *Minn. Med.,* 57:195–198.
5. Martini, E., Gualtierotti, T., and Marzorati, A. (1943): Die Rükkenmarkelektronarkose. *Pflügers Arch. Ges. Physiol.,* 246:585.
6. Melzack, R., and Wall, P. D. (1965): Pain mechanism: A new theory. *Science,* 150:971–979.
7. Ray, C. A. (1975): Control of pain by electrical stimulation. A clinical follow-up review. In: *Brain Hypoxia, Pain,* edited by H. Penzholz, M. Brock, J. Hamer, M. Klinger, and O. Spoerri, pp. 216–224. Springer-Verlag, Berlin.
8. Shealy, C. N., and Maurer, D. (1974): Transcutaneous nerve stimulation for control of pain: Preliminary technical note. *Surg. Neurol.,* 2:45.
9. Shealy, C. N. (1974): Transcutaneous electrical stimulation for control of pain. *Clin. Neurosurg.,* 21:269.
10. Shealy, C. N., and Shealy, M. C. (1975): Behavioural techniques in the control of pain: A case for health maintenance vs. disease treatment. In: *Pain: New Perspectives in Therapy and Research,* edited by M. Weisenberg and B. Tursky, pp. 21–33. Plenum Press, New York.
11. Thornsteinsson, G., Stonnington, H. H., Stillwell, G. K., and Elveback, L. R. (1977): Transcutaneous electrical stimulation: A double-blind trial of its efficacy for pain. *Arch. Phys. Med. Rehabil.,* 58:8–13.
12. Ventafridda, V., Fochi, C., and Sganzerla, E. P. (1977): L'Elettrostimolazione transcutanea nel trattamento del dolore oncologico. *Anest. Rianim.,* 18:87–97.
13. Ventafridda, V., Sganzerla, E. P., and Fochi, C. (1979): Considerazioni sull'uso di sostanze psicotrope ad azione antidepressiva in terapia antalgica. *Minerva Med.,* 70 (*in press*).

Discussion

Part II. Management of Pain of Advanced Cancer: Ablative Neurosurgical Procedures and Augmentative (Stimulating) Neurosurgical Procedures

Siegfried (Zürich): I would like to reply to what Pagni said about the utility of percutaneous combined rhizotomy of the trigeminal nerve and glossopharyngeal nerves. I would like to emphasize again that we are talking about cancer patients who are in very poor condition, and I think that open surgery on a posterior fossa carries with it a very high operative risk. I agree that many times pain is outside the trigeminal and glossopharyngeal domain, but we are proposing the percutaneous rhizotomy just for pain of the face. And once you achieve a good relief of pain in the face, you can also perform cervical root rhizotomy if pain is spreading beyond the face.

Broggi (Milano): Dr. Lipton, in my experience, out of 142 cordotomies at the C_1-C_2 level, I had only one paralysis and 6 cases of leg weakness, but 15 of walking ataxia that faded away in 7 to 10 days. Does your experience agree with mine?

Lipton (Liverpool): Our figures vary slightly, I had a paralysis also, a few unexpected cases of leg weakness, and two ataxias, one in the arm, one in the leg. Rosomoff mentions about a 20% incidence of ataxia.

Questioner: Dr. Loeser, have you observed worsening of pain during or after dorsal column stimulation?

Loeser (Seattle): Yes. There is a significant number of patients who usually 6 months to a year after dorsal column stimulation complain that they develop a new sensation when the stimulator is turned on and that that sensation is in itself painful. There is no remedy for that other than not using the stimulator.

Bonica (Seattle): I think it is most appropriate to make a comment about the use of acupuncture for pain management in cancer because it is related to electrical stimulation. I have just reviewed the American literature for some review article and could not find that anyone was using it, and there are, therefore, no statistics. In my 3-week visit to the People's Republic of China, I was very surprised to learn that this is one of the few areas in which the Chinese do not use acupuncture. So, apparently they have tried it and it is no longer used.

Questioner: Dr. Richardson, do you see tolerance with brain stimulation or with central nervous system stimulation for pain-relief?

Richardson (New Orleans): Yes, you do see tolerance to stimulation, Yoshio Hosobuchi has been working with tolerance for some time. We have seen it in a few of our patients. It can be held down to a minimum by using the least amount of stimulation that is effective for pain-relief. And it also can be obviated by the use of drugs.

I have some questions regarding the use of conjoint drug therapy. Almost all of our patients are on tricyclic antidepressives that increase the amount of serotonin in the central nervous system and also obviate sleep problems. These drugs will decrease the amount of stimulation necessary. We have also used antinorepinephrine agents, such as disulphone, which in the U.S.A. is called Antabuse® and is used for alcoholism. It inhibits norepinephrine and will increase the effectiveness of stimulation by blocking an antagonist modulation system. It will also produce serotonin mania if you use it in conjunction with tricyclics in large doses, and we have had one patient who had serotonin mania and required 2 weeks of hospitalization and treatment with phenothiazenes. We also have a trial going with the FDA on the use of tryptophan as an antitolerance drug. We have little data, but it seems to be more effective than anything else we have.

Questioner: Dr. Richardson, have you measured endogenous opiate levels in relation to stimulation?

Richardson: Yes, we have measured endogenous opiates in ventricular fluid but not in peripheral blood. John Adams has done that and found that there is an increase in opiate-like substances in peripheral blood during central gray stimulation. We have found a marked rise in opiate-like substances in the third ventricular fluid during stimulation, reaching a maximum peak at about 50 min and then gradually decreasing.

Questioner: Dr. Richardson, what is the scientific basis for the assumption that the opiates and paraventricular gray stimulation are mediated through the same system?

Richardson: (a) They are both blocked by nalaxone, a specific morphine antagonist. (b) They are both dependent on serotonin. (c) Dorsal lateral cordotomies in the rat and the cat block the effect of central gray stimulation below the level of the cordotomy in the rat. An animal who has had section of the dorsal lateral column on one side, if given morphine, will show analgesia in the other three extremities and no analgesia in the extremity below the dorsal lateral section. It has also been shown in rats that spinal cord reflexes are released from the effect of morphine by sectioning the cord at the C_1 level.

Questioner: Dr. Richardson, have you noted any behavioral changes?

Richardson: Yes, we have noted very mild but easily observable behavioral changes. Some patients become less depressed. Other patients have had a fright reaction during stimulation. Now, we think this is probably related to having the electrode placed a little too deeply in the hypothalamus, but many patients have excellent pain inhibition with no other side effects. They also will have an obvious elevation of mood apparently unrelated to the pain-relief.

Questioner: Dr. Richardson, is the procedure effective for deafferentation pain, that is, pain in an area of numbness?

Richardson: In some patients, yes; in other patients, we have to use either VLP or internal capsule stimulation. And we have some patients with mixed pain in whom central gray stimulation relieves their chronic mechanical back pain but does not relieve the area of burning pain in their leg caused by nerve injury.

So in some patients you have to choose which pain you are going to attack because you don't want to do two procedures on the same patient at the same time.

Questioner: What is the mortality rate in cordotomy and myelotomy operations, Dr. Papo?

Papo (Ancona): In the past when these operations were performed with broad indications, the mortality rate was about 2 to 4%. Today these operations are reserved for special cases, and mortality rate should be practically negligible. Regarding myelotomy, it is difficult to say. It certainly is very low.

Questioner: Dr. Papo, what is the incidence and mechanism of painful dysesthesia in the lower unilateral limb after cervical cordotomy?

Papo: The current hypothesis is that these are mainly deafferentation pains. The incidence depends mostly on how long the patients survive. In some studies by Guillot, several years ago, all patients operated on for coxalgia and coxarthosis had painful dysesthesias of this kind.

Questioner: Dr. Papo, what do you recommend for cordotomy, local or general anesthesia?

Papo: I believe that general anesthesia is best, because data obtained with local anesthesia have no value since one may be misled by contused fibers that temporarily don't transmit anymore.

Pagni (Torino): Dr. Papo, what about cingulumotomy?

Papo: I performed it some years ago on two groups of patients: some psychiatric patients and some patients in pain; and I noticed that the main difference was in the intensity of psychic deterioration that I could see in the two groups.

While the psychiatric patients tolerated the operation well and the therapeutic results were sometimes useful, in the patients with pain, especially when due to neoplasia, the psychic deterioration was terrible, so I completely abandoned this type of operation.

I recently met Eldon Folz, who introduced this type of operation, and he, too, doesn't perform it anymore.

Loeser: In some of our stimulation procedures for pain-relief, our approach has been to try to reduce the magnitude of the surgical procedures for pain-relief, especially in terminal cancer patients. The selection of the specific procedure should be based on the location of the pain, the prognosis for the particular patient involved, and the extent of the procedure that will be selected.

Problems of Cancer Pain in the Head and Neck

Roberto Molinari

Oncology Department, Istituto Nazionale Tumori Milano, 20133 Milan, Italy

Only 35% of head and neck malignant tumors (with the exception of cancer of the lips and larynx) can be successfully treated and cured of the disease. The rest will develop recurrences or metastases or both. Of these 50 to 60% will develop pain. Head and neck cancers usually recur locally and spread to the regional lymph nodes. Distant metastases occur in only 5 to 15%, and only cancer of the nasopharynx and tonsil show general metastases in about 30 to 35%. Pain due to cancer growth tends to be localized in the head and neck, and its pathogenesis depends on the site more than on the histology of the tumor. Epidermoid cancer tends to ulcerate and deeply infiltrate surrounding structures, whereas glandular tumors and lymphomas generally grow by enlargement, so that pain is less frequently encountered in the latter type of tumors. On the whole, histological types of malignant tumors in decreasing order of their importance in causing pain are:

1. Epidermoid squamous carcinoma
2. Undifferentiated carcinoma
3. Adenoid cystic carcinoma
4. Bone sarcoma
5. Fibrosarcoma
6. Condrosarcoma
7. Lymphoma
8. Melanoma

PATHOGENESIS OF THE PAIN

The mechanisms by which head and neck cancer can cause pain include: (a) stimulation of mucosal and submucosal nerve endings, (b) ulceration and superinfection, (c) compression and involvement of sensitive nerve branches, and (d) bone invasion.

Stimulation of Mucosal and Submucosal Nerve Endings

This mechanism is specific for the initial phases of cancer growth. It can be considered to be mainly responsible for local burning sensations, superficial pain, and reflex neuralgic pain, such as otalgia in exophitic or erosive lesions.

Ulceration and Infection

Most of the cancers that arise from mucosal membranes (squamous cancer) of the mouth and pharynx tend to ulcerate, because of both central necrosis and microtraumatisms. Ulceration is not always painful per se, at least in the absence of local irritant agents, such as alcohol or acids, but the ulcer paves the way for infection by the microorganisms that are abundantly present in these cavities. Necrotic tissue and alimentary deposits are excellent culture grounds for bacteria, which can develop and cause subsequent inflammation and edema. Pain due to ulceration is markedly increased by movement of the involved part, and it therefore varies from site to site. Exacerbation by function is minimal in static regions such as cheek, floor of mouth, hard palate, nasal and paranasal cavities, and nasopharynx and is severe in the dynamic structures such as the tongue, soft palate, and faucial arch.

Involvement of Nerve Branches

The deeply infiltrating component of head and neck cancer frequently involves important nerve branches and trunks whose location is constant. Because of this, painful symptoms generally correspond to the anatomic site of the tumor. The most frequently involved nerves are: the lingual nerve by cancer of the mobile part of the tongue and floor of the mouth; the mandibular branch of the fifth nerve by cancer of the inferior gum and of the retromolar space and glossopalatine arch; the glossopharyngeal nerve by cancer of the tonsil and the lateral part of the base of the tongue.

Important sensitive nerve branches are not present in the laryngeal and hypopharyngeal regions, so that problems of pain are unusual in these regions. On the contrary, malignant tumors of nasal and paranasal cavities with particular locations can involve branches of the maxillary nerve, such as the infraorbital or, more often, the superior alveolar nerves. Advanced nasopharyngeal cancers cause mainly palsy of motor nerves, but also serious trigeminal neuralgias when the bone barrier is crossed. Lymph node metastasis causing marked enlargement with the mechanism of direct involvement of nervous branches is practically the only one that can induce severe pain in the neck.

Bone Invasion

Direct involvement of the bone is not painful per se. Pain arises when tumor progression involves nerve branches (as occurs in cancer of the alveolus) or when the path of neoplastic infiltration is followed from the surface by bacterial infection, with consequent osteomyelitis as occurs in alveolar tumors and in cancer of the maxillary antrum, where a superimposed obstructive sinusitis feeds the bone infection.

Adjuvant Factors

The above-mentioned mechanisms can obviously combine themselves in various ways and be all concomitant. Their effects, and consequently the importance of the problems of pain, can be made worse by other factors that are independent of the tumor but that are connected with often unavoidable consequences of the treatment or with functional and psychologic problems.

Post-radiation Damage

These range from simple mucositis to radionecrosis, by many intermediate degrees. When associated with persistence or recurrence of cancer (and consequently with the above-described mechanisms) they give rise to the most distressing situations. More frequent than spontaneous necrosis of a tumor mass is necrosis induced by radiation, which constitutes a rich ground for superimposed infection. Furthermore, it involves healthy tissues that contain sensitive nerve structures that have not been previously destroyed by the cancer. Apart from this extreme complication, radiation induces reactive fibrosis, which can cause more or less painful muscular contractions (trismus). On the whole, the combination of neoplastic recurrence with radionecrosis represents about 70% of the major problems of pain in cancer of the head and neck.

Functional Problems

Functions such as phonetics, breathing, and deglutition are frequently affected in cancer of the larynx and hypopharynx, where, on the contrary, problems of pain are rarely present. In cancer of the nasal and paranasal cavities, pain is mainly due to involvement of bony structures and branches of the fifth nerve; in cancer of the nasopharynx it is very frequently associated with palsy of one or more cranial motor nerves (and functional disorders make persistent pain less tolerable). However, the worst combination of pain and functional trouble is seen in cancer of the mouth and oropharynx, where bouts of hyperalgesia and neuralgia during chewing and swallowing can severely compromise the eating process.

Psychological Problems

All the above-mentioned mechanisms are often intensified by particular psychologic reactions, both basic and progressively acquired.
1. The great majority of the patients with cancer of the mouth and pharynx are heavy drinkers and smokers, with their basic psychologic problems.
2. Combination of pain and functional disorders make the psychologic conditions worse; all these symptoms influence one another in a sort of vicious cycle.

3. A particularly negative effect on the psychologic effects of cancer of the head and neck comes from the fact that these tumors can be seen, so that the patient can personally follow, day by day, the progress of his illness.

SPECIFIC PAIN SYNDROMES

Many pain syndromes associated with head and neck tumors can be listed; some of the most frequent and serious are:

Site and Type of Lesion	*Mechanism of Pain*
Cancer of the floor of the mouth, with bone involvement, with or without radionecrosis	Lingual or mandibular neuralgia complicated by pain caused by the superimposed infection
Cancer of the glossopalatine arch, with involvement of the tongue and the tonsil with or without trismus	Glossopharyngeal neuralgia, with mandibular nerve involvement
Cancer of the maxillary antrum	Maxillary neuralgia
Cancer of the nasopharynx, with invasion of the base of the skull	Dull painful syndrome in the nape of the neck and occipital region
Cancer of the nasopharynx, with invasion of the ethmoidal structure	Trigeminal pain
Advanced neck node metastases or recurrences	Cervical plexus and/or Arnold's nerve neuralgia
Postirradiation "wooden neck"	

Oncologic Therapy of Pain in Cancer of the Head and Neck

Roberto Molinari

Head and Neck Oncology Department, Istituto Nazionale Tumori Milano, 20133 Milan, Italy

More than half of the patients with cancer of the head and neck will sooner or later experience pain due to local or regional progress of their illness or, less frequently, to distant metastases. Apart from the latter, which are not specific to these tumors, the present report deals with the etiologic treatment of pain that is strictly localized in the head and neck region.

The weapons at our disposal are traditional: radiotherapy, surgery, and chemotherapy, alone or combined. Since the greatest majority of the problems of pain arise from recurrences after previous treatments, these are to be carefully taken into account for oncologic therapy. It is therefore necessary to consider every treatment not only as an isolated symptomatic measure for palliation, but also as a part of a general therapeutic plan in which we must always remember that progress of the tumor and severity of pain are related. In other words, pain can be frequently expected and avoided in many cases.

Pain can obviously occur in every phase of the illness, but the more advanced the tumor is, the more serious the problems of pain. At the beginning of the illness, every oncologic treatment can and must aspire to cure cancer and prevent pain. In advanced cases, a cure is not the main goal, although it is not to be renounced. However, an active antineoplastic therapy can often represent a valid alternative to a merely passive management of the pain.

RADIOTHERAPY

Radiotherapy is generally the first treatment used in cancer of the head and neck. In very advanced cases that are not suitable for other therapy, radiation therapy alone can often resolve problems of pain, especially when the tumor is highly radiosensitive. These include undifferentiated carcinoma of the nasopharynx and tonsil, ulcerating carcinoma of the tongue and floor of the mouth, and undifferentiated tumors of the nasal and paranasal cavities. In the great majority of cases, however, persistent pain is the consequence of recurrent cancer previously treated with surgery or radiotherapy (2,5). In the latter case, a new course of radiotherapy can hardly achieve consistent results from both an oncologic and a symptomatic viewpoint. On the contrary, the unavoidable overdosage can more often induce radionecrosis and finally increase the pain. Therefore, repetition of radiation therapy must be carefully thought over and performed only if very poor results can be expected from alternative treatments or when there is still some possibility for a cure. This is the case in nasopharyngeal cancer, where intraosseous recurrences are quite frequent and painful and where therapeutic alternatives are not possible. Great caution is needed in order to avoid damage to the spinal cord and to not make the condition of the patient worse by causing mandibular necrosis or trismus. With these precautions and by using different fields, the results are often satisfactory.

Recurrence with consequent pain after surgery represents the larger field of application of radiotherapy. This often happens in cancer of the paranasal cavities, mouth, and oropharynx, where surgery is frequently used as first treatment. On the other hand, in cancer of the larynx and hypopharynx, which is mostly treated with surgery, problems of pain are very rare, both at the initial stage of the disease and after recurrences.

Nevertheless, radiotherapy is a useful means in these cases. The task of the radiotherapist sometimes can be complicated by problems of dosimetry due to modifications resulting from surgery, such as removal of the jaw or other bony structures or removal of muscles such as the sternomastoid. On the other hand, these same changes sometimes facilitate the treatment by making possible and safer the choice of particular techniques not previously usable, such as interstitial radiotherapy or moulded radium apparatus.

It is extremely difficult to quantify the results on the pain of this kind of treatment separately from the oncologic ones. Remission of pain actually comes from the objective neoplastic regression, but the former is not a compulsory consequence of the latter. Radiotherapy pursues certain aims, but these are not always attained; furthermore, it can sometimes cause undesirable side effects, which can undo or even make worse the results achieved.

SURGERY

Symptomatic and Palliative Surgery

Surgical removal of lesions that were previously treated with radiotherapy and have recurred forms part of a combined treatment, even if not planned. This type of recurrence can actually give rise to pain or not, but, apart from oncologic results, remission of pain is a goal that is more frequently and consistently achieved by surgery than by radiotherapy (4).

Recurrence with bone invasion, especially when combined with radionecrosis, is one of the most frequent causes of pain. In this case the removal of bone involved by cancer is the most rapid and direct means of resolving this otherwise difficult problem. When feasible, surgery is repeated if necessary; our duty is only to carefully weigh the pros and cons of this treatment. Postoperative complications due to previous radiotherapy are to be considered in order to avoid life-threatening situations or too-protracted postoperative periods. The evaluation of these risks depends on the personal experience of the surgeon, who must sometimes reject a radical treatment in favor of a shorter and uneventful course with an acceptable expectancy of life with no problem of pain.

Surgery after radiotherapy is applicable and useful in many clinical situations, but mainly in case of:

1. recurrence of cancer of the oral cavity with radionecrosis;
2. osteoradionecrosis of the jaws, with or without neoplastic recurrence;
3. recurrence of oropharyngeal cancer (tonsil, base of the tongue, retromolar space, or anterior pillar);
4. recurrence of tumors of the nasal and paranasal cavities; and
5. recurrence of neck node metastases, after both radiotherapy and surgery.

In case of tumors initially advanced (T_3, T_4) and not previously treated, destructive surgery can be chosen as the first therapy when alternative treatments offer poor chances of resolving pain, independently of purposes of a cure.

Prevention of Problems of Pain

Major problems of pain in cancer of the head and neck can also be prevented by a careful choice of the initial treatment, not only by taking into account the anticipated results of the treatment but also by bearing in mind the future of the patient. When the expected cure-rate is statistically poor, the probabilities that progress of the tumor will cause pain are to be evaluated. As a consequence, we can be induced to modify our therapeutic plan and to choose different approaches, such as surgery instead of radiotherapy. In fact, surgery brings about section of nerve branches and trunks, which is tantamount to a real denervation. Consequences of surgery, such as cosmetic and functional damages, are often more willingly accepted than is the persistence of severe pain; and also an operation is an active therapeutic procedure that provides at least a psychologic relief to the patient, who is aware of his illness. It is often thought that these patients prefer less aggressive treatments, but this is not always true.

In my experience there are three main clinical situations in which the occurrence of severe pain syndromes is strongly affected by the choice of the first treatment:

1. Extended cancer of the mobile tongue and floor of the mouth. If interstitial radiotherapy is not feasible, external conventional irradiation has little chance of success in curing the patient. On the contrary, it

can result in many problems of pain, through radiomucositis or radionecrosis.
2. Cancer of the gums and retromolar space or adjacent structures involving the bone. In these cases, external radiotherapy can only rarely cure the patient but, on the other hand, is able to frequently induce trismus and very painful radionecrosis.
3. Very-large neck node metastases. Except for the more radiosensitive histotypes, such as undifferentiated carcinoma of the nasopharynx or tonsil, lymph node metastases are generally resistant to radiation therapy. Their progress can involve cervical nerve roots and cause severe pain. Very high doses of radiotherapy are to be given to these nodes; if radiotherapy does not succeed in curing them, the so-called "wooden-neck syndrome" often takes place, and in this case any form of curative or palliative surgery is no longer feasible. In all these cases, the initial treatment should be surgery whenever possible, because whatever the oncologic result may be, it is the same as prevention of pain (1).

CHEMOTHERAPY

The rationale of anticancer chemotherapy in patients with severe pain is the assumption that a correlation does exist between regression of the tumor and reduction of the pain. In head and neck cancer this correlation has been clearly demonstrated and is probably due to the fact that the tumor mass is generally smaller than it is in other regions of the body.

Chemotherapy with a palliative purpose has been used for many years in head and neck cancer. Many drugs have been tested including methotrexate, bleomycin, adriamycin, and hydroxyurea. Unfortunately, results have been inconsistent and quite poor. Better results, on the tumor and on the pain, can be achieved by combining different drugs (polychemotherapy) or by increasing the dose of single drugs. The latter was also pursued by using intra-arterial administration to reach the maximum concentration of the drug in a reduced area with no need for a general administration in too high a dose. In this method a catheter is placed in the external carotid artery via its superficial temporal branch; the drug is introduced by slow infusion in 8 to 20 hr daily in 10 to 15 days. Immediate results are very satisfactory: Remission of pain is generally prompt even when the objective regression of the tumor is partial or absent. Tumor regression is achieved less frequently and depends on the type of schedule used (Table 1).

However, intra-arterial chemotherapy cannot be employed in all of the patients because of anatomical or surgical reasons. Moreover, generally it can not be used for more than 15 to 25 days and requires hospitalization. As a consequence, this type of administration is not very suitable for palliative purposes; in addition, it requires further treatment by general administration in order to delay the unavoidable rapid relapse.

TABLE 1. Immediate results of intra-arterial chemotherapy using different single drugs at the Instituto Nazionale Tumori, Milano (INTM)

Drug dosage (per day for 10–15 days)	Total cases	% Tumor regression							Overall > 50%	
		< 50%		50%–>90%		Complete				
		No.	%	No.	%	No.	%	No.	%
MTX[a] 5 mg	26	20	77	5	19.2	1	3.8	6	23
ADM 0.3/kg	9	5	55.5	4	44.5	0	0	4	44.5
MTX 50 mg + CF	11	4	36.4	7	63.6	0	0	7	63.6
BLM 15 mg	30	12	40	14	46.7	4	13.3	18	60
VCR + BLM	27	8	29.6	12	44.4	7	26	19	70.4

[a] MTX = methotrexate; ADM = adriamycin; BLM = bleomycin; CF = citrovorum factor; VCR = vincristine.

General or systemic chemotherapy is more simple and has less risk, at least when drugs are not administered at very high doses. Results on both tumor and pain are not satisfactory when single drugs are used, and only methotrexate causes regression in many cases when it is administered at high doses with Leucovorin® rescue; regressions achieved, however, are rarely very significant (Table 2). Combinations of various drugs have been used by many investigators with better results, but also in this case a strict correlation was observed between clinical response and the number and amount of the drugs used. Severe toxicity is often encountered and is the main limitation of these palliative treatments, which cannot be employed for a long period of time and generally require hospitalization.

In order to overcome this obstacle, we have recently tested a new schedule of low-dose chemotherapy that was expressly set up for palliative, protracted treatments. This schedule is based on some concepts of synchronization of the cell cycle and uses vincristine, bleomycin, and methotrexate (VBM) in a particular sequence (3). In our experience, toxicity was almost negligible and not so different as was expected; oncologic results were very satisfactory in terms of frequency and importance of the regressions achieved (62% of tumors regressed more than 50%, and 32% of the tumors almost completely regressed (Table 3). Patients not previously treated with radiotherapy showed the best results, with 88% of regression greater than 50% of the initial size and 41% of complete regression (Table 4).

The most impressive finding was a clear correlation between clinical objective response and remission of pain; this was almost constant in responsive patients but was also observed in the absence of a significant objective regression (Table 5). The length of the remission was correlated with the importance of the initial response: The mean duration was 2.2 months in the group of less-responsive patients; 4 months in good responders (from 50 to 90% of regression); and 6.6 months among total responders. In 4 of 60 cases the regression achieved lasted 12 to 13 months. When there was a relapse, in 20% of the patients the pain did not occur again, and in 50% it required only simple, conventional treatment. In a certain number of cases we were able to profit from the regression achieved, since it was then possible to employ analgesic procedures (surgery, radiotherapy, or other oncologic treatments), with a palliative purpose.

In conclusion, by applying these principles of oncologic therapy to impending or expected problems of pain, we have noticed during the past 8 years a progressive reduction in the number of patients who require specific major analgesic treatment: 27% of those with head and neck cancer in 1970, 18% in 1973, 13% in 1975, and 10% in 1977. These results can be achieved only by means of a strict cooperation among the surgeon, radiotherapist, and chemotherapist; each must be aware of the limits of his own treatment and of the possibilities of the others.

TABLE 2. *Immediate results of general chemotherapy using different single drug schedules in palliative treatment of head and neck cancer (INTM experience)*

Drugs and schedules	Total cases	% Tumor regression						Overall > 50%	
		< 50%		50%->90%		Complete			
		No.	%	No.	%	No.	%	No.	%
CCNU[a] 130 mg/sq m/6 weeks p.o.	11	10	90.9	1	9.1	0	0	1	9.1
MTX 25 mg ×2/week p.o.	14	12	85.7	1	7.1	1	7.1	2	14.3
ADM 60–75 mg/sq m/3 weeks i.v.	35	30	85.7	1	2.9	4	11.4	5	14.3
BLM 10 mg/sq m/×2/week i.v.	14	12	85.7	1	7.1	1	7.1	2	14.3
BLM 15–30 mg/sq m/week i.v.	29	20	68	7	24.1	2	6.9	9	31
MTX 40–60 mg/sq m/week i.v.	23	15	65.2	8	34.8	0	0	8	34.8
BLM 10 mg/sq m ×2/week i.v.	16	14	87.5	2	12.5	0	0	2	12.5
MTX 40 mg/sq m/week i.v. + VCR 1 mg/week + BLM 30 mg/week (sequential) + MTX 20 mg/sq m/week	60	23	38.3	18	30	19	31.7	37	61.6

[a] CCNU = chloroethyl-cyclohexyl-nitrosourea; MTX = methotrexate; ADM = adriamycin; BLM = bleomycin; VCR = vincristine.

TABLE 3. Results of general chemotherapy with VBM: regression achieved in cancer of the head and neck, by site of the tumor

Site	Total cases	0%–< 25% No.	%	25%–< 50% No.	%	50%–< 90% No.	%	90%–< 100% No.	%	Overall > 50% No.	%
Oral cavity (post.)	12	0	0	2	17	5	41.5	5	41.5	10	83.3
Oral cavity (ant.)	22	6	27	3	14	4	18	9	41	13	59
Oropharynx	11	2	18	3	27	4	37	2	18	6	54.5
Larynx-hypopharynx	12	5	41	1	8	4	34	2	17	6	50
Lips, skin	3	1	33	0	0	1	33	1	33	1	33.3
Totals	60	14	23	9	15	18	30	19	32	37	62

TABLE 4. Results of general chemotherapy with VBM: regression according to previous treatment

Previous treatment	Responses			
	<50%		>50%	
	No.	%	No.	%
Radiotherapy Surgery + radiotherapy	21	48.8	22	51.2
No treatment Surgery alone	2	12	15	88
Totals	23	38	37	62

TABLE 5. Relationships between objective regression and remission of pain in 27 patients with problems of pain, using VBM

Remission of pain	Objective regression							
	0–25%		25%–50%		50%–90%		Complete	
	No.	%	No.	%	No.	%	No.	%
No remission	2/6	33	1/4	25	1/9	11	0/8	0
Slight	2/6	33	1/4	25	0/9	0	0/8	0
Important	1/6	17	2/4	50	5/9	55	0/8	0
Complete	1/6	17	0/4	0	3/9	33	8/8	100

REFERENCES

1. Badellino, F. (1977): Terapia palliativa delle metastasi linfonodali nei carcinomi della testa e del collo. *Nuovo Arch. Ital. Otol.,* 5:561.
2. Hayward, M. (1977): Headache and pain in the head and neck. In: S. Lipton: *Persistent Pain: Modern Methods of Treatment, Vol. I.* Academic Press, London.
3. Molinari, R., Mattavelli, F., Chiesa, F., Cantu', G., Costa, L., and Tancini G. (1978): Results of palliative treatment of advanced or recurred head and neck squamous carcinoma using a sequential low dose combination chemotherapy (V B M), (*in press*).
4. Richard, J., Vandebrouck, C., Lefur, R., and Cachin, Y. (1971): Que faut-il penser de la bucco-pharyngectomie transmaxillaire de rattra-page? *Ann. Otolaryngol. (Paris),* 88:663.
5. Wolff, H. G. (1963): *Headache and Other Head Pain.* Oxford University Press, London and New York.

Cancer Pain in the Head and Neck: Role of Analgesics and Related Drugs

Raymond W. Houde

Department of Medicine, Memorial Sloan-Kettering Cancer Center, New York, New York 10021

Systemic analgesics of some type are virtually always employed at some stage in the management of pain due to head and neck cancer. The choice of a particular drug, of a particular class of drugs, or of additional adjuvant symptomatic drugs will rest on a number of considerations relating to the patient's present status and past medical history. Head and neck cancer is comprised on a wide diversity of neoplasms which, to name but a few, include the various intracranial and cranial neoplasms, cancers of the mouth, tongue, nasopharynx, oropharynx, larynx, cervical esophagus, salivary glands, thyroid glands, lymph nodes, and skin and underlying soft tissues. The extent to which these cancers produce pain, disability, disfigurement, and suffering is also subject to considerable differences in the clinical evolution of each of these neoplasms, what medical intervention has been undertaken or is being done, and a number of complications which can occur, such as necrosis, ulceration, infection, occlusion of blood vessels or lymphatics, and fractures occurring as a consequence of either the disease or its treatment.

To be considered in decisions of management, particularly as they relate to the use of systemic drugs, are factors relating to the patient's age, social habits, and the social consequences of a disease which may be so visible to one's family, friends, and associates. Some types of cancer, such as those of the brain, eye, thyroid, and blood and lymphatic systems are not uncommonly encountered in the young, but most head and neck cancers, particularly that of the skin and mucous membranes of the upper respiratory system and the upper digestive tract, are chiefly diseases of the middle-aged and the elderly. Patients with cancer of the oral cavity, pharynx, larynx, and esophagus also often give a history of heavy smoking or drinking, or both, and the consequences of these in terms of respiratory or metabolic impairment can be important determinants in the choice of drugs for the management of pain. Finally, the emotional impact of cancer, which may be disfiguring, give rise to offensive odors, or interfere with one's power of speech or ability to communicate cannot be underestimated. Many of these patients present formidable challenges in medical management.

In its varied forms, head and neck cancer can give rise to virtually any type of pain, or none at all. The extent to which pain gives rise to suffering will be influenced, to a great extent, by the presence or absence of other signs or symptoms, such as intractable cough, respiratory distress, nausea and vomiting, profuse or foul-smelling secretions, profound weakness, or even severe anxiety and fear of further disfigurement, invalidism, or death. Depending upon how the patient views these as threats to his being and to his self-esteem, they may take precedence over pain or conversely, and more commonly, they may make any pain worse.

The choice of analgesic medications or adjuvant drugs to control pain, anxiety, insomnia, or any of the other symptoms contributing to suffering must, of necessity, be individualized. Some routes of drug administration will be found to be either impossible or inadvisable, and some drugs and drug combinations contraindicated. The nonnarcotic analgesics of the antipyretic-antiinflammatory type are most frequently employed, primarily because they are less apt to suppress cough and respiration, to cause secretions to become thickened and more troublesome, or to cause an increase in intracranial pressure. Although cancers of the head and neck can be extremely painful, the majority of patients generally respond to the administration of aspirin or acetaminophen, administered either by mouth or crushed and given by nasogastric tube. Mixtures containing other simple analgesics, such as APC tablets and aspirin with antacids, have also been employed, although there is no reason for using them in preference to the simple analgesics. On the other hand, mixtures of simple analgesics with propoxyphene or phenobarbital have been effective when the antipyretic-antiinflammatory drug was not. Consideration must be given to the fact that many of these patients have ulcerations of the mouth or pharynx, severe dysphagia or obstruction, or lesions which are apt to bleed easily and would, accordingly contraindicate aspirin either because of its local effects or antithrombotic effects.

If the pain cannot be controlled with these agents, more potent drugs such as indoprofen appear to be more effective and may make possible the postponement of narcotics. However, if pain is not otherwise controlled, there is no reason to withhold narcotics. Customarily, the milder, orally administered narcotics such as codeine, propoxyphene, or pentazocine are given along with aspirin or acetaminophen. In some patients, codeine's antitussive effects are also a desired attribute of that drug.

With persisting pain and repeated administration of even mild narcotics, some tolerance may develop and require appropriate adjustments in the dose of the narcotic. In some patients with more severe pain, particularly deep in the ear or in the head, it may, in fact, be necessary to use the more potent orally effective narcotics and, if possible, in combination with a simple analgesic.

Many patients with head and neck cancer are quite depressed and can benefit from an antidepressant such as imipramine, amitriptyline, or clomipramine. Tranquilizers, primarily of the phenothiazine type, are occasionally advisable, although some caution should be taken with patients with a history of alcoholism or liver disease. Some head and neck pains are neuralgic in type or lancinating, and in these patients, the use of carbamazapine and/or phenytoin may be indicated. Care should be taken not to administer carbamazapine to patients receiving monoamine-oxidase inhibitors. Both carbamazapine and phenytoin are capable of precipitating a number of hypersensitivity reactions, so that patients should be monitored for the possibility of hematopoietic reactions. In patients with intracranial lesions, steroids primarily in the form of dexamethasone may prove of some benefit.

In summary, the problems of pain in head and neck cancer are extremely complex and generally require some form of combined management directed not only at relieving pain but also at other causes of suffering so commonly encountered in these patients.

ACKNOWLEDGMENT

Supported in part by a Grant from the National Institute on Drug Abuse #DA 01707.

Cancer Pain in the Head and Neck: Role of Nerve Blocks

John J. Bonica and Jose L. Madrid*

*Department of Anesthesiology, University of Washington School of Medicine, Seattle, Washington 98195, and *Department of Anesthesiology and Pain Clinic, Ciudad Sanitaria "10 de Octobre," Madrid, Spain*

In patients with moderate to severe pain due to cancer of the head and neck, nerve blocks can be used as diagnostic or prognostic tools or to control the pain for a prolonged period of time. Diagnostic blocks are used to determine the mechanism and pathways of the pain, whereas prognostic blocks are used to predict the effects of neurolytic block or neurosurgical section. The basic principles, advantages, and disadvantages of therapeutic blocks for pain in this region are similar to those mentioned in the panel on nerve blocks.

Pain in the face is often caused by tumors which commonly arise from structures about the mouth, nose, and paranasal sinuses. The physician should not hesitate to inject the gasserian ganglion, because relief of pain must be obtained for the patient even at the price of producing keratitis from block of the ophthalmic branches of the trigeminal nerve. The problem here is quite different from that in patients who have tic douloureux or other benign, chronic pain in whom the life-expectancy is long and a corneal ulcer is a serious complication. Gasserian ganglion block is particularly useful if the lesion involves structures which are supplied by more than one of the major divisions of the fifth cranial nerve. In such cases, it is preferable to carry out a gasserian ganglion block at the onset to produce a widespread field of analgesia into which the cancer can spread without producing more pain subsequently.

Severe pain which often accompanies cancer of the posterior mouth and throat is most effectively relieved by neurosurgical section of the sensory roots of the glossopharyngeal and part of the vagus nerves, a procedure best achieved by the posterior intracranial root (Dandy technique). Blocks of these nerves with local anesthetics may be used as diagnostic and prognostic tools; but, since such blocks also involve motor nerves, neurolytic blocks are contraindicated because they produce prolonged paralysis of pharyngeal and laryngeal muscles, resulting in the loss of the patient's ability to swallow and phonate. This is an especially serious complication if the block is done bilaterally. Unilateral neurolytic block of the glossopharyngeal nerve of the most painful side may be considered in patients with excruciating pain not adequately relieved by narcotics and whose physical condition is too poor to permit neurosurgical section. Pain in the back of the head and upper neck may require block of C_2 and C_3, first with a local anesthetic to ascertain the pain pathways and subsequently with a neurolytic agent. In many instances, cancer of the mouth, tongue, or lower jaw spreads laterally and posteriorly to produce moderate to severe pain and sometimes trismus, which can be effectively relieved by block of the mandibular nerve combined with paravertebral block of the upper two cervical nerves.

Occasionally, tumors of the face and head cause a burning discomfort in addition to the severe neuralgia and deep, aching pain. The burning pain is usually located over one side of the head, the eye, and teeth, and lower and sometimes the upper jaw, the temporal region, and the nape of the neck which is not relieved by block of the somatic nerves. In such cases, cervical sympathetic block should be carried out, first with a local anesthetic; and if it relieves the burning pain, the procedure is repeated with phenol or alcohol as a supplement to somatic block.

Figures 1 through 7 show nerve block procedures used for various types of cancers that produce pain in the face and neck. Figure 1 shows a patient with fibrosarcoma of the left orbit with invasion of the maxilla which produced severe pain in the left eye and ipsilateral side of the face, especially the cheek, which could not be relieved with large doses of morphine. Injec-

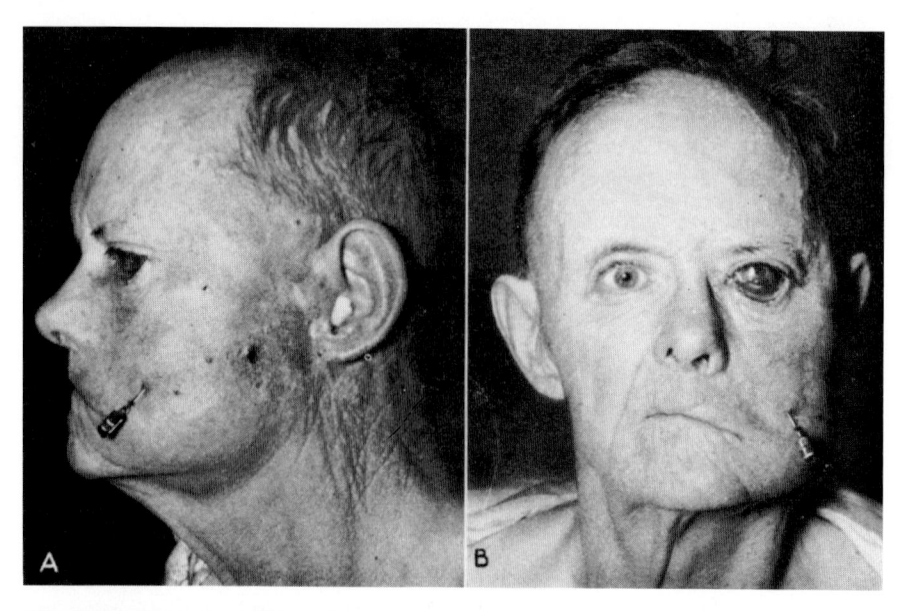

FIG. 1. Fibrosarcoma of the left orbit with invasion of the maxilla. Pain relieved with alcohol block of gasserian ganglion.

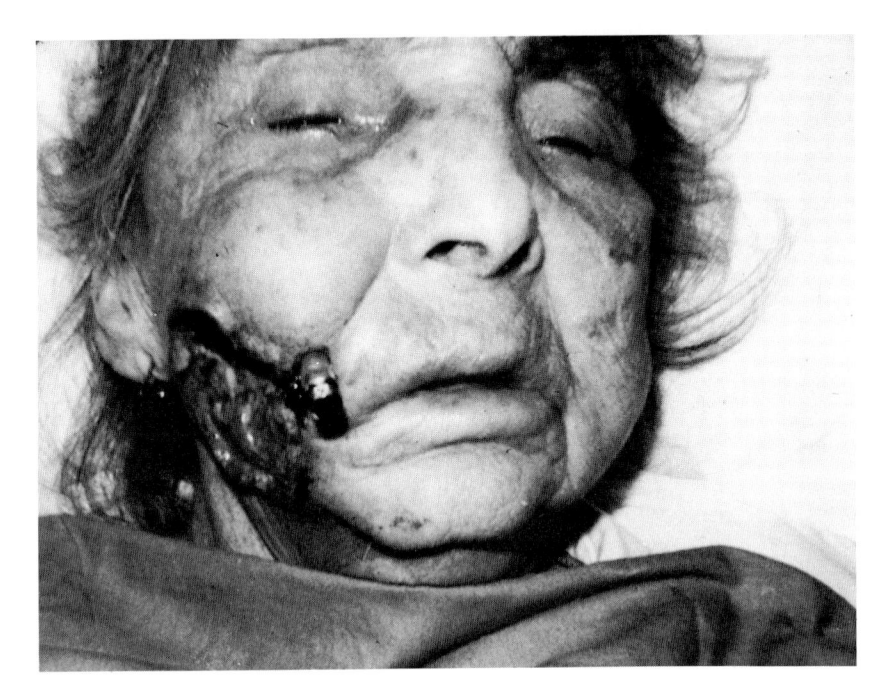

FIG. 2. Invasive epidermoid carcinoma on the skin of the cheek which required an extensive block at the gasserian ganglion level to provide complete analgesia.

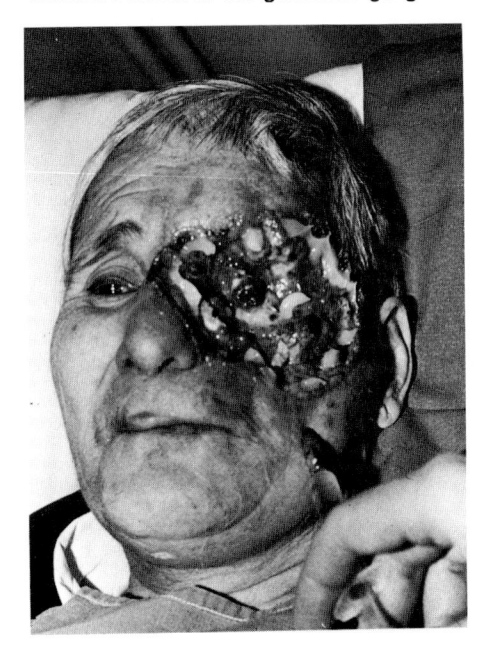

FIG. 3. Advanced carcinoma of the orbit which could not be blocked at the trigeminal division affected by the tumor and also required a gasserian ganglion block.

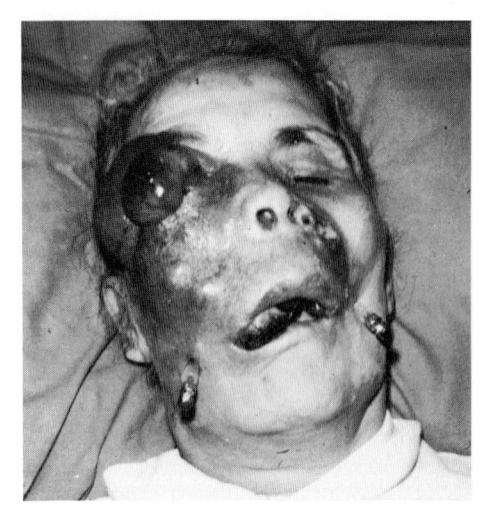

FIG. 4. Advanced cancer which originated in the upper half of the maxillary antrum involving malar, ethmoidal, and orbital structures, and expanding past the midline. In this case it was necessary to block the gasserian ganglion on both sides.

tion of 1 ml of absolute alcohol into the gasserian ganglion produced complete relief. Three months after the block, the patient began to experience diffuse, burning pain over the ipsilateral side of the face. Examination at this time revealed that he still had anesthesia in the distribution of the trigeminal nerve. After three separate cervical sympathetic blocks produced adequate, though not complete, relief of the burning pain, the procedure was repeated with alcohol. By supplementing the blocks with relatively small doses of narcotics several times daily, the patient remained virtually pain-free until he died 5 months later.

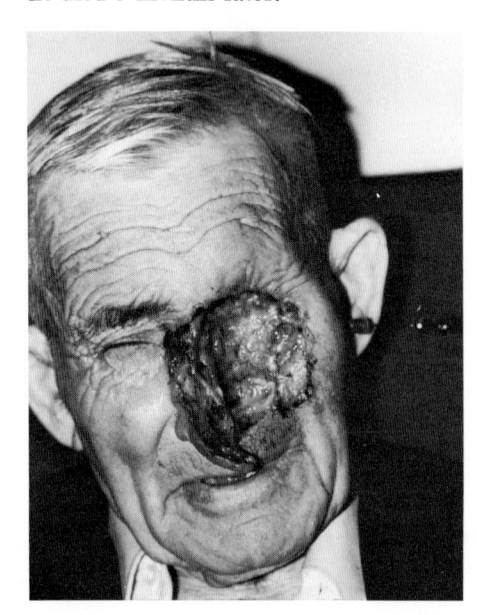

FIG. 5. Invasive and destructive carcinoma treated with alcohol maxillary nerve block by the lateral extra-oral route. Curiously this patient developed a phantom pain at the tip of the nose.

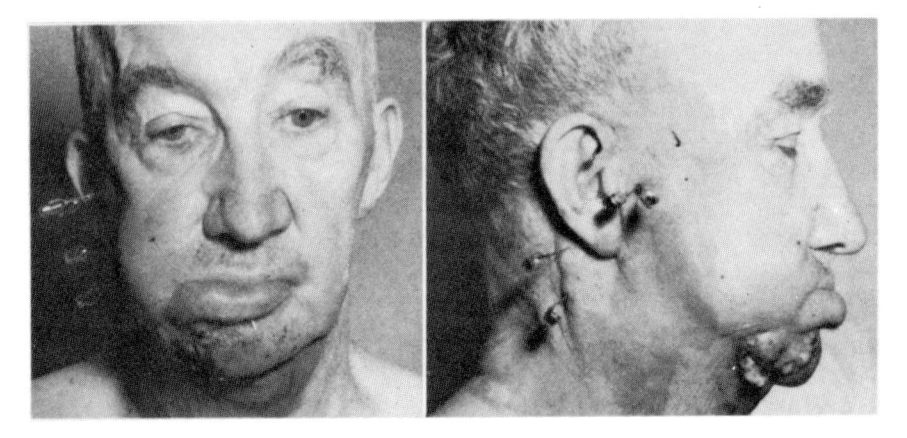

FIG. 6. Patient with cancer of the tongue with invasion of the cheek, lower jaw and chin. Severe pain not relieved by intensive radium and roentgen therapy and large doses of narcotic analgesics, but relieved with alcohol block of the right maxillary, mandibular, and second and third cervical nerves.

When the tumor is localized in the skin of the face, usually it is painless until there is extensive ulceration. Epidermoid carcinoma in the skin of the cheek usually is accompanied by local and referred pain (Fig. 2).

Advanced cancer of the orbit usually spreads to the entire area supplied by the ophthalmic and maxillary divisions of the trigeminal nerve. When the division affected can not be blocked, it is necessary to perform a block at the gasserian ganglion level (Fig. 3).

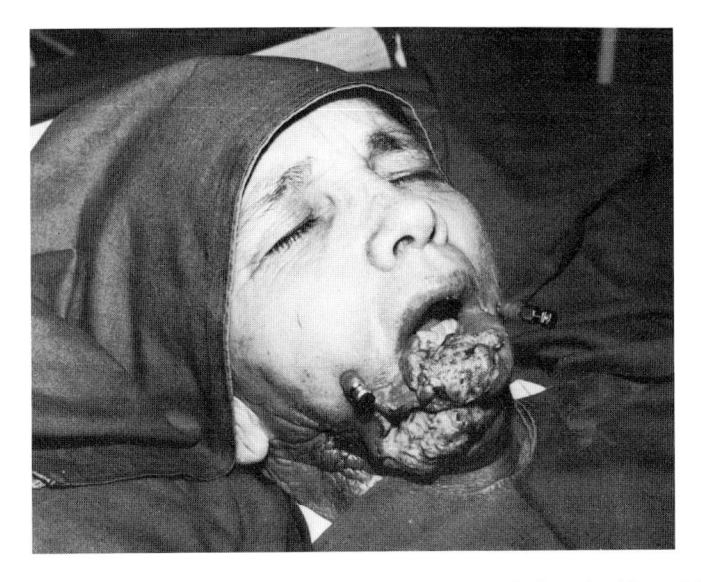

FIG. 7. Epidermoid carcinoma of the lower jaw which invaded both sides of the face. Bilateral gasserian ganglion block.

Advanced cancers originating in the upper half of the maxillary antrum can expand laterally to involve the malar bone, expanding medially to invade the ethmoidal and orbital structures. Moreover they can pass the midline, affecting practically the entire face and requiring a bilateral gasserian ganglion block (Fig. 4).

Block of the branches of the trigeminal nerve can be done in advanced cancer pain of the face. The patient can be blocked by the lateral extra-oral route if the anatomical landmarks are not distorted (Fig. 5).

Figure 6 shows a patient with cancer of the tongue with invasion of the cheek, lower jaw, and chin. Severe pain never relieved by radiation therapy and large doses of narcotic analgesics was effectively relieved with alcohol block of the right maxillary and mandibular nerves and of the second and third cervical nerves.

Epidermoid carcinoma of the lower jaw involves structures supplied by the mandibular nerve and not infrequently invades other areas, requiring block of the cervical nerves to afford relief of pain (Fig. 7).

REFERENCES

1. Bonica, J. J. (1953): *The Management of Pain,* pp. 1445–1466. Lea & Febiger, Philadelphia.
2. Madrid, J. L. (1975): Exference de 363 cas d'analgesie par alcool et phenol. *Cah. Anesthesiol.,* 23:825–827.

though it is not possible to exclude that in some cases paroxysmal pain could be referred from the ear and throat to the face.

Cancer Pain in the Head and Neck: Role of Neurosurgery

Carlo A. Pagni

2nd Chair of Neurosurgery, University of Torino, Torino, Italy

Patients with malignancies of the face, head, and neck often suffer severe pain. Commonly, at the beginning, pain is associated with enlargement of the tumor; and surgery, chemotherapy, and radiotherapy usually afford relief of pain. Intense intractable pain, as a rule, arises only in advanced stages of the disease. When tumor growth can no longer be controlled by anticancer modalities, pain becomes one of the main problems for the patient. Pain is due to various mechanisms: peripheral stimulation of nociceptors due to ulcerative and inflammatory processes; pressure on nerve trunks engulfed by the tumor and fibrosis consequent to surgery and repeated radiation of neoplastic infiltration of nerve trunks and of the base of the skull; and radiodermitis (10,44,60).

At this advanced stage, pain usually is referred to large areas in the peripheral fields of multiple cranial or cervical nerves, bearing no relation to the original tumor site. Sometimes pain is bilateral. Patients usually complain of persistent, progressively increasing pain. A rather common feature is paroxysmal bouts of pain in the face, throat, and ear, which is provoked by talking, mouth movements, or swallowing (preventing food-intake, which worsens the condition of the patient). These agonizing outbursts recall the paroxysmal pain of trigeminal and glossopharyngeal neuralgias. Burning sensations are frequent. Deep-seated pain in the ear is one of the most serious complaints. Other distressing symptoms include difficulty in swallowing, breathing, and talking; loss of taste; dread of repeated bleedings, suffocation, and imminent death. These cause the patient to be depressed and anxious. In spite of these miserable conditions survival is often protracted.

The progressive loss of efficacy of analgesic drugs and the impracticability of peripheral nerve blocks due to the lack of diffusion of drugs in the scleroneoplastic tissues are the causes for referral to the neurosurgeon. Many procedures have been attempted to relieve cancer pain in the head and neck.

TRIGEMINAL OPERATIONS

In pain confined to the trigeminal area, alcohol or phenol blocks of trigeminal branches or ganglion and trigeminal rhizotomy have been attempted (4,18,28,44,54,63). About 50% of patients have satisfactory relief, but detailed information on duration of follow-up and results usually are not reported by the authors. White and Sweet (63) obtained satisfactory relief to time of death or to long follow-up in 17 out of 36 cases. However, partial trigeminal denervation has been shown to have limited efficacy in this kind of cancer pain. In fact, except for very selected cases, patients after trigeminal operation keep complaining of pain in the spared trigeminal areas or in extratrigeminal territories.

MULTIPLE RHIZOTOMIES

Dandy, in 1929 (9), proposed combined rhizotomy of the 5th and 9th root, and if necessary of the upper cervical ones. This method has been used quite extensively with fair results (4,18,30,42,43,44,59,60,63). Advances in anesthesiology and postoperative care permit good results with this operation, which formerly carried a very high operative mortality. Nonetheless, mortality shortly after operation is still high, especially if patients are elderly and in a poor condition. In my series of 12 patients, 1 patient died in the immediate postoperative period, and 4 patients died 15 to 32 days after surgery.

Complete section of the trigeminal and glossopharyngeal nerves is usually successful in affording relief of pain in the face, tongue, jaw, and throat, so that, as White (61) states, this seems not to be the major problem. The rapid disappearance of dysphagia makes swallowing easier and patients quickly gain weight. High cervical and occipital pain is easily controlled by section, bilateral if possible, of the upper cervical roots. Careful search for the second cervical rootlets (which can emerge from the cord above the arch of the atlas) and for a fairly common C_1 root must be made, because both may be easily missed by the unaware surgeon (59,60). Their section is essential for high occipital and submandibular pain-relief.

Deep ear pain is difficult to control. Section of the 5th and 9th nerves is insufficient since the middle ear, tympanic membrane, and external auditory canal are also supplied by the nervus intermedius and by the upper vagal rootlets (45), which must be cut. The use of the operative microscope makes easier identification and section of these rootlets.

Everybody who has used combined rhizotomy agrees that section which includes the 5th, 7th, 9th, upper rootlets of the 10th and upper cervical roots is essential for ample and persistent pain-relief. Unsatisfactory results are usually inadequate denervation of the algogenic areas. Sometimes patients with very long survival, and free from paroxysmal pain, still complain of some discomfort produced by unpleasant sensations in the denervated areas and dryness of the mouth. These and dread of bleeding, suffocation, and death cause the patient to remain anxious and depressed. Therefore, combined therapy with psychotropic drugs may be necessary after rhizotomy.

TRIGEMINAL TRACTOTOMY

Section of the descending root of the trigeminal according to Sjöqvist (51) should block all the pain afferents from the face, because the pain fibers of the 7th, 9th, and 10th enter the descending trigeminal tract collected behind the fibers of the mandibular division of the 5th (29). A few case series have been reported in the literature (18,19,23,29,31,35,38,52,56,62). Usually tractotomy was combined with section of the upper cervical roots to control neck and occipital pain (20,21,56). Gros et al. (20,21) added glossopharyngeal rhizotomy to tractotomy in 27 out of 29 cases, division of the upper rootlets of the 10th in another 7 cases, and cervical rhizotomies in every case.

The reported mortality ranges from 46% (23) to 0% (38). Low mortality is due to better selection of patients, advances in anesthesiology and intensive care, and more frequent use of tracheostomy before operation. Results regarding pain-relief seem to be quite different in the different series. The differences could be due to the different levels of incision, which makes comparison of results difficult; incisions a few mm rostral to the obex could be more effective in producing persistent relief and analgesia than the lower ones, because some fibers of the 5th, 7th, 9th, and 10th might terminate rostral to the obex (62).

In a series of 19 cases, White and Sweet (62), made the incisions above, below, or at the obex level. There were 5 operative deaths, and among the 12 survivors, 7 had recurrence of pain which persisted until death. Subsequent trigeminal rhizotomy did not improve results in some cases. Thus in the opinion of White (61), "medullary tractotomy . . . has not proved to be a successful solution for relief of pain from cancer in the oro-pharynx even if combined with division of the upper cervical sensory roots."

Mracek (38), on the other hand, "successfully performed" medullary tractotomy combined with upper-cervical root section in 12 patients; no other information is given in his short report. Gros et al. (20) reported satisfactory results in a group of 21 patients: 8 of 18 survivors had recurrence of pain or painful dysesthesia, but good relief was obtained by the other 10 patients. In 1969, Gros et al. added 16 new cases of trigeminal tractotomy with satisfactory results (21). It seems to me, however, the good results reported by Gros et al. (20,21) might be due to the fact that in most of the patients they added section of glossopharyngeal nerve, upper rootlets of the vagus, and cervical nerve roots. This emphasizes the need for multiple rhizotomy in order to do ample and sustained pain-relief.

Recently Crue et al. (8) and Hitchcock (26) attempted stereotaxic percutaneous lesion of the trigeminal tract in a few cases. Localization of the tract was based on radiological coordinates, recording of evoked potentials, and clinical effects of stimulations. The procedure produced good results, and it seems indicated in patients in very poor condition.

MESENCEPHALIC TRACTOTOMY

In 1936, Serra and Neri (49) made the first section of quintothalamic fibers at the level of the pons for cancer pain of the face. Then Dogliotti (11,12) introduced spino- and quintothalamic tractotomy at the mesencephalic level. However, the procedure was employed only in a few cases (1,5,13,58). Open mesencephalic tractotomy, in spite of the fact it seemed appropriate to control face and head pain, was abandoned because of the high operative mortality and complications.

The operation was attempted again after the introduction of stereotaxic technique by Spiegel and Wycis (53). Stereotactic mesencephalic tractotomy seems devoid of high operative risks and complications. Only series of a few cases, however, have been reported (25,35,64). Furthermore, results seemed generally very poor (25,64). In 1976, Mazars et al. (37) reported excellent results in an impressive series of 76 cases of head cancer pain. There were neither major complications, nor operative mortality; the risk of occurrence of central pain was minimal (37). Suppression of pain was achieved in 68 out of 76 patients (89%). Unfortunately, detailed results of long-term follow-up are not available. Mazars et al. (37) state categorically that stereotaxic mesencephalotomy is the procedure of choice for pain of the head and neck, and only the lack of experience with it led to the introduction of other less-valuable procedures. Nashold (39) and Voris and Whisler (57) share this opinion and say they prefer mesencephalotomy to multiple rhizotomy.

STEREOTACTIC THALAMOTOMY

Stereotaxic lesions were produced simultaneously at thalamic level in the VPM and CM-Pf-intralaminar nuclei by many surgeons (24,32,40,41,42). The purpose was to block nociceptive impulses bound for the VPM and for so-called "polysynaptic pathways" with the hope of obtaining more-lasting analgesia and relief of pain. Everybody reported "inadequate pain-relief" or "some subjective relief from pain;" every surgeon, however, treated usually only a few cases.

According to Mark et al. (33,34) lesions of the CM-Pf-intralaminar complex which did not produce sensory defects or central pain were sufficient to suppress pain in 12 out of 13 patients. Fairman (14) obtained similar results in 9 cases. In my experience (40,41,42) unilateral lesions exactly targeted on the CM-Pf-intralaminar complex, with minimal involvement of the VPM or other thalamic nuclei, yield only very transient results with recurrence of pain usually in a few days. Voris and Whisler (57) reported similar experience. Careful review of the case reports of Mark et al. (33) reveals that psychic disturbances (confusion, disorientation, memory loss) were recorded. Furthermore their anatomic studies (34) indicated lesions involved the CM nucleus. I wonder whether pain-relief in their patients might have been due to minor leukotomy effects.

I achieved somewhat better results (40,41,42) with combined destruction of the VPM, VPL, CM-Pf-intralaminar and limitans nuclei; the lesions included the thalamo-midbrain junction impinging on the midbrain, the PO region, and the pulvinar. Only patients who died within 2 months of the operation obtained permanent relief; otherwise, there was recurrence of pain (40,41). Lesions including the VPM-VPL nuclei of course entailed the risk of occurrence of central pain (6,40). Tasker (55) obtained permanent relief in 14 out of 19 patients, whose average survival was 4 months, with combined lesions of the VPL, VPM, CM-Pf-intralaminar complex; in 5 cases there was recurrence in a few weeks or months. Thus it seems thalamotomy can afford relief of pain in patients with short life-expectancy, usually for no longer than a few weeks.

Therefore I read with the highest interest the papers of Fairman (15) and Sano (48). Fairman (15) submitted 104 patients to (apparently unilateral) CM-Pf-intralaminar thalamotomy. Sano (48) performed bilateral destruction of the CM-Pf-intralaminar complex ("thalamolaminotomy"). In both series incidence of complications was very low and there was no operative mortality. Mild psychic disturbances cleared up in a few days. "Satisfactory relief of pain—without sensory disturbances—i.e., no pain at all or some tolerable pain no longer requiring narcotic analgesics was obtained in 70% of all the patients. The pain-relief lasted for the entire period of survival, which ranged between 2 and 12 months. . . ." (15); pain was liable to recur only "several months later" (48). In spite of these extraordinarily valuable results, not yet duplicated by others, both Fairman (15) and Sano (48) introduced unilateral or bilateral destruction of the posterior hypothalamus, which is believed to play an important role in the emotional-motivational aspects of pain. This "posteromedial hypothalamotomy" produced results which were better than those achieved with "thalamolaminotomy."

Richardson (47) and Cooper et al. (7) reported excellent pain-relief could be achieved by means of pulvinar lesions. Since then, some cases of head cancer pain were submitted to unilateral or bilateral pulvinectomy (41,50). Experience is limited, but so far it seems pulvinectomy does not improve upon the results of thalamic surgery for pain (17,41,50).

PSYCHOSURGERY

Leukotomy was employed in small series of cases, especially for bilateral pain (63). Pain-relief was very satisfactory, both with large, bilateral transection of the frontal white matter, or with transection limited to the lower frontal quadrants. Sadly, "although these subjects were relieved of pain and suffering . . . apathy and psychologic deterioration were severe" (63). In unilateral extensive leukotomy, too, pain-relief was accompanied by some degree of mental confusion and apathy (63). Large frontal lesions made in a one-stage procedure, make the patient disoriented and apathetic. If lesions of the same size are made in increments over a period of days, or if small lesions are made at short intervals, it is possible to obtain relief of pain without sensibly handicapping the patient's mentation (22). Thus White and Sweet (63) introduced graduated bilateral coagulation of medial frontal white matter. By means of implanted unipolar electrodes an area of frontothalamic projection fibers, a centimeter in diameter, is destroyed on both sides. Another two or three such lesions are made at intervals of several days. The patient may be made free from concern about pain, dread of strangulation, death, etc. Destruction of the frontal white matter can be stopped before severe mental deterioration ensues.

Cingulotomy was introduced by Folz and White (16). In the cingulum run pathways mediating activities of the limbic system to the anterior thalamus and the forebrain, which play a major role in emotional behavior. The hope was to modify the patient's emotional response to pain, thus relieving suffering, with only minor psychic impairment. The changes effected by cingulotomy seem identical to those effected by leukotomy; however, these effects appear less damaging to the intellectual faculties (2,27). Folz and White (16) obtained excellent relief, at 6- to 18-months follow-up, with unilateral or bilateral lesions of the cingulum in a group of patients who showed marked emotional reaction to pain with enhancement of their complaints of pain. Rétif et al. (46) obtained poor results in 1 patient.

Bertrand et al. (3) introduced the stereotaxic section of the frontothalamic pathways, on one or both sides, as they lie in the anterior limb of the internal capsule. The operation was performed on 5 patients; all were free from pain and "well oriented" some weeks or months after the operation.

The conservative methods of modern psychosurgery seem to allow good control of pain with moderate psychic impairment. In my own limited experience, however, pain-relief has always been associated with psychic disturbances.

FINAL REMARKS

In head and neck cancer pain, extension of painful areas to territories of multiple cranial and cervical nerves, bilaterality of pain, and psychologic distress due to a devastating disease making patients anxious and depressed make treatment one of the most arduous problems that the neurosurgeon has to cope with. Many surgical procedures have been attempted. There is no consensus about the efficacy and limitations of various methods.

In my opinion two factors should guide the surgeon in the choice of operation: the patient's condition and life-expectancy. If the patient's condition is good and life-expectancy long, multiple rhizotomy is the most useful operation because it assures long-lasting relief. In spite of advances in anesthesiology and intensive care, multiple rhizotomy always carries a certain operative risk. Therefore in the patient in a poor condition with short life-expectancy (limited to 2 or 3 months) stereotaxic surgery is to be preferred, as operative risks are minimal and patients can expect relief as long as they will survive.

Thalamic lesions should be large enough to affect a major part of the VPM-VPL, CM, Pf, intralaminar and limitans nuclei contralateral to the painful side. Such large lesions usually involve the lower part of the dorsomedial nucleus, adding a minor leukotomic effect which may play an important role in producing relief of pain and suffering. Bilateral "thalamolaminotomy" or "hypothalamotomy" (15,48), as well as mesencephalotomy (37) might be more rewarding, but I have no experience with them.

Trigeminal tractotomy either by open or stereotaxic technique in my opinion can be abandoned; the best results are achieved only in association with rhizotomy of the cervical, glossopharyngeal, and vagal rootlets (20, 21,56).

In bilateral pain, psychosurgery, by means of graduated bilateral coagulation of medial frontal white matter (63) or of cingulotomy (16,27) seems to allow good control of pain with moderate psychic impairment.

REFERENCES

1. Bailey, R. A., Glees, P., and Oppenheimer, D. R. (1954): Midbrain tractotomy: A surgical and clinical report with observations on ascending and descending tract degeneration. *Mschr. Psychiat. Neurol.,* 127:316–335.
2. Ballantine, H. T., Cassidy, W. L., Flanagan, N. B., and Marino, R. (1967): Stereotaxic anterior cingulotomy for neuropsychiatric illness and intractable pain. *J. Neurosurg.,* 26:488–495.
3. Bertrand, C., Martinez, N., and Hardy, J. (1966): Frontothalamic section for intractable pain. In: *Pain,* edited by R. S. Knighton and P. R. Dumke, pp. 531–535. Little, Brown, Boston.
4. Botterell, E. H. (1961): Discussion to Parsons H., Opérations sur les nerfs craniens et les racines cervicales postérieures pour d'autres formes de névralgie et de douleur dans des affections malignes. *Excerpta Med. Intern. Congr. Series,* 36:31.
5. Brihaye, J., Thiry, S., LeClercq, R., Rétif, J., and Grégoire, A. (1962): Le traitement chirurgical de la douleur. *Acta Chir. Belg.* [Suppl.], 2:255–457.
6. Cassinari, V., and Pagni, C. A. (1969): *Central Pain. A Neurosurgical Survey.* Harvard University Press, Cambridge, Mass.
7. Cooper, I. S., Amin, I., Chandra, R., and Waltz, J. M. (1973): A surgical investigation of the clinical physiology of the LP-Pulvinar complex in man. *J. Neurol. Sci.,* 18:89–110.
8. Crue, B. L., Todd, E. M., and Carregal, E. J. A. (1970): Percutaneous radiofrequency stereotaxic trigeminal tractotomy. In: *Pain and Suffering: Selected Aspects,* edited by B. L. Crue, pp. 69–80. Charles C Thomas, Springfield, Ill.
9. Dandy, W. E. (1929): Operative relief from pain in lesions of the mouth, tongue, and throat. *Arch. Surg.,* 19:143–148.
10. Dodd, G. D., Dolan, P. A., Ballantyne, A. J., Ibanez, M. L., and Chau, P. (1970): The dissemination of tumors of the head and neck via the cranial nerves. *Radiol. Clinics North Am.,* 8:445–461.

11. Dogliotti, A. M. (1937): Trattamento del dolore nei tumori. *Min. Med.*, 28:455–461.
12. Dogliotti, A. M. (1938): First surgical sections in man, of the lemniscus lateralis (pain-temperature path) at the brain stem, for treatment of diffused rebellious pain. *Anesth. Analg.*, 17:143–145
13. Drake, C. G., and McKenzie, K. G. (1953): Mesencephalic tractotomy for pain. Experience with six cases. *J. Neurosurg.*, 10:457–462.
14. Fairman, D. (1966): Evaluation of results in stereotactic thalamotomy for the treatment of intractable pain. *Confin. Neurol.*, 27:67–70.
15. Fairman, D. (1976): Neurophysiological basis for hypothalamic lesion and stimulation by chronic implanted electrodes for the relief of intractable pain in cancer. In: *Advances in Pain Research and Therapy. Vol. 1: Proceedings of the First World Congress on Pain*, edited by J. J. Bonica and D. Albe-Fessard, pp. 843–847. Raven Press, New York.
16. Folz, E. L., and White, L. E. (1966): Rostral cingulotomy and pain "relief." In: *Pain*, edited by R. S. Knighton and P. R. Dumke, pp. 469–491. Little, Brown, Boston.
17. Fraioli, B., and Guidetti, B. (1975): Effects of stereotactic lesions of the pulvinar and lateralis posterior nucleus on intractable pain and dyskinetic syndromes of man. *Applied Neurophysiol.*, 38:23–30.
18. Grant, F. C. (1943): Surgical methods for relief of pain. *Bull. N.Y. Acad. Med.*, 19:373–385.
19. Gros, Cl., Vlahovitch, B., Jourdan, D., and Solassol, A. (1954): Traitement neurochirurgical des algies cranio-faciales d'origine cancereuses. *Sem. Hôp.*, 30:1947–1949.
20. Gros, Cl., Cordier, M., Vlahovitch, B., and Roilgen, A. (1963): Neurotomie combinée et traitement des algies cervico-cranio-faciales d'origine neoplasique., *Ann. Chir.*, 17:533–539.
21. Gros, Cl. (1969): *Montpellier Chir.*, 15:53
22. Hackett, T. P., White, J. C., and Sweet, W. H. (1966): Leukotomy for the relief of pain: The selection of cases and psychological hazards. In: *Pain*, edited by R. S. Knighton and P. R. Dumke, pp. 461–467. Little, Brown, Boston.
23. Hamby, W. B., Shinners, B. M., and Marsh, I. A. (1948): Trigeminal tractotomy. Observations on forty-eight cases. *Arch. Surg.*, 57:171–177.
24. Hassler, R., and Riechert, T. (1959): Klinische und anatomische Befunde bei stereotaktischen Schmerzoperationen im Thalamus. *Arch. Psychiat. Nervenkr.*, 200:93–122.
25. Helfant, M. H., Leksell, L., and Strang, R. R. (1965): Experiences with intractable pain treated by stereotaxic mesencephalotomy. *Acta Chir. Scand.*, 129:573–580.
26. Hitchcock, E. (1970): Stereotactic trigeminal tractotomy. *Ann. Clin. Res.*, 2:131–135.
27. Hurt, R. W., and Ballantine, H. I. (1974): Stereotactic anterior cingulate lesions for persistent pain: A report on 68 cases. *Clin. Neurosurg.*, 21:334–351.
28. Jefferson, A. (1963): Trigeminal root and ganglion injections using phenol in glycerine for the relief of trigeminal neuralgia. *J. Neurol. Neurosurg. Psychiatry*, 26:345–352.
29. Kunc, Z. (1964): *Tractus spinalis nervi trigemini. Fresh anatomic data and their significance for surgery.* Nakladatelství Ceskoslovenské Akademie. Vêd, Praha.
30. Lapras, C., Fisher, G., and Trouillias, P. (1968): Radicotomie combinée dans le traitement des douleurs cervico-faciales d'origine neoplasique. *Lyon Chir.*, 64:548–556.
31. Le Beau, J., and Billet, R. (1953): Tractotomie bulbare trigeminale et nevralgie du glossopharyngien. *Rev. Neurol.*, 88:265–271.
32. Le Beau, J., Lecasble, R., Choppy, M., and Dondey, M. (1966): Stéréo-thalamotomies localisées pour le traitement des douleurs irréductibles. *Confin. Neurol.*, 27:56–62.
33. Mark, V. H., Ervin, F. R., and Hackett, T. P. (1960): Clinical aspects of stereotactic thalamotomy in the human. I. The treatment of chronic severe pain. *Arch. Neurol.*, 3:351–367.
34. Mark, V. H., Ervin, F. R., and Yakovlev, P. I. (1963): Stereotactic thalamotomy.

III. Verification of anatomical lesion site in the human thalamus. *Arch. Neurol.,* 8:528–538.
35. McKenzie, K. G. (1955): Trigeminal tractotomy. *Clin. Neurosurg.,* 2:50–69.
36. Mazars, G., Rogé, R., and Pansini, A. (1960): Stereotactic coagulation of the spinothalamic tract for intractable trigeminal pain. *J. Neurol. Neurosurg. Psychiatry,* 23:352.
37. Mazars, G., Merienne, L., and Cioloca, C. (1976): État actuel de la chirurgie de la douleur. *Neuro-Chir.* 22, *Suppl.* 1:1–164.
38. Mracek, Z. (1977): Surgical management of intractable pain due to malignant tumors in the face and neck. *J. Neurosurg. Sci.,* 21:123–125.
39. Nashold, B. S. (1972): Extensive cephalic and oral pain relieved by midbrain tractotomy. *Confin. Neurol.,* 34:382.
40. Pagni, C. A. (1966): Discussion to Ervin, F. R., Brown, C. E., and Mark, V. H. Striatal influence on facial pain. *Confin. Neurol.,* 27:88–89.
41. Pagni, C. A. (1974): Place of stereotactic technique in surgery for pain. In: *Advances in Neurology, Vol. 4: International Symposium on Pain,* edited by J. J. Bonica, pp. 699–706. Raven Press, New York.
42. Pagni, C. A., and Maspes, P. E. (1970): Problems in the surgical treatment of pain in malignancies of the head and neck. In: *Current Problems in Neurosciences,* edited by H. T. Wycis, pp. 138–153. Karger, Basel.
43. Pagni, C. A., Maspes, P. E., Visca, A., and Bollati, A. (1969): Riflessioni sul problema del trattamento chirurgico delle algie cranio-cervico-faciali da neoplasia maligna mediante radicotomie multiple. *Min. Neurochir.,* 13:29–33.
44. Parsons, H. (1961): Opérations sur les nerves crâniens et les racines cervicales postérieures pour d'autres formes de nevralgie et de douleur dans les affections malignes. *Excerpta Med. Int. Congr. Ser.,* 36:30–31.
45. Peele, T. L. (1954): *The Neuroanatomical Basis for Clinical Neurology.* McGraw-Hill Book Co., New York.
46. Rétif, J., Crahay, S., and Brihaye, J. (1966): Leucotomie frontale a minima avec interruption sélective du faisceau cingulaire, uni o bilatérale, dans le traitement chirurgical de la douleur. *Acta Neurol. Psych. Belg.,* 66:499–513.
47. Richardson, D. E. (1967): Thalamotomy for intractable pain. *Confin. Neurol.,* 29:139–145.
48. Sano, K. (1977): Intralaminar thalamotomy (Thalamolaminotomy) and posterior medial hypothalamotomy in the treatment of intractable pain. In: *Pain—Its Neurosurgical Management. Part II: Central Procedures,* edited by H. Krayenbühl, P. E. Maspes, and W. H. Sweet, pp. 50–103. Karger, Basel.
49. Serra, A., and Neri, V. (1936): Die elektro-chirurgische Unterbrechung der Zentralbahnen des V Paares am lateralen ventrale Rand des Pons Varoli als erster Behandlungsversuch von hartnätigen Neuralgien des Trigeminus durch Tumoren des Schadelbasis. *Zbl. Chir.,* 63:2248–2251.
50. Siegfried, J. (1977): Stereotactic pulvinarotomy in the treatment of intractable pain. In: *Pain—Its Neurosurgical Management. Part II: Central Procedures,* edited by H. Krayenbühl, P. E. Maspes, and W. H. Sweet, pp. 104–113. Karger, Basel.
51. Sjöqvist, O. (1938): Studies on pain conduction in the trigeminal nerve. A contribution to the surgical treatment of facial pain. *Acta Psychiatr. Scand.* [*Suppl.*], 17:1–139.
52. Sjöqvist, O. (1950): La section chirurgicale des cordons et des voies de la douleur dans la moelle et le tronc cerebral. *Rev. Neurol.,* 83:38–40.
53. Spiegel, E. A., Wycis, H. T., Marks, M., and Lee, A. J. (1947): Stereotaxic apparatus for operations on the human brain. *Science,* 106:349–350.
54. Sweet, W. H. (1976): Controlled thermocoagulation of trigeminal ganglion rootlets for differential destruction of pain fibers: Facial pain other than trigeminal neuralgia. *Clin. Neurosurg.,* 23:96–102.
55. Tasker, R. R. (1975): Neurological concepts of pain management in head and neck cancer. *Can. J. Otolaryngol.,* 4:480–484.
56. Vlahovitch, B., Fuentes, J. M., Choncair, Y., Moreau, P., and Pascal, M. (1976):

Gestes complementaires à l'operation de Sjöqvist dans les algies cancéreuses cervico-faciales. *Neuro-chir.*, 22:503–515.
57. Voris, H. C., and Whisler, W. W. (1975): Results of stereotaxic surgery for intractable pain. *Confin. Neurol.*, 37:86–96.
58. Walker, E. A. (1942): Relief of pain by mesencephalic tractotomy. *Arch. Neurol. Psychiatry*, 48:865–883.
59. Wetzel, N. (1959): Neurosurgical procedures for the control of intractable pain in malignancies of the head and neck. *Am. J. Surg.*, 98:800–804.
60. Wetzel, N. (1966): The relief of pain in malignant disease in the head and neck by sensory root section. In: *Pain,* edited by R. S. Knighton and P. R. Dumke, pp. 431–437. Little, Brown, Boston.
61. White, J. C. (1962): Evaluation of operation for relief of pain. *Neurol. Med-Chir.*, 4:1–28.
62. White, J. C., and Sweet, W. H. (1955): *Pain. Its Mechanisms and Neurosurgical Control*. Charles C Thomas, Springfield, Ill.
63. White, J. C., and Sweet, W. H. (1969): *Pain and the Neurosurgeon. A Forty Years Experience*. Charles C Thomas, Springfield, Ill.
64. Wycis, H. T., and Spiegel, E. A. (1962): Long-range results in the treatment of intractable pain by stereotaxic midbrain surgery. *J. Neurosurg.*, 19:101–106.

Discussion

Part II. Management of Pain of Advanced Cancer: Therapy of Cancer Pain in the Head and Neck

R. Molinari and M. Tiengo (Moderators)

Questioner: Dr. Molinari, what are the complications of intra-arterial administration in chemotherapy of tumors of the head and neck?

Molinari (Milano): The main risk is of pushing the catheter too low, causing the passage of the dose into the internal common carotid and cerebral complications that are, nevertheless, reversible. The most frequent complication is local arteritis. In about 15% of cases, one cannot cannulate the artery for anatomic reasons.

Questioner: Dr. Pagni, what is your experience with the technique of cisternal infusion with cold hypertonic salt solution?

Pagni (Torino): I have used cold salt solution and hypertonic salt solution for pain of the lower limbs, not for this type of pain, with relief never lasting longer than 3 weeks. Many people perform instead a phenolic block with intracisternal phenol. Personally, I have never done a phenolic block of the nerves of the posterior fossa.

Questioner: Dr. Houde, what is your experience in using corticosteroids, notably solumedrol, to control pain?

Houde (New York): We use the corticosteroids as an adjuvant in patients who have special forms and types of problems, primarily associated with increased intracranial pressure or massive edema; and, in these circumstances, you have to recognize the dangers of using steroids, particularly in patients in whom there may be a risk of producing or precipitating a gastric hemorrhage. The drug we use is dexamethazone in fairly high doses, going up to about 16 mg a day and tapering off during the course of a few weeks.

Role of Oncologic Therapy in Pain Involving the Chest and Brachial Plexus

Georges Brulé

Medical Oncology Unit, Institut Gustave-Roussy, 94800 Villejuif, France

Pain in the chest may become manifest by major functional signs, e.g., cough, dyspnea, dysphagia, pain either localized in the precordial or in the pleural region. Bone metastasis or infiltration of the brachial plexus by the tissue may cause cervicobrachial or intercostal neuralgia or pain spread over the ribs, the shoulder blade, or the upper limb. Compression of large veins occurs, leading to edema of the face or arms. All these manifestations appear either as an initial sign of the disease or more often at the terminal phase when the patient has already received numerous courses of treatment.

At this stage, the three main therapeutic weapons available in the oncologic armamentorium may still be used: surgery, radiation, or various medical disciplines such as chemotherapy, hormone therapy, or adjuvant medication. The contribution of each of these approaches is discussed briefly.

SURGERY

In case of recurrent and ulcerated breast tumor with involvement of radionecrosis, instead of attempting a radical extensive surgical excision, it seems preferable to proceed with an epiploplasty. The procedure implies stemming the epiploon under the skin and filling up the loss of tissue (following excision of the tumor and radionecrosis) and covering the flap with a dermoepidermal graft. Over the last few years, at Institut Gustave-Roussy, some 50 patients (11) have undergone this type of surgery followed by extremely satisfactory results occurring either immediately or after a period of time. Most patients who died some months after the procedure remained comfortable, and death was not due to local or regional recurrence, but a result of distant complications.

The chest surgeon may also have to interfere in case of isolated pulmonary metastases, particularly if the latter occurs distally near the pleura causing either unceasing bouts of cough or pain. Surgery may extend from partial resection of an isolated metastasis to pneumonectomy or lobectomy.

The neurosurgeon may also become involved in patients manifesting signs of intraspinal neoplastic lesion by performing a laminectomy, which at times prevents paraplegia and relieves the patient's pain.

For carcinoma of the esophagus which despite radiation therapy progresses to the final stage of dysphagia, two techniques may be used. One is the simple Fontan-type gastrostomy which involves opening of a cone of gastric wall sutured to the skin. Special attention must be paid to make sure that reflux through the slit of anastomosis does not occur. Such a direct gastrostomy makes frequent and easy change of the sound possible. With endoscopy, an attempt may be made to insert a cannula through the tumor.

Finally, mention must be made of the value of emergency low tracheotomy for patients showing a high compression of the trachea. The ideal incision is made between the 2nd and 3rd tracheal cartilage under the cricoid cartilage at one finger's breadth above the upper edge of the sternum with the patient's head extended. In case of tracheal tumor, the incision must be made lower, after sternotomy is done and a long cannula is inserted.

Major surgical interventions for tumors of the posterior mediastinum, such as neurinomas, which are usually cured by the operation done before intense pain occurs have not been included. Finally, it may be mentioned that some clinicians still use pleural talc-dusting in recurring metastatic pleural discharge. After drainage of the pleural fluid, the pleura is sealed by the injection of talcum via a trocar. The success of this technique depends on the flexibility of the pleura. Previous radiation therapy of the thoracic wall is a contraindication to the technique.

RADIATION

In regard to the use of radiation therapy, I will discuss exclusively cases involving recurrent or metastatic cancers. Two questions usually arise:

1. Is it possible to resume radiotherapy for a previously irradiated zone?
2. What are the various methods and procedures for palliative irradiation of antalgic interest?

The protocols of irradiation which have been used in the past for treating patients showing recurrence were often crude, and the pattern of dose distribution could be considerably improved by more sophisticated techniques (12). These include individualized beam-shaping by especially tailored lead blocks, by combination of various types of radiation (for instance, photons and electrons), or association of beam therapy and interstitial therapy, a combination that has been made more reliable through the help of computer dosimetry.

The use of a large number of fields (of various sizes, shapes, weight, etc.) considerably improves the dose distribution, but there is an increased risk of errors during the set-up of the patient.

In our institute, radiotherapists have worked out a particular type of palliative irradiation composed of 2 sessions of 8.50 greys (or 850 rads or

650 rads) or 6.50 greys delivered at 48-hr interval. This concentrated irradiation is well tolerated and is most useful for palliative radiotherapy (7). Without considering the radiobiologic problem, it may be said that 3,000 centigreys (15 × 200) in 3 weeks is equivalent to 2 × 850 centigreys in 2 days or 3 × 635 centigreys or 4 × 500 centigreys. Clinical experience shows good tolerance of the normal tissues. Skin and mucosal reactions appear 1 week earlier than for fractionated irradiation, but their maximum is the same and their repair takes no longer. This technique is very handy for carcinoma of the esophagus with very poor prognosis. Over a group of 44 patients, dysphagia was definitely improved in 65% of cases and gastrotomy could be delayed.

Mediastinal Compression

Mediastinal compression due to tumor is managed differently by different radiotherapists. Because of fear of edematous reactions, it is often advised to carry out irradiation with small doses over a long period of time. However, severe compression with vascular and respiratory obstruction requires very prompt relief even at the risk of the use of concentrated radiation therapy. Clinical experience with 14 patients with severe mediastinal compression has shown that these risks are actually limited when doses of 2 × 6.50 centigreys (equivalent to 22.50 greys in 3 weeks) are used.

Of the 14 patients, 13 improved rapidly. Improvement was evident during the first week and in 50% of cases it was evident on the third day. Moderate reactions (nausea in 2 patients, thoracic pain in 4 cases, and marked dyspnea in 2) appeared within a few hours after the first session and lasted about 3 hr. They were less frequent after the second session. The most interesting results concern 7 patients with alarming symptoms of severe respiratory obstruction. In 6, concentrated irradiation caused an immediate relief. Mean survival time was 4 months, extending to a maximum of 12 months.

Bone Metastasis

Concentrated irradiation was used for patients with multiple, painful metastasis of the spine, the ribs, or other sites in order to obtain rapid relief of pain and avoid long-term treatment. The doses used were 2 × 6.50 greys or 2 × 8.50 greys, depending on the extent of the treated volume, the site, and the general condition of the patient. No major side effects were noticed even upon treatment of 3 sites simultaneously. Pain was completely relieved in 35% of patients and significantly 1 week after irradiation. The average duration of the remission lasted 2 months. A second irradiation for recurring pain was usually less effective than the first.

CHEMOTHERAPY

Intra-arterial chemotherapy, a technique which has been widely used, may be employed for lesions of the upper limb, including osteosarcoma, melanoma, or any conjunctive tumor. It may also be injected via the external mammary route when the neoplasm is located in the thoracic wall or the breast (1).

Our own experience at Institut Gustave-Roussy, which dates back 10 years, and the published report on the use of the regional chemotherapy reveal that this has no advantage over the systemic route. Moreover, this procedure is difficult and requires complex equipment. It keeps the patient in bed and leads to complications which are not only systemic but also local, vascular, or cutaneous disorders. For all these reasons, this method was definitely given up.

On the other hand, local or regional chemotherapy is still being successfully used for the treatment of pleural discharge. In this case, local therapy is easier to apply than talc-dusting. I will not consider intrapleural injection of colloidal gold, which has been used for some 10 years. Because of the high cost and special care required for the life-duration of this isotope, therapy with colloidal gold has been abandoned, except maybe in some centers in Switzerland. Intrapleural injections of drugs may be highly effective, provided the proper agent is chosen. Alkylating agents are among the most active drugs, and two of them appear much better than average. The first is Thiotepa® and the second Mannomustine® or Degranol® (1). Easy to handle, these products cause local necrosis at injection-site less frequently than pure nitrogen mustard and unlike cyclophosphamide do not need to be metabolized hepatically to be active.

New liposoluble derivates of podophyllotoxin have been recently introduced. Vehem 26 and VP16 offer the advantage of crossing the seromeningeal or pleural barrier and seem to be as active by the systemic route as by the local route (2). Local intrapleural chemotherapy has considerable advantages; it is not toxic because the product does not diffuse through the pleura and therefore does not cause general hematologic or digestive toxic manifestations as alkylating agents do.

Amongst the increasing number of antimitotic agents available to the oncologist, for therapy of recurrent cancer it is essential to choose the substance which shows the least crossed resistance with previously used drugs. Subcutaneous injection of methotrexate, 6 mg/m^2/day × 4 injections at exactly 6-hr intervals gives satisfactory results in intradermal or cutaneous local or regional recurrence of breast cancer, by reducing the lesion and producing relief of local pain (3). In extended forms of breast cancer, with bone and lymph node involvement, adriamycin-vincristine-methotrexate seems to be the most effective therapeutic combination. It is also used as the initial treatment in breast cancer in preparation for irradiation and possibly surgery. In over 35% of the patients, the primary tumor and nodes are considerably reduced by decreasing the inflammatory reactions of these very rapidly growing tumors (6).

Unfortunately, no chemotherapeutic combination with marked activity in bronchial cancer is available. This also holds true for the resultant compression phenomena, which are usually better controlled by radiotherapy. Nonetheless cyclophosphamide seems to be the most frequent treatment for bronchial oat-cell carcinoma and the local phenomena which they cause. Cyclophosphamide may be used either alone or in combination with nitrourea derivatives.

Mediastinal compression linked with hematosarcoma, particularly immunoblastic lymphosarcomas at times react dramatically with vincristine, a derivative of periwinkle. This response is so consistent that some writers have used it as a therapeutic test if histologic examination proves doubtful. Unfortunately, this dramatic action does not last long and relapse occurs rapidly. The same applies for the effectiveness of bleomycin, mithramycin, and possibly *Cis*-platinum (diamine dichloride) in very rapidly growing pulmonary metastasis of embryonic carcinomas. Often these three products give dramatic results, but unfortunately the benefit is of short duration. Mithramycin has been given up by most clinicians because of its toxicity when administered in effective doses. The combination of bleomycin-*Cis*-platinum and vinblastine seems to give somewhat longer and more frequent remission than when each product is used separately (8).

Combined treatment with radiation and drugs is often used in the treatment of breast cancer, in severe forms of Hodgkin's disease, and in embryonic malignant tumors of the mediastinum in both children and adults. Without going into very complex radiobiological explanations, it is known that cells under formation are radioresistant and yet very sensitive to antimitotic drugs, whereas cells in phase G 1 and not under multiplication are chemoresistant but may be destroyed by radiation. Unfortunately, while this combination is highly effective in damaging tumoral tissues, it also increases normal tissue reaction leading to intense skin or pulmonary manifestations.

Finally, it must be pointed out that addition of heparin to antimitotic drugs, particularly in case of bronchopulmonary cancer seems to potentiate significantly the action of chemotherapy without aggravating the toxicity of these substances.

HORMONE THERAPY

Most forms of pain in the chest and cervicobrachial region in the female result from terminal stages of breast cancer. Therefore reference to hormonal treatment must be made when discussing this subject.

Without discussing the physiology of hormone therapy, hormones may be classified into three groups, each apparently acting specifically on a certain type of lesion. In the elderly female, estrogens, diethylstilbestrol in particular, often exert a striking effect on large, ulcerated and painful lesions. Within 6 to 8 weeks this medication causes disappearance or marked regression of ulcerative and painful lesions extending over a large surface.

Androgens, particularly synthetic androgens, are indicated for younger females. At Institut Gustave-Roussy, we use drostalonone propionate which has the least-virilizing side effects. These synthetic androgens are remarkably effective, especially on bone metastatic lesions of ribs, vertebrae, etc. (4).

High doses of progestational agents, particularly medroxyprogesterone acetate, which is the best tolerated of all such agents and which may be given at high dose by the oral route, often cause complete disappearance of intrapulmonary parenchymatous nodules (10).

Anti-estrogen agents form the latest introduction in hormone therapy. Tamoxifene is by far the easiest to handle. An extensive study of this product during the last few years has revealed that it is somewhat less effective in bone metastasis than are androgens. On the other hand, it is most effective for all metastatic skin nodes and bone lesions of breast cancer. In particular, in the female with primary tumor containing progesterone and estrogen receptors, dramatic results are frequently obtained by combining drostalonone propionate and tamoxifene in case of chemoresistant metastatic dissemination (5).

Major endocrine surgery (i.e., adrenalectomy or hypophysectomy) may yield dramatic relief of bone pain, especially in patients in whom metastasis occurs long after the primary lesion and who have become resistant to hormone therapy.

Finally, as a last resort in the terminal stage, high-dose corticoid medication may improve the patient's general condition. Amongst corticoids prescribed by us, methylprednisolone is particularly well tolerated with hardly any side effects (9). The product is given as a single intravenous injection in the morning, the dose varying between 40 and 300 mg. As reported by other writers, methylprednisolone exerts palliative effects not only on pain but also on dyspnea and cough. This may last several weeks, so that some bed-ridden patients do get up and resume normal life for some time. No satisfactory physiologic explanation seems obvious to justify this beneficial action which other corticoids, being more toxic in equivalent doses, fail to manifest. It seems that in addition to the anti-inflammatory action common to all corticoids, methylprednisolone exerts an effect on the hypothalamus. Several other writers, particularly in France, have noted this effect.

CONCLUSION

In conclusion, pain involving the chest and brachial plexus is a major problem. The oncologist often has to treat a patient who has received several other therapies and who knowingly will not be cured. But there still exist tools which in many cases will give long periods of remission. These tools will delay the terminal stage and the use of major narcotic agents and substances which modify the patient's behavior.

REFERENCES

1. Brule, G., Eckhardt, S. J., Hall, T. C., and Winkler, A. (1973): *Drug Therapy of Cancer,* edited by World Health Organization, Geneve.
2. Brule, G., Chauvergne, J., Guerrin, J., and Klein, T. (1974): Clinical study of new derivatives of podophyllotoxin. *Proceedings of the XI International Cancer Congress,* Florence, Vol. 5. Excerpta Medica, Amsterdam.
3. Brule, G. (1970): Le traitement des tumeurs solides par le Methotrexate Estratto da: *Corso Superiore sulla Chemioterapia dei Tumori,* Milano, 23–27 Marzo, 1970.
4. Brule, G. (1970): Chimiotherapie et hormonotherapie. *Revue du Praticien,* XX, 27:4259–4270.
5. Brule, G. (1976): Cooperative clinical study of 178 patients treated with Tamoxifene. *Symposium on the Hormonal Control of Breast Cancer,* Manchester.
6. Chauvergne, J., Gary-Bobo, J., Pommatau, E., Carton, M., Brule, G., Clavel, B., Guerrin, J., and Berlie, J. (1977): Polychimiotherapie des cancers mammaries en phase avancée. Association ternaire avec doxorubicine. Analyse de 209 observations. *Bulletin du Cancer,* 64,4:667–680.
7. Dutreix, J., Schlienger, M., Chauvel, C., and Daguin, R. (1971): Concentrated irradiation: Concentrated palliative radiotherapy for tumours affecting the oesophagus, brain, bones and mediastinum. *Ann. Clin. Res.,* 3:9–15.
8. Einhorn, L. H., and Donohue, J. (1977): Cis-diamminedichloroplatinum, Vinblastine, and Bleomycin combination chemotherapy in disseminated testicular cancer. *Ann. Intern. Med.,* 87:293–298.
9. Happert, J. L., Catel, P., Allin, O., Bouslama, A., and Engel, J. C. (1973): L'action antalgique du 6 alpha méthyl-prednisolone hémisuccinate de sodium en carcérologie pratique. *Médecin de Paris,* 45–50.
10. Londner, J. (1973): Etude de l'utilisation de la Medroxyprogesterone per os en carcinologie: A propos de 40 observations. *Thèse Paris.*
11. Petit, J. Y., Lasser, P., and Fontaine, F. (1977): Indications de l'épiplooplastie au cours de l'évolution du cancer du sein traité. A propos de 20 épiplooplasties faites à l'Institut Gustave-Roussy. *Bulletin du Cancer,* 64,4:659–665.
12. Tubiana, M. (1974): Achievements to be expected from new developments in tumour radiotherapy. *Europ. J. Cancer,* 10:373–380.

Role of Analgesics and Related Drugs in Pain Involving the Chest and Brachial Plexus

H. U. Gerbershagen

Institut für Anaesthesiologie, Univ-kliniken, Langenbeckstrasse 1, Mainz, West Germany

In many countries cancer patients are not informed of the etiology and prognosis of their disease process. The psychologic, emotional, and behavioral aspects of cancer pain are frequently discussed among physicians. With cancer patients, however, this discussion is avoided. Thus, many physicians misjudge the despair and the anxiety of cancer pain patients even if the clinical picture is impressive, e.g., with difficulty in swallowing, dyspnea, lymphedema, postradiation paralysis, etc.

The psychologic and psychotherapeutic guidance of these patients is often wanting. These patients should at least benefit from the selective action of psychotropic drugs. Even in the absence of detectable psychic distress or alteration we do start patients with painful tumor growth of the chest and upper extremities on low dose *phenothiazines* (e.g., thioridazine), *thioxanthenes* (e.g., chlorprothixene), or *butyrophenones* (e.g., haloperidol). The mode and site of action have been aptly described by Halpern and Kocher.

Some patients require *tricyclic antidepressants with anxiolytic properties* (amitriptyline) in addition to neuroleptics. Tumor infiltration of blood and lymph vessels often induces the symptomatology of reflex sympathetic dystrophy. Its typical signs and symptoms are: severe, constant, burning pain; neurovascular instability (e.g., vasoconstriction with cyanosis, edema, cold extremity or vasodilatation); and sudo- and pilomotor alterations. A general hyperactivity of the autonomic nervous system is usually present. *Sedative phenothiazines* (chlorpromazine, thioridazine) or *thioxanthenes* (chlorprothixene) combined with antidepressants like amitriptyline will achieve fair to good relief. According to the pathogenesis of pain, acetylsalicylic, metamizol, and indomethacin are effective analgesics. For intractable pain of reflex sympathetic dystrophy, cervicothoracic sympathetic blocks are highly effective. In addition a 2-week trial of *cortisone derivatives* is indicated prior to any narcotic administration.

The dull, compressing, tightening pain of lymphedema or solid tumor infiltration into nerve sheaths and blood and lymph vessels is difficult to treat. Repeated or continuous nerve blocks frequently decrease the edema and provide relief. Amitriptyline (30 to 75 mg/day) and levomepromazine (75 mg/day) are the most effective drugs in our experience. If inflammatory processes are present or only a short time has elapsed after radiation therapy, nonnarcotic analgesics with strong antiinflammatory properties will reduce this constant pain. Vasodilators and high-ceiling diuretics (e.g., furosomide) do not reduce edema or pain and should not be given.

Pain in and around inflamed and necrotizing tumor tissue is effectively treated with aspirin-like drugs and antibiotics. Narcotic analgesics are used only if other methods fail or cannot be used.

Neoplastic disease of the chest and brachial plexus is frequently accompanied by muscle hypertonicity and muscle spasms. In most cases this severe, dull pain is induced by positive feedback mechanisms associated with cancer pain and is not due to tumor infiltration of muscle tissue. Centrally acting relaxants (e.g., orphenadrine citrate) administered simultaneously with pharmacological doses of aspirin, paracetamol, or indometracin will control this muscular pain. Due to the interruption of motor reflex mechanisms nonmuscular pain is often reduced reflexly. If these prove ineffective, regional blocks should be used.

Many cancer patients develop a typical protective posture of the upper extremity and neck. This reflexly induces muscle-hypertonicity, muscular contraction, and typical dull, aching pain. As far as drug treatment is concerned, anxiolytic and sedative minor tranquilizers (e.g., diazepam), centrally acting muscle relaxants, and nonnarcotic analgesics are the drugs of choice.

Radiating, sharp pain in the thoracic region and upper extremity is most often considered to be due to tumor-induced nerve compression. Without careful examination many patients are started on narcotic analgesics, and the physician is awaiting total nerve compression. However, this radiating pain might be caused by muscular, ligamentous, or joint trigger-point syndromes with their pseudoradicular symptomatology. These can be most effectively relieved with infiltration of a local anesthetic into the trigger point. Depending on the patient's pain reaction, an anxiolytic phenothiazine (levomepromazine) or a more sedative drug (e.g., thioridazine) will enhance the effects of nonnarcotic analgesics and muscle relaxants.

In proven painful nerve compression, antiepileptics like carbamepazine (up to 800 mg/day) or phenytoin (diphenylhydantoin, up to 600 mg/day) and thioridazine (90 mg/day) will often reduce this sharp pain. In these patients we prefer a rapid increase in carbamepazine dosage to the normal, creeping administration. Until effective blood levels are attained nefopam, 90 to 120 mg, is given orally. If additional analgesics are required, a short-term application of phenylbutazone (600 to 800 mg/day) or nefopam (360 to 450 mg/day) is justified. With inadequate pain-relief the physician might have to fall back on tilidin (250 to 300 mg/day) or narcotic analgesics.

The dull, intrathoracic visceral pain associated with neoplastic disease of the esophagus and mediastinal structures can be controlled for a long period of time with metamizol.

The throbbing, boring, sometimes sharp pain of tumor invasion of bone and periosteum often becomes unbearable at night. Drug treatment consists of mood-elevating drugs and *sleep-inducing butyrophenones* (e.g., haloperidol 0.6 to 0.9 mg/day). Metamizol as a nonnarcotic analgesic often reduces pain to a tolerable degree. If a more potent analgesic has to be applied, tilidin is the most effective in this type of pain and has the advantage of long effective duration.

In my opinion, patients suffering from cancer pain of the chest and upper extremities should be carefully examined physically *and* psychologically. Severe cancer pain is often controlled by a combination of tricyclic antidepressant plus neuroleptic. It is a matter of course that nefopam, tilidin, and narcotic analgesics should be administered whenever other pain develops and other drug therapy is insufficient. We always give psychotropic medications with these potent drugs. Thus, we reduce the requirement for narcotics. In addition, we do rotate nefopam, tilidin, and narcotic analgesics administration every 3 weeks. It is our impression that with pain-relieving doses of each drug, the doses and adverse effects can be kept low.

Role of Nerve Blocks in Pain Involving the Chest and Brachial Plexus

M. Swerdlow

Regional Pain Relief Centre, University of Manchester School of Medicine, Salford, M6 8HD, Lancashire, England

Patients with severe cancer pain in the thorax, with or without involvement of the brachial plexus, are frequently presented for treatment of the pain. Types of cancer causing the pain vary considerably.

Etiologic Factors

Thoracic-wall pain may result from pleuromesothelioma, pleurocarcinoma, or sarcoma of the spine. Chest-wall pain may also be due to pleural irritation or erosion of ribs and involvement of intercostal nerves, which causes severe, radiating pain along affected dermatomes. Sharp, localized, unilateral chest pain or dull, aching pain often results from extension of a tumor onto the chest wall. On the other hand pleural or pericardial fluid-formation due to carcinomatosis is not commonly associated with pain (14).

Cancer in the *mediastinum* can occur from direct spread of lung, breast, or esophageal cancer and thoracic nerves, pleura and the sympathetic chain may be involved. Mediastinal pain may also result from secondary involvement of mediastinal glands. It produces a dull, burning or boring, central, persistent pain. Tumors arising in the mediastinum are very common. Many are benign; of the malignant ones many are in lymph nodes (either reticuloses or secondary from carcinoma bronchus or esophagus) or from primaries outside the chest such as breast or stomach.

Slow-growing, space-occupying lesions within the thorax may reach a considerable size before producing any symptoms other than vague restosternal pressure, perhaps with discomfort in the back and between the shoulder blades; the advent of severe chest pain usually signifies invasion of the chest wall. Malignant deposits involving cervical nerve roots or the brachial plexus may cause severe, intractable pain in the arm of mysterious origin. Cancer of the lung and breast are the two commonest causes of involvement of cervical nerve roots and the brachial plexus. The first thoracic nerve is often involved secondary to vertebral involvement and is difficult to

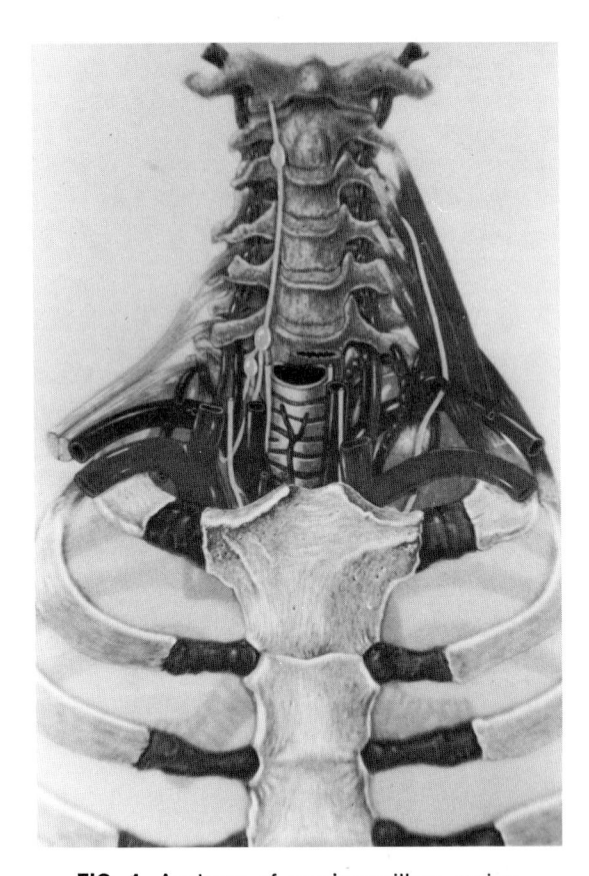

FIG. 1. Anatomy of cervico-axillary region.

visualize on X-ray; suggestive is a hard mass above clavicle together with a Horner's syndrome.

Tumors at the apex of the chest are commonly accompanied by Pancoast syndrome (the superior pulmonary sulcus syndrome)—unilateral pain in the upper chest, axilla, and arm, Horner's syndrome with some weakness of the arm. Study of the anatomy of the apex of the thorax demonstrates the large number of nerves which are at risk in this region (Fig. 1). Neuritic radiation is almost always at first in the distribution of the lower roots of the brachial plexus (16), sometimes limited to the ulnar nerve only. The cause is usually carcinoma bronchus, which as it spreads encroaches on the upper thoracic somatic and sympathetic nerves and on to the brachial plexus. Rarely the same syndrome can be caused by osteogenic sarcoma of the vertebrae or by upwardly extending mediastinal tumors.

Pain in the arm may also be caused by: (a) metastatic lesions of lower cervical or upper thoracic vertebrae or primary tumors of these vertebrae; (b) pressure on the brachial plexus, either supraclavicular, infraclavicular, or axillary; (c) pressure on large vessels by lesions in the axilla or root of neck.

Carcinoma Lung

The presenting symptoms and signs may have been present for 4 to 6 months with epidermoid cell tumor, which tends to cause local pulmonary symptoms and is the commonest cell type to cause the Pancoast syndrome. In contrast, small-cell carcinoma shows rapid growth and very early metastatic dissemination.

Lesions of the periphery of the lung which involve parietal pleura give rise to sharp neuralgia in the distribution of the intercostal nerves or dull, boring pain. If the central portion of diaphragmatic pleura is involved, pain is referred to the shoulder and neck. If sympathetic fibers are involved, there is diffuse, burning pain. Secondaries in the lungs most commonly originate from kidney, breast, thyroid, and prostate.

The median survival time after diagnosis is reported to be less than 6 months and the 5-year survival barely approaches 10% (16); however in the case of well-differentiated tumors the patient may live for many years.

Carcinoma Breast

Pain consequent to breast cancer usually results from bone metastases. According to Brennan (2), the amount of pain correlates with the rate of progression of the tumor rather than the extent of skeletal involvement.

Cancer of the breast is rarely the cause of local pain. However, advanced local breast cancer may be painful when inflammatory reaction distends the breast, when local infiltration of chest wall occurs, or if the tumor ulcerates. Secondaries in a rib or the sternum frequently cause intractable pain either from pressure on periosteum or on intercostal nerves or from pathologic fracture or involvement of pleura. Pain from such bone involvement may be alleviated by radiation.

Primary or secondary spread from breast cancer may reach the brachial plexus or major vessels of the arm causing edema, cyanosis, and burning pain in the limb. Stellate ganglion block will be necessary in addition to somatic block to provide pain-relief.

Development of bone pain in patients after mastectomy is difficult to attribute with certainty to metastases because osteoporosis and osteoarthritis are common in this age of patient; a bone scan may help in diagnosis (5). Local recurrence at the site of mastectomy may produce pain due to ulceration and secondary infection. Lymphedema of the arm may follow with severe shoulder-arm pain. The lymphatic spread to neighboring lymph nodes may also result in pressure on nerves and vessels.

Esophageal Cancer

Dysphagia is outstandingly the most common symptom in *esophageal* cancer. Carcinoma of the esophagus does however frequently cause retrosternal discomfort or aching pain in the back. Occasionally there is severe retrosternal pain, sharp or burning in nature, and usually only occurring on swallowing; it may radiate to the neck, shoulder, or between the scapulae. Occasionally also the vagus nerve may be involved, with pain referred to the ear or pharynx.

Skeletal Cancer

Pain from bone metastasis may be caused by stretching of periosteum, fracture of a rib, or collapse of a vertebral body. Primary or secondary cancer of the vertebrae produces pain which is at first localized but may spread to involve intervertebral nerves and produce root or girdle pain. Fibrosarcoma and chondrosarcoma of the upper ribs are uncommon causes of nerve involvement and pain. The development of back pain may be the first indication of metastasis to the spine. X-ray and bone scan may establish the diagnosis; if radicular pain is present it will help with localization. If no deposits are seen on X-ray, the pain should nevertheless be treated.

Spinal cord compression should be suspected in any patient with severe localized back or radicular pain especially if associated with sensory changes or motor weakness. Myelography should be carried out and, if necessary, urgent surgical or radiotherapeutic decompression of epidural metastases. Severe girdle-type back pain can result from extradural spinal metastases which can cause compression of the cord and spontaneous relief of pain.

TREATMENT

It will be clear from the above discussion that there are many different causes for thoracic pain in the cancer patient and a correspondingly wide range of treatments in relation to the nerves involved, the virulence of the growth, and the condition of the patient. In deciding on the type of pain treatment to be carried out the cell type and likely survival time will be important data. Needless to say the procedure must be carried out with full aseptic precautions, and the patient's informed consent should be obtained before commencing treatment. Pain sometimes becomes prominent at a time when the advent or existence of metastases is difficult to ascertain. Assuming that the state of the cancer coincides with the type and distribution of the pain and that possible coincidental causes for the pain (e.g., spondylolisthesis) are excluded, I believe it is reasonable to go ahead and treat the pain. To wait until it is proved beyond doubt that the pain is due to progress of the disease would often subject the patient to quite unnecessary suffering.

Pain of localized bone secondaries can often be easily controlled by radiation. Pain from nerve involvement however usually calls for relief by neurolytic methods, although it can sometimes be relieved by radiation, cytotoxic drugs, or antiinflammatory agents such as the corticosteroids (7) and the value of these various measures should be considered before proceeding to surgical or chemical neurolysis. The best treatment for pain from primary involvement of the chest wall is surgical excision as long as not more than two ribs are involved. Unfortunately Pancoast tumor is not amenable to palliative surgery.

The patient with thoracic pain should be referred as early as possible to an oncologist or radiotherapeutist if he has not already seen one. When the oncologists are unable to provide adequate pain-relief, some form of neural blockade may well provide the best possibility of relief. However, in a patient with a long life-expectancy (such as some patients with carcinoma of the breast) a cordotomy might well be the treatment of choice, or with localized pain a posterior rhizotomy. At the other extreme, a terminal patient with a very short survival expectancy might well be managed with appropriate analgesic and allied drugs if these can be made to provide adequate pain-relief. However, in patients with lung carcinoma, dyspnea may rule out cordotomy and may make narcotic drugs inadvisable; nerve blocking, with its minimal effect on respiration, will obviously then be advantageous.

Subarachnoid Neurolytic Blocks

In providing pain-relief by nerve blocking, by far the most useful measure in general is intrathecal neurolysis. In relation to the lower thoracic segments (i.e., caudad to T_5) this provides no real problems, and in fact this is the safest part of the cord to inject with little risk of producing bladder or limb paresis. Most workers report good results with the use of intrathecal neurolysis for the lower thoracic dermatomes. However, the spines of the vertebrae are very oblique in the mid-thoracic region, and the performance of spinal puncture can be very difficult; it is sometimes necessary to introduce the spinal needle at a technically easier spinal level (See Fig. 2) and then apply a corrective tilt of the operating table to "run" the solution towards the desired nerve root level; a somewhat larger volume of solution may be necessary (i.e., 1 to 1.5 ml).

When it comes to pain in the upper thoracic segments, particularly with Pancoast syndrome, the position is neither so simple nor so safe. The reason is by no means clear. There is a divergence of opinion on the value of subarachnoid neurolysis for pain in the upper chest and shoulder. Those who employ phenol or chlorocresol in glycerine find that the results in the cervical and upper thoracic levels are inferior to those obtained with these agents at lower spinal levels (13,15,18). On the other hand Kuzucu and his colleagues (10) and others who employ alcohol (8) report better results at high than at low spinal levels. This difference requires investigation.

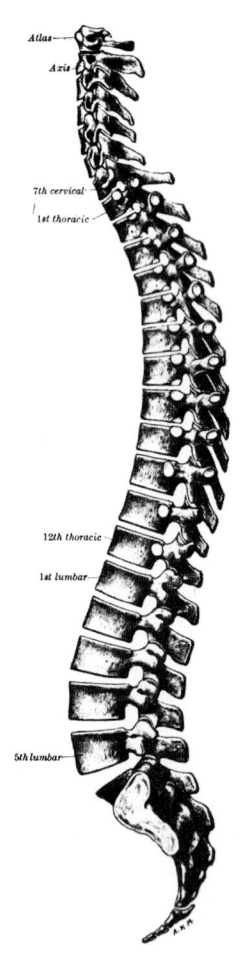

FIG. 2. Anatomy of spinal column.

Papo and Visca (15) found that of 21 patients with apical and upper chest pain, only 3 obtained good results and 9 fair; whereas of 17 patients with lower chest pain (caudad to T_6) 6 had good pain-relief and 5 obtained moderate pain-relief from intrathecal phenol. Kuzucu et al. (10) report that in 73% of their 322 patients pain was cervical or thoracic and results were very satisfactory. Katz (8) found that with intrathecal alcohol, thoracic pain was more easily treated than pelvic pain. Maher and Mehta (13) employed intrathecal 5% phenol or 2% chlorocresol in 235 cases of carcinoma shoulder, arm, lung, or breast and report that 72 were significantly relieved. Ventafridda and Martino (19) report "good" results in 71% with cancer pain in upper chest wall and in 56% with upper lung plus brachial plexus pain, but the duration of relief was only about 3 weeks.

Of the latest 140 cases in the author's series treated by intrathecal phenol or chlorocresol, 35 had pain in the thorax, of whom 15 had associated brachial plexus pain. Twenty-nine had lung cancer, 5 breast cancer, and 1 had a melanoma. Of the patients with lung cancer 15 had good or moderately good pain-relief up to death, but death occurred within a week in 4, within a month in 3 and within 3 months in 4 patients. The remaining 14 lung cancer patients obtained little or no relief from the subarachnoid neurolysis.

When there is widespread bilateral pain, it is worth trying the effects of intrathecal hypertonic saline which, however, frequently fails to give an adequate duration of relief. Papo and Visca (15) warn that "one stage bilateral phenolization should never be done at T_{5-10} because of risk of hypotension."

In the event of unsuccessful intrathecal block, there are a number of alternative techniques which may be tried including subdural, extradural, and paravertebral blocks.

Subdural Blocks

Subdural injection is carried out with the aid of an image-intensifier. A spinal needle is inserted and advanced to the epidural space. It is gently advanced until it impinges on the dura and then pushed forward a fraction. Injection of a small amount of iophendylate will show when the tip of the needle is subdural; X-ray shows myodil in line between dura and arachnoid. One to three ml of 5 to 8% phenol in glycerine are now injected; injection is slightly resisted. The technique is not easy, and the relief is often of inadequate duration. The cervical nerve roots on both sides can be covered from a centrally placed needle, or the lower cervical plus upper thoracic nerve roots can be blocked at one session. Maher suggests that alternate injection of phenol and air will provide greater spread.

Extradural Blocks

Extradural injection of 5 to 10% phenol in glycerine may be employed in the upper thoracic and the cervical segments and has the advantage that there is no risk of its spreading beyond the foramen magnum and that severe headaches will not occur. The author has sometimes found extradural neurolytic block to give effective and lasting results. Others (11,12) report similar findings. Continuous or intermittent injection of local anesthetic via an indwelling extradural catheter should be considered in terminal cases.

Paravertebral Blocks

Paravertebral somatic nerve block is rarely used. As Bonica (14) points out, intrathecal or extradural block is preferable to paravertebral neurolysis because they act proximal to the site of the bony pressure on the nerve and because they spare the motor fibers of the nerve. *Intercostal* block is only useful for anterior and anterolateral metastases and, in my experience, neurolytic block of intercostal nerves usually does not last long enough. It can be used as an interim measure, while intrathecal, subdural, or rhizotomy/cordotomy is being planned. Intercostal neurolysis is useful in pathologic rib fractures; phenol or chlorocresol is injected between the fracture faces.

Pain in the distribution of the intercostal nerves due to invasion of the paravertebral chest wall may require paravertebral block not only of the affected roots but also of the adjacent ones caudal and cephalad. It is easier for the patient (and for the physician) to do an intrathecal rhizotomy of a number of posterior nerve roots. However, in some patients, pain in the shoulder from involvement of lower cervical roots can be effectively relieved by paravertebral block of the appropriate cervical nerve roots. The block is carried out at the tip of the transverse process(es), and it is advisable to perform a prognostic local anesthetic block before employing a neurolytic agent.

Brachial Plexus Blocks

When none of the above methods is satisfactory, Bonica (1) recommends that alcohol block of the brachial plexus should be performed if necessary. Brown (3) reports that when the brachial plexus is infiltrated with cancer cells, relief can be obtained "in a reasonable proportion of patients" by infiltrating the plexus with 1 or 2% aqueous phenol using not more than 20 ml of the solution. The procedure may cause severe pain for up to 48 hr after injection.

However, glandular infiltration in the supraclavicular region may make access to the brachial plexus (and to the stellate ganglion) difficult or impossible.

Sympathetic Block

Because of the invasive nature of many intrathoracic tumors, visceral fibers of the sympathetic nervous system may become involved. It is as well, therefore, in cases where somatic block does not produce complete pain-relief to try the effects of an appropriate sympathetic block with a local anesthetic solution such as bupivacaine or lignocaine. As an alternative to sympathetic nerve block, intravenous guanethidine may be tried for upper-limb pain (6).

Carcinoma of the breast is often accompanied by edema of the arm and severe, burning pain in the shoulder and arm. Stellate block may be helpful—it should be performed with local anesthetic first, before contemplating neurolytic block (17).

When treating pain due to carcinoma of the esophagus, thoracic sympathetic ganglion block of 2–5 T should be used for upper esophagus and block of 5–7 T ganglia for lower esophagus. If this doesn't relieve all the pain, vagus block should be performed just above the clavicle. A prognostic local anesthetic block should be performed prior to bilateral vagal section.

Invasion of the subclavian vessels will result in edema of the arm, which is objectively cool but subjectively has a burning sensation. These symptoms will be relieved by stellate ganglion block with local anesthetic, which should be tried before somatic block; as Challenger (4) points out, sympathetic block has the advantage of not producing paresis or sensory disturbance.

PAIN FOLLOWING ANTICANCER THERAPY

In addition to the pathological causes described above, the cancer patient may have pain in the thorax for a number of different reasons. Pain or discomfort in the chest and/or arm can occur as a result of surgical or radiation therapy.

Radiation fibrosis in the pectoral axillary area used to be a problem, but my colleagues at the Christie Cancer Hospital tell me that this rarely creates difficulties nowadays. However, irradiation therapy of carcinoma breast can cause brachial plexus neuropathies. Kiff (9) reports such a case successfully relieved by intravenous regional sympathetic block with guanethidine. However, frequently the pain of fibrosis of the brachial plexus requires neurosurgical pain-relieving operations.

Lymphedema in patients who have undergone axillary dissection can cause arm heaviness which may be accompanied by pain in the neck and shoulder region due to tissue traction by the weight of the arm. It is important to see to restoration of upper-limb function as well as reduction of lymphedema.

Pain in the scar of a mastectomy or lobectomy operation is not uncommon and may interfere with simple daily actions, such as washing. It may be a symbol of resentment of the scar itself and of the mastectomy, and this must be borne in mind when considering pain-relieving therapy.

Finally beware of post-herpetic neuralgia obscuring the onset of cancer pain. Cancer is one of the conditions which is thought to occasionally light up the dormant varicella virus. I have seen two patients with post-herpetic neuralgia which proved resistant to treatment, and in whom it became clear (fortunately without too much delay) that, in fact, cancer was causing pain in the same dermatomes as the herpetic rash.

REFERENCES

1. Bonica, J. J. (1953): *The Management of Pain.* Lea & Febiger, Philadelphia.
2. Brennan, M. J. (1973): In: *Cancer Medicine,* edited by J. F. Holland and E. Frei. Lea & Febiger, Philadelphia.
3. Brown, A. S. (1976): Pain relief in malignant disease. In: *Symposium on Malignant Disease.* Roy. Coll. Physicians Edinb. Publication No. 47.
4. Challenger, J. H. (1978): Sympathetic nervous system blocking in pain relief. In:

Relief of Intractable Pain, 2nd ed., edited by M. Swerdlow. Excerpta Medica, Amsterdam.
5. Creech, R. H. (1976): In: *Oncologic Medicine,* edited by A. I. Sutnick and P. F. Engstrom. University Park Press, Baltimore.
6. Holland, A. J. C., Davies, K. H., and Wallace, D. H. (1977): Sympathetic blockage of isolated limbs by intravenous guanethidine. *Can. Anaesthetists' Soc. J.,* Vol. 24.
7. Jackson, S. M. (1978): Radiotherapy, anticancer drugs and hormones. In: *Relief of Intractable Pain,* 2nd ed., edited by M. Swerdlow. Excerpta Medica, Amsterdam.
8. Katz, J. (1975): Subarachnoid alcohol injections for the management of chronic pain. In: *Recent Progress in Anaesthesiology and Resuscitation.* Excerpta Medica, Amsterdam.
9. Kiff, J. G. H. (1974): *Pain Relief.* Heinman, London.
10. Kuzucu, E. Y., Derric, W. S., and Wilber, S. A. (1966): Control of intractable pain with subarachnoid alcohol block. *JAMA,* 195:133.
11. Lourie, H., and Vanasupa, P. (1963): Comments on the use of intraspinal phenol-pantopaque for relief of pain and spasticity. *J. Neurosurg.,* 20:60.
12. Madrid, J. (1975): *Proceedings of Symposium on Cancer Pain.* Florence, Italy.
13. Maher, R., and Mehta, M. (1977): Spinal and extradural analgesia. In: *Persistent Pain,* edited by S. Lipton. Academic Press, London.
14. Olson, K. B., (1973): Pain. In: *Cancer Medicine,* edited by J. F. Holland, and E. Frei. Lea & Febiger, Philadelphia.
15. Papo, I., and Visca, E. (1976): Intrathecal phenol in the treatment of pain and spasticity. *Prog. Neurol. Surg.,* 7:56.
16. Selawry, O. S., and Hansen, H. H. (1973): Lung cancer. In: *Cancer Medicine,* edited by J. F. Holland and E. Frei. Lea & Febiger, Philadelphia.
17. Swerdlow, M. (1977): Peripheral nerve blocking in the relief of pain. In: *Persistent Pain,* edited by S. Lipton. Academic Press, London.
18. Swerdlow, M., editor (1978): *Relief of Intractable Pain,* 2nd ed. Excerpta Medica, Amsterdam.
19. Ventafridda, V., and Martino, G. (1976): Clinical evaluation of subarachnoid neurolytic blocks in intractable cancer pain. In: *Advances in Pain Research and Therapy, Vol. 1, Proceedings of the First World Congress on Pain,* edited by J. J. Bonica and D. Albe-Fessard, pp. 699–703. Raven Press, New York.

Role of Neurosurgery in Pain Involving the Chest and Brachial Plexus

Donald E. Richardson

Department of Neurological Surgery, Louisiana State University School of Medicine, and Hotel Dieu Hospital Pain Rehabilitation Unit, New Orleans, Louisiana 70112

Carcinoma-induced pain involving the chest and brachial plexus can be one of the most rewarding types of pain for control by neurosurgical techniques. With rare exceptions, gratifying results can usually be obtained in a large number of patients and with minimal side effects and relatively low complication. The most common etiology of chest wall and brachial plexus pain in men is recurrent carcinoma of the lung, and it usually produces symptoms by invasion and contiguous spread. In women, the most common cause is recurrent carcinoma of the breast with either regional node metastasis or contiguous spread.

Pain in patients with recurrent carcinoma of the upper quadrant of the body may be caused by invasions of the pleura, the periosteum, or nerves involving the chest wall or brachial plexus. In addition to tumor invasion, however, benign causes of pain must be considered. Postsurgical changes, such as partial nerve injury, perineural scarring, loss of sensation with deafferentation pain, and occasionally radiation neuropathy are other causes for the pain which are not directly related to the patient's disease. One of the most common types of chest wall pain occurring in patients who have had thoracotomies for lung lesions is incisional pain or pain caused by damage to the intercostal nerves at the time of thoracotomy. This has been greatly reduced recently by the use of well-padded retractors or by the section of the intercostal nerves at the time of the primary surgery. Brachial plexus pain can be a difficult differential diagnosis in an occasional patient who has pain beginning a few weeks following surgery with dissection about his brachial plexus, either in the axilla or supraclavicular fossa. Fortunately for the neurosurgeon, the control of pain does not always require a specific diagnosis, except for the patient who continues to complain of pain that is primarily due to emotional factors and who is being treated for organic pain.

A rare cause of pain in the upper extremities and chest wall in patients with carcinoma is invasion of the spine itself with nerve root compression or localized bone pain. In these patients, the pain can be either midline or often bilateral, which not only produces a difficult pain syndrome to control surgically, but also may indicate impending spinal cord compression with paraplegia. Obviously, the prevention of spinal cord compression and paraplegia would be of primary importance, and the pain would have to be placed secondary in the line of treatment.

The two things that patients with terminal cancer fear the most are pain and loneliness. One must remember that, in patients with terminal disease, appropriate discussions with the patient regarding his treatment and his disease, a realistic but supportive attitude, psychiatric consultation, religious counseling, and a careful explanation to the patient and his family that pain-relieving procedures do not improve or retard the underlying disease process are a necessary part of treatment. The treatment of underlying depression and anxiety will greatly enhance the treatment of the pain problem itself and, at times, has provided enough pain-relief that the patient did not have to have a neurosurgical procedure carried out at all. The use of narcotics for the control of anxiety and depression can be misleading as an indication of the degree of the patient's pain.

TIME AND SELECTION OF THE PROCEDURE

In our clinic we consider pain-relieving neurosurgical procedures to be indicated when the patient has begun to require potent narcotic medications, that is, when the patient changes from codeine and propoxyphene to morphine, or other potent narcotics. The reason for this is that we believe tolerance to narcotics occurs fairly rapidly, making it necessary to increase the dosage to control the patient's pain. Moreover, in our experience, narcotics add to the anorexia, weight loss, and to the general debility of the patient with terminal cancer and often produce apathy, lethargy, and chronic depression.

Selection of procedures, of course, requires sophisticated consideration of the patient's problem. The most difficult consideration is the prognosis for life. Patients with very short life-expectancies can be adequately managed with nerve blocks or maintained on narcotics. Trying to provide an adequate prognosis on patients with terminal cancer is fraught with many problems and often is misleading. Our present recommendation is that, if the patient's life-expectancy is longer than 3 to 4 months, a neurosurgical pain-relieving procedure is indicated. In patients who have a very short life-expectancy, nerve blocks or large doses of narcotics or both are usually effective. If the patient's pain, however, is excruciating and cannot be controlled by nerve blocks, or is accompanied by much suffering and loss of emotional control, a saline lobotomy would be offered the patient with a prognosis of less than 3 to 4 months.

In patients with terminal cancer, there is always the question of how long one should wait for positive anticancer therapy, such as radiation or chemotherapy, to produce pain-relief before proceeding with neurosurgery. Waiting 3 to 5 weeks for a patient to respond to radiation therapy or chemotherapy is not an unrealistic consideration, but allowing continuation of pain and suffering while a series of chemotherapeutic agents are tried without considerations for the patient's comfort is without merit. It is our policy not to wait longer than 3 to 4 weeks following the termination of radiation therapy or a course of chemotherapy before offering the patient a pain-relieving procedure if his pain is not significantly improving at that time. It is unlikely that significant reduction of pain will occur later than 3 to 4 weeks following a course of such therapy.

PREOPERATIVE WORK-UP AND EVALUATION

The basic work-up required prior to pain-relieving neurosurgical procedures can be quite minimal. However, there are some specific indications and procedures that should be carried out in a reasonable attempt to ascertain whether the patient has a potentially complicating factor prior to surgery. In addition to the usual blood count, cardiogram, urinalysis, biochemical profile, and chest X-ray which are carried out on every patient, there are specific indications for further studies. Cervical and thoracic spine films should be obtained in patients if there is any reason to think that the patient may have spine invasion and potential spinal cord compression. In addition, isotope bone scans and soft tissue scans can be obtained to accurately delineate the degree of the patient's tumor recurrence and invasion. If there is significant question as to whether the patient has spinal cord invasion with potential spinal cord compression, a preoperative myelogram can be done without great difficulty. In patients with a large amount of pulmonary metastasis, postoperative pneumonectomy, radiation pneumonitis, or possible phrenic nerve palsy, pulmonary function studies and fluoroscopy of the diaphragms should be carried out before surgery to ascertain the potential for respiratory insufficiency, especially if a chordotomy or extensive rhizotomy is being planned.

In addition, in patients who have extensive tumor recurrence and who are to have general anesthesia, it is our policy to have a preoperative isotope blood volume carried out, because they often have a depleted blood volume and may need to have blood replacement with either whole blood or packed cells prior to any surgical procedure. In any patient with personality change that cannot be explained on the basis of medication or other central nervous system symptoms or manifestations, both isotope cerebral scans and computerized axial tomography are carried out to rule out the possibility of cerebral metastases. We have had 1 patient who had the diagnosis of cerebral metastasis made at the time of ventriculography before stereotaxic procedure for relief of his brachial plexus pain. Although this situation can usually be managed by use of large doses of steroids, it is obviously preferable to have a diagnosis prior to surgery and to avoid intercranial operations for pain-relief on patients with cerebral metastasis.

SELECTION OF THE SPECIFIC PROCEDURES

The selection of procedures for pain-relief are based on the location of the patient's pain, anticipated duration of life, and general condition of the patient. Obviously, an extensive rhizotomy with section of the sensory portions of the nerve roots involving the entire arm is not acceptable, since patients will not have the use of the extremity due to the loss of position sense and sensory feedback required for motor function of the extremity. An amputation of the extremity usually follows such ill-advised procedures. Time-consuming and extensive procedures on patients with only a few weeks to live are undesirable.

Below, are listed the procedures that we are using most commonly at the present time for pain involving the chest wall and brachial plexus in patients with recurrent cancer. This outline is then matched with the type of pain that each procedure can be used for in most cases. This outline does not take into consideration the longevity of the patient, which is discussed further in the discussion of each procedure, and leaves out some procedures that are rarely performed. Moreover, in each type of pain only one of these is indicated.

The procedures include: (A) sensory rhizotomy or neurectomy; (B) anterolateral cordotomy; (C) thalamotomy; (D) stimulation of periventricular gray; (E) hypophysectomy; (F) saline lobotomy.

Location of pain	Procedures applicable
Small area of chest pain	A, B
Large area of chest wall	B, C, D, E, (F)
Lower brachial plexus (and chest)	B, C, D, E, (F)
Upper brachial plexus (and neck)	C, D, (E), F
Bilateral chest and brachial plexus	C, D, (E), F

SPECIFIC PROCEDURES

Sensory Rhizotomy or Neurectomy

Use of spinal sensory rhizotomy can be extremely rewarding in patients with fairly well-localized chest wall pain. It is ideally suited for patients with postthoracotomy incisional pain due to damage to the intercostal nerves. In addition, relatively small areas of pain involving the chest wall can be quite adequately controlled with rhizotomy with minimal morbidity to the patient. It is one of the most easily tested procedures since, prior to operative rhizotomy, temporary paravertebral or intercostal nerve blocks can be carried out with relative ease with X-ray control. The diagnostic block helps to predict the amount of pain-relief the patient will derive from the surgery, allowing both the patient and the surgeon to be reasonably sure of his results prior to operation.

At the present time, we are using percutaneous X-ray controlled radiofrequency coagulation of nerve roots at the neural foramen. Stimulation of the nerve root can produce paresthesias in the area of the patient's pain. Once this is done, brief general anesthesia with intravenous Brevital® is given and the nerve root is then coagulated, either at 70°C or at 90°C. The 70°C coagulation is used in an attempt to differentially destroy the small, unmyelinated pain fibers and leave other sensation otherwise intact, and 90° coagulation for complete destruction of the nerve root. In patients with pain secondary to cancer, I have not attempted to do a differential rhizotomy, but have usually totally destroyed the nerve root. Usually, 1 min of coagulation at 90°C, if the electrode is well-placed against the nerve root, is sufficient for its complete lysis (9).

Anterolateral Cordotomy

Percutaneous, high cervical cordotomy is the procedure of choice in patients who have unilateral, lower brachial plexus and chest wall pain or a large area of chest wall pain that would require an extensive rhizotomy for control. Percutaneous, high cervical cordotomy between the lamina of C_1 and C_2 vertebrae carried out under local anesthesia has given excellent results if the patient is cooperative enough to allow the procedure to be done. Insertion of a small needle electrode into the anterior quadrant of the cord with stimulation followed by slowly increasing radiofrequency lesions will give good analgesia involving the lower brachial plexus and chest wall as well as the abdomen and leg if necessary. However, an attempt to raise the cordotomy to the upper brachial plexus or cervical plexus levels may cause extension of the lesion into the motor fibers of the spinal cord with contralateral weakness and can produce respiratory weakness or hemiparesis. In addition, in patients with bilateral pain, a bilateral cordotomy is considered highly dangerous owing to the production of sleep apnea with respiratory arrest.

In some patients, it is difficult to do a percutaneous cordotomy, either for anatomic reasons or because of poor cooperation on the patient's part. In these patients, we still use open high cervical cordotomy under general anesthesia. Our technique for this is quite simple and requires only 1 hr of operating time. A small, midline incision is made from the base of the skull to the C_3 spinous process, and the muscles are reflected unilaterally on the side opposite the pain so that the C_2 lamina is exposed on that side. A self-retaining retractor is placed between the lamina and against the muscles laterally, and when open, usually rotates the spine considerably. The C_2

lamina is then removed, and the dura is opened in a horseshoe-shaped fashion to hinge laterally and is sutured to the paraspinous muscles. The denticulate attachment is then sectioned, and the cord is rotated by grasping the dentate ligament. Low magnification with loops or the operating microscope can then be used with excellent visualization of the anterior quadrant of the spinal cord. Section of the anterior quadrant, beginning 1 or 2 mm anterior to the dentate ligament and carried to just medial to the exit of the ventral rootlets, is then carried out with ease.

In our experience, failures of pain control from chordotomy have been primarily due to late development of pain on the opposite side of the body or upward extension of tumors through the brachial plexus, reaching levels above the chordotomy sensory level. Thus, some consideration of the potential for further tumor invasion and spread of pain should be considered along with the other factors involving the selection of this procedure for pain control. In addition, chordotomy does not usually relieve disagreeable paresthesias and numbness. Careful discussion with the patient regarding the character of his discomfort and pain should be carried out, since some patients describe paresthesias and numbness as being painful (8), which is not relieved by chordotomy.

Thalamotomy

The advantages of radiofrequency-induced destruction of the medial thalamus are that the procedure can be carried out under local anesthesia, it carries minimal morbidity and mortality, it will control pain over the entire opposite side of the body, and it results in no detectable sensory loss.

On the other hand a disadvantage of thalamotomy is that pain-relief cannot be expected to be maintained for more than 6 months to 1 year. Most of the patients who have had thalamotomy for pain control have had excellent relief for at least 6 months but, between 6 months and 1 year, the pain recurs. In addition, an acutely painful experience, such as a pathologic fracture, may cause the previous chronic pain to return.

Lesions placed in the medial thalamus, including the centrum medianum, parafascicularis, and medial pulvinar will usually control contralateral pain quite well. Care should be taken with the placement of the lesion not to allow the destruction to extend laterally into the main sensory nucleus, since patients will complain bitterly of numbness and may have dysmetria following lateral extension of their lesion. Bilateral lesions can be carried out if carefully done for patients with bilateral pain with good results and no significant side effects. Patients who have thalamotomy for pain usually have a transient period of euphoria lasting a week to 10 days which then resolves (6).

This procedure can be very useful in patients with brachial plexus and upper chest wall pain who have had a previous pneumonectomy and have borderline pulmonary function and who might have further compromise of pulmonary function secondary to chordotomy or extensive rhizotomy.

Stimulation of Periventricular Gray

The technique of periventricular gray stimulation, while not widespread at this time, is very efficacious for relief of pain in any area of the body. The advantages of this procedure are that it can be carried out under local anesthesia, it does not produce a lesion of the nervous system with potential for complications from neural destruction, it is under the patient's control so that it can be used when needed, and it will control pain in any area of the body, including extensive unilateral pain or bilateral pain.

A detailed description of the procedure and its results are in a separate section of this volume ("Central Gray Stimulation for Control of Cancer Pain") (4,5). Briefly the procedure is carried out by stereotaxically inserting a stimulating electrode into the periventricular gray just anterior to the posterior commisure. Stimulation is then carried out using percutaneous leads until reassurance is obtained that the procedure is effective for relieving the patient's pain. Then, at a second procedure, the radiofrequency induction receiving device is placed under the skin and connected to the electrode pairs to be used for stimulation. The patient then uses a radiofrequency coupled transmitter to self-stimulate when necessary for pain control.

In most patients, continuous stimulation is not necessary, since intermittent stimulation may be effective for many hours. The secondary gain from this procedure is that patients who use ventricular gray stimulation seem to have an elevation of their mood with consequent relief of chronic depression. We have found that, with periventricular gray stimulation, some of the other side effects of tumor growth are not controlled. It will often control dysesthesias, paresthesias, and complaints of numbness associated with nerve destruction. However, in patients with burning pain secondary to deafferentation, the procedure may not be effective. Pressure sensation or discomfort secondary to tumor mass also is not relieved by these procedures and, if a patient is habituated to narcotics, it may not relieve the patient's pain completely.

Hypophysectomy

The usefulness of hypophysectomy for the control of carcinoma of the breast, prostate, and endometrium is widely recognized and is used extensively. Metastatic carcinoma of the prostate to the dorsal spine and ribs or cervical spine with secondary pain can be quite readily controlled with either a transnasal hypophysectomy, alcohol injections of the hypophysis, radiofrequency coagulation of the hypophysis, or transfrontal removal of the hypophysis. The results with carcinoma of the breast are somewhat less gratifying in that only about 50 to 60% of the patients have significant control of their disease with hypophysectomy. The use of hypophysectomy for endometrial carcinoma has been utilized in only a small number of cases in our experience, but excellent results were obtained by this procedure.

Hypophysectomy for pain of nonhormonal-dependent tumors has recently been utilized, and there is some early clinical evidence that control of pain from any cause can be relieved by hypophysectomy. The mechanism for control of pain by hypophysectomy is apparently by interference with an inhibitory mechanism for the endogenous opiate system. It has been well established that naloxone, a morphine antagonist, when given after hypophysectomy, causes immediate return of pain in patients who have received excellent pain-relief by this technique. At the present time, the selection of patients for hypophysectomy, the expected results, and the indications and contraindications for its use are not well established and will have to await further clinical trials (2,3).

Saline Lobotomy

The technique of saline lobotomy has not been utilized widely for pain control, though it is an excellent technique for relieving pain in patients who have a short life-expectancy of less than 4 months. It is also an excellent procedure in patients who have marked suffering and emotional stress associated with their illness and pain. The procedure can be easily done on patients who are quite ill and who have pain in any area of the body (chest, neck, brachial plexus, and bilaterally). The disadvantages of this procedure are that, if it has to be repeated over a period of time, as in cases where the patient has lived longer than anticipated, the patient will develop progressively more severe frontal lobe damage and personality changes that are undesirable from the point of view of maintenance of his personality and relationships with his family and friends. In patients with relatively short life-expectancy, however, the procedure gives excellent pain control with pain asymbolia and the alleviation of suffering with the ability to withdraw, or greatly reduce, large doses of narcotics rapidly with minimal side effects except physiological withdrawal symptoms.

This procedure, done under local anesthesia, entails placing bilateral trephines approximately 2 cm from the midline just anterior to the coronal suture line. A #20 spinal needle is then inserted into the frontal lobes bilaterally or, in most cases, unilaterally at the first injection; 8 to 10 cc of sterile saline are injected as the needle is slowly withdrawn from the frontal white matter. Usually, injections of 1 to 2 cc of saline every centimeter as the needle is removed produces an excellent result. The procedure can be titrated by talking to the patient during the injection and discontinuing the injection when there is an obvious change in the patient's affect or mood. It has been our experience that injections only on one side is all that is necessary at the initial time of treatment and, later, the second side may be added if necessary (1).

As the patient's pain begins to return, the procedure can be repeated percutaneously by simply inserting the #20 needle through the scalp over the burr holes after sterilizing the skin. Injections of saline, either unilaterally or bilaterally, can then be repeated as needed. Patients usually require injections at 6-week to 2-month intervals and, if no more than two or three injections are required, personality defects are relatively mild. However, the longer the patient survives, and the more injections required, the more permanent the frontal lobe effects become. At the present time, we reserve this procedure for patients who have a very short life-expectancy and who have severe pain and suffering not controlled with narcotics (7).

SUMMARY

An attempt has been made to present in a concise review the procedures that have been found to be efficacious and are currently in use in our clinic for the control of cancer pain in the area of the brachial plexus and chest. The development of newer procedures is continuing at a rapid pace at this time, and it is understood that these procedures will obviously be modified by newer techniques and by the experience of the surgeon involved. Emotional support for the patient and his family, as well as the recognition and treatment of underlying depression and anxiety regarding his disease and ultimate death are necessary for optimum control of the patient's pain. The procedures of sensory rhizotomy, anterolateral cordotomy, thalomotomy, periventricular gray stimulation, hypophysectomy, and saline lobotomy offer the neurosurgeon a wide armamentarium for the control of almost all types of pain involving the neck, arm, and chest wall. The indications for surgery at this time are pain that has not responded to radiation or chemotherapy and that has increased in severity to the point where the patient is requiring potent narcotics for pain-relief. The avoidance of narcotic tolerance, anorexia, weight loss, and suffering secondary to chronic pain, and the avoidance of the use of narcotics for a period of time longer than 3 to 4 months is thought to justify the performance of the procedures described.

REFERENCES

1. Bridges, T. J., and Liss, H. R. (1958): Saline lobotomy for relief of pain due to advanced cancer. *Cancer* (VI) 11:322.
2. Moricca, G. (1974): Chemical hypophysectomy for cancer pain. In: *Advances in Neurology Vol. 4, International Symposium on Pain,* edited by J. J. Bonica, pp. 707–714. Raven Press, New York.
3. Richardson, D. E. (1967): Recent advances in the neurosurgical control of pain. *So. Med. J.,* 60:1082–1086.
4. Richardson, D. E. (1974): Thalamotomy for control of chronic pain. *Acta Neurochir.,* [Suppl.], 21:77–88.
5. Richardson, D. E., and Akil, H. (1977): Long term results of periventricular gray self-stimulation. *Neurosurg.,* 1:199–202.
6. Richardson, D. E., and Akil, H. (1977): Pain reduction by electrical brain stimulation in man, Part 2: Chronic self administration in the periventricular gray matter. *J. Neurosurg.,* 47:184–194.

7. Rosomoff, H. L., Carroll, F., Brown, J., and Sheptak, P. (1965): Percutaneous radiofrequency cervical cordotomy: Techniques. *J. Neurosurg.*, 23:639–644.
8. Tindall, G. T., Nixon, D. W., Christy, J. H., and Neill, J. D. (1977): Pain relief in metastatic cancer other than breast and prostate gland following transsphenoidal hypophysectomy. *J. Neurosurg.*, 47:659–662.
9. Uematsu, S., Udvarhelyi, G. B., Benson, D. W., and Siebens, A. A. (1974): Pericutaneous radiofrequency rhizotomy. *Surgical Neurol.*, 2:319–325.

Discussion

Part II. Management of Pain of Advanced Cancer: Pain Involving the Chest and Brachial Plexus

B. R. Fink (Moderator)

Questioner: Dr. Swerdlow, do you think that extradural neurolytic block is less harmful than subdural, and is it effective in relieving cervical pain?

Swerdlow (Manchester): Extradural block is certainly likely to cause less damage than intrathecal block, and in the cervical region it is certainly safer. Because so many of the patients we have treated have lived for a very short time, we found that very often extradural neurolytic block has been effective in this region. Elsewhere in the spinal cord we are less inclined to use it.

Questioner: How many milliliters of phenol do you use in performing extradural block?

Swerdlow: We usually use phenol aqueous solution and, of course, you have to be very careful indeed, ensuring that the tip of the needle is not within the theca. I use about 2 ml for each nerve segment that I want to block.

Sapio (Taranto): You mentioned three types of blocks: intrathecal or subarachnoid, extradural or peridural. What is the third type?

Swerdlow: The third type is subdural. That is to say, injection of the chemical between the dura and the arachnoid. There is a potential space between the dura and the arachnoid; and it is possible, using image-intensification and radio-opaque dye, to get the tip of the needle into this subdural space and then inject the phenol into the space. When this procedure is successful, it is very good because you can get a block of both sides with one injection and because it is very safe.

Rampulla (Urbino): I would like to know something about supraclavicular neurolysis of the brachial plexus.

Swerdlow: I should tell you that both alcohol and phenol when applied to the brachial plexus will give a period of 24 to 48 hr of agony to the patient, and it is important to give them sufficient analgesia medication. It depends on how infiltrated the area is. Of course, glandural infiltration in the supraclavicular region can sometimes make this procedure difficult; it can sometimes make cervical nerve blocks difficult.

Scalabrin (Padova): Dr. Brulé, you talked about the chemotherapic combination of neomicyn, *cis*-platinum, and vincristine. Do you have other data on the single or combined use of *cis*-platinum in the palliative or curative chemotherapy of thoracic neoplasia?

Brulé (Villejuif): I cannot give you any precise data yet. But we are studying *cis*-platinum as one of a small group of European chemotherapists, and we have made some screening. As you know, we already know that it is effective in testicular tumor and mainly on pulmonary metastasis of testicular tumor. But the action is very brief. You may have a complete disappearance of all metastatic lesions, but they will reappear in about 6 weeks to 2 or 3 months later. So the problem is to have a long remission. That is the reason why we are trying a combined therapy.

Graziussi (Napoli): Dr. Richardson, do you use local or general anesthesia in placing the cannula for percutaneous rhizotomy? And would you tell us the percentage of success in pain-relief according to your experience?

Richardson (New Orleans): We do it with local anesthesia. It should always be done with local anesthesia. We sometimes use intravenous Brevital,® which is a very ultra-short-acting barbiturate, during the period of coagulation to reduce the patient's discomfort. I cannot give you a percentage but, in general, we select rhizotomy for patients who have the least amount of pain, and our results have been excellent because we can always test for the effect of the rhizotomy by doing a temporary nerve block prior to the procedure. So our results are almost 100% successful, at least temporarily. We may have to do something else later if the patient's cancer spreads and involves a larger area.

Porges (Vienna): You did not mention the endoscopic thoracic sympathectomy for treatment of irradiation pain of the arm or of thoracic secondaries involving the sympathetic system.

Richardson: The main reason I did not mention it is that I have never done one. We do very few sympathectomies. We have sympathetic blocks done, and if the patient has good results, then we do sympathectomy. Most of the sympathectomies in my area are done by the transaxillary approach by the thoracic surgeons. I also find a very small number of patients who require sympathectomy.

Questioner: Dr. Swerdlow, do you have any experience with barbotage of spinal fluid in alleviation of cancer pain?

Swerdlow: It is by no means sure to produce any pain-relief, but it is pretty sure to produce a good headache.

Murri (Reggio Emilia): Dr. Gerbershagen, what are the advantages or disadvantages of tilidine in regard to morphine?

Gerbershagen (Mainz): The greatest advantage is that the effective duration is longer than that of morphine, about 6 to 8 hr on the average. As to addiction, dependence is no problem in cancer patients, otherwise I would say it is, in our experience, just about as addictive as morphine. In Germany it is not yet considered to be narcotic because of the structural formula, but I am pretty sure that in a couple of years it will be treated just as a narcotic.

Richardson: We have done hypophysectomy routinely, and we find it extremely effective for carcinoma of the prostate and moderately effective for carcinoma of the breast. And we are not trying to use hormone assays with tumor cell banning of estrogens to select patients for hypophysectomy of the breast. This has all been well established. My point was that hypophysectomy for non-hormonodependent tumors is still considered an experimental procedure. And I do not have reliable figures on efficacy, failure rate, and complication rate in non-hormonodependent tumors. We have a tremendous amount of data on patients with carcinoma of the breast and of the prostate. In my experience, hypophysectomy for carcinoma of the prostate with bone pain has been about 95% effective. With carcinoma of the breast, it has been about 50 to 60% effective.

Gerbershagen: In our Institute we have done over 400 hypophysectomies, and for 5 or 6 years we have not been doing them anymore or we are doing them very seldom—about 10 or 15 each year. That is due to better manipulating of medical hormonal treatment. At the very beginning, we did not have a good compound.

Role of Analgesics and Related Drugs in Visceral and Perineal Pain

Raymond W. Houde

Department of Medicine, Memorial Sloan-Kettering Cancer Center, New York, New York 10021

Cancer involving the abdominal viscera and pelvis, and perineum, include a wide variety of neoplasms, both primary and metastatic, which can produce pain in a multiplicity of ways related either directly to the tumor itself or to complications of the disease or its treatment. Often the sources of pain are multiple and may involve both visceral and somatic afferent neural pathways for pain. The systemic analgesics, in particular the centrally acting drugs, are nonselective as to the site or source of pain, and thus provide an advantage over methods of controlling pain which rely upon precise identification of the involved pain pathways. This is especially true when both visceral and somatic structures are involved, or when the cause of the pain is in the midline or bilateral.

Centrally acting drugs such as the narcotics and their congeners are generally employed for the management of visceral and pelvic pain, although, contrary to popular opinion, the antiinflammatory-type analgesics are also effective and may be used to advantage in combination with other drugs. However, when there is gastrointestinal ulceration, bleeding, or the risk of perforation, salicylates and other antiinflammatory drugs are contraindicated. Since most nonnarcotics are also commonly administered by the oral route, they are obviously of little value when there is bowel obstruction or serious malabsorption.

The narcotic-type analgesics are also not without shortcomings, for most of these drugs will increase the tone of smooth muscle and of the sphincters; and they have hormonal effects, which can lead to urinary retention, obstipation, and fluid retention. Hepatic dysfunction can interfere with the metabolic disposition of most narcotics, although this does not commonly occur except in very far advanced disease of the liver. On the other hand, when hepatic function is intact and there is marked impairment of drug elimination by the kidney, active metabolites may accumulate and, as is the case with meperidine, lead to serious toxic reactions (1).

Most of the narcotic agonist-antagonists have effects similar to those of the narcotic agonists, to which they are most closely related. However, as partial agonists, these drugs tend to have ceiling effects, so that their effects may not be so intense as those of the typical narcotic agonist, particularly on the bowel.

The choice of an analgesic should be based on the nature and the quality of the pain and what is known of the extent of the disease. Pains may be dull and persistent, or intermittent and sharp, or cramp-like. If the patient is able to take medication by mouth, the combined administration of a narcotic and a nonnarcotic analgesic such as aspirin is generally indicated. For more severe pain, it may be necessary to employ parenteral medications but again, if it is not contraindicated, the concurrent administration of a simple analgesic by mouth may help to stay the too-rapid development of tolerance.

The indications of employing adjuvant drugs such as the anxiolytics, tranquilizers, and antidepressants are essentially the same as they would be in other clinical situations. With the exception of methotrimeprazine, there is no good substantial evidence that the phenothiazines or any of the other psychotropic drugs have any analgesic properties of their own, or that they are capable of enhancing the effect of standard analgesics in the absence of severe anxiety or depression, or symptoms contributing to suffering, such as nausea and vomiting. All of the narcotic analgesics increase the tone of smooth muscle including that of the intestine, and decrease peristalsis, so that one must be alert to the possibility of obstipation and obstruction. Commonly these patients do require stool softeners and cathartics to be taken on a fairly regular basis. The narcotic agonist-antagonists such as pentazocine have less of an effect on the bowel, but this drug is a somewhat shorter-acting drug than the morphine agonist analgesics, and there is a relatively high risk of psychotomimetic reactions. Methotrimeprazine, on the other hand, is a phenothiazine analgesic which has little effect on the bowel but can produce obstructive jaundice typical of the phenothiazines. Methotrimeprazine also has appreciable sedative and hypotensive actions, so that it is generally wise to start it at a lower dose than would be expected to be necessary for pain control. Methotrimeprazine may also be employed to supplement a narcotic analgesic, although there is an increased risk of precipitating both its hypotensive and sedative effects. Neither methotrimeprazine nor pentazocine will substitute for a narcotic in a narcotic-dependent patient, and, in fact, the pentazocine may precipitate abstinence.

In summary, the systemic analgesics and, in particular, the potent, centrally acting analgesics can play an important role in managing patients with intra-abdominal and pelvic pain. However, assessment for the possible causes of pain should always be done before prescribing any analgesic regimen, for many of these drugs may mask signs or symptoms which could delay the institution of definitive measures to prevent serious or life-threatening complications.

ACKNOWLEDGMENT

Supported in part by a Grant from the National Institute on Drug Abuse #DA 01707.

REFERENCE

1. Szeto, H. H., Inturrisi, C. E., Houde, R. W., Saal, S., Cheigh, J., and Reidenberg, M. M. (1977): Accumulation of normeperidine, an active metabolite of meperidine, in patients with renal failure or cancer. *Ann. Intern. Med.,* 86:738–741.

Role of Nerve Block with Neurolytic Solutions for Pelvic Visceral Cancer Pain

Daniel C. Moore

The Mason Clinic, Seattle, Washington 98195

ANATOMICAL CONSIDERATIONS

Pain fibers from the pelvic viscera pass through the pelvic plexus, the hypogastric plexus, the aortic plexus, and the pelvic nerve. Pain fibers from the lower portion of the colon enter the spinal cord at the level of the first and second lumbar nerves and the second, third, and fourth sacral nerves. Those from the bladder enter at the level of the eleventh and twelfth thoracic and first lumbar nerves, as well as the second, third, and fourth sacral nerves. And those of the male and female reproductive systems enter at the tenth thoracic through the second lumbar nerves, as well as the second, third, and fourth sacral nerves (1).

The location of the plexuses prohibits safe, accurate placement of needles in or in close proximity to them. Therefore, block of the pain fibers from the pelvic viscera must be done where they, along with somatic nerves, enter the central nervous system—namely, paravertebrally or in the epidural or subarachnoid spaces (1,3,4,8,9,11,17,19,20). The injection of neurolytic solutions at these locations often results in incontinence of urine or feces and varying degrees of paralysis of the lower extremities.

An alternative method of eliminating pain, particularly when the male and female reproductive organs are its source, is ablation of the pituitary gland, which also has undesirable complications (2,10,12).

DIAGNOSTIC BLOCK

Seldom does cancer of the pelvic viscera remain within a single organ. Often it metastasizes to other intra-abdominal organs, and it frequently invades bone. These metastases exert pressure on somatic nerves, and this intensifies the pain. Therefore, prior to injection of a neurolytic solution for a lumbar sympathetic or epidural block, a diagnostic block using a long-acting local anesthetic drug—preferably 0.5% bupivacaine (Marcaine®) with 1:200,000 epinephrine—is advisable. However, diagnostic blocks are not used prior to ablation of the pituitary gland, where accurate needle placement presents problems initially and where a second placement would increase complications, or for subarachnoid block, where small quantities of local anesthetic drugs would not give a definitive result.

THERAPEUTIC BLOCKS

With the exception of lumbar sympathetic and unilateral subarachnoid block, the patient experiences intense, unbearable pain during administration of these blocks. Therefore, the patient must be anesthetized. During ablation of the pituitary, light general anesthesia or topical anesthesia with local infiltration usually suffices.

Lumbar Sympathetic Block

If pain is limited to the fundus of the bladder, bilateral block of the first through the third lumbar sympathetic ganglia with 5 ml of 50% to absolute alcohol or 6 to 7% phenol may give temporary pain-relief for 1 to 4 weeks, with no or minimal alteration in bladder, rectal, or lower extremity function. However, as the tumor grows and/or metastasizes and the pain recurs, final attempts to relieve pain with neurolytic drugs must involve more aggressive therapy—that is, placing of a neurolytic solution in the epidural or subarachnoid space.

Epidural Block (Lumbar or Caudal)

Weak solutions of alcohol, such as 30%, as well as 6% aqueous phenol, and volumes from 10 to 30 ml, have been injected with partial to complete relief of pain. The degree of dysfunction of the bladder, rectum, and lower extremities is usually proportionate to the volume and concentration employed. Relief from such an injection seldom has a prolonged duration.

Subarachnoid Block

Hypertonic saline. The neurolytic solution least likely to cause motor and sensory loss in the bladder, rectum, and lower extremities is hypertonic cold or partially frozen normal saline injected subarachnoidally (3,4,19,20). This technique involves removal of 30 to 60 ml of cerebrospinal fluid and replacement of it with 30 to 60 ml of partially frozen 7 to 15% normal saline. The higher volumes and the stronger concentrations result in the maximum pain-relief, the longest duration of action, and the most severe complications. The hazards of this technique range from reversible complications, such as severe pain during injection, hypotension, nausea and vomiting, and convulsions, to life-threatening or permanent ones, such as cardiac failure, pulmonary edema, incontinence of urine and feces, and paresis of the lower extremities.

Unilateral blocking of one to three dermatomes with alcohol or phenol. When the pain from the pelvic viscera is unilateral, blocking of one to three posterior spinal roots with 0.5 to 0.75 ml of absolute alcohol or 6 to 7% phenol (plain or in glycerine) may provide relief ranging from a few days to 2 to 3 weeks. Usually if more than two of the lumbar or sacral spinal roots are blocked unilaterally, weakness of the extremity can be expected, with or without incontinence of urine or feces. If bilateral block is attempted, one side should be done and then at least 24 hr should pass before the opposite side is blocked. Even if no complications result from the first injection, they are likely to occur following the second injection, particularly if more than two or three roots are blocked.

Transection of the spinal cord with alcohol. When the patient (a) is incontinent of urine and feces, (b) is not ambulatory, (c) has excruciating pain, or (d) preferably experiences all three, definitive treatment is subarachnoid injection and complete transection of the spinal cord with 10 to 15 ml of absolute alcohol at the first or second lumbar interspace (1,11). Prior to the injection of the alcohol, a similar amount of cerebrospinal fluid is withdrawn.

Pituitary Ablation with Alcohol

Certain primary cancers (male and female reproductive organs) and their metastases, which are susceptible to hormonal influence, can be treated with pituitary ablation employing 1.0 to 2.0 ml of absolute alcohol, depending on the size of sella (2,10,12). Pain-relief ranging from a few days to over 4 months results. The pain-relief varies from complete to partial in 70% of the patients, while the pain remains unchanged in 30% of the patients. Pain from other types of cancer has been treated with ablation of the pituitary with some success.

With this technique the bladder, rectum, and lower extremities are not affected, but rhinorrhea, nasal hemorrhage, leakage of cerebrospinal fluid, diplopia, hemianopia, and infection, as well as death from the injection, may occur. Also, as would be expected, diabetes insipidus, with or without hypopituitarism, ensues.

CONCLUSIONS

Treatment of cancer pain of the pelvic viscera with neurolytic drugs is a "trade-off" between pain-relief and complications—with or without pain-relief. Percutaneous or surgical cordotomy, myelotomy, and lobotomy usually are more accurate and effective (5,6,7,14,15,16,21). They are preferred to neurolytic, chemical sectioning techniques for they seldom require repeating, as is the rule with neurolytic drugs. However, these procedures too are associated with complications, such as lymphedema of the legs, partial to complete urinary and fecal incontinence, respiratory difficulties, and so forth; and they can be totally unsuccessful (13,14,18,21).

Block with a neurolytic drug should be done only when: (a) the patient and/or the family knows the consequences, (b) pain-relief, even for short periods of time, is desired, and (c) life-expectancy is limited.

The physician who does the block should: (a) have mastered the block technique, preferably learning it from an expert; (b) be skillful in its performance; (c) have the facilities and knowledge to cope with its complications; and (d) not become frustrated by less than optimal results—that is, partial to complete failures.

REFERENCES

1. Bonica, J. J. (1953): *The Management of Pain.* Lea & Febiger, Philadelphia.
2. Corssen, G., Holcomb, M. C., Moustapha, I., Langford, K., Vitek, J. J., and Ceballos, R. (1977): Alcohol-induced adenolysis of the pituitary gland: A new approach to control of intractable cancer pain. *Anesth. Analg.,* 56:414.
3. Hitchcock, E. (1967): Hypothermic subarachnoid irrigation for intractable pain. *Lancet,* 1:1133.
4. Hitchcock, E., and Prandini, M. N. (1973): Hypertonic saline management of intractable pain. *Lancet,* 1:310.
5. Lin, P. M., Gildenberg, P. L., and Polakoff, P. P. (1966): An anterior approach to percutaneous lower cervical cordotomy. *J. Neurosurg.,* 25:553.
6. Lipton, S. (1968): Percutaneous electrical cordotomy in relief of intractable pain. *Br. Med. J.,* 2:210.
7. Lipton, S., Dervin, E., and Heywood, O. B. (1974): A stereotactic approach to the anterior percutaneous electric cordotomy. *Adv. Neurol.,* 4:689.
8. Maher, R. M. (1955): Relief of pain in encurable cancer. *Lancet,* 1:18.
9. Mehta, M. (1973): *Intractable Pain.* W. B. Saunders Co., Ltd., London.
10. Miles, J., and Lipton, S. (1976): Mode of action by which pituitary alcohol injection relieves pain. In: *Advances in Pain Research and Therapy, Vol. 1: Proceedings of the First World Congress on Pain,* edited by J. J. Bonica and D. Albe-Fessard, p. 867. Raven Press, New York.
11. Moore, D. C. (1976): *Regional Block,* 4th ed. Charles C Thomas, Springfield, Ill.
12. Moricca, G. (1974): Chemical hypophysectomy for cancer pain. In: *Advances in Neurology, Vol. 4: International Symposium on Pain,* edited by J. J. Bonica, p. 707. Raven Press, New York.
13. Mulland, S., and Hosobuichi, Y. (1968): Respiratory hazards of high cervical percutaneous cordotomy. *J. Neurosurg.,* 22:291.
14. Rifkinson, N. (1978): Neurosurgery and pain control. *Anesthesiology News,* 4:11.
15. Rosomoff, H. L. (1969): Bilateral percutaneous cervical radiofrequency cordotomy. *J. Neurosurg.,* 31:41.
16. Rosomoff, H. L. (1974): Percutaneous radiofrequency cervical cordotomy for intractable pain. *Adv. Neurol.,* 4:683.
17. Stovner, J., and Endresen, R. (1972): Intrathecal phenol for cancer pain. *Acta Anesthesiol. Scand.,* 16:17.
18. Tenicela, F., Rosomoff, H. L., Feist, J., and Safar, P. (1968): Pulmonary function following percutaneous cervical cordotomy. *Anesthesiology,* 29:7.
19. Thompson, G. E. (1971): Pulmonary edema complicating intrathecal hypertonic saline injections for intractable pain. *Anesthesiology,* 35:425.
20. Ventafridda, V., and Spreafico, R. (1974): Subarachnoid saline perfusion. In: *Advances in Neurology, Vol. 4: International Symposium on Pain,* edited by J. J. Bonica, p. 477. Raven Press, New York.
21. White, J. C. (1965): Relief of terminal cancer pain. *Surg. Gynecol. Obstet.,* 120:115.

Neurolytic Blocks in Perineal Pain

V. Ventafridda, C. Fochi, E. P. Sganzerla, and M. Tamburini

Department of Pain Therapy and Rehabilitation, National Cancer Institute, Milan, Italy; and Department of Anesthesiology, Universita degli Studi, 20133 Milan, Italy

Perineal pain due to neoplastic disease manifests itself as three different types of sensation which can be either separated or associated: a "burning sensation," tenesmus, and somatic pain without trigger points. In order to comprehend the intensity of this painful syndrome and the alteration which it can cause in the patient's personality, we report the results obtained from a study carried out in our Pain Therapy Department.

We have submitted two groups of patients affected by cancer of the rectum to a psychometric test (MMPI) (6): the first (control) group was composed of colostomy patients who were free from pain and disease; the second group consisted of 25 patients with perineal pain in an evolutionary stage. In the second group (Fig. 1) we observed a marked increase in all clinical personality scales; in particular 40% of such subjects (against the 12% of the patients in the first group) present a remarkable increase (scores superior to 70 T.) of the neurotic scales (hysteria, hypochondriasis, and depression) (Fig. 1).

Because these personality alterations cause a drop in the pain threshold, it is important to start therapy as soon as possible at the time the pain symptomatology is still localized and the usual nonnarcotic analgesic drugs are no longer sufficient. The simplest and most suitable treatment of these painful syndromes are neurolytic subarachnoid sacral blocks or chemical rhizotomy and peridural caudal block.

Neurolytic hyperbaric solutions offer some advantages over hypobaric solutions with alcohol, because it is easier technically to block the lower area affected by pain and it is less discomforting for the patient during the procedure.

Several authors have achieved good results with classic Maher's technique, which consists of performing subarachnoid infiltration with hyperbaric phenol in glycerine at the level of the L_5-S_1 interspace (9). Lifshitz et al. (8) reported that out of 90 patients with perineal pain due to gynecologic malignancy treated with one or more sacral phenol blocks, 77% of them derived satisfactory to excellent results. Using this technique, Stovner and Endresen (13) produced analgesia for almost 1 month for 83% of the patients affected by cancer of the rectum, anus, and external genitalia.

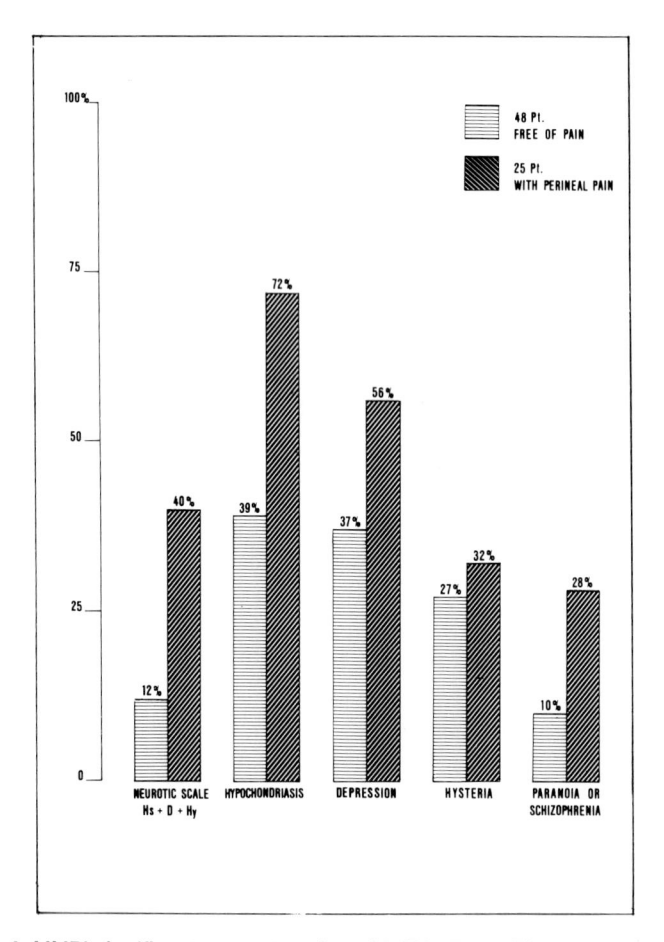

FIG. 1. MMPI significant percent scales with T > 70 on 73 ostomy patients.

Papo and Visca (11) also reported that 30 of 35 patients affected by cancer of the rectum derived good and fair pain-relief.

In 1975, Kuhner and Assmus (7) published the results of a study of 596 patients treated with hyperbaric phenol. They noted that the best results were obtained in patients with pain due to cancer of the rectum, 79% of whom derived complete relief and 13% partial relief of pain, and in patients with urogenital tumors of whom 67% obtained complete relief and 23% partial relief.

All of the authors who have reported on the technique mentioned bladder sphincter complications as being present in most patients.

In regard to perineal pain in patients treated with repeated peridural injection of bupivacaine, different authors reported prolonged analgesia in patients with nonmalignant pain (2,3,4,5). Furthermore, caudal blocks with bupivacaine and corticoid compounds have produced beneficial effects in patients with low back pain (1–14).

MATERIAL AND METHODS

We have treated 47 patients with pain caused by the following neoplastic primary tumors: 36 with cancer of the rectum; 4 with cancer of the uterus; 2 each with cancer of the vagina and prostate; 1 each with cancer of the vulva and sigmoid; and 1 with a cordoma. For these patients, two techniques were used: caudal blocks with local anesthetic and corticoids and chemical rhizotomy.

Technique of Caudal Epidural Block

The standard technique of caudal epidural block was used (Fig. 2A). Following placement of the needle into the sacral canal, 10 ml of 0.25% bupivacaine combined with 80 mg of methyl-prednisolone were injected. This procedure was repeated on an average of 6 times at intervals of 3 to 4 days.

Chemical Rhizotomy

The technique of chemical rhizotomy is as follows: With the patient in a sitting position, a 23-gauge needle was introduced through L_5-S_1 interspace (Fig. 2B) into the subarachnoid cavity. Once this was done, the point of the needle was carefully withdrawn posteriorly until CSF flow was reduced to a trickle in order to try to avoid the roots which lie more ventrally. A solution of 0.8 ml of 7.5% phenol in glycerine was injected slowly using two different positions:

1. *For bilateral pain,* the patient was in a sitting position, tilted backward at an angle of 15 to 30° to the edge of the table.
2. *For unilateral pain,* the patient was made to lie on the painful side with the head of the table raised 30°.

The patients kept these positions for 30 min.

An immediate indication of the extent of chemical rhizotomy was the appearance of an area of hypesthesia from S_2 to S_5 which was reduced to S_4-S_5 during the ensuing 48 hr. Each of these procedures was repeated as soon as the pain occurred.

The caudal epidural block with local anesthetic and corticoid was used when: (a) There was no clinical data indicating spread of the disease; (b) micturition was normal; (c) there was no skin erosion or trigger points; and (d) the patient was complaining of a burning sensation or tenesmus.

We used chemical rhizotomy when the patient affected by the perineal

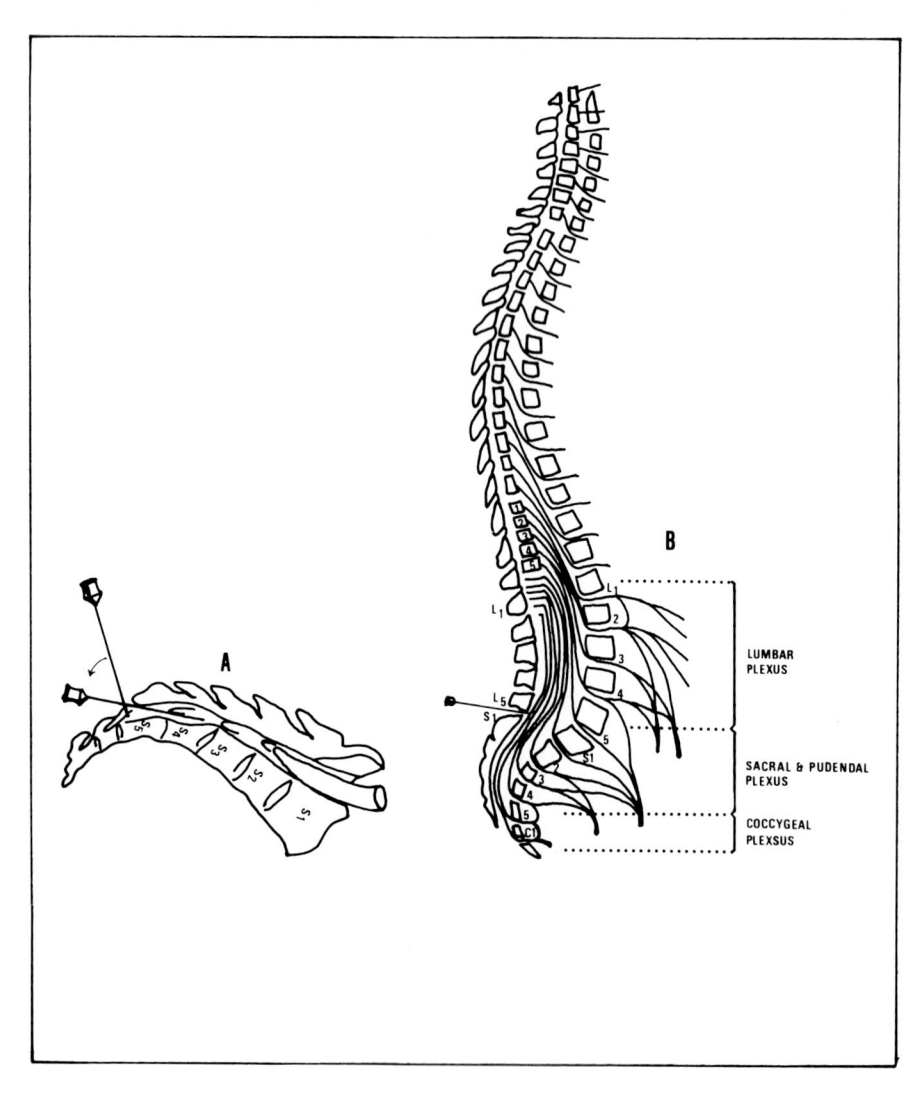

FIG. 2. A. Caudal-epidural blocks. **B.** Subarachnoid sacral blocks.

pain showed: (a) suspicious signs of recurrence of the disease; (b) macroscopic areas of vulvovaginal or pararectal erosions and evident "trigger points"; and (c) trouble with micturition or preexisting bladder dysfunction.

The follow-up of these patients was carried out every month until death of the patient or the further spreading of the pain. In addition, another group of 13 patients including 8 treated with caudal epidural blocks and 5 with chemical rhizotomy have been followed for 4 weeks using a weekly chart filled in by the patients and which included: (a) evaluation of pain intensity using the visual analogue of Scott and Huskisson (12); and (b) the total amount of time the patient spent standing, lying, sitting, and sleeping.

RESULTS

Of 47 patients affected by perineal pain due to neoplastic disease (Table 1), 39 have been treated with chemical rhizotomy. A total of 77 neurolytic blocks were performed for an average of 1.97 blocks for each patient. The average duration of pain-relief was 5.43 months. Bladder sphincter complication was noted in 19 patients (49%).

We carried out 48 caudal epidural blocks in 8 patients, averaging 6 blocks for each patient. In this group the average duration of pain-relief was 3.5 months.

The average time of pain-relief after chemical rhizotomy in 14 patients with trigger points was 5.92 months. In 14 patients with evident erosion areas, it was 8.35 months; and in 11 patients without trigger points or erosion areas but with pain spreading to S_{2-3} areas, the pain-relief lasted only 1.09 months (Table 2).

Among the 5 patients who underwent chemical rhizotomy and were followed with the weekly pain charts, the visual analogue showed an average reduction of pain of 71.4%. The total number of hours the patient was up and about increased by 204%, while the time the patient spent sitting and lying down was diminished by 36%, and the total number of hours asleep were increased by 25%. Less favorable, though still-significant results were reported in 8 patients treated with caudal blocks: Pain was reduced by 47.4%, and the total hours the patient was active were increased by 37% (Fig. 3).

COMPLICATIONS

Prolonged muscle weakness in the lower limbs did not develop in any of our patients. We believe that this complication can be obviated with a correct technique.

Meningeal reactions and low pressure headaches may also be avoided with prophylactic measures such as the use of a fine spinal needle (21 to 23 gauge), bed rest, oral and parenteral administration of fluids (10).

TABLE 1. Results with block therapy of perineal pain

	Number of patients	Number of treatments	Mean N° of treatments	Mean analgesic time (months)	Bladder impairment
Caudal-epidural blocks	8	48	6	3.5	—
Chemical rhizotomy	39	77	1.97	5.4	19 (49%)

TABLE 2. Duration of pain relief

	N° of patients	Mean analgesic time (months)
With trigger points	14	5.9
With macroscopic ulcerations	14	8.35
Without trigger points or ulcerations with spreading	11	1.09

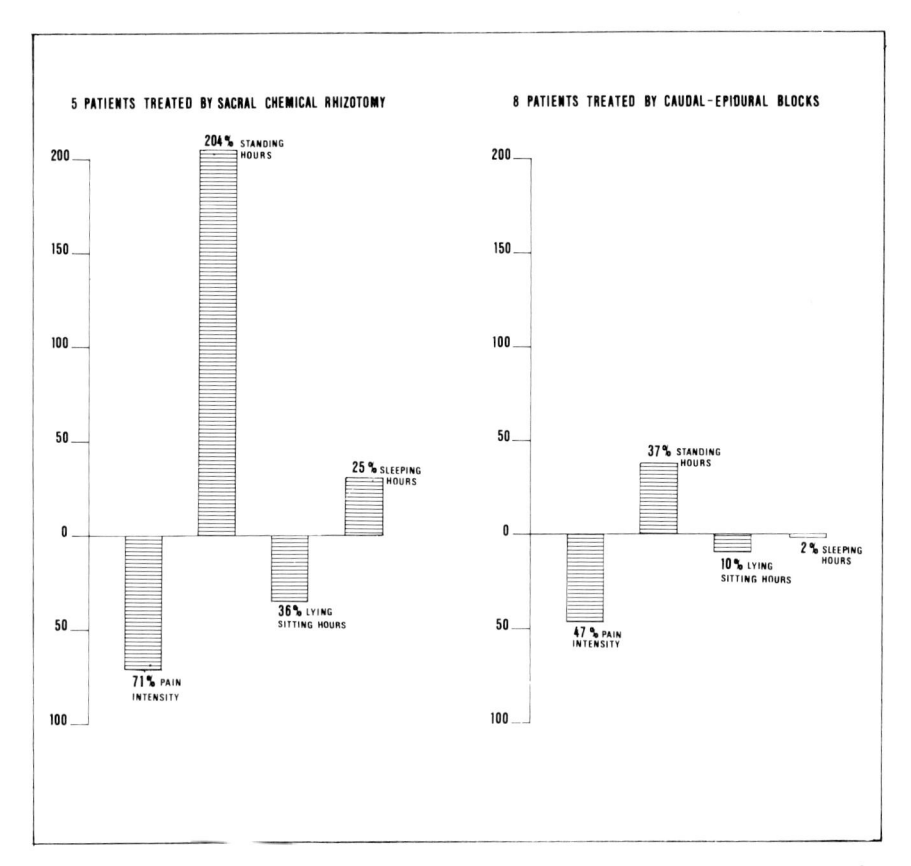

FIG. 3. Percent change of perineal pain intensity and some living activity data after one month on 13 patients affected by cancer of the rectum.

Problems concerning rectal dysfunction did not develop in our patients because 79% of them had a colostomy. Impotence, with loss of penile erection has also been reported after treatment in advanced cases (10). Bladder complications, such as incontinence or, more frequently, retention, are rather common, because among the roots affected by the chemical lesion are S_2-S_3-S_4, which contribute to the nervi erigentes and pudendal nerves with consequent relaxation of external and internal sphincters of the bladder. This kind of complication may be partially avoided when the pain is unilateral and the neurolytic block is performed with the patient lying on the painful side.

Of the group treated with chemical rhizotomy, 19 (49%) patients developed difficulties with micturition. A bladder rehabilitation, preceded by urodynamic tests, is important in such cases. Bladder retention, which often occurs, can be cured by inserting a urethral catheter right after the procedure. A few days later, the catheter is removed and the patient is encouraged to urinate at regular intervals by using manual suprapubic compression and by giving subcutaneous injections of 5 mg of urocoline for the first 5 days and the same dose orally for the following week.

CONCLUSIONS

Our experience and that of other writers (7,8,10,11,13) suggest that subarachnoid phenol block at level L_5-S_1 is useful, simple, and a very efficacious method in relieving perineal neoplastic pain. The best results are obtained in patients having tumors which involve peripheral nerve fibers. We noted the longest pain-relief in patients with trigger points, or perineal skin and mucous erosion, or necrosis due to neoplastic process or radiation therapy (tenesmus and burning sensation were partially relieved). Bladder dysfunction, the most common complication of neurolytic blocks, may be controlled by prompt rehabilitation.

Follow-up of patients must be performed at least monthly, and blocks must be repeated immediately as the pain develops in adjacent areas. In such instances, before undertaking cordotomy or an enlarged chemical rhizotomy, a scintigraphic study is useful to ascertain if there are further involved areas to treat with radiation therapy.

Pain control may be achieved for a significant period of time and in some patients it lasts until death. For those patients having perineal pain due to side effect of local radiation or surgical scar by Miles operation, the repeated caudal epidural anesthetic block is a practical tool free of complications in order to get a good and sometimes prolonged analgesia.

Our experiences lead us to conclude that pain-relief obtained by neurolytic block in perineal cancer pain improves the daily living activity of the patient and therefore, even for a short period, the quality of his life.

REFERENCES

1. Breivik, H., Hesla, P. E., Molnar, I., and Lind, B. (1976): Treatment of chronic low back pain and sciatica: Comparison of caudal epidural injections of bupivacaine and methyl prednisolone with bupivacaine followed by saline. In: *Advances in Pain Research and Therapy, Vol. 1, Proceedings of the First World Congress on Pain,* edited by J. J. Bonica and D. Albe-Fessard, pp. 927–932. Raven Press, New York.
2. Ciocatto, E. (1964): The management of pain. In: *International Anaesthesiology Clinics, Vol. 2.* Little, Brown, Boston.
3. Dogliotti, A. M., and Ciocatto, E. (1955): Method of differential block in pain relief. *Anesthesiology,* 16:623–626.
4. Defalque, R. J. (1974): Treatment of chronic pain with bupivacaine epidural block. *Anesth. Analg.,* 53:841–843.
5. Hannington-Kiff, J. G. (1971): Treatment of intractable pain by bupivacaine nerve block. *Lancet,* 2:1392–1394.
6. Hathaway, S. R., and McKinley, J. C. (1967): *Minnesota Multiphasic Personality Inventory: Manual for Administration and Scoring.* Psychological Corporation, New York.
7. Kuhner, A., and Assmus, H. (1975): Intrathecal application of phenol in the treat-

ment of intractable pain. In: *Brain Hypoxia-Pain: Advances in Neurosurgery, Vol. 2,* pp. 256–263. Springer-Verlag, Berlin, Heidelberg, New York.
8. Lifshitz, S., Debacker, L. J., Buchsbaum, H. J. (1976): Subarachnoid phenol block for pain relief in gynecologic malignancy. *Obstet. Gynecol. (N.Y.),* 48:316–320.
9. Maher, R. M. (1966): Phenol for pain and spasticity. In: *Pain—Henry Ford Hospital International Symposium,* edited by R. S. Knighton and P. R. Dumke. Little, Brown, Boston.
10. Mehta, M. (1973): *Intractable Pain.* W. B. Saunders Company, Ltd., London, Philadelphia, Toronto.
11. Papo, I., and Visca, A. (1974): Phenol rhizotomy in the treatment of cancer pain. *Anesth. Analg.,* 53:993–997.
12. Scott, J., and Huskisson, E. C. (1976): Graphic representation of pain. *Pain,* 2:175–184.
13. Stovner, J., and Endresen, R. (1972): Intrathecal phenol for cancer pain. *Acta Anesth. Scand.,* 16:17–21.
14. Swerdlow, M., and Sayle Creer, W. (1970): A study of extradural medication in the relief of the lumbosciatic syndrome. *Anaesthesia,* 25:341–345.

Role of Neurosurgery in Visceral and Perineal Pain

John D. Loeser

Department of Neurological Surgery, University of Washington, Seattle, Washington 98195

Neoplasms of the abdominal and pelvic viscera are not uncommon causes of chronic pain, although the actual incidence of pain associated with individual neoplasms is hard to determine. Those tumors which are locally invasive seem to be the more customary producers of visceral and perineal pain. It is also difficult to determine what percentage of cancer patients will endure chronic pain in the perineal or abdominal regions. Not only does the malignancy itself have the potential for causing pain, but the aftereffects of surgery and radiation therapy can also lead to chronic pain.

It may be very difficult in a particular patient to ascertain what the contribution of any one of these three may be to the patient's pain problem. We must also be aware of the possibility that a patient's complaint of pain may also be due to depression, fear, or feelings of isolation. While surgical measures are likely to alleviate pain due to noxious stimulation, cutting nerves is not a good way to relieve depression or fear. Careful patient-selection is clearly the single most important factor. Although much has been written on this topic, predictors of surgical outcome are still not well-established.

In general, the cancer patient is more likely to be relieved of pain by a surgical procedure than is a patient with chronic pain due to a nonmalignant disease process. It is ironic, then, that surgical relief of pain is often deferred far too long in the cancer patient and utilized far too quickly in the patient with a nonmalignant disease. The presence of narcotic addiction should not be a factor in determining who is offered neurosurgical relief of pain: If the operation is successful, it is not difficult to withdraw the patient from narcotics (8).

NEURECTOMY

A logical place to begin my discussion of neurosurgical therapy for visceral and perineal pain is in the periphery. Although neurectomies would appear to be a rational approach to discrete pain, they are rarely successful. The propensity of the neoplastic process to spread beyond the denervated zone is one reason not to consider peripheral neurectomy. To reach the involved nerve it may be necessary to operate through a previously irradiated field or traverse the neoplasm itself. In addition, visceral pain is notoriously diffuse. I can see almost no role for peripheral neurectomy in cancer pain.

DORSAL RHIZOTOMY

Pelvic and perineal pain may be alleviated by the appropriate dorsal rhizotomies (2,4,11,16,17,20,23,25,28,30). Midline pain requires bilateral rhizotomies; unilateral pain is often well-controlled by this procedure. The major problem with sacral dorsal rhizotomies for pelvic and perineal pain is the impairment of urinary and anal sphincters which follows extensive sacral denervation. Unilateral rhizotomies are usually well tolerated; bilateral rhizotomies will cause loss of voluntary control of bowel and bladder. This restricts bilateral sacral rhizotomies to patients who have already had a colostomy and a urinary diversionary procedure or a catheter (4).

Bilateral sacral rhizotomies are most easily performed via a midline incision from L_4 to S_2, a laminectomy of L_5, S_1, and S_2 and exposure of the dura at its caudal termination. The dura is opened and the roots identified by both morphology and the response to stimulation. All of the roots caudal to S_1 may be divided without compromising leg function. Unilateral rhizotomies may be done through the same incision or may be performed extradurally by exposing the roots through the sacral foramina. This procedure may also be accomplished with a radiofrequency probe passed percutaneously; reliable data on the efficacy of this method is not available.

If the pain involves segments higher than S_2, dorsal rhizotomy is likely to lead to significant difficulty with lower-extremity function. Although a single root of the lumbosacral plexus may be divided with impunity, one cannot totally denervate the extremity without causing paralysis and loss of protective reflexes. To the extent, therefore, that the pain involves the lumbar roots, dorsal rhizotomy is usually not a satisfactory mode of therapy. Since the origin of the pain is usually neoplastic involvement of nerves or viscera, the operative field for sacral rhizotomy is usually free of tumor. When the neoplasm has invaded the sacrum, dorsal rhizotomy is probably not a wise surgical choice.

The surgeon must be cognizant of the fact that pelvic and abdominal visceral pain may be transmitted via the autonomic nervous system and may not be relieved by sacral rhizotomy. Preoperative assessment with appropriate nerve blocks will indicate the sites of origin of the pain and the role of the autonomic and somatic afferent systems. Nerve blocks do not seem to be a reliable predictor of the long-term efficacy of a surgical procedure, however. Data on the efficacy of dorsal rhizotomy for visceral and perineal pain due to cancer are contained in Table 1.

TABLE 1. *Dorsal rhizotomy for visceral and perineal pain*

Author	Year	No.	% Success[b]
Barrash & Leavens (2)[a]	1973	71	70
Bohm & Franksson (3)	1958	7	100
Crue et al. (4)	1970	18	72
Loeser (11)[a]	1972	7	43
Onofrio & Campa (15)	1972	18	28
Paillas (17)[a]	1972	6	0
Ray (20)[a]	1943	?	?
Scoville (23)[a]	1966	2	100
Sindou et al. (25)	1974	12	75
White & Sweet (30)[a]	1969	35	58

[a] All patients had malignancies, percentage success for pain in this site uncertain.
[b] Pain-relief for 3 months or longer or until death if survival less than 3 months.

CORDOTOMY

Cordotomy is a particularly effective surgical therapy for visceral and perineal pain (5,7,10,12,15,19,21,23,28,29). There are many methods of sectioning the anterolateral quadrant of the spinal cord; common operative sites are upper thoracic and upper cervical. When the pain is midline, bilateral cordotomies will be required. Frequently, the patient reports unilateral pain; but, after a cordotomy, pain is found to be present on the other side as well. This is probably due to masking of a minor pain by a more severe one. When the major pain is relieved, the minor one becomes recognized.

A cordotomy will markedly reduce pain and temperature sensation on the contralateral side of the body. There is no nerve block which simulates this lesion, so preoperative testing of efficacy cannot be carried out. Unilateral cordotomies carry a low risk of bladder dysfunction; bilateral cordotomies will impair male sexual function and bladder control in either sex in about 10% of the patients. Leg weakness should be an uncommon complication. One of the major drawbacks of cordotomy is that the sensory loss and pain-relief may disappear months or years after the original operation. Repeat cordotomy is rarely effective. Of course, the short life-expectancy of most patients with pain due to cancer tends to reduce the likelihood of late cordotomy failure. Since the operation is performed in the cervical or thoracic regions, it is well removed from the neoplasm and radiation effect; wound healing is less likely to be compromised. Cordotomy is frequently the operation of choice for patients with visceral and perineal pain due to cancer (Table 2).

One of the most significant advances in the surgical management of pain due to cancer was the development of percutaneous techniques for cordotomy (10,15,21). These have made it possible to offer cordotomy to any

TABLE 2. Anterolateral cordotomy for visceral and perineal pain

Author	Year	Number	Type	Site	Mortality	Success[b]	Complications
Diemath et al. (5)	1961	50	O	C,T	8	82	~20
Frankel & Prokop (6)	1961	59	O	T	11	67	~20
French et al.	1966	103	O	C	0	96	~25
Lin et al. (10)[a]	1966	39	P	C	0	74	~5
Nathan (12)	1963	77	O	C,T	0?	77	~15
Nolan & Peyton (13)	1956	40	O	C,T	2.5	75	~10
Onofrio (16)[a]	1970	41	P	C	2	85	~5
Raskind (19)	1969	190	O	C,T	3	92	~15
Rosomoff (21)[a]	1974	1279	P	C	?	84	~5
Schwartz (22)	1960	73	O	C	12	70	~20
Simionescu (24)	1957	62	O	T	?	74	?
White & Sweet (29)[a]	1969a	271	O	T	8	77	~10
(29)[a]	1969b	28	O	C	?	75	~10

[a] Number of patients with visceral and perineal pain uncertain, all patients had cancer.
[b] Pain-relief for 3 months or longer or until death if survival is less than 3 months.

patient, regardless of cachexia or debilitation. A needle is placed in the cervical spinal cord under X-ray control, and its position verified by the responses to electrical stimulation; a lesion is made using radiofrequency current. Surgeons who utilize percutaneous cordotomy regularly have reported excellent relief of pain and few complications. The procedure is deceptively simple, and the inexperienced operator will have a significantly lower success rate and more complications.

Each neurosurgeon has his preferred site and method for performing a cordotomy. There seems to be no published evidence that one form of this operation is more likely to succeed than another or that one technique has fewer complications.

MYELOTOMY

Midline myelotomy is another surgical procedure that can be performed either open or percutaneously; a limited number of patients have been re-

TABLE 3. Commissural myelotomy for visceral and perineal pain

Author	Year	Number	Type[a]	Site[b]	Mortality	% Success[c]
Armour (1)	1927	1	O	TL	100	
Hitchcock (9)	1970	2	P	C	0	100
Papo & Luongo (18)	1976	4	O	C	0	25
Sourek (26)	1969	19	O	TL	0	100
Wertheimer (27)	1953	93	O	TL	7	65

[a] O = open; P = percutaneous.
[b] C = cervical; TL = thoracolumbar.
[c] Pain-relief for 3 months or longer or until death if survival is less than 3 months.

ported but pain-relief can be excellent. Most neurosurgeons have little experience with myelotomy, although this operation seems to be gaining popularity. It is designed to interrupt a multisynaptic, diffusely projecting system that is distinct from the spinothalamic pathways transected during a cordotomy (9,18,26,27). This can be accomplished in the thoracolumbar region on a segmental basis or in the high cervical region where more diffuse pain loss will ensue (9). Myelotomy seems to have a low complication rate and deserves further trial in patients with pain due to cancer. The available data on myelotomy are contained in Table 3.

SYMPATHECTOMY

Sympathectomy can effectively relieve pain originating in thoracic and abdominal viscera (28). Nerve blocks are most helpful in delineating the exact structures involved in the transmission of noxious stimuli; neurolytic blocks are often superior to surgical resection. Splanchnectomy or ganglionectomy may be required to denervate the involved viscus. The vagus nerve may also carry afferents from the upper abdominal viscera (14). When a malignancy spreads from a viscus and involves parietal peritoneum or body wall, sympathectomy alone will not effectively relieve the pain. For this reason, cordotomy is usually superior to either dorsal rhizotomy or sympathectomy when visceral or perineal pain is due to cancer. No one procedure seems clearly superior. Meaningful contrasts between these operations are difficult because of unknown factors in patient-selection and differing criteria for pain-relief.

HYPOPHYSECTOMY

A few unfortunate patients with cancer have pain syndromes which are not amenable to any local denervating procedures. When prostatic carcinoma metastasizes widely to bone, for example, no local operation is likely to provide significant relief. Some of these neoplasms are responsive to hypophysectomy; both rate of tumor growth and pain are favorably altered (West, *this volume*). Of course, replacement hormone therapy is required. Nonetheless, excellent palliation can be obtained with some endocrine-sensitive neoplasms. The methods of destroying the pituitary gland are many; once again the surgeon's choice seems to be the relevant variable.

BRAIN OPERATIONS

Other patients with uncontrolled visceral and perineal pain may be candidates for *thalamotomy*. This stereotaxic procedure can effectively eliminate pain; unfortunately, the beneficial effects rarely last more than 1 year. A cancer patient with such a short life-expectancy might be a candidate for this operation, however. *Cingulumotomy* or selective mesial frontal lobotomy also has a place in the management of cancer pain. This operation markedly reduces the affective response to noxious stimulation without producing much change in actual sensory thresholds. It seems to be particularly valuable in the patient who is depressed and anxious as well as in pain. It is unfortunate that the furor about psychosurgery has limited so severely the availability of cingulumotomy for the small number of patients who have no other reasonable method of obtaining pain relief.

SUMMARY

Visceral and perineal pains due to cancer are often not well managed. Neurosurgical therapy is often delayed until after trials of chemotherapy, local surgery, and radiotherapy, all of which may be known to be of little value in the management of a particular neoplasm. Patients are placed on debilitating medications to control pain, because their physicians are unaware of the chronic effects of the drugs and the potential advantages of neurosurgical therapy. When survival for more than 3 months seems likely, pharmacotherapy is unlikely to be the optimal treatment modality. Prompt neurosurgical intervention can offer the patient complete relief of pain without the mind-clogging effects of narcotics. When survival is likely to be less than 3 months, percutaneous surgical or neurolytic techniques are usually superior. If survival is likely to be less than 1 month, pharmacotherapy is usually appropriate. Each patient's disease, personality, and environment must be carefully considered to plan optimal therapy.

REFERENCES

1. Armour, D. (1927): Lettsomian lecture on the surgery of the spinal cord and its membranes. *Lancet,* 1:691–697.
2. Barrash, J. M., and Leavens, M. E. (1973): Dorsal rhizotomy for the relief of intractable pain of malignant tumor origin. *J. Neurosurg.,* 38:755–757.
3. Bohm, E., and Franksson, C. (1958): Coccygodynia and sacral rhizotomy. *Acta Chir. Scand.,* 116:268–274.
4. Crue, B. L., Jr., Todd, E. M., Wright, G. H., and Maline, D. B. (1970): Sacral rhizotomy for pelvic pain. In: *Pain and Suffering,* edited by B. L. Crue, pp. 20–34. Charles C Thomas, Springfield, Ill.
5. Diemath, H. E., Heppner, F., and Walker, A. E. (1961): Anterolateral cordotomy for relief of pain. *Postgrad. Med.,* 29:485–495.
6. Frankel, S. A., and Prokop, J. D. (1961): Value of cordotomy for the relief of pain. *NEJM,* 264:971–974.
7. French, L. A., Chou, S. N., and Story, J. L. (1966): Cervical tractotomy: Technique and clinical usefulness. In: *Henry Ford Hospital International Symposium,* edited by R. Knighton, pp. 311–319. Charles C Thomas, Springfield, Ill.
8. Hall, T. C. (1970): Philosophy of pain control in cancer patients. *Postgrad. Med.,* 48:223–227.
9. Hitchcock, E. R. (1970): Stereotactic cervical myelotomy. *J. Neurol. Neurosurg. Psychiat.,* 33:224–230.
10. Lin, P. M., Gildenberg, P. L., and Polakoff, P. P. (1966): An anterior approach to percutaneous lower cervical cordotomy. *J. Neurosurg.,* 25:553–560.
11. Loeser, J. D. (1972): Dorsal rhizotomy for the relief of chronic pain. *J. Neurosurg.,* 36:745–750.
12. Nathan, P. W. (1963): Results of antero-lateral cordotomy for pain in cancer. *J. Neurol. Neurosurg. Psychiat.,* 26:353–362.
13. Nolan, Robert K., and Peyton, William T. (1956): Cordotomy for relief of pain in incurable squamous-cell carcinoma of the cervix uteri. *Am. J. Obstet. Gynecol.,* 71:790–792.
14. Oi, M., and Kobayashi, K. (1963): Vagotomy as a surgical procedure for relief of pain. *Am. J. Surg.,* 106:49–56.
15. Onofrio, B. M. (1970): Recent results with percutaneous cordotomy. *Mayo Clin. Proc.,* 45:689–694.
16. Onofrio, B., and Campa, H. K. (1972): Evaluation of rhizotomy. Review of 12 years' experience. *J. Neurosurg.,* 36:751–755.
17. Paillas, J. W., and Pellet, W. (1972): Dorsal nerve root section in the treatment of refractory peripheral pain. In: *Pain,* edited by R. Janzen et al., pp. 209–213. William & Wilkins, Baltimore.
18. Papo, I., and Luongo, A. (1976): High cervical commissural myelotomy in the treatment of pain. *J. Neurol. Neurosurg. Psychiat.,* 39:705–710.
19. Raskind, R. (1969): Analytical review of open cordotomy. *Int. Surg.,* 51:226–231.
20. Ray, B. S. (1943): The management of intractable pain by posterior rhizotomy. *Res. Publ. Assoc. Res. Nerv. Ment. Dis.,* 23:391–407.

21. Rosomoff, H. L. (1974): Percutaneous radiofrequency cervical cordotomy for intractable pain. *Adv. Neurol.*, 4:683–688.
22. Schwartz, H. G. (1960): High cervical cordotomy—technique and results. *Clin. Neurosurg.*, 8:282–293.
23. Scoville, W. B. (1966): Extradural spinal sensory rhizotomy. *J. Neurosurg.*, 25:94–95.
24. Simionescu, M. D. (1957): The management of pain due to pelvic malignancy: A follow-up of 122 cases. *Zlb. Neurochir.*, 17:284–287.
25. Sindou, M., Fischer, G., and Mansuy, L. (1976): Posterior spinal rhizotomy and selective posterior rhizidiotomy. *Prog. Neurol. Surg.*, 7:201–250.
26. Sourek, K. (1969): Commissural myelotomy. *J. Neurosurg.*, 31:524–527.
27. Wertheimer, P., and Lecuire, J. (1953): La myelotomie commissurale postérieure. *Acta Chir. Belg.*, 52:568–574.
28. White, J. C. (1968): Operations for the relief of pain in the torso and extremities: Evaluation of their effectiveness over long periods. In: *Pain,* edited by A. Souilairac et al., pp. 503–519. Academic Press, London.
29. White, J. C., and Sweet, W. H. (1969): *Pain and the Neurosurgeon,* pp. 678–767. Charles C Thomas, Springfield, Ill.
30. White, J. C., and Sweet, W. H. (1969): *Pain and the Neurosurgeon,* pp. 633–660. Charles C Thomas, Springfield, Ill.

Discussion

Part II. Management of Pain of Advanced Cancer: Viscereal and Perineal Pain

L. Gennari and J. Loeser (Moderators)

Frova (Milano): Dr. Houde, what do you think about drug treatment for visceral pain in children?

Houde (New York): At our Institution we apply the same rules to children that we do to adults. If they have pain that can be controlled with simple analgesics, those are the drugs that we employ. If they require more potent drugs, we go to more potent drugs, generally in combination with the simple analgesics, and more often than not by administering them by oral route. Our biggest problem, I think, in dealing with children is that doses have to be adjusted to their body size. Our biggest problem actually is in teenagers because they seem to be under the greatest psychological turmoil having pain and cancer. They tend to be the patients in whom we use the largest amounts of drugs including narcotics.

When we use narcotics and tranquilizers or the anxiolitic drugs, we frequently run into complications, and I think that we have generally found that the narcotics are actually good tranquilizers in themselves. Most people who misuse narcotics are those who try to combine them with other drugs.

Madrid (Madrid): Dr. Moore, could you describe your technique for spinal cord transection with absolute alcohol?

Moore (Seattle): The patient is placed in the jackknife position, the level of the injection is the second lumbar interspace, the level of the neurolysis is from the second lumbar interspace caudad, and the complications are those that you would expect; the block is not done unless the patient is incontinent of feces and urine and also has an involvement of the somatic nerves of the lower extremity with severe pain. It is a final and drastic procedure that is used to relieve pain.

Nicosia (Catania): Dr. Ventafridda, is the continuous epidural still an indication in pain treatment? Has anybody experienced a long-lasting continuous epidural by chronic infusion?

Ventafridda (Milano): The continuous epidural, the introduction of a foreign body for a long time, always gives a patient affected by a tumor some complications. The pain gets worse and is long-lasting. For this reason, we no longer use this technique. We have seen major cases of infection, and there is not anything worse than aggravating the condition of these patients.

Rampulla (Urbino): Dr. Moore, do you have experience of transsacral neurolysis with phenol in water? If you do, what are your impressions?

Moore: We have done a few cases of transsacral block. I assume that this is a question regarding the injection of the third sacral nerve at the foramina. They are, in our experience, not too effective. Furthermore, one cannot be selective in doing so, and, therefore, you may expect bladder, rectal and, to some extent, lower extremity involvement. So we have not used any technique of this nature in treating these patients.

Overview of Analgesia

Robert G. Twycross

The Churchill Hospital, Headington, Oxford OX3 9EJ, England

A recent report has emphasized that many patients dying of cancer do so only after weeks or months of uncontrolled pain. Parkes (7) compared hospital-centered and home-centered terminal care by means of post-bereavement visits to the surviving spouse, and found that about 20% of the hospital patients died with their severe and mostly continuous pain unrelieved. A similar percentage of patients experienced pain of comparable intensity before admission to the hospital, which suggests that the hospital stay did not lead to improved relief. Of those who died at home, 10% had severe pain pre-terminally, but terminally the proportion rose to almost half. In contrast, following admission to St. Christopher's Hospice—a unit specializing in symptom control in far-advanced cancer—the percentage of patients with severe pain fell from 36% to 8%.

In the home-based patients, the main reason for poor pain control appeared to be a failure on the part of the general practitioner to ensure that regular doses of an appropriate analgesic were given in sufficient quantity to alleviate the pain. One man of 54 became totally demoralized and for several months spent much of the time crying. He was so frightened that he clung to his wife and became "hysterical" whenever she left the room. He received an injection each *week* and was not able to go into hospital as there was no bed available. Similar accounts given by other respondents suggested that neurotic exaggeration was not the explanation. Several patients put up with their pain without complaint on the supposition that nothing could be done to relieve it or that their chances of recovery would be enhanced if they refrained from taking powerful analgesics.

The medical profession has a lot to learn before it can confidently assure patients that severe pain in advanced cancer can be controlled. Reasons for inadequate relief are many, but more fundamental than the incorrect use of analgesics is the tendency for a doctor to cease to be systematic when confronted with a dying patient. Instead of carefully analysing the cause(s) of the patient's pain(s), the doctor prescribes a fixed dose of a standard preparation or, worse, underrates the intensity of a patient's discomfort and does nothing.

ASSESSMENT OF THE PAIN

Pain may be limited to one site or be multifocal. Each site where pain is felt should be recorded. The use of a body image to record the site(s) of pain is a great help. It acts as a base line for future reference, facilitates patient management in situations where several doctors are involved, and helps in the consideration of underlying mechanisms (Fig. 1). Descriptions of pain being "like raving toothache" and "stabbing, especially when I move" point to nerve compression and influence the course of treatment should analgesics alone fail to relieve (Table 1). A diagnosis of cancer does not, however, mean that the malignant process is necessarily the cause of the pain. As in other areas of medicine, diagnosis must precede treatment. Bedsores, constipation, peptic ulcer, cystitis, or musculoskeletal disorders may prove to be the cause, and are all conditions that benefit from specific treatment.

Intensity of pain is assessed not only by the patient's description but also

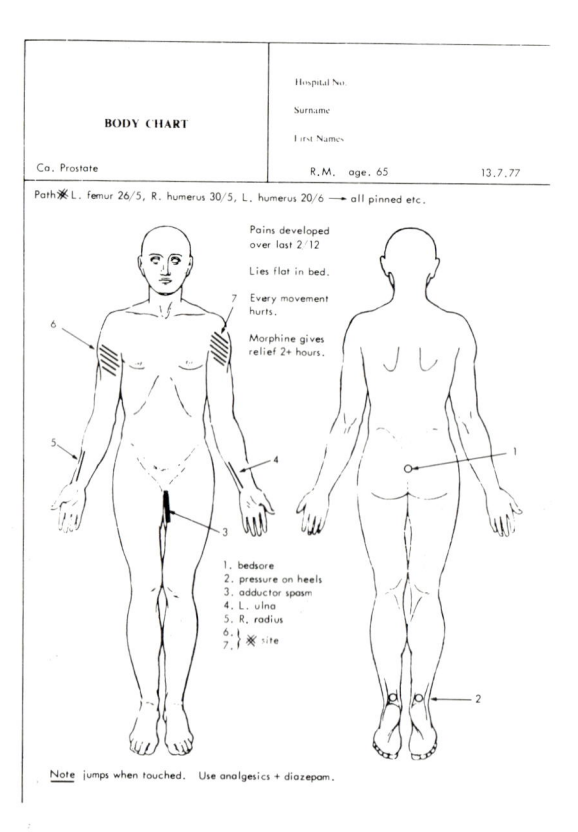

FIG. 1. Pain chart of 65-year-old male with carcinoma of prostate. Adductor spasm is usually protective, i.e., secondary to involvement of the pubis; treatment is as for bone pain, though sometimes diazepam may be necessary.

TABLE 1. *Treatment of pain in advanced cancer*

Mechanism	Analgesic adjuvants	Co-analgesic	Nondrug treatment	Other measures
Soft-tissue infiltration	aspirin (mild) — codeine (moderate) — morphine (severe)	Aspirin	Radiotherapy	diversion — heat — massage
Bone involvement				
Nerve compression		Prednisolone	Nerve block	
Raised cerebral pressure		Dexamethasone		
Lymphedema		Diuretic	Compression sleeve	modification of lifestyle
Abdominal visceral epigastric	? antiemetic ? anxiolytic ? laxative		Celiac axis ganglion block (Presacral block)[a]	
hypogastric				
Ulceration—infection		antibiotic		
Constipation	Specific treatment			
Second pathology				

[a] The use of nerve blocks for lower abdominal pain is limited by probability of causing urinary retention.

TABLE 2. *Factors affecting pain threshold*

	Threshold lowered		Threshold raised
Discomfort		Relief of symptoms	
Insomnia		Sleep	
Fatigue		Rest	
Anxiety		Sympathy	
Fear		Understanding	
Anger		Diversion	
Sadness		Elevation of mood	
Depression			
Mental isolation		Analgesics	
Introversion		Tranquillizers	
(Past experience)		Antidepressives	

by discovering what drugs have failed to relieve, whether sleep is disturbed, and in what way activity is limited ("How long is it since you went out?", "What are you doing around the house?", etc.) In addition, the patient's spouse should be interviewed; generally speaking, one finds that the patient has made light of his suffering. A patient may be in severe pain without looking distressed. With an obviously distressed patient who says or implies, "It's all pain, doctor," detailed assessment is impossible. In this situation the pain is compounded by anxiety and fear, and the patient should be reviewed after an initial injection of diazepam and diamorphine or morphine. The dose will depend on the patient's previous medication and general condition, but 10 mg of each is usually not excessive in a young or middle-aged patient. In some patients, pain is minimal at rest but intolerable on movement.

A 4-year-old child with an inoperable pontine glioma experienced increasing pain in the head and occipital region. She lay flat all the time because elevation of the head caused a marked increase in pain. With this history it was necessary to postulate a local source of pain (possibly caused by postradiation meningeal adhesions) in addition to the diffuse headache of secondary hydrocephalus (which would have been helped by a more erect posture). The diffuse pain was relieved by small, regular doses of morphine, but not until she was transferred from a King's Fund to an Ellison bed (which elevates head, neck, and trunk in unison) was it possible for the child to sit up without pain. Subsequently, it became possible to transfer the child from bed to a high-backed reclining chair and, eventually, to lift her onto her mother's lap. This suggested that some of the pain had been caused by spasm of the neck muscles, and that the confidence engendered by the ability to sit up in bed allowed additional maneuvres to be undertaken without pain.

The probability of the initial prescription's being inadequate increases with the intensity of pain. Patients should, therefore, be reassessed within hours if the pain is overwhelming, or after 1 or 2 days if severe or moderate. If troublesome or unacceptable side effects result, treatment may need to be modified. In addition, the relief of the major pain may allow a second, less severe pain to become apparent.

An 85-year-old man with carcinoma of the prostate and pain in the right femur caused by a metastasis was treated with aspirin and morphine. Casual questioning the next day indicated that, although it was less severe, he was still in pain. Further questioning revealed that the site of pain was now retrosternal and epigastric; he had no femoral pain at all. The dose of morphine was, therefore, left unaltered, and the prescription of an antacid resulted in complete relief.

PAIN CONTROL

Relief of pain may be achieved by one or more of the following methods: (a) modification of the pathologic process; (b) elevation of the pain threshold; (c) interruption of pain pathways; and (d) immobilization.

Modification of Pathologic Process

Osseous metastasis is the main cause of pain in the majority of patients with carcinoma of the breast, bronchus, or prostate. Bone pain is also common in carcinomata of the kidney and thyroid and in multiple myeloma. Modification of the pathology by radiation, chemotherapy, or hormone treatment should always be considered even in far-advanced cancer, though it is important to ensure that the treatment is not worse than the disease. Moreover, because androgens or estrogens have been prescribed, this does not mean that analgesics should be withheld. A combined approach should be employed. If relief is obtained and there are no complaints of "breakthrough" pain, then the analgesic regimen can be modified—a less potent analgesic prescribed or the treatment withdrawn completely.

Radiation therapy gives partial or even complete relief in 90% of patients experiencing bone pain, and generally may be administered in a single, nonfractionated dose. A recent study showed that, although patients treated by a single dose commonly had more nausea and vomiting, many of those receiving fractionated treatment were exhausted by the end of the course (8). Fractionation is probably necessary only when there is a high risk of nausea and vomiting despite prophylactic anti-emetics, e.g., when irradiating in the region of L_1 and when treating half or more of the pelvis.

Elevation of Pain Threshold

Pain is a dual phenomenon, one part being the perception of the sensation and the other the patient's emotional reaction to it. This means that attention must be paid to nondrug factors that modulate pain threshold, such as anxiety and depression, as well as to the correct use of analgesics and other drugs (Table 2). Most patients fear the process of dying—"Will it hurt?", "Will I suffocate?"—and many fear death itself. Many of these fears remain unspoken unless the patient is given the opportunity to express them. The doctor needs to give time and opportunity for the patient to talk about his progress or lack of it. Tranquilizers have only a limited place in terminal cancer care. Patients who are markedly anxious or agitated usually need a combination of a tranquilizer and an analgesic; so does the patient with overwhelming pain.

Depression not only can, but frequently does, supervene in patients receiving so-called "euphoriant" drugs. The likelihood of this occurring increases the longer a patient is maintained on a narcotic analgesic (14). An antidepressant should be prescribed in these circumstances, starting with half the usual adult dose, as debilitated patients often become confused if a higher dose is given, particularly when other psychoactive drugs are being taken concurrently. Support and companionship are always necessary, particularly in cases where the depression is more properly described as sadness at the thought of leaving behind one's family, one's friends, and all that is familiar.

The use of analgesics is best seen as but one way—generally a powerful way—of elevating the pain threshold, though a failure to allow the patient to express his fears and anxieties can cause otherwise relievable pain to remain intractable.

Use of Analgesics

To allow pain to re-emerge before administering the next dose not only causes unnecessary suffering but encourages tolerance. "Four-hourly as required" or PRN medication has no place in the treatment of persistent pain; whatever its etiology, *continuous pain requires regular preventive therapy*. The aim is to titrate the dose of the analgesic against the patient's pain, *gradually increasing the dose until the patient is pain-free*. The next dose is given before the effect of the previous one has worn off and, therefore, before the patient may think it necessary. In this way it is possible to erase the memory and fear of pain. As patients do not like constantly taking tablets or receiving injections, a 4-hr interval between doses should be regarded as the norm though sometimes more frequent administration may be necessary. Many patients do not require a dose in the middle of the night though, if necessary, a patient should be awakened to take it (or set his alarm) rather than let him wake later complaining of pain.

The effective analgesic dose varies considerably from patient to patient; *the right dose of any analgesic is that which gives adequate relief for at least 3, preferably 4 or more hr*. "Maximum" or "recommended" doses, derived mainly from postoperative parenteral single-dose studies, are not applicable in advanced cancer. For example, the effective dose of *oral* morphine ranges from as little as 5 mg to more than 100 mg every 4 hr. Patients will usually accept two, sometimes three, analgesic tablets per administration, together with additional medication; four or more tablets of the same preparation are not often acceptable. Generally, if two tablets are not adequate, the patient should be transferred to a more potent alternative. Pain unrelieved by other measures, not short life-expectancy, is the primary criterion for prescription of morphine or other narcotic analgesics.

Anti-inflammatory Drugs

The importance of aspirin in the relief of bone pain has recently been reemphasized (13). Many osseous metastases produce or induce the production of a prostaglandin, probably PGE_2, which causes osteolysis (2) and also lowers the "peripheral pain threshold" by sensitizing free nerve endings (3). Aspirin (in high dosage) and other nonsteroidal anti-inflammatory drugs (NSAID) inhibit the synthesis of PGs and by so doing alleviate pain. This suggests that, compared with morphine, NSAID should be relatively more efficacious in bone pain than in pain caused by soft-tissue infiltration. Our experience in Oxford would support such a hypothesis (Fig. 2).

Response to PG inhibitors is, however, variable; a fact which can be explained if certain cancer-cell types synthesize osteolytic agents other than or in addition to PGE_2. It has been shown, for example, in patients with hypercalcemia in association with multiple myeloma or a reticulosis, that the urinary excretion of PG metabolites is normal and that bone resorption appears to be due to secretion of "osteoclast activating factor" by tumor cells (6). Other candidates include ectopic parathyroid hormone and active vitamin-D metabolites or related sterols.

Despite the variable response, it should now be regarded as a general rule that aspirin and other potent NSAID should be used either alone or in combination with a narcotic analgesic when seeking to relieve bone pain by pharmacologic means (13). Aspirin in a dose of between 3 and 6 g a day has much to commend it and is available in a variety of preparations. Phenylbutazone commonly causes fluid retention and, in the elderly and debilitated, indomethacin is prone to cause or exacerbate neuropsychiatric disturbances. Newer agents such as flurbiprofen and diflunisal appear promising, and it is possible that they may prove useful in patients who fail to respond to aspirin.

Corticosteroids

Corticosteroids prevent the release of PGs by exerting a "stabilizing" effect on cell membranes; they do not inhibit PG synthesis. They do, however, have an impact on elements of the inflammatory process not connected with PGs and commonly stimulate appetite and elevate mood (1). Even so, clinical impression suggests that corticosteroids are not so effective as aspirin in relieving bone pain, though they are probably more effective in alleviating

BODY CHART

Hospital No.
Surname
First Names

Ca. Vagina   O.C. age 69   10.9.77

Several weeks
* Worse on Movement
  eased by DG
3. Produced on palpatation

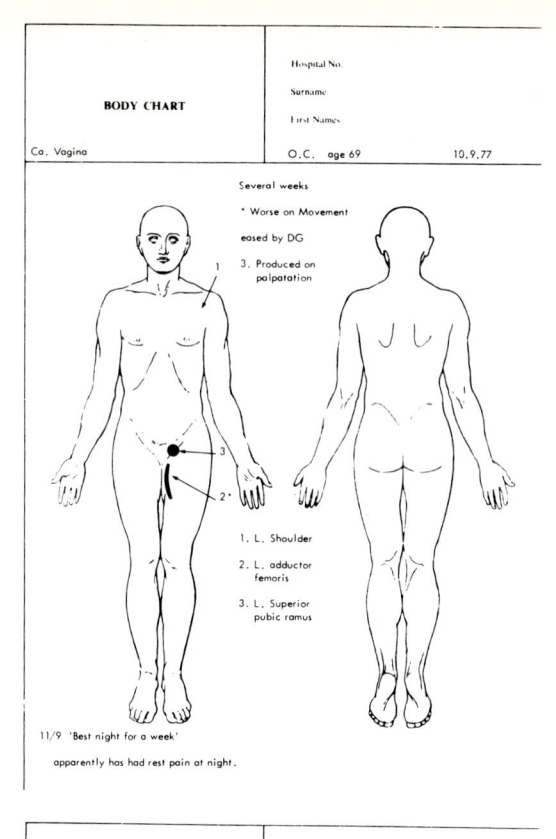

1. L. Shoulder
2. L. adductor femoris
3. L. Superior pubic ramus

11/9 'Best night for a week'
apparently has had rest pain at night.

BODY CHART

Hospital No.
Surname
First Names

Ca. Prostate   G.B. age 81   8.12.76

Path ✳ 6/75 ⟶ Pin & Plate

1. Constant Poor Nights
   Worse on Movement
   Little benefit from fortral 6-8 day.

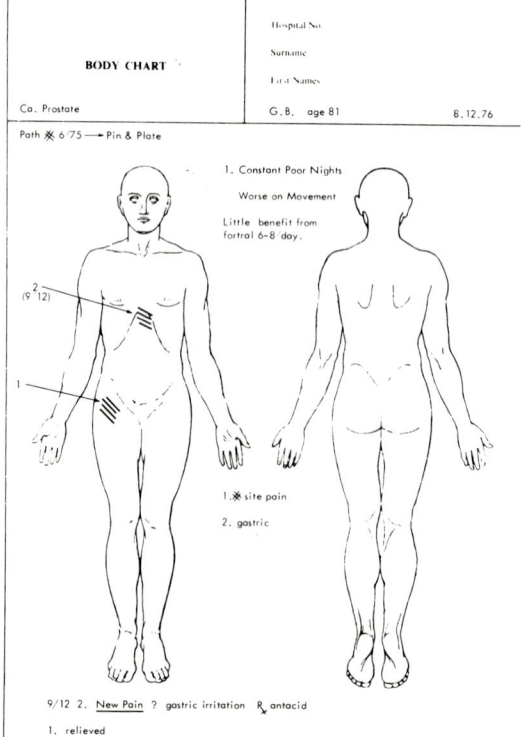

2 (9/12)

1. ✳ site pain
2. gastric

9/12 2. New Pain ? gastric irritation ℞ antacid
      1. relieved

pain associated with extensive soft-tissue infiltration in relatively circumscribed areas, e.g., head and neck cancers or pelvic malignancy and with massive hepatic metastases. Sometimes, particularly with pelvic malignancy, greater relief is obtained by using both aspirin and prednisolone in association with a narcotic analgesic.

The usual starting dose is prednisolone 10 mg t.i.d., reducing to 10 mg b.i.d. or 5 mg t.i.d. after a week. Prednisolone should also be used when pain is caused by nerve compression (*vide infra*). With headache caused by raised intracranial pressure, the more potent dexamethasone is often necessary, together with an analgesic. The usual starting dose is 4 mg t.i.d. reducing, if possible, to 2 mg t.i.d. or less when the headache has been controlled satisfactorily.

Narcotic Analgesics

When the nonnarcotic analgesics (aspirin and paracetamol/acetominophen) fail to relieve, a weak narcotic such as codeine or dihydrocodeine should be prescribed alone or with aspirin or paracetamol. Pentazocine, a partial agonist, has no place in the treatment of cancer pain. By mouth it is not a potent analgesic; 50 mg of pentazocine is less effective than two tablets of aspirin-codeine (Codis®) or of paracetamol-propoxyphene (Distalgesic®) (9). Moreover, the proportion of patients experiencing psychotomimetic side effects is unacceptably high and, although such side effects tend to be dose-related, they have been observed after even small doses by mouth. Similarly, orally administered pethidine/meperidine should not be regarded as a potent analgesic and, by injection, acts only for some 2 to 3 hr.

Papaveretum and dipipanone are useful intermediates between weak narcotics and morphine. Dipipanone is available only with cyclizine as Diconal®, though there is no evidence that it causes more nausea than other narcotics. Alternatively, aspirin and opium (Nepenthe®) may be used; each 1 ml of undiluted Nepenthe® contains about 10 mg of morphine and is usually supplied as a 10% (1 ml in 10) or 20% (2 ml in 10) solution in chloroform water. Precipitation occurs when stronger solutions are dispensed. Dextromoramide (Palfium® 5 and 10 mg) although potent is relatively short-acting; it is, however, useful as "top up" medication for patients who experience occasional exacerbations of pain but whose pain for the most part is well controlled.

The top of the analgesic ladder is not reached simply by prescribing morphine or diamorphine (diacetylmorphine, heroin). Both may be given in

←

FIG. 2. Pain charts of 2 patients with bone pain. Complete relief was obtained using morphine and aspirin. In both morphine was subsequently stopped without a return of pain, though after several weeks it became necessary to represcribe it. Virtually bedfast when admitted, both patients became fully mobile.

a wide range of oral doses, from 5 to 100 mg every 4 hr though, in fact, it is unusual to need more than 30 mg. By mouth, morphine and diamorphine have similar actions and unwanted effects but, owing to more complete absorption, oral diamorphine is about 1½ times more potent than oral morphine (12). Both opiates are commonly dispensed with cocaine in a vehicle containing alcohol and syrup ("The Brompton Cocktail"). Some patients, however, complain about the "sickliness" of such mixtures, while others dislike the alcoholic "bite." Moreover, the benefit of a small, fixed dose of cocaine is probably slight and has, on occasion, caused restlessness and hallucinations in the elderly. It is my practice, despite the recent inclusion of a convenient formulation in the British National Formulary, to dispense morphine in chloroform water alone, the patient adding blackcurrant juice or other flavoring as desired. If dispensed in combination with prochlorperazine or chlorpromazine, the incorporation of one of the flavored proprietary syrups usually circumvents the need for additional flavoring.

When regular injections are required I use diamorphine hydrochloride, available in ampoules as freeze-dried pellets. It is considerably more soluble than morphine sulphate—100 mg will dissolve in 0.2 ml. This means that the volume injected need never be large, an important consideration when repeated injections have to be given to a cachectic patient (Table 3). It should be emphasized that most patients can be maintained on oral medication. The main indication for parenteral administration, apart from the last few hours of life, is intractable nausea and vomiting despite the prescription of antiemetic.

The need for injections may sometimes be avoided by using morphine suppositories. Several strengths are available ranging from 10 to 60 mg Proladone® suppositories, which contain 30 mg of oxycodone pectinate are also available; after administration the oxycodone is slowly released from the pectin core over several hours. Thus one or two suppositories every 6 or 8 hr may be adequate. Fifteen mg of oxycodone is equivalent to 10 mg of morphine. Alternatively, round-the-clock relief may be maintained by using Duromorph®, a microcrystalline suspension of morphine, 2 or 3 times a day. It is available as an intramuscular preparation in capped vials each containing 70.4 mg of morphine base in 1.1 ml (64 mg/ml). The dose will depend on the patient's previous medication. For example, assuming a 1:3 oral to parenteral potency ratio for morphine, 32 mg of Duromorph® (0.5 ml) bd will probably substitute adequately for 30 mg of oral morphine 4-hourly.

Levorphanol (Dromoran® 1.5 mg) and phenazocine (Narphen® 5 mg) should be regarded as alternatives to morphine and diamorphine (Table 4). By mouth on a weight-for-weight basis, both are approximately 4 to 5 times more potent than morphine and have a longer duration of action. Methadone (Physeptone®) may also be useful in these circumstances but, because of its prolonged plasma half-time (15), should be used with care, if at all, in the elderly or extremely debilitated.

TABLE 3. *Injection volume of equi-analgesic doses of diamorphine and morphine*

Preparation	Solubility in water at 25°C (1 g in × ml)	Potency relative to diamorphine	Available ampoules (mg/ml)	Volume of equi-analgesic doses (ml) 30	60	90	120 mg
Diamorphine hydrochloride	1.6	1	(Freeze-dried)	0.1	0.1	0.15	0.2
Morphine sulphate	21	½	15[a]	4	4	12	16
			30[b]	2	4	6	8

[a] Maximum strength available in the United States
[b] Maximum strength available in the United Kingdom

TABLE 4. *Approximate oral analgesic equivalence of potent narcotics*

Analgesic	Tablet	Dose of diamorphine hydrochloride	Dose of morphine sulphate
Dipipanone (Diconal®)	10 mg (+30 mg cyclizine)	3 mg	5 mg
Papaveretum (Omnopon®)	10 mg	3 mg	5 mg
*Levorphanol (Dromoran®)	1.5 mg	5 mg	8 mg
*Phenazocine (Narphen®)	5 mg	15 mg	25 mg
Nepenthe (undiluted)	1 ml	8 mg	12 mg

Note: i. *Dextromoramide* (Palfium®)—single 5-mg dose is equivalent to diamorphine 10 mg/morphine 15 mg in terms of PEAK effect but acts only for 1–2 hr. Useful as an additional "as required" analgesic for intermittent, severe, breakthrough pain.

ii. *Methadone* (Physeptone®)—single 5 mg dose is equivalent to diamorphine 5 mg/morphine 7.5 mg. Has a prolonged plasma half-time, which leads to *accumulation* when given repeatedly. Thus, it is several times more potent when given *regularly.*

iii. *Often satisfactory 6-hourly.

Adjuvant Medication

Most patients with terminal cancer have more than one symptom. Nausea and vomiting are both common and the use of a narcotic analgesic tends to precipitate or exacerbate these symptoms, particularly if the patient is ambulant. Patients prescribed a narcotic analgesic should be questioned about nausea and vomiting and either have an antiemetic (e.g., prochlorperazine; metoclopramide, cyclizine) prescribed simultaneously or the need for one reviewed 2 or 3 days later. Constipation almost always occurs when a narcotic is taken regularly, but generally responds to the *regular* use of an appropriate aperient.

The value of diversional activity should not be forgotten. It ranges from back-rubs to craft work, talking books, access to radio and television, someone to talk to, and dayroom activities. Pain is worse when it occupies the patient's whole attention. Diversional activity does much more than just "pass the time;" it also diminishes the pain.

Narcotic Addiction and Tolerance

Although the term *drug addiction* has been replaced officially by *drug dependence,* unofficially it continues to be used. Drug dependence is currently defined as:

"A state, psychic and sometimes also physical, resulting from the interaction between a living organism and a drug, characterized by behavioural and other responses that always include a compulsion to take the drug on a continuous or periodic basis in order to experience its psychic effects, and sometimes to avoid the discomfort of its absence. Tolerance may or may not be present" (17).

This is a broader definition than that of 1964, which emphasized the need for both tolerance and an early development of physical dependence in addition to strong psychologic dependence (16). The term *drug dependence* now more closely approximates to the popular conception of addiction—a compulsion or overpowering drive to take the drug in order to experience its psychologic effects. Occasionally, a patient is admitted who appears to be addicted, demanding "an injection" every 2 or 3 hr. Typically such a patient has a long history of poor pain control and will for several weeks have been receiving fairly regular (4-hourly as required) but inadequate injections of one or more narcotic analgesics. Given time, it is usually possible to control the pain adequately, prevent clock-watching and demanding behavior, and, sometimes, transfer the patient to an oral preparation. But even here, it cannot be said that the patient is addicted, as he is not demanding the narcotic in order to experience its psychologic effect but to be relieved from pain for at least an hour or two.

Even so, many doctors are reluctant to use narcotic analgesics, particularly diamorphine or morphine, because they assume that tolerance will result in the medication's becoming ineffective. This is understandable as little information has been available concerning the long-term effects of narcotic analgesics when administered regularly to relieve persistent pain. The lack of data resulted in predictions being made on the basis of animal and human volunteer studies. However, in the studies using ex-addicts at the Addiction Research Center in Lexington, the emphasis has been on *inducing* tolerance and physical dependence as rapidly as possible by using maximum tolerated doses rather than administering the drugs in doses and at intervals comparable to a clinical regimen (5). Although such studies have been useful in predicting abuse liability, their relevance to clinical practice is questionable.

To allow predictions to be made on the basis of clinical experience, the notes of 500 patients admitted consecutively to St. Christopher's Hospice were reviewed (10). A total of 218 patients received diamorphine regularly for at least 1 week. By grouping the patients according to survival after commencing diamorphine, it was demonstrated that *the longer the duration of treatment the slower the rate of rise in dose*. In a second review (14), 115 patients who had received diamorphine regularly for at least 12 weeks were selected from approximately 3,000 patients admitted over 7 years. Dose-time charts were prepared. Visual analysis indicated that in many there was an initial phase when the dose was increased several times within 1 or 2 weeks followed by a prolonged phase when the dose was increased less often or not at all (Fig. 3). It was also clearly demonstrated that *the longer a patient survived after prescription of diamorphine, the greater the likelihood of a reduction in dose*.

Dose reductions were made on a trial and error basis in patients who had improved generally over a number of weeks and who had had no recent episodes of "breakthrough" pain. Reductions were also made after successful

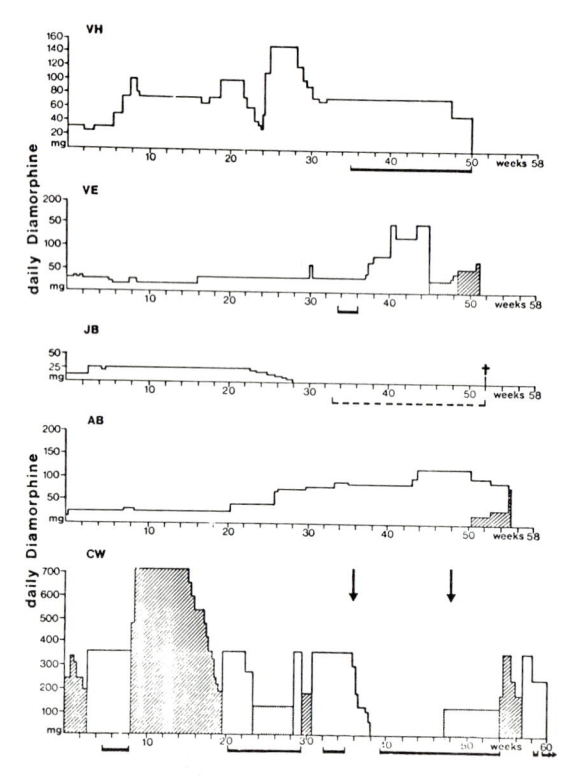

FIG. 3. Dose-time charts of 5 patients with advanced cancer (14). *Open areas,* diamorphine by mouth; *hatched areas,* diamorphine by injection; *dotted areas,* other narcotic analgesic (V. E., C. W.): *arrow,* phenol-in-glycerine nerve block; *horizontal bar,* time spent at home. V. H., V. E., and A. B. received diamorphine up to the time of death; C. W. is still alive.

intrathecal nerve blocks in 5 patients and after treatment with a cytotoxic agent or radiation in a number of others. A total of 9 patients stopped receiving diamorphine; 3 stopped taking diamorphine altogether; 4 patients stopped for more than 4 months; and 2 stopped for approximately 3 weeks.

It was concluded that, when used as part of a pattern of total care, diamorphine may be used for long periods without concern about tolerance. Moreover, although physical dependence probably develops in most patients after several weeks of continuous treatment this does not prevent the downward adjustment of dose when considered clinically feasible. Experience with methadone, levorphanol, and phenazocine suggests that the "natural history" of their long-term use in patients in pain is similar to that of diamorphine and morphine.

Interruption of Pain Pathways

The place of peripheral and intrathecal nerve blocks and neurosurgical procedures has been discussed elsewhere in this volume. It should be noted, however, that analgesics alone are often effective in relieving pain due to nerve compression. If the response is poor, however, the use of prednisolone 5 to 10 mg 3 times a day is recommended. By reducing inflammatory swelling around the growth, the effective tumor mass is reduced and the compression alleviated. In patients with a prognosis of only a few weeks, this may be sufficient to circumvent the need for chemical neurolysis. In those with a longer life-expectancy, the pain may return as the tumor continues to grow; in these a nerve block will be required. In patients whose morale is low or precarious, it is advisable to warn that a block may become necessary, in order to avoid loss of confidence should the pain return.

Modification of Lifestyle

Some patients continue to experience pain on movement despite analgesics, other drugs, radiotherapy, and nerve blocks. In these, the situation may be improved by suggesting commonsense modifications to daily activity. For example, a man may continue to struggle to stand when shaving unless the doctor suggests that sitting would be a good idea. Such a suggestion is accepted more readily if accompanied by a simple explanation of why weight-bearing precipitates or exacerbates the pain. Individually designed plaster or plastic supports for patients with multiple collapsed vertebrae or Thomas splints for femoral pain are occasionally necessary to overcome intolerable pain on movement in bedfast patients.

Internal fixation or the insertion of a prosthesis should be considered if a pathological fracture of a long-bone occurs, as these measures obviate the need for prolonged bed rest and pain is usually relieved. The decision whether or not to treat surgically depends on the patient's general condition; but, whereas in bronchial carcinoma or malignant melanoma pathological fracture often presages death, in breast cancer this is not generally so, particularly if the tumor is hormone-sensitive. The median survival after the first or only pathological fracture associated with breast cancer is about 6 months ranging from 2 months to 4 years (11).

EXPECTATIONS

A recent survey of patients with persistent pain suggested that patients' expectations in relation to relief are lower than they need be (4). However, whereas relief is obtained within 2 or 3 days in some patients, in others, particularly those whose pain is made worse by movement and in the very anxious and depressed, it may take 3 to 4 weeks of inpatient treatment to achieve satisfactory control. Even so, it should be possible to achieve some improvement within 24 to 48 hr in all patients. Although the ultimate aim is complete freedom from pain, we will be less disappointed but, paradoxically, more successful if in practice we aim at "graded relief." Further, as some pains respond more readily than others, improvement should be assessed in relation to each pain. The initial target should be a pain-free, sleep-full night. Many patients have not had a good night's rest for weeks or months and are exhausted and demoralized. To sleep through the night pain-free and wake refreshed is a boost to both the doctor's and the patient's morale. Next, one aims for relief at rest in bed or chair during the day; finally, for freedom from pain on movement. The former is always eventually possible; the latter is not. However, the encouragement that relief at night and when resting during the day brings, gives the patient new hope and incentive and enables him to begin to live again despite limited mobility. Freed from the day- and nightmare of constant pain, his last weeks or months take on a new look.

The doctor must be determined to succeed and be prepared to spend much time assessing and reassessing the patient's pain and other symptoms. Decisive action is needed to avoid the situation reported recently of a 90-year-old man, admitted to a London teaching hospital with bone pain, who died still in pain 3 months later (4). With cancer one is dealing with a progressive pathological process. This means that new pains may develop or old pains re-emerge. It should not be assumed that a fresh complaint of pain merely calls for an increase in a previously satisfactory analgesic regimen; it demands reassessment, an explanation to the patient and, only then, modification of drug therapy or other intervention.

ACKNOWLEDGMENTS

Tables 1 and 4 and Figs. 1 and 2 are reproduced by permission of Pitman Medical, Tunbridge Wells, England.

REFERENCES

1. Anonymous (1974): Corticosteroids in terminal cancer. *Drug Ther. Bull.,* 12:63–64.
2. Editorial (1976): Osteolytic metastases. *Lancet,* 2:1063–1064.
3. Ferreira, S. H. (1972): Prostaglandins, aspirin-like drugs and analgesia. *Nature New Biol.,* 240:200–203.
4. Hunt, J. M., Stollar, T. D., Littlejohns, D. W., Twycross, R. G., and Vere, D. W. (1977): Patients with protracted pain. *J. Med. Ethics,* 3:61–73.
5. Isbell, H. (1948): Methods & results of studying experimental human addiction to newer synthetic analgesics. *Ann. N.Y. Acad. Sci.,* 51:108–122.
6. Mundy, G. R., Raisz, L. G., Cooper, R. A., Schechter, G. P., and Salmon, S. E. (1974): Evidence for the secretion of an osteoclast stimulating factor in myeloma. *N. Engl. J. Med.,* 291:1041–1046.
7. Parkes, C. M. (1976): Home or hospital? Terminal care as seen by surviving spouses. *J. Roy. Coll. Gen. Pract.,* 28:19–30.
8. Penn, C. R. H. (1976): Single dose and fractionated palliative irradiation for osseous metastases. *Clin. Radiol.,* 27:405–408.
9. Robbie, D. S., and Samarasinghe, J. (1973): Comparison of aspirin-codeine and paracetamol-dextropropoxyphene compound tablets with pentazocine in relief of cancer pain. *J. Int. Med. Res.,* 1:246–252.
10. Twycross, R. G. (1974): Clinical experience with diamorphine in advanced malignant disease. *Int. J. Clin. Pharmacol.,* 9:184–198.

11. Twycross, R. G. (1977): Care of the terminal patient. In: *Breast Cancer Management—Early and Late,* edited by B. A. Stoll, pp. 157–163. Heinemann Medical Books Ltd., London.
12. Twycross, R. G. (1977): Choice of strong analgesic in terminal cancer: diamorphine or morphine? *Pain,* 3:93–104.
13. Twycross, R. G. (1978): Bone pain in advanced cancer. In: *Topics in Therapeutics 4,* edited by D. W. Vere, pp. 94–110. Pitman Medical, Tunbridge Wells.
14. Twycross, R. G., and Wald, S. J. (1976): Long-term use of diamorphine in advanced cancer. In: *Advances in Pain Research & Therapy, Vol. 1: Proceedings of the First World Congress on Pain,* edited by J. J. Bonica & Albe-Fessard, pp. 653–661. Raven Press, New York.
15. Verebely, K., Volavka, J., Mule, S., and Resnick, R. (1975): Methadone in man: Pharmacokinetics & excretion studies in acute & chronic treatment. *Clin. Pharmacol. Ther.,* 18:180–190.
16. World Health Organisation (1964): Expert Committee on Drug Dependence, 13th Report. *Technical Report Series,* No. 287.
17. World Health Organisation (1969): Expert Committee on Drug Dependence, 16th Report. *Technical Report Series,* No. 407.

The Nature and Management of Terminal Pain and the Hospice Concept

Cicely Saunders

St. Christopher's Hospice, 51–53 Lawrie Park Road, Sydenham, S.E.26. 6DZ, England

Continuity of care for people suffering from persistent cancer aims to ensure that throughout the whole course of the disease they receive treatment appropriate to each stage and that, as far as possible, this is carried out in the place that accords best with their own way of life and its commitments. In this presentation I will consider this type of care as given at St. Christopher's Hospice.

We owe our patients the attempt to decide when our management has finally turned into care for their dying, even though this may be a difficult moment to identify. We define it as occurring when all active treatments only hold out diminishing returns coupled with increasing morbidity, when the incidence of side effects or the management required by the treatment itself serve only to isolate the patient from those around him and hinder him from completing life in his way.

Some may believe that both patient and doctor should fight for life until its end; but to talk of accepting death when its approach is inevitable is not mere resignation on the part of the patient, nor is it defeatism or neglect on the part of the doctor. For both of them it is the very opposite of doing nothing. If the doctor and his whole team play their part in managing pain and other problems, the patient will be given the opportunity to manage this part of his life himself. He may well make an intensely individual achievement of great importance to him and to his family.

It should never be said that *no* treatment is being offered. Much can be done in general management and in detailed medication, and at no time in the total care of a cancer patient is the awareness of him as a person of greater importance.

HOSPICE CARE

This phase of treatment and the attitude that should underlie it has recently attracted much professional and public interest and is frequently discussed under the title "Hospice Care." Although neither the traditional nor the modern hospices concern themselves exclusively with the needs of people

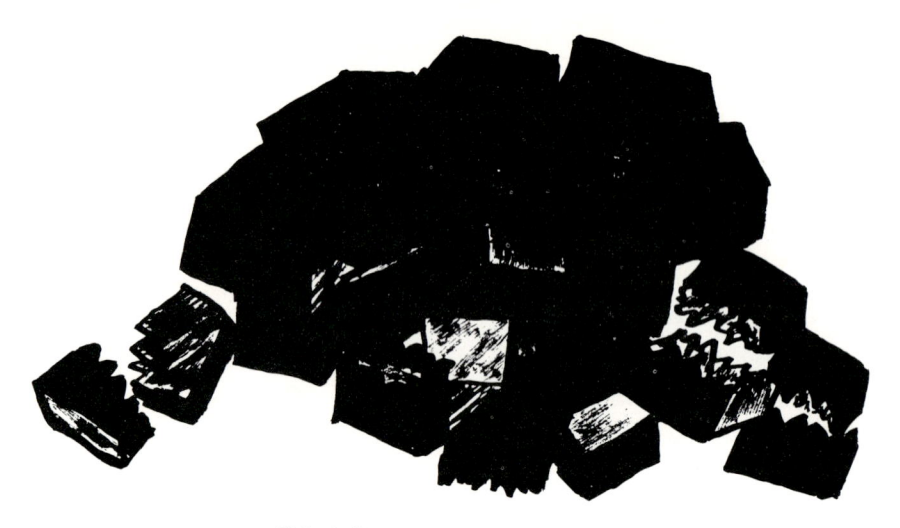

FIG. 1. "I am a scrap heap."—E. S.

with terminal malignancy, this has always been a major part of the work done in these facilities. The professional personnel in hospices set out to diagnose and treat what can often be termed *total pain,* for it includes physical, emotional, social (both interpersonal and financial), and spiritual aspects. In many such centers it has been impressively shown how this pain can almost always be relieved, while the patient remains alert until the disease process itself finally clouds his consciousness.

A series of pictures painted by St. Christopher's patients illustrate how they saw their terminal pain. They show the feeling of being impaled by a red-hot iron, of being totally isolated from the world by the encircling "muscles of tension," the sudden jab on movement, the implacable heaviness of pain, the conviction that one *is* a kind of scrap heap, the endless questions "Why?" and the fears of a lonely, threatening journey.

One woman, with a year's history of unrelenting pain from a carcinoma of the pancreas, drew it as a small rodent boring into the side of a tree trunk. A few traces of green at the top were described to me as, "My life, trying to get through." She was in St. Christopher's for 11 weeks and a friend wrote to me after her death:

> It was nothing short of a miracle. When I last visited her in a previous hospital she was like a demented animal—consumed with pain, incoherent of speech, and quite vicious. I was very frightened, not knowing how to cope, and felt unable to face another visit. Words cannot describe my reaction when I saw her in St. Christopher's—restored to the dignity of a calm, rational human being again. . . . From then on I was able to remain with her for hours at a time, instead of minutes, holding conversation and discussing things of interest dear to her heart. . . . By so doing, I too have gained in spiritual strength. I can only thank you for making my friend's last days bearable when once they were unendurable.

Vital signs in a ward specializing in the control of terminal pain include the hand steady enough to draw, the mind alert enough to write poems and to play cards, and above all the spirit to enjoy the family visits and spend the last weekends at home.

Incidence and Magnitude of Pain

Reports from several studies suggest that approximately half of those who die from various forms of cancer are likely to suffer terminal pain and that a great deal of this is not adequately relieved. Parkes (9) summarized the memories of more than 270 people 1 year after the death of a spouse from cancer in the area of St. Christopher's Hospice. Defining the terminal period as the time between the end of active treatment and death (average about 6 weeks), he divided his patients into home-, hospital-, or hospice-centered. Although the home-centered patients had less pain during the pre-terminal period (5% of some 130 patients), during the terminal period 28% of them were said to have had severe pain which remained unrelieved to the time of death. Of over 90 hospital-based patients 20% had pre-terminal pain, and this figure did not alter for the terminal period. In contrast, 36% of the 42 patients referred to the Hospice had unrelieved pre-terminal pain, but the figure dropped to 8% after admission. The amount of pain reported was the most significant finding of his study. All of these figures should, we hope, have been improved after 10 years of experience, and the survey is being repeated as part of the evaluation of the practice and teaching of St. Christopher's Hospice.

The following related case histories describe the pain suffered by 3 patients and illustrate their general management and the individual achievements and family reconciliations that were made possible:

Case 1. Mr. John G., aged 61, a self-employed retailer of wine-making supplies, came to St. Christopher's Hospice with a history from his doctor of 18 months of severe spinal pain from a carcinoma of bronchus unrelieved by laminectomy, radiotherapy, and increasing doses of morphine and chlorpromazine. He knew that he was terminally ill, and both he and his family were feeling exhausted and bitter after months of obviously intense suffering. His drugs were not altered for the first 48 hr because he began to respond immediately to the atmosphere of security and friendly activity in the ward.[1] After a few days a combination of anti-inflammatory drugs (prednisolone and phenylbutazone) produced a dramatic change in pain and mood. The 4-hourly dose of oral morphine was reduced from 150 mg to 120 mg, where it remained. Mr. G. took part fully in the life of the ward: he organized the raffle of a toy made by his sister and began occupational therapy. Two weeks later he was less well and was often drowsy and occasionally somewhat confused, but he continued to enjoy frequent visits from his family and

---

[1] "The importance of morale and sympathetic understanding in a unit devoted to the care of dying people cannot be over-emphasised, and added to this major contribution to their psychologic comfort may be an enhanced subjective effect of drugs. In assessing pharmacological efficacy in these circumstances the group effect should be considered." (4)

visits to the Hospice Bar. He was entirely clear-headed when he sent for his family and announced to them that he did not think he would be alive the next day. He handed over his raffle to another patient, thanked all the staff, and had farewell drinks with his family before he lapsed into unconsciousness and died peacefully 36 hr after he had called them in.

After his death his wife wrote to the ward: "I thank you from the bottom of my heart for the kindness, compassion and caring which you gave to my dear husband. The last month of his life was an unexpected bonus, which turned out to be pain-free, care-free and restored his faith—I would add—mine also. I will never forget. God bless you all."

His sister wrote to me:

". . . Please find money order. My wreath of flowers to my dear brother, John.

He had all his wreaths of flowers while at St. Christopher's through the very great kindness shown by the doctors and staff, so feel the money is more beneficent than flowers.

I experienced something wonderful during the month I visited John. Three men who had never met before got together as brothers. I used to call them the three Js, two Johns and a Joseph: They worked together side by side, helping each other and Joe sat by my brother's bed the whole day he was dying, fetching cloths as he needed them and talking to him.

Something else I witnessed that day also. During the early evening I saw John look straight ahead on two occasions and give the most wonderful smile; there was no one at the foot of the bed or opposite, for John H. had passed on a few hours before. . . .

If it hadn't been for St. Christopher's our family would never have had this last happy month together with our loved one.

Now the three Js have gone together in peace. May God bless your Christian belief and work always."

Case 2. Mr. John H., an accountant aged 56, was admitted a week after Mr. G. and died the day before him. His pain had also been persistent and poorly controlled ever since a laparotomy and colostomy had been performed 6 months before. At the time he was admitted neither dihydrocodeine by mouth more or less regularly nor pethidine by injection 3 times daily were relieving it. He was still hopeful that something might be done to close the colostomy. He also said he felt better immediately after he was welcomed into the ward community, but he never talked much about his illness. His unsatisfactory medication was immediately altered to a morphine mist every 4 hr with prochlorperazine by day (5 mg) and chlorpromazine at night (25 mg). The dose of morphine alternated between 20 and 30 mg during his 3-week stay as his pain occasionally broke through the constant level of control. During this time five injections of diamorphine (5 to 10 mg) were given with the phenothothiazine because of episodes of vomiting. He needed one injection of diamorphine 20 mg during the afternoon he died.

Mr. H. was able to complete some accountancy a few days after his admission; he joined his friends with occupational therapy and entertained his large family who came with him to Chapel and to other Hospice functions. Four days before he died he was still working, he celebrated his wedding anniversary with his family and came with Mr. G. and Mr. C. to the Hospice Pilgrim Club evening.

His family spent his last day at his side, and nine of them were present as he died. A staff nurse said prayers with them all (a St. Christopher's custom which is practically never refused by the family). Several of Mr. H's family came back to the Chapel for the Sunday morning service 2 days later.

His wife wrote to me: "For me, he kept a diary. . . . All my prayers were answered after my husband entered your hospice. He was completely without hope, yet he recovered to such an extent that he was able to enjoy happiness, friendship, and love for his fellow man."

Case 3. Mr. Joseph C., aged 68, a retired painter and decorator, was admitted to St. Christopher's Hospice with a history of several months' severe, left-sided and back pain from a metastatic carcinoma of kidney. He was loath to admit how much he had suffered during the months when he had been in and out of a local hospital until we had demonstrated that we could relieve his pain while he still remained alert and active. He was given a mist morphine 20 mg with prochlorpromazine 5 mg every 4 hr with almost complete pain control and, as he later told us, his first night's sleep for months. After 48 hr he allowed us to increase his dose of morphine, and it remained at 30 mg until his death 4 weeks later. He also was given prednisolone 5 mg and indomethacin 25 mg q.d.s. Soon after admission Mr. C. became active, performing surprisingly vigorous physio- and occupational therapy and completing a large number of mosaic trays. After 2 weeks he recorded a television interview for a National network in which he said that he felt that he and the Hospice were fighting his advanced cancer together, that he now no longer even thought of pain and hoped to have a little more life ahead.

As his two friends began to fail, he took charge of Mr. G's raffle, completed Mr. H's last mosaic tray and sat and talked with them and their families throughout their last day. He himself developed a chest infection during the 12 hr in which his two friends died, and he was very upset and grieved together with the staff at their loss. His condition deteriorated rapidly from then on; but his usual medication, now given by injection, controlled all physical distress, and he died peacefully in the middle of the night with his wife and her sister at his side. He had been in the Hospice for 5 weeks.

One of his friends wrote to me:

"In the early hours of this morning my friend Joe C's earthly sojourn ended. Joe was a down to-earth man, a heart of gold, a comedian and often a "gor blimme" bloke. Please, will you and your ministering angels accept my heartfelt thanks for making the evening of his life a happy event, I repeat, A Very Happy Event. If there is another world, then Joe was living to go to it, an example I shall keep to the end—or my beginning."

These three men had a quiet, rather ill companion in their four-bed bay. Mr. M. watched their activities in a somewhat detached manner. He spoke little but obviously felt drawn to some extent into the ward "Club." He had expected the first two deaths but was more shocked when Mr. C also died. He told us that he missed them, but he was able to welcome two new patients with his usual quietness and at present is considerably better than on admission. All three families called back to see him.

These family groups made full use of the time given to them by the relief of the pain of terminal malignant disease. All three patients had suffered months of unrelieved distress, yet none of them presented physical problems that could not be tackled quickly and effectively by the specialist team of the Hospice. We could not take away the pain of parting; but the mental suffering of each patient was alleviated by the physical ease, which at the same time greatly decreased much of the exhaustion and anxiety of their families. Each of the three groups found new meaning in life and faith, and their spiritual pain was also comforted.

These patients lived and died in the small community of an open ward bay, part of the larger community of the Hospice. This way of sharing their experience made a major contribution to the control of pain and also to the support of the grieving families. The letters illustrate the nature of hospice care for terminal pain and provide reasons why the local registrar of deaths has stated that she can recognize by their peace the Hospice families in her waiting rooms.

Mr. G's family expressed what we must surely all feel, "Why could he not have had this help before?" Too many patients reach those who can offer them proper understanding and management of their pain late in its crippling course, or not at all. Their families are left with haunting memories, and from them comes the almost-universal public fear of the inevitability of pain in terminal malignant disease. We owe them better than this. Every hospice will have such stories, and in order to set them in context with ascertained facts concerning randomly selected families who have experience of hospice care, the reader is referred to the report of the Newhaven Hospice to the National Cancer Institutes on two years' experience (7) and to Parkes (9) report on some of his psychosocial studies at St. Christopher's.

Results of Comparative Study

Findings from a comparative study of 34 families of cancer patients who died at St. Christopher's Hospice matched with 34 families of patients who died elsewhere showed statistically significant differences favoring the group from the Hospice in ways which have already been illustrated in the story of the three men given above. The families of patients managed at the hospice recalled the following:

1. Greater mobility of the patient.
2. Less pain rated as severe (but not bought at the cost of greater drug-induced confusion).
3. Less anxiety among spouses during the period of terminal care with fewer somatic symptoms.
4. Spouses spent much more time at the patient's bedside and very much more time talking to staff, other patients, and visitors. They were more likely to have helped to care for the patient and more likely to know a doctor's name.
5. Doctors and nurses at St. Christopher's were less likely to be seen as "busy" or "very busy" than staff elsewhere.
6. Despite the fact that 2 or 3 patients died each week on each floor of the Hospice, only 6% were said to have been upset by the death of another patient. The same figure was given for those in other wards, none of which were for "terminal care."

In addition, 27 families from each setting completed a check-list which allowed them to agree or disagree with general statements regarding the hospital. The statement which best characterized St. Christopher's was, "The hospital is like a family," which was checked by 78% of the St. Christopher's families and only 11% of the rest. It was also shown that St. Christopher's families were no more likely to be active in their religion than the other families; but many recognized the existence of the Christian foundation, and all who did reacted positively to it.

Development of Hospices

St. Christopher's Hospice was established in 1967 to relieve suffering by developing methods of care, analyzing knowledge and carrying out research into the control of the physical, mental, and social distress of chronic and long-term illness. It has helped to establish a code of practice that can be shared with all those caring for patients with similar problems. Some patients will need the experienced and confident care of a separate, specialized unit, but for the majority this will not be an available option. Nor should it be necessary.

The attitudes and skills which are being developed have already been shown to be eminently transferable. From experience at St. Christopher's and elsewhere came the pioneering work of the Symptom Control Team of St. Luke's Hospital, New York, which has now been adapted by the Support Team of St. Thomas' Hospital, London. Similarly, the Continuing Care Units in the United Kingdom and the Palliative Care Unit and Service of the Royal Victoria Hospital, Montreal (also related to St. Christopher's) have already been replicated both in the U.S.A. and elsewhere. The Home Care Team in New Haven (Connecticut, U.S.A.) has roots in both St. Christopher's and St. Joseph's Hospices. Historically these are all related through the author's initial experience at St. Luke's Hospital, London which was developed during 7 year's work at St. Joseph's Hospice (10).

The Home Care and Symptom Control Teams have shown that the control of terminal pain does not have to be carried out in a geographically separate unit, though there are some patients and families who need the expertise and the space they should find there. A few such hospices will be needed for patients with intractable problems, for research, and for teaching in terminal care; but most patients will continue to die in general hospitals, cancer or geriatric centers or, best of all, in their own homes. The staff they will find there should be learning how to meet their needs.

GENERAL PRINCIPLES OF HOSPICE CARE

The following list of the essential components of terminal care is the fruit of years of working and visiting in different units and of discussions with others working and interested in this field (6,11). Above all, it is the outcome of the good fortune which gave me the opportunity of listening to patients and their families during the 30 years since a dying patient said to me that he wanted, "What is in your mind and in your heart."

Management by an Experienced Clinical Team

The team or unit for terminal care must carry out its practice in such a way as to earn the respect and cooperation of the doctors who refer their patients. A multidisciplinary medical approach is as important in the later stages of cancer management as in the earlier phases of the disease. Moreover, this concept applies to other patients who may present with terminal pain. Consultation will often be needed between physician, surgeon, radiotherapist, chemotherapist, and sometimes the psychiatrist and the clinician who runs the local Pain Clinic. It is no longer adequate medicine to try to cope alone with difficult decisions in terminal cancer management, even though the needs of many patients have been and still will be dealt with successfully by their own family doctors, single-handed.

A group of consultants in a unit or team may act merely as a resource while the patient remains in the care of his family doctor or of the specialist who was involved with his initial treatment. The team may, however, take over his care completely, particularly if there is some special need such as intractable pain and distress, which is still all too often most ineptly treated in acute care units as well as in the patient's own home. There should be no feeling of failure on the part of the doctor whose experience is other if transfer to a special ward or hospice is carefully discussed and planned. Whenever the original doctor keeps in touch, his visits are likely to have a special place in maintaining a patient's morale. Few patients expect miracles at this stage, but they are all prey to feelings of failure and rejection and respond to a gesture that implies continued concern.

Understanding Control of the Common Symptoms of Terminal Disease, Especially Pain in All Its Aspects

Doctors and nurses need to concentrate on the development of these skills and special units should initiate research and share their knowledge. Terminal pain is so different in character and meaning from most pain met in a teaching hospital that the methods of giving relief and the standards of comfort and alertness that should be expected are sometimes difficult to establish in a general ward. This has to be demonstrated to both doctors and nurses if their patients are to have adequate treatment for the many symptoms that often accompany this usually generalized disease.

Terminal care is being increasingly recognized as a facet of oncology, but it is not always recognized that symptom control and general support should accompany the chemotherapy of advanced disease.

Attention to this part of the patient's therapy brings staff of all kinds closer to the often isolated patient and brings him the personal support he may so greatly need. Once such an attitude and regime is established, it should then be easier to desist from inappropriate treatments.

Skilled and Experienced Team Nursing

These patients need the stability and continuity of an experienced nursing team built up of members with varied trainings and backgrounds. This demands confident leadership from the ward sister and close communication both among the nursing staff. Moreover, it requires close communication between the nurse and others who will be involved with their patients, including social workers, physiotherapists, occupational therapists and, of course, the doctors.

The flexible staffing pattern needed cannot always be established in a general ward, and lack of time is a constant problem. This can, however, be exaggerated: An attitude can be conveyed in a brief meeting or in the way in which procedures are carried out. Student and auxiliary nurses frequently bring a special contribution. Odd moments spent with the patients instead of in a Nurses' Station are an irreplaceable part of their care. The chaplain's place in the whole team may begin from his support of the nursing staff who, most of all, bear the daily burden of relationships with dying and sorrowful people.

A Full Interdisciplinary Staff

This is not the field for total individual involvement, which can be most unhelpful for both patient and staff member. It takes time to build the ways of working together but such teams are to be found in other specialized units, for example, those for Intensive Care or Renal Dialysis. They are particularly needed by staff members who are grappling with emotional as well as with practical demands. Psychiatrists and social workers have frequently been involved as support. Such a team, together with all its professional members, should be seen to include the ward orderlies, domestics, and porters, often the people to whom hospital patients turn to most easily. Their support should not be underestimated or ignored. Students of all kinds may also assume this role.

It is important that as many different members as possible should meet for frequent discussion. Though the clinician does not abrogate his clinical responsibility, each member should be ready to assume a degree of leadership concerning an individual patient or family. St. Christopher's has been open for less than 11 years and approximately one-third of the nursing staff have worked 5 years or more, one-third between 1 and 5 years and one-third are in their first year. There is very little unplanned turnover. All of the doctors, except for one rotating Junior Doctor, and most of the other staff and the volunteers have made a long-term commitment.

A Home Care Program

A Home Care Program involving all the different disciplines among the staff must be developed according to local circumstances and be integrated with the hospitals, the family practices of the area, and the inpatient unit. Patients can then be admitted at the moment of their choice and of accurately defined medical need, and they will also be able to move easily to and from the wards for periods varying from days to weeks or months as short-term improvements are fully exploited. The way home, like the way back to the "Acute Care System" must always remain open.

Relief of pain in itself may make possible unexpected progress in these directions. Confidence may enable a family to keep a patient at home, often confounding all predictions. Where patients have access to adequate nursing, a 24-hour on-call service and other support, which may well include good neighbours and volunteers, home is likely to remain their choice. Even so, many people who have said they would like to die in their own homes need inpatient care, if only for the last few days. Some families find much greater relief and unity in a professional milieu in the last hours, and others realize that they cannot face the thought of death at home after all. They must be enabled to accept the help of admission without feelings of guilt. Those who manage to the end have a great feeling of satisfaction to ease their bereavement but once again, this is only possible if pain is controlled. Half of St. Christopher's patients are being nursed in their own homes at any one time.

Recognition of the Patient and Family as the Unit of Care

Families should have every available option open to their choice and expect recognition of their cultural and individual needs. Once this has become part of the ethos of a ward it becomes largely self-perpetuating. Occasional visits by ward staff to a patient's home with a family doctor or a domiciliary team member will emphasize the importance of including the family in the care of any seriously ill person. Not everyone will have the time or the understanding to embark on long family discussions, but everyone can recognize the family by name and accept them as an integral part of the team caring for the patient.

We should aim to give the maximum privacy to those who need it for peace and for the expressions of tenderness which are inhibited in a general ward. Separate units usually have more opportunity to give a special welcome to the solitary, but I have often seen how nurses in a general ward are able to do this and to make the distinction between the lonely, who welcome their friendship and the isolate, to whom this may well be an intrusion.

Admission to a hospice does not mean the expectation of inevitable death, and some patients and families wish to maintain their denial of the likely outcome. The staff will accept this if it is a consistent choice but find that in most cases a more realistic sharing of the situation will develop. At St. Christopher's Hospice a sheet is kept in the notes for any member of staff to note relevant comments made by patients concerning their illness. Not all of these are used, as some patients just cannot discuss these matters and not all comments get recorded. Most of those that are completed (more than half of all patients) show a developing realization of the situation and acceptance of it.

A Mixed Group of Patients

Although the homes or hospices that welcome only dying patients have given superb care for many years and by doing so, have frequently outweighed any fear locally of a "death house," yet we do not believe that this should now be the ideal. A good community is usually a mixed one, as is pointed out by a letter from a patient in St. Christopher's Hospice with Motor Neurone Disease:

I was very interested in the article about the death of Jane Zorza (February 25) but would like to say that the impression given, although accurate for the particular patient, does overstress the aspect of painless dying.

As a patient who has been in a hospice for nearly 18 months my view is that this impression is far too narrow. The hospice is a caring community for anyone in need of total support, and provides the opportunity for patients to live in pleasant surroundings in the knowledge that every assistance will be given both to family and patient whenever and however it is required. Some, like Jane Zorza, are only helped to die painlessly but many live hopefully and often happily for long periods.

As a patient I can give my own experience and also my observation of many other patients where the multi-sided care and treatment offered by the hospice have improved the quality and extended the length of life beyond any imaginable expectation. I have seen many patients enter the hospice, apparently near death and completely without hope, who have after a few weeks recovered to such an extent that they have been able to return home—in some cases for many months—to live happily with their families, knowing that they have the full support of the hospice home care team at all times.

For those of us not able to be cared for outside the hospice there is an atmosphere of caring and living which is the point that needs to be stressed. We do not enter a hospice to die but to live what is left of our time as happily and fully as possible." (5)

St. Luke's Nursing Home Day Centre, Sheffield and most of the new Continuing Care Units include a proportion of patients with nonmalignant diseases of a longer-term nature. St. Christopher's Hospice has welcomed 10 to 20% of its ward patients from this group, and from the beginning there have been a number of elderly people who live in their own bedsitting rooms in a separate Wing. Transfers to and from the wards are fairly common, and there is no doubt that the Hospice will extend its longer-term accommodation when it becomes possible. The person with the prognosis of some 2 years has often more difficult problems to handle than the one with only a few months to live and may greatly need the support of a suitable community or a Home Care Team.

Bereavement Follow-up

Many hospitals make special arrangements for families who come to collect certificates and property, but our work should not end there. Family pain is part of terminal pain, and the family has to recover. A bereavement follow-up will identify and support those in special need, working in cooperation with the family doctor and any local services which can be involved. Many doctors give such support as part of their service to the families they have known over the years. Most of the bereaved are not so fortunate and a follow-up may fill this gap and ease the tragedy and long morbidity.

Social workers and chaplains have initiated such work from general hospitals, but normally a team, usually of volunteers, will be required to meet with all those in need, with a leader to train and support the visitors themselves. There is no doubt that many families suffer from the sudden break from a staff who have cared for the patient and who have perhaps for a long time been a great part of their lives. In a small unit the families will be recognized as they enter the door, and reception staff have a special role in this part of care for the bereaved. An informal welcome back may be all that is needed. It has been found that only a small proportion of the bereaved will remain dependent upon either this support or the more formal program for more than a few months.

Methodical Recording and Analysis

Detailed recording and analysis make possible the evaluation and monitoring of clinical experience and the establishment of soundly based practice. St. Christopher's Hospice now has nearly 6,000 detailed and analyzed records retrievable for its retrospective surveys.

Hinton's (3) important study of the physical and mental distress suffered by 102 patients in the general wards of a teaching hospital is a definitive work and essential reference point. From the enormous volume of writing now available we can still turn for enlightenment to the pioneer work of Worcester (12), who published the lectures he had been giving to the medical students of Harvard from his background of family practice. This classic is still in print (13), but gradually the anecdotal approach is being supplemented by the more analytical (8). This is a challenge to those who feel that "tender, loving care" is all that is needed. Nothing can take its place but terminal care of the 1970s developed from previous experience, but now it should not be the same as that of the 1900s or even the 1950s. "Efficient loving care" is our aim, and every resource of clinical and social medicine has to be exploited.

Teaching in All Aspects of Terminal Care

Teaching in this field is much in demand by students and graduates of all the disciplines concerned. This is being given in conferences and seminars, in rounds and visits, and in outside lectures by members of the staff. We find that lectures and ward rounds of this kind are likely to be overcrowded. Besides the encouraging comeback, often years later, of those who have attended only one session, there should be reinforcement of such teaching for medical and nursing students in their own hospital wards. One of many groups of medical students who visited the hospice at their own request wrote afterwards: "It was a relief to be able to discuss freely a subject which is usually actively avoided in a large teaching hospital." Another student said on a teaching round: "In our hospital the patients have to earn their morphine."

Much of the future growth must be more closely integrated with general teaching centers, and the development of specialist teams within them must be encouraged. Nevertheless, the special units are likely to maintain their role of stimulating initial interest and of organizing courses for those who will in their turn be moving into this field. This is no longer a discipline in which no past special experience need be required.

Imaginative Use of the Architecture Available

In planning and building these facilities it is essential to have rooms for families to visit in groups; windows for patients to look from, and opportunities for them to move around; room for staff to work easily and to relax and for anxious visitors to take time off or to brace themselves for a meeting. Beauty is healing, and a feeling of openness and access to the world outside are chief among the needs of a unit for terminal and long-term care. Some of us have been fortunate enough to plan purpose-built hospices; others have learned to adapt whatever they could find, and successful practice has often arisen from the imaginative use of structural peculiarities. Emphasis should be given to the need for rooms for private talk; these must be found, whatever the area offered.

The proportion of single rooms to bays or wards dictates the way a ward team handles the patient's last hours and the needs of his family at that time.

Some feel strongly that no patient should be expected to witness the death of another person dying in the same room or bay. Others, mainly those with fairly generous space, find that this can almost always be managed so that the reaction of most patients and their families is almost entirely positive (as in the case of the group of patients described above). The peaceful death of a patient who shows no distress in breathing or in any other way, who is not left alone and, above all, one who is not hidden behind screens and curtains, repeatedly enables other patients to feel more confident about their own end. A distressing death would indeed have the opposite effect, but those who are expert in such care should not let this occur. Families in the bays talk with each other and with other patients, and it is rare for them to return for the practical business of the next day without going to see those they have known to give thanks for the friendship that has comforted them all. A patient's widow wrote to us:

> One thought that I would like to pass on to you. I think one of the greatest aids I personally received from St. Christopher's was being able to watch other patients die peacefully and easily without being shuffled off behind curtains and so on. I think those experiences have been of great therapeutic value to me so that when the time came for Eric to die, I felt no panic or even great distress and consequently was able just to concentrate on sharing his last moments. My son and I have spoken of this, and he says that he felt exactly the same way.

Longer-stay patients play a special role in the life of a ward for they are part of its hospitality and support, although, like the staff, they will need a holiday from it at times. Patients admitted within a short time of death and certain others will require single rooms. As St. Christopher's Hospice enlarges from 6 single rooms in 54 beds to 18 single rooms in a total of 62 beds, it has these groups specially in mind.

An Efficient Administration

Efficiency is very comforting, and competence in administrative detail gives security to patients, families, and staff. It also eases the liaison with outside contacts that is so essential for the small, specialized unit.

What are the economics of the provision of such care? St. Christopher's Hospice has close links with the National Health Service and has contractual arrangements for the majority of its beds. This means that there is no financial barrier between any of its patients and their care, and it has been shown that the cost to the National Health Service of a hospice bed will be no more than 50 to 70% of the cost of a teaching hospital bed and 70 to 80% of a general hospital bed in the same area. Moreover, the modern hospice is likely to have at least half of its patients in their own homes. It offers specialist consultations and support on referral from the patients' own doctors, district nurses, and other community services.

The high nurse-patient ratio in a hospice is more than compensated for, not only by the less complex overhead costs of such a unit, wherever it is situated, but also by the omission of tests and treatments that are no longer appropriate. (The cost-effectiveness of hospice care is currently being studied by the National Cancer Institutes, U.S.A. which has contracts with three of the many hospice units opening in the United States.) Above all, the hospice movement sets out to ensure that every person who can no longer benefit from the increasing complexity of the general hospital will have the support he and his family need in the right place, whether it be in his own home (if he has one), his treatment hospital, a cottage or community hospital, or a hospice.

The Cost of Commitment and the Search for Meaning

Members of staff will at times become drained by the work of the wards and in other contacts with the families of patients, and some are at risk of developing what has been described as the "Staff Burn-out Syndrome" (2). Informal safety valves should arise spontaneously according to local personalities and surroundings, but care must be taken to see that regular discussions, off duty, study leaves, and extra time off are arranged before a crisis is reached. Staff members must be prevented from investing all their emotional commitment in their work.

The management of terminal pain in all its aspects will at times cause pain and bewilderment to all members of the staff. If they do not have the opportunity of sharing their griefs and their questions, they are likely to leave this field or find a method of hiding behind a professional mask. Those who commit themselves to remaining near the suffering of dependence and parting find they are impelled to develop a basic philosophy, part individual and part corporate. This grows out of the work undertaken together as the members find that they each have to search, often painfully, for some meaning in the most adverse circumstances and gain enough freedom from their own anxieties to listen to another's questions of distress.

Most of the early homes and hospices were Christian foundations, their members believing that if they continued faithfully with the work to which they felt called, help would reach their patients from God. Some of the traditional ways of expressing this faith are being interpreted afresh today, but there are also many people entering this field who have still to consider their own religious or philosophical commitment. This is not an optional extra; it has a fundamental bearing on the way the work is done.

In considering these essential components of terminal care, it is important to distinguish between the general principles being interpreted at St. Christopher's Hospice and its own peculiar characteristics, stemming from the personalities of its staff and, above all, from its Christian foundation. The seed from which the Hospice grew was a gift of £500 left by a man from the Warsaw Ghetto who died of cancer in a London hospital in 1948. His promise, "I'll be a window in your Home" was fulfilled 19 years later when the first patients were admitted. That phrase and his other request, "I want what is in your mind and in your heart," sum up the need of all patients for the skill combined with friendship that make up terminal care. The original gift of £500 had grown to £500,000 when the community of the Hospice was opened in 1967. Now, 11 years later, the need to extend further its research into the control of pain in all its aspects and the ever-increasing demands for teaching have grown far beyond its original ideas—but they have still to be balanced to the daily needs of each patient, family, and staff member.

The patients have always been the central members of the community. Every day they bring their pain and their feelings of anger, bitterness, and grief into the Hospice as they are admitted. Yet the overwhelming majority find the atmosphere is peaceful, welcoming, and often joyful, for their pain is relieved and most of these feelings are transformed. We believe this is the work of the spirit of the God who is in all men, however they may seek for truth.

It seems to us that only the belief that all men belong to the family of a God who shared and shares their death can bring an answer not only to those whom we try to help but to the millions of the deprived and wronged, above all to those who have never had any chance of finding either a worthwhile life *or* death. That all wrongs will be righted and all the comfortless comforted should be the perspective of the individual, personal care that is offered in a hospice.

This is also the perspective in which the St. Christopher's Hospice staff are able to say to those of different beliefs or of none who face the problems of terminal pain, together with the atheist doctor and the priest in Camus' novel *The Plague* "We're working side by side for something that unites us beyond blasphemy and prayers" (1).

REFERENCES

1. Camus, A. (1948): *The Plague.* Hamish Hamilton, London.
2. Freudenberger, H. J. (1975): *The Staff Burn-Out Syndrome.* Drug Abuse Council Inc., 1828 1st St., N.W., Washington, D.C.
3. Hinton, J. (1963): Mental and physical distress in the dying. *Q. J. Med.,* 32:1.
4. Hinton, J. (1964): Editorial problems in the care of the dying. *J. Chronic Dis.,* 17:201.
5. Holden, E. (1978): Letter in *The Guardian.* London, March, 1978.
6. Kastenbaum, R. (1976): Towards standards of care for the terminally ill. Part III. A few guiding principles. *Omega,* 7:191.
7. Lack, S. A., and Buckingham, R. (1977): *Final Report. A Continuing Care at Home Program for Patients with Terminal Cancer and Their Families.* Hospice, Inc., New Haven, Connecticut.
8. Mount, B. M. (1976): The problem of caring for the dying in a general hospital. The Palliative Care Unit as a possible solution. *Can. Med. Assoc. J.,* 115:119.
9. Parkes, C. M. (1977): Evaluation of family care in terminal illness. In: *The Family and Death,* edited by E. R. Pritchard et al. Columbia University Press, New York.

10. Saunders, C. M. (1967): *The Management of Terminal Illness.* Hospital Medicine Publications Ltd., London (Available from St. Christopher's Hospice).
11. Wald, F. (1976): Report of International Work Group in Death, Dying and Bereavement. "Proposed Standards for Terminal Care." *Personal communication.*
12. Worcester, A. (1935): *The Care of the Aged, the Dying and the Dead.* Charles C Thomas, Springfield, Ill.; Blackwells, Oxford (1961).
13. Worcester, A. (1977): *The Care of the Aged, the Dying and the Dead.* Re-printed by Arno Press, New York.

Terminal Care from the Viewpoint of the National Health Service

Gillian Ford

Department of Health and Social Security, Alexander Fleming House, London SE1, England

This paper describes the management of the final stages of malignant disease within the context of the National Health Service (NHS) of Great Britain. This is not the place to embark on a detailed description of the vast organization for providing health care which is the British National Health Service. But there are one or two important points about it which need to be remembered. It differs from insurance-based systems in that it is not a mechanism for paying bills, or reimbursing bills paid by patients. It is a system which requires the Secretary of State to provide such services as he considers appropriate for the purpose of discharging duties laid upon him by various Acts of Parliament and to meet all reasonable requirements for hospital accommodation, medical and other professional services, the care of expectant mothers and young children, facilities for the prevention of illness, aftercare of those who have suffered illness and so on. The list is not quite endless but comprehensive enough to explain why more than 750,000 people are employed by the NHS in England, the total for Great Britain reaching over 900,000. Although the Secretary of State's responsibilities are thus far-reaching and comprehensive, he does not have the power to direct individuals who work within it to practice in any particular specialty or in any particular geographical area. His task is to make the service possible by providing the facilities, and employing staff—both of which are carried out through the health authorities to whom the Secretary of State delegates his powers.

Thus there are powers to provide services but not to direct individuals, either in the sense described (such as might occur in the armed forces) or as to the standard or type of clinical treatment provided. In this the members of the medical, nursing, and dental professions and physiotherapists are deemed to be the only arbiters. The concept of clinical freedom is zealously guarded both by those who practice within the NHS and those who administer it.

DEVELOPMENTS OUTSIDE THE NHS

In spite of the comprehensive nature of the NHS, some patients seek treatment as private individuals from privately-run institutions. A number of charitably-run homes supplement NHS or local authority accommodation for those who, because of age or disability, need a sheltered milieu. New developments in medical care often emerge from academic departments or research institutes, and generally such developments are absorbed into the NHS as their value is recognized; but occasionally the private/charitable sector makes a sustained contribution to care or treatment or both. Terminal care is an important example. Of the 40 or so special units for those with terminal malignant disease, only about 10 are wholly within the NHS although most of the others receive some financial support from health authority sources. The special units for terminal care have a unique approach to death and dying which does not deny the fact of death but sees that the troubles that precede it, whether these be of body, mind, or spirit, receive attention and care.

ESTIMATES OF NEED

A responsibility of those who are concerned with running and administering the NHS is to look at developments outside, in University Departments, or the private or charitable sectors, or in other countries and to try to assess the impact on the NHS. What, for example, is the population's need for kidney machines or for early detection of fetal abnormality? More particularly, what measures are there of the need for special facilities for the treatment of terminal malignant disease? In the U.K. details are, of course, collected for all deaths by diagnosis. Details are shown for 1973, in the following tables (5). (The large totals have been rounded.) Table 1 shows the total of all deaths by age group. Table 2 shows deaths in the same year from neoplastic disease in the same age groups and the percentage that these form of all deaths. Thus, totals are reached of about 120,000, or a fifth of all deaths, occurring from cancer. The majority of these take place in hospitals rather than at home—the proportion has been rising for cancer as it has for all causes. This is shown in Table 3. The proportion of deaths occurring in

TABLE 1. *Total deaths in the United Kingdom in 1973*

Sex	0–4	5–24	25–64	65+	Totals
Males	7,802	4,840	86,000	198,000	297,000
Females	5,704	2,324	50,000	233,000	291,000

TABLE 2. Deaths from neoplastic diseases in the United Kingdom in 1973

Deaths	Sex	0–4	5–24	25–64	65+	Totals
Number of deaths from neoplastic disease	Male	172	642	24,000	41,000	65,000
	Female	124	438	21,000	35,000	56,000
Percent of total deaths due to neoplastic disease	Male	2%	11%	28%	21%	22%
	Female	2%	19%	41%	15%	19%

private institutions, which would include hospices outside the NHS, was 10% in 1974.

As far as sheer numbers are concerned, the tables show something of the problem. But illness, symptoms, distress, and pain are not revealed by such data. A recent article by Parkes (4) recounted a survey of 276 married patients under the age of 65 with cancer. Particular attention was paid to the amount and duration of pain, because this was the most prominent cause of distress. Of the sample, 60% of the patients died in hospitals, but the amount of time spent at home during the terminal stage was 3½ times that spent in the hospital by the sample as a whole. Table 4 shows the interviewer's assessment of two features of the final illness.

Since patients who had less pain *before* the terminal period were most likely to go home and remain there, the finding that a high proportion ultimately experienced severe to very-severe pain underlines the need for active treatment of pain in this group. The findings are not dissimilar from those of Cartwright and associates (2) who reported pain present in 66% of a stratified sample of 785 deaths from all causes studied by interview of relatives within 9 months. Pain was reported in 87% of those whose death was due to cancer, although the extent to which this remained unrelieved was not known.

TABLE 3. Place where deaths occurred

| | All deaths ||| Cancer deaths |||
Year	Home	Hospital[a]	Other	Home	Hospital[a]	Other
1965	38%	50%	12%	37%	60%	3%
1970	33%	54%	13%	33%	62%	5%
1974	31%	56%	13%	31%	64%	5%

[a] Non-psychiatric hospitals. Includes NHS and non-NHS facilities.

TABLE 4. *Interviewer's assessment of two features of the final illness*

	Home-centered (65 patients)	Hospital-centered (100 patients)
Mobility		
Confined to bed	6	45
Intermediate	45	43
Fully up	12	0
Pain		
None to mild	19	34
Moderate	13	32
Severe to very severe	29	19

Dr. Parkes also compared three groups of patients and the extent to which pain was relieved. The conclusions from this part of the study were that, of hospital-centered patients, 20% were said to have suffered severe and mostly unrelieved pain and this state did not change during the final phase of care in hospital. Those patients who were confined at home showed that pain became an increasing problem. Six percent experienced unrelieved pain prior to the final period, but this proportion rose to 42% during the final phase of care at home. Those patients admitted to St. Christopher's Hospice showed a reduction in severe and unrelieved pain from 36% in the pre-terminal period to 8% in the terminal phase. This clearly has implications for pain control irrespective of where the patient is being cared for.

SERVICES FOR PATIENTS WITH CANCER

There can be no doubt of the size of the problem. What is our capacity for tackling it?

The central core for the provision of medical and surgical services is the district general hospital. An urban population of 100,000 to 150,000 will almost certainly have such a general hospital, and there most treatment for cancer begins after referral from the patient's own general practitioner. But such a hospital is unlikely to have radiotherapy services or specialists in the use of cytotoxic therapy, or a clinical pharmacologist. These more specialized services are centralized within hospitals—often teaching hospitals—which serve a much bigger population than their immediate district. This means that some patients requiring prolonged treatment have to travel for radiotherapy or other cancer therapy. The annoyances of this have been partly eased in some places by building hostel-type accommodation so that patients can stay overnight without being admitted to a hospital bed. Treatment with cytotoxic drugs may be available in the same hospital as radiotherapy, but in only a few places are the cancer specialists grouped together in one unit for treatment of cancer as such. Only a few departments within hospitals and even fewer whole hospitals are designated for treatment of cancer alone. However, there is an increasing trend towards grouping together the various specialties concerned in it. In four NHS Regions experimental "Regional Cancer Organizations" have been established. These have the aim of providing high standards of diagnosis and coordinated treatment for all cancer patients throughout the Region. It is hoped that medical staff in other Regions will watch with interest the evaluation of this combined approach.

It has been shown that the majority of patients with cancer die in NHS hospitals in ordinary general wards. In some hospitals teams of specialists from different disciplines plan the management of the individual patient throughout the course of his or her illness. Most hospitals do not set aside a whole or part of a ward for those who are terminally ill. This may be a deliberate decision to avoid the stigma of the "death ward." It may be a deliberate decision by medical staffs, that they as individuals are each responsible for the total care of their own patients from beginning to end, even though other disciplines may be involved at intermediate stages. This may require a deliberate undertaking given to relatives or to the family doctor that admission to the acute ward is possible if symptoms or social conditions require it.

Community Services

Patients who are in their own homes will receive care from a number of sources; indeed, some patients will have reached hospitals because the community services will have provided screening procedures such as those for cancer of the cervix or lung cancer. More commonly, general practitioners dealing with patients who they regard as "at risk" because of their age, lifestyle, or symptoms will have initiated the sequence which leads to hospital treatment and continuing surveillance.

Both the community services of the health authority and those of the local authority will be involved in the care of patients in their own homes when hospital treatment has ceased. The objective of this care will be the sustaining both of the patient and the family. The family doctor is a key member in the organization of this. He may have a nurse working within his practice, or he may call upon the community staff or services run by health authorities, e.g., health visitors, home visits from occupational therapists or physiotherapists. Home helps provided by the local authority may be assisted by volunteers from the Womens' Royal Voluntary Service, who provide a service which delivers hot meals to patients' homes.

The social worker, also employed by the local authority, may assess the situation, which will include the need for practical services, walking aids, commodes and so on. This category of somewhat mundane objects and services may seem irrelevant to the pain of terminal malignant disease, but it must be remembered that the pain of a bedsore may be the most dominant feature in a patient's list of problems and maintenance of mobility is thus very important.

Care from the NHS primary health team comes from medical and district nursing staff, and health visitors. In addition there may be home visits from occupational therapists and physiotherapists. NHS staff may be supplemented by Marie Curie Foundation nurses and other helpers—some local authorities provide night sitters and laundry/incontinence services. The most sustained support comes from relatives and neighbours, and this has been described as "often remarkable" (6).

Teamwork

The teamwork of care at home is just as necessary as that within the hospital because of the multiple ills and sorrows which require attention. If symptoms are ignored, the problems of pain are likely to become worse—as later are those of bereavement. The advantages of teamwork in hospital and in the community are the mix of skills, personalities, and temperaments. The disadvantages are difficulties in establishing clear lines of communication and the diffusion of contacts which any one patient may have. If he feels that nobody is in charge, he is bound to experience *fear*. The hospital will offer an outpatient appointment—but it may be some weeks ahead. But if the family doctor has been kept fully in touch with the patient's progress and the plans for further treatment, if any, he has an invaluable role. Apart from mobilizing both health and social community services he may be the first person to whom the patient reveals the full extent of his pain, and he may need to consider more treatment deliberately aimed at pain, including further radiotherapy or changes or increases in analgesics.

Home, Hospital or Hospice?

Unfortunately, as we have seen, patients' needs for pain-relief are not always met. It is also clear that medical staff, hospital, and family doctors alike do not know the scope for pain control which is already available.

This is no fault of the NHS as a system of providing care. But the bigger the framework the more difficult for those operating within it to keep in touch and to know what the plan of management is, whether at home, in hospital or at home *and* hospital. The NHS provides community and specialist services in a unique way but combining the best elements of both takes patience and perseverance, as a general practitioner knows. Community care is not in itself necessarily better than hospital care. But because it is familiar to the patient it is believed to be what he would prefer, and so it will normally be until he sees his family using all their energies, and more, in looking after him. Hospital specialist services are not necessarily failing in their provision for terminal care, but the patient may not wish to be there.

A precise or absolute policy for terminal care is doomed to fail. It is a matter on which the patient's circumstances and preferences will have a profound influence. Certainly some staff feel that an acute general ward is not the ideal place to care for a dying patient, because its pace and atmosphere are geared for the acutely ill. The regular drug round may inadvertently be late because of an emergency admission. A 4-hour interval may be stretched to 6. Special arrangements for an evening at home or an outing to the "pub" consume staff time and may be trivial and burdensome to those who are responsible for order within the ward.

Patients too are often slow to bring their needs to staff busy with patients whose needs seem to be more pressing. Nevertheless, a patient may welcome a return to the ward where there are familiar faces and routine and, as the tables show, the majority of patients who die from cancer do so in ordinary general hospitals. Hospice care is often combined with a domiciliary team which provides experts who assist the general practitioner to care for patients in their own homes. This seems to provide the best answer in certain circumstances. Through the focused nature of their work, hospice staff became skilled at managing pain and other symptoms. Because hospices are small care given has a tailor-made quality, comforting to patient and family alike.

CONCLUSIONS

Future Developments Within the National Health Service

It goes without saying that ideally those who are experiencing their terminal illness should have no less attention and care paid to them than if there were a possibility of cure. But health services, insurance systems, and individuals have also to weigh the economic aspects of treatment. While "good health" may be the aim of a State for its population or a family for its members, a good death is not yet in the same category. In the light of the evidence of need, both measured and suspected, it is possible that there will be a conscious effort to include terminal care as one of the many priorities for NHS expenditure. Exactly how this will be accomplished is for health authorities to determine.

Hospice care is not cheap, but it appears to be considerably less expensive than care in a general hospital providing all acute services. Hospices for patients with terminal illness and with pain problems have tended to develop with substantial NHS support and sometimes even wholly within it. The National Society for Cancer Relief and the Marie Curie Memorial Foundation have also made very substantial contributions in this field. The NHS has looked to the hospices to pioneer developments in pain and symptom management, and they have became foci of excellence and a milieu for staff of all the different disciplines to receive training and to carry back to their own hospitals the essential features of hospice care.

Most staff working within the NHS will continue to be mainly occupied with primary care, or medical and surgical specialist services, or long-term care of the elderly, but many are realizing that the patient with terminal malignant disease, whether at home or in a hospital ward, has needs which should be met. Transfer to a special unit may not be possible or desirable, but the assurance of a hospice or hospital bed, when necessary, is an important factor in managing patients at home. For the future one looks at the following possibilities. The growth in the hospice movement suggests that most of the big centers of population in the U.K. may, by the next century, have such a development. In addition to the 40 or so already in existence, another 20 are planned. Ideally these would be closely associated with academic departments, that is, hospitals teaching undergraduates so that this subject may be taught in the early part of the curriculum, not left to postgraduate activities. It seems essential that such hospices should run or actively participate in home care schemes. These provide learning and teaching experience of care in the home and show clearly that it is not home care *versus* hospital/hospice care—the two are complementary.

Where care is being provided in a big general hospital a degree of skill may be acquired by a team of staff (the symptom control team) who provide the expertise within that hospital. Whether they have a part of the hospital, or part of a ward, solely for their own patients under their care is a matter for local agreement. It may be preferable to keep the patient in a ward with which he is familiar and use the team when and wherever they are needed. In the smaller hospitals outside the major conurbations the mixture of skills and specialties may not be diverse enough for it to be possible to set up such a team. For some particular types of pain the local hospital may provide a specialist service such as a pain clinic where nerve blocks and other surgical procedures may be carried out. These may be a small but very important part in the management of pain in the terminal and pre-terminal stages.

Patients living in towns or rural areas served by smaller hospitals may not have ready access to expert terminal care either while they are at home or when they are admitted to hospital. Fortunately there is not only an increasing interest in the subject, but also it is hoped that opportunities for postgraduate experience for medical and nursing staff, though few at the moment, will multiply as the number of units increase and more courses can be offered. Interested staff from a variety of disciplines are taking notice of developments and patients are benefiting as a result. But even so, a few informed professional staff scattered sparsely amongst a population of 100,000 to 200,000 people do not add up to a focus of skill and experience which can be recognized and drawn upon by doctors suddenly faced with problems of pain which appear insoluble. Patients are quick to realize when their medical advisors are becoming fearful that they will be unable to negotiate the next bend in the pain spiral. There is much anxiety about creation of addiction, of causing stupor alternating with pain. Since any family doctor will only have 4 or 5 patients a year who die of cancer, he is unlikely to become skilled at managing all the pain problems which may be present. But a very great deal can be done by frequent discussion in postgraduate medical centers (where hospital medical staff and general practitioners meet) and articles in the medical press. The Department of Health held a symposium in 1972, on Care of the Dying, and many helpful ideas were aired at that time (6).

Perhaps the most necessary adjunct at this stage, to patient-care and the continuing process of education, is the availability somewhere of expert advice when the doctor feels he has come to the end of his therapeutic armamentarium. The symptom control team of a big hospital may be miles away, the nearest hospice even further, but it is unlikely that they cannot be reached by telephone. Most of the hospices already offer this kind of advisory service for practitioners, and it is much appreciated and effective in instilling professional confidence.

A recent leading article in the *British Medical Journal* (1) concluded with a quotation from Hinton (3): "We emerge deserving of little credit; we who are capable of ignoring the conditions which make muted people suffer. The dissatisfied dead cannot noise abroad the negligence they have experienced." I would add that I believe that fear of inadequacy has caused professional staff to wear a mask of indifference and that this fear is unnecessary. Many have now demonstrated that though the home or the hospital may be far from ideal, it is possible to cope with patients' pain. It does not require a million pounds, or magic, but confidence that pain control is possible, with detailed attention to a variety of therapeutic measures coupled with that attitude which accepts the whole patient and his needs but sees him as a person.

REFERENCES

1. *Br. Med. J.* (1978): Pain and the dissatisfied dead. 25:459–460.
2. Cartwright, A., Hockey, L., and Anderson, J. L. (1973): *Life Before Death*. Routledge and Kegan Paul, London, Boston.
3. Hinton, J. (1972): *Dying*, 2nd ed. Penguin Books Ltd., Harmandsworth, Middlesex, Baltimore.
4. Parkes, C. M. (1978): Home or hospital? Terminal care as seen by surviving spouses. *J. R. Coll. Gen. Pract.*, 28:19–30.
5. *Registrar General's Statistical Review of England and Wales Tables (Medical)* (1973): Her Majesty's Stationery Office, London.
6. Silver, C. P. (1976): Terminal care. *Br. J. Hosp. Med.*, 16:579–584.

Discussion

Part II. Management of Pain of Advanced Cancer: Continuing and Terminal Care

Questioner: Dr. Ford, what is the cost of patients managed in hospices compared to those patients managed in general hospitals?

Ford (London): It is considerably cheaper to provide care in a separate unit than in an acute hospital providing the full range of special services.

Questioner: Dr. Saunders, do you think that respiratory depression due to high doses of narcotics necessary to control severe pain of a terminal cancer patient makes it impossible to use them for adequate pain-relief?

Saunders (London): I have had 30 years experience with such patients and have found that side effects of narcotics are very much less when these drugs are given to control severe cancer pain than when they are given to normal volunteers. We do not find that the respiratory depression is a clinically difficult problem to handle. Remember that as tolerance to analgesia increases so does their tolerance to side effects.

Twycross (Oxford): I'd go along with that. In practice when morphine is given by mouth there is no problem with respiratory depression. Indeed we sometimes use morphine purposely to lower the respiratory rate in some of our patients who have respiratory distress, and this can be of great benefit to the patient.

Questioner: Dr. Saunders, what are the psychologic reactions of the medical and paramedical staff to the continuous and exclusive contact with patients who suffer and die?

Saunders: The nurse that I showed you with the patient near the end showed a degree of grief and affection for that patient. Like many of us she moved into this field because of knowing personally the problem of pain and bereavement in her own family. She is able to see that patient relieved of the pain and making something creative out of his time. That is totally different from walking up and down at the end of a bed and seeing a patient with unrelieved pain and despair. Even so the staff grieve when a patient who has become very much a part of the ward dies. And I'll certainly never stop feeling sad when I see a family member walking alone out of the house.

Questioner: Dr. Saunders, are the patients dismissed from St. Christopher's with antalgic therapy followed by the Hospice's staff? What relationship is there between the Hospice's staff and the family doctor?

Saunders: Our work is integrated with that of the ordinary community services. We keep in constant communication with the family doctors who have the responsibility of the patient. We work alongside. We will have made recommendations and give support in prescribing, and be ready for consultation and may be called to the home, but not need to bring the patient into the Hospice.

Iacono (Ragusa): Dr. Saunders, what is the numerical ratio between patients and medical and paramedical staff in the Hospice?

Saunders: We have at the moment 54 beds, and we are going to increase this to 62 leaving aside the wing for old people. At any time we will also have about 60 patients at home. For this patient population of about 120 we have 40 doctor's sessions a week, that is 20 half-days of which 12 are at least taken in straight teaching. We are going to increase our doctor coverage as the number of beds increase. We also have one whole-time-equivalent nurse in the establishment for each patient bed. That means day duty, night duty, study leave, and all the rest

DISCUSSION

of it. For example, if we have an 18-bed ward we will have 7 or 8 nurses on duty in the morning, 4 or 5 in the afternoon, with an overlap for discussions, and 2 or 3 on duty at night. Roughly one-half of our nurses are trained and one-half untrained. Our tendency is to move to having more trained nurses in proportion.

Lipton (Liverpool): Dr. Ford, why do you believe that pain-control methods cannot be spread throughout the British hospital service?

Ford: What I said was that I believe there would be centers where some highly specialized procedures for controlling pain were carried out but that it would be up to the local hospital staff to acquire the knowledge which will permit them to refer patients for specific procedures. I emphasized the need for treatment to be available locally, because the nature of terminal care is such that patients usually are unwilling to remain away from their families and friends for very long. The onus then is on the medical staff to provide the best personal care and the best pain-relief. Doctors used to know which patients might benefit from nerve block, neurosurgery, or other modalities and to refer them to the right facility. I did not say that pain control would not spread because of the nature of National Health Service, but rather because of the nature of terminal care, which precludes that these procedures would be on everybody's door step.

Questioner: Dr. Twycross, are not oral preparations of morphine in the homes of patients easily obtained by addicts who have ready access to such patients?

Twycross: As far as I know no solution of morphine in any home in Britain has ever fallen into the hands of an addict. We do not have a big addict problem fortunately, and certainly we have had no alarms on this score.

Ford: I should add that a dilute solution of morphine is not going to be of very great interest to an addict.

Twycross: That is right. The solution of morphine is generally not stronger than 10 mg. It may be weaker but usually not stronger in the majority of patients.

Bonica (Seattle): Dr. Saunders, how many hospices are there in Britain?

Saunders: Between 38 and 40, but the impact these hospices are having is very much greater and more widespread than the number of patients managed in them would suggest.

Bonica: Dr. Saunders, what percentage of patients with advanced cancer are managed in hospices?

Saunders: Very small number because we have 600 admissions a year in this 60-bed facility. Altogether, there are something like 800 beds in hospices, so that if we use St. Christopher's data a total of about 8,000 patients are managed in hospices. This is a very small percentage of the 820,000 patients with cancer, but the effect of what we are doing, although difficult to assess accurately, involves many more patients. Many family doctors in our area, after having shared care of a patient with us once or twice will then take care of patients themselves and call us only if we are needed for special consultation.

Bonica: Dr. Saunders, what percentage of patients outside hospices are managed properly with pain-relief?

Saunders: I think that Dr. Parkes' figures give us the feeling that roughly 50% of patients who die of cancer are likely to experience moderate to severe pain. And if we take Dr. Parkes' figures which are more optimistic than Dr. Cartwright's, we can expect that half of those are going to die with unrelieved pain. In other words, 25% of cancer patients continue to have pain which remains unrelieved until they die. I am afraid we are not doing well and have a long way to go to provide good pain-relief to terminal cancer patients.

Fink (Bethesda): In the United States of America, there has been some interest in the hospice concept for several years, and there has been a fostering of the development of hospices by the National Cancer Institute, which is the primary agency of our Federal Government responsible for cancer research and therapy. However, recently, through the interest of our President, Mr. Jimmy Carter, and his medical advisor, Dr. Peter Bourne, and much interest on the part of our media, newspaper, television, and public interest groups, there is a rising awareness of the kinds of concepts which have been discussed and relate to hospice. At the current time, hospices or organizations called hospices are springing up all over the U.S. In some instances the hospice concepts are much as has been discussed by Saunders and colleagues. In others these are simply names used for the typical nursing homes which exist in our country. From the point of view of the Federal Government we are most interested in evaluating the hospice in the U.S. to determine its efficiency and effectiveness in dealing with the type of symptoms that have been discussed by our colleagues of the United Kingdom. It is also fair to point out, however, that in the United States the practice of medicine is generally a private practice. Therefore, before laws become firm we must ascertain how the hospice concepts will be handled in the United States.

Fontanella (Milano): Dr. Twycross, have you ever encountered a patient with such severe pain that it could not be relieved? If you have, and his life-expectancy was very short, do you think it would be better for him to live or to die early?

Twycross: We approach pain control on a sort of graded scale. First of all, we set out to achieve freedom from pain at night and assure the patient of a good night's rest, and that we achieve with 99.5% of our patients. We then try to produce ample pain-relief during the day, with the patient at rest, sitting or lying. The round figures from several institutions including St. Christopher's would be 98%. In other words, we are highly successful in producing pain-relief at rest during the day. The third stage is pain-relief on movement during the day. This is where we have to compromise a bit, and the figure is probably about 80% success. But even in those who do not get complete relief on movement during the day, the pain is reduced. Moreover, we introduce what I call "modification of lifestyle" or relative immobilization to help reduce pain on movement from an intolerable to an acceptable level. There have been 1 or 2 patients where we have really been in trouble; those have been patients with paraplegia due to spinal cord compression and nerve root infiltration. The situation was resolved by doing a spinal cord transection. On occasion it is necessary to reduce the level of consciousness in order to achieve good pain-relief. Just what percentage of patients require this I can't say, but these constitute a small number of patients. I emphasize a small number of patients in whom a combination of physical, spiritual, and psychologic factors prevent us from producing ample pain-relief without reducing the level of consciousness. Of course when that happens, one is hastening the development of terminal hypostatic pneumonia, but this is a very small percentage of our patients.

Saunders: I think that the question being asked is really, "Do we think that there does come a time for any number of terminal cancer patients when it would be better to kill them rather than to go on trying?" And it is some form of legalized euthanasia that is perhaps in his mind. I would like to say that in the very great number of years that I now have known these patients, the number who have consistently asked to be permitted to die is very small indeed, and their reason has not been pain, but despair or just anger in a person who has had previous emotional problems. I am not saying that we can absolutely produce complete pain-relief while the patient is alert; I would say that we can always relieve pain at the expense of some alertness. But I would like to add one more thought about this. If, because of previous treatment the patient's pain is very difficult or impossible to control, and the patient asks you to kill him, you are going to be in a very difficult position, and you are going to need to call in the expert. Let us suppose for the moment that active euthanasia is part of the law in one of our countries, and consequently some patients will demand it and say this is a personal freedom they should have, but it would take away the right of every other patient on long-term care. But we are offering a positive alternative of producing ample pain-relief. We should be reaching the stage at which nobody needs to make the desperate request for death, and I believe we can.

Moricca (Rome): With regard to euthanasia I would like to remind all of us that we are not responsible for the disease. We are responsible for the therapy. Therefore we must not kill, but we must fight pain and effectively relieve it. And there are many possibilities against pain. Some are offered during the terminal phase of the disease, others are those that have been discussed and explained during this symposium. I therefore think that the problem of euthanasia doesn't exist and should not exist.

Panel: Future Needs, Goals, and Directions

J. Bonica and V. Ventafridda (Moderators)

Bonica (Seattle): Ladies and Gentlemen, after 3½ days of long and extensive discussions on almost every aspect of pain of advanced cancer, we have reached the focal point of this international symposium: consideration of future goals. We must set a direction and consider actions we must take to improve the control of pain of advanced cancer. For this portion of this program we have gathered an outstanding panel of experts. I regret that Prof. Veronesi was unable to remain for this session because, as current President of the International Union Against Cancer (UICC), he has been in a position of making suggestions in setting goals for the management of pain of cancer patients everywhere. Fortunately, Prof. Pietro Bucalossi, President of the Italian League Against Cancer and former Director of the Milan Cancer Institute, has graciously agreed to give his thoughts about this problem. Moreover, we are fortunate in having Professor Emilio D'Ambrogio, representing the Minister of Health of Italy, and Dr. Diane Fink, Director of the Division of Cancer Control and Rehabilitation of the National Cancer Institute of the United States. Both will be able to present the current and future position of the governments of these two countries regarding this problem of cancer pain.

Prof. Loeser will discuss the neurosurgical aspects, Prof. Bond will represent psychology and psychiatry, Profs. Houde and Twycross will consider future needs regarding systemic drugs, Professors Pannuti and Gennari will discuss the needs in anticancer modalities, while Prof. Ventafridda as co-Chairman of this panel will make the closing remarks. It is hoped that each member of the panel will consider future goals, directions, and needs within the framework of the current status of each area, particularly regarding the deficiencies which exist.

I will start the discussion by making certain general observations and remarks. The presentations made in this symposium have substantiated and confirmed my conviction about the current deficiencies that exist in the management of patients with pain of advanced cancer. As I have listened to each speaker and the informal discussions of the panels, certain points have emerged which impressively emphasize the critical need for much greater research and educational efforts, and consequently improvement in the control of pain of cancer.

In regard to research, I wish to stress my strong conviction that one of the first orders of business is to carry out comprehensive national and regional epidemiologic studies to ascertain the incidence and magnitude of pain in cancer in general, and the incidence, severity, and duration of pain with each specific type of tumor in particular. Data presented here has confirmed the suspicion of many of us that pain develops much more frequently in cancer patients than most people believe. Moreover, it is clear that in most instances it is not effectively relieved. I believe we have reached the consensus that the multidisciplinary approach for team management of the pain of cancer, which I have suggested for many years, is one of the most effective, if not the most effective way, of dealing with this serious health problem.

Another area of research that needs to be done urgently, is to study the basic biochemical, neurologic, and psychologic mechanisms of cancer pain. Why and how do large tumors pressing on major nerves or plexuses produce pain? Is it stimulation of axons, lowering of nociceptor thresholds, or increased sensitivity to norepinephrine as occurs with other types of peripheral nerve injuries, or is it due to production of pain-producing substances? What role does block of large fibers with consequent loss of their pain-inhibitory action play in this type of pain? Why and how do bone tumors produce pain which is usually excruciating? How does infiltration of cancer cells in perineural, perivascular, and perilymphangetic tissue cause pain? Is it a biochemical, neurologic, or pathological process?

Does ischemia consequent to obstruction of large arteries by tumors really produce pain by producing asphyxia, cellular breakdown with the liberation of pain-producing substances? Is the pain of venous engorgement edema caused by compression of large veins due to primarily mechanical or biochemical nociceptor stimulation? How does fibrosis of the brachial plexus or the lumbosacral plexus that follows cancer therapy produce pain?

What role do the recently discovered endorphins play in cancer pain and its relief? How can we manipulate them to achieve maximum analgesia? I am convinced that once we obtain answers to these basic questions, we have the science and technology to produce agents or techniques, or both, with which we'll be able to exert exquisitely specific anti-pain action to produce relief.

Still another extremely important area of research is in the psychologic, psychosocial, and behavioral aspects of cancer pain. Although hundreds of studies have been directed to the problem of cancer per se, very few have looked at the impact of the pain. What influence does the pain of cancer have on the emotional and behavioral condition of the cancer patient and conversely, what impact do psychologic, personality, environmental, and psychosocial factors have on the pain experienced by the cancer patient. I hope Prof. Bond will suggest future activities in this area.

In my introduction to this symposium I emphasized, and indeed almost belabored, the critical need to improve the education of medical, dental, nursing, and psychology students, and students from other health professions to become involved in the management of patients with cancer. Equally important is the education or reeducation of graduate physicians and other health professionals in the basic principles of cancer pain diagnosis and therapy. All members of the oncology team should become appreciative of the importance of optimal cancer-pain control. By the same token, pain therapists who become involved in managing cancer pain must also become fully acquainted with the other aspects of oncologic process. In other words, we must develop well-integrated multidisciplinary teams, each member of which knows "all of the plays" of the game and not just his or her field.

Although during this symposium we have achieved greater interaction and communication among participants from various disciplines than has been the case heretofore, it is clear that we still have some way to go before we have the optimal integrator approach. For example, in discussing the application of various therapeutic modalities, there is still a tendency to consider each by itself and not as part of a combined pain therapy. Moreover, with some exceptions, there was the tendency to extol the virtues and the advantages of each technique while its disadvantages, limitations, and complications were not given due emphasis. These are reflective of the tubular vision I spoke about in my introductory remarks.

Now for a few comments on particular topics. In regard to the anticancer modalities I was pleased to learn of the comprehensive data on the incidence and magnitude of pain of cancer presented by Foley and Pannuti. I hope other oncologists follow their example and collect and publish data on the problem of pain as well as other aspects of cancer treatment.

In regard to the systemic analgesics there is an obvious need for well-controlled studies of large doses of aspirin and other nonnarcotic analgesics in a sufficiently large number of cancer patients in order to more accurately define their efficacy and limitations. Moreover, in view of the significant incidence of depression, it is surprising to note the very meager amount of data from control studies of psychotropic drugs. Similarly, in view of the significant role played by psychologic factors in chronic pain, it is surprising that there are virtually no data on large numbers of patients managed with hypnosis, biofeedback, and/or behavioral modification techniques for cancer pain.

Although nerve blocks and neurosurgical procedures have been used extensively in patients with cancer pain, there have been very few controlled clinical trials on sufficient numbers of patients to permit us to define the role of each of these techniques in managing cancer pain. In addition to the use of these techniques in a sufficiently large number of patients, it is essential to apply the basic principle of the controlled clinical trial in evaluating each of the methods for the type or types of cancer pain for which the specific technique is indicated. Only with these types of data will it be possible for us to define more precisely the indication and advantages, as well as limitations and disadvantages and complications of each procedure for each type of pain (i.e., considering the mechanism, intensity, site, degree of spread, and other characteristics of the pain).

These are some of the many factors which must be considered in the future. And now, let me call upon Prof. Bucalossi to make some general comments on the symposium and some suggestions for future goals and activities.

Hon. Prof. Pietro Bucalossi

President, Italian League Against Cancer; Vice-President, House of Representatives of the Republic of Italy

When Professor Bonica asked me to take part in this meeting I think he did so because of my 30 years' experience at the Milano National Cancer Institute—the second such facility created in the world (after the one in Leningrad) for the specific treatment of cancer. I was sent to this Institute, then a place for terminal patients, from a general surgery hospital and it was quite different from today.

I often remember the terrible screams of a poor woman who was suffering from cancer of the pelvis with excruciating pains. At the time there was a solid obstacle that did not permit the use of the drugs and other modalities that have been rightly emphasized at this symposium. Then pain was considered from a religious point of view, an instrument for the spiritual life of the individual. Therefore, the use of drugs was banned, because it was believed that it accelerated the death of the patients. These notions were discounted in part by the late Pope Pius XII in the early 1950s.[1] Subsequently, this first battle was won, and the result was that by eliminating or reducing pain in those patients, it was possible to lengthen their lives and permit them to live more comfortably until their deaths. Since then there has been an impressive evolution in the specific treatment of pain in cancer. In these patients tragic factors, such as unbearable pain, together with the physical disability caused by the tumor or the anticancer therapy, produce a progressive deterioration of the personality.

The first experiences in our Institute (I say "our" fondly, but I am no longer part of the Institute) were directed toward neurosurgery applied to pain. The Department that is now directed by my friend, Ventafridda, with competence and passion, and to whom much is owed for the success of this meeting, was created in our Institute.

This symposium is a very special one and has the entirely new characteristic of having gathered here physicians and scientists of different disciplines: Oncologists are meeting and interacting with physiologists, neurologists, pharmacologists, anesthesiologists, and those of other disciplines and comparing their experiences with those of investigators. I have had this type of experience, and I wish to make a consideration regarding a certain attitude that I had towards cancerology. I have heard my colleague, Bonica, who is

---

[1] See p. xxix in Introduction.

the most prominent person in the organization of this symposium, point out the necessity of an interdisciplinary character of our medical and paramedical knowledge. I agree wholeheartedly on this point if it means that from these meetings questions are posed and ideas emerge which stimulate more and better research by those who are qualified in investigation, and hopefully this will produce new knowledge which then can be applied to the care of patients with cancer pain.

I would have some doubts, and I say this quite frankly, if the decision of the application of such knowledge for the care of patients were to be made by an assembly of this kind. And this goes for all problems connected with cancerology where we have seen and still see the prominence of technical factors over clinical ones. My dear departed friend, D'Argent, Professor of Clinical Oncology in Lyon, France, in his lessons said something regarding cancerology and cancer pain treatment with which I completely agree. That is: At a certain point a decision must be made regarding the patient, and this decision can be made only by the person who knows the possibilities of treatment the particular form of cancer requires. He further stated that the oncologist must be like a conductor who knows perfectly well what the violin, the brass, and the drums can produce and who is able to harmonize these sounds and to use them to create a concert that is the expression of perfect harmony. I believe in the treatment of cancer pain this consideration has its importance, because in the treatment of pain in cancer we have to deal not only with the pain and the associated psychologic effects present in all kinds of illnesses, but must consider that elements which are both curative and exclusively palliative intertwine. Obviously, the doctor who must prescribe the therapy must be fully aware of the advantages, disadvantages, limitations, and complications of a large number of interventions proposed to him so he can judge and decide, based on his own experience and the information provided by consultants, the application of the most effective therapy at the right time and in the right sequence so as to provide optimal pain-relief.

I agree with what Dr. Ford said about the creation of special centers qualified to give information regarding what should be done, because it is impossible to have in each and every hospital one or more persons who can solve these problems promptly and effectively.

I would like to end my short discourse by emphasizing that the Floriani Foundation has taken the initiative on this very important topic and has had great success which is due not only to its generosity but to the intelligence with which this initiative has been realized. I think that when we ask what should and can be done in the future, I think that this Foundation could represent a standard of reference for this type of meeting and the notions presented that there should be continuous interaction of researchers of various disciplines in order to conduct a strategy of the fight against cancer pain. So, in the future let's not leave it a dream but make it become a reality by creating these centers for the study and treatment of cancer pain from which indications of the strategy that is to be applied can be diffused out.

Bonica: I very much appreciate the comments made by my esteemed colleague, Professor Bucalossi, not only because he is one of the great pioneers of cancerology and has had vast experience in this field, but also because of his sustained interest and the national and international prestige and influence he has acquired. The doubt he expressed about who should make the final decision about the most appropriate therapy for each patient is both of theoretical and clinical importance. Professor Bucalossi, perhaps you are not aware that in conceiving and espousing the multidisciplinary approach to the management of chronic pain (including cancer pain) during the past three decades, one of the crucial points I've made is that no matter how many other physicians and health professionals are included in the decision-making process about mechanisms of diagnosis and therapy, each patient must have one and *only one* physician whom I have called "the manager." It is the responsibility of the managing physician not only to carry out the basic principles of diagnosis and therapy inherent in medical practice, but also to coordinate in an exquisite manner the consultations and to collect the information which will permit him to decide what is the correct diagnosis and what is the most appropriate therapeutic strategy. In the case of patients with cancer, it is the oncologist who should assume this responsibility. In order to "orchestrate" the actions of various consultants and put their ideas together so as to produce a "concert," it is essential for the oncologist not only to know all about the disease (tumor) but also to know well the mechanisms of the pain associated with cancer and to know all about the various modalities available for its relief, i.e., indications, advantages, limitations, complications, and contraindications. Unfortunately, in the past, with the exception of you and a few of your colleagues working in cancer who have had the precocious foresight and perspicacity, most oncologists have neglected the problem of pain or at least given it low priority in their consideration of the problem as a whole. Earlier, I presented evidence that in the past and even currently, cancer pain is usually badly managed and many patients continue to suffer moderate to severe pain until they die.

I have also presented the various reasons for this sad state of affairs and these need reemphasis here. For one thing, in virtually all of the exhaustive studies on virtually every aspect of cancer, the pain has received little or no attention. For another, with the exception of persons in some comprehensive cancer centers, oncologists have not interacted with neurologists, physiologists, pharmacologists, anesthesiologists, and all of the other people who could provide expert advice to permit the oncologist to make the right decision as to what is the most effective therapy for the pain (in contrast to the cancer). Because unfortunately no one person can have all of the knowledge, skills, and expertise to know all about each of the many therapeutic modalities and apply them effectively, it is essential for the oncologist to consult these various individuals and to obtain and collate the information they provide him and then make the right decision as to which therapy will be most effective for a particular patient. I hope that this symposium will serve as a stimulus for oncologists to collaborate and work in "concert" with other health professionals who have expertise in pain management so that in the future *all* cancer patients will be provided with maximum relief of their pain and suffering.

I now call upon Dr. Diane Fink, Director of the Division of Cancer Control and Rehabilitation of the National Cancer Institute of the United States, to tell us about the plans of the American Government to help solve the serious problem of cancer pain.

Diane Fink

National Cancer Institute, Bethesda, Maryland

My remarks will be divided into three major areas: (a) general areas of concern in the U.S.; (b) specific areas of concern of the National Institutes of Health (NIH); and (c) areas of concern and future directions for the National Cancer Institute (NCI).

In my comments during the discussion of terminal care I mentioned that there is a great interest in the U.S. in the problems of chronic pain and suffering and death and dying not only in cancer but in all of the major diseases. This interest is at the highest legislative level from our President, Mr. Jimmy Carter, to many of our congressional leaders within the Congress of the United States. In addition, we are seeing a great deal of interest manifested by the general public of our country as reflected by activities of many groups representing consumer interests, the news media, and by the many articles and discussions about the critical need to improve the care of patients with chronic pain and the problem of suffering. And quite amazingly much interest in improvement in the care of the dying patient.

Based on these kinds of interests and others, Dr. Donald Fredrikson, Director of the National Institutes of Health, has organized a study team composed of representatives from all governmental agencies that might be involved in the areas that I have mentioned and specifically in pain research. The purpose of this study team is to coordinate the federal government's approach to the problems of pain and suffering. This group plans to make a number of recommendations to Dr. Fredrikson, who will then make determinations along with the heads of other agencies within our government as to directions and future support, primarily for pain research but also for improving patient-care. The recommendation will include greater support for pain research and other needs for experimental studies in the area of pain.

I won't go into specific detail because I am really quite amazed, John, that as you went through your list of future goals and needs, the thinking of the NIH team is along these lines. In addition to pain research there will also be recommendations regarding needs for studies in the problems of terminal care and the need for demonstration programs in terminal care. And perhaps most importantly, programs to facilitate research in pain in its broadest sense. These considerations will include the very important allocations of funding and the development of specifically related study sections which we use to judge applications that will be concerned with pain research. Recommendations will also include greater needs in training of scientists for pain research and of physicians in the proper care of patients with cancer pain. I am speaking in rather broad terms.

We will also recommend centers for pain research and therapy whether these be in Comprehensive Cancer Centers, as described by Dr. Bonica, or perhaps in other institutions which have the kinds of expertise that would be necessary to deal with pain problems. And then also procedures to allow the rapid development and clinical experimental use of investigations of new drugs that might fall under what we call "Schedule One" of our narcotic laws, so that we can allow the proper pharmacologic and clinical studies to be undertaken of such agents. These recommendations will be presented to Dr. Fredrikson within the next several weeks. The Pain Study groups have been meeting every week since last fall, and since I serve on many of them I know that we hope to have our work finished in the very near future. Now from this we expect to hold a national conference in the U.S. on issues of pain and suffering, to look not only at research and demonstration needs but also health-care-delivery type issues. We have found that such National Conferences to raise awareness are exceedingly important to stimulate the various members of our scientific community to areas of importance found by groups such as Dr. Fredrikson's study group.

With regard to the National Cancer Institute, which is part of the NIH, we have the major responsibility for cancer research and demonstration, but the overall view of needs by the NIH in all areas of pain research we feel is exceedingly important for cancer pain, because these will help to elucidate certain basic mechanisms of pain. Whether this is done in the categorical institutes such as ours, or these discoveries come from institutes like the National Institute for Neurological and Communicative Disease and Stroke, or the National Institute of General Medical Sciences, does not matter, as long as it has applicability to the cancer patient. We consider this cross-fertilization among the various institutes and among the many parts of the government exceedingly important. As Dr. Bonica has mentioned, my own Division of Cancer Control and Rehabilitation has supported the majority of cancer-related pain research, psychological research and terminal-care activities of the National Cancer Institute. However, the Division of Cancer Treatment Research is becoming increasingly involved in the problems of pain research, and through its drug development program it can deal with our problems of assessing new analgesic drugs. It can also set the stage for development of new drugs and the kind of pharmacologic studies that will be required. In addition it has a large network of investigators throughout the U.S. that have dealt with oncologic treatment, and currently it is seeking ways of including pain research and clinical trials into this network. This division has at its disposal a large hospital service in the Washington, D.C. area. With regard to our own activities our primary responsibility is dealing with that large percentage of cancer patients who are seen in community hospitals. In addition to the research we have described, our major activity has been in attempting to set up a hospice program, not necessarily of the type of St. Christopher's because of the difference in medical practice, economic factors, and other considerations in the United States. However, we plan to set up a program that can be evaluated in a scientific way so that eventually we will know what it will take to deal with terminal care in a hospice-like atmosphere.

In addition we are quite concerned about the problems Dr. Bonica has talked about, such as how is cancer pain handled by the average practitioner in the U.S. and the so-called patterns of cancer care for pain. We are exceedingly interested in the epidemiologic studies dealing with the incidence, severity, and magnitude of cancer pain as national and regional health problems and its psychologic, physiologic, sociologic, and economic impact on the patient, the family, and society. The continuing education of physicians, nurses, and other health professionals is an important task ahead; but perhaps most importantly it is conferences of this type that make the interest of our federal government in an area as broad as chronic pain research known to the people and to the biomedical community. You can help us disseminate the word that there is great interest within the U.S. federal government of the development of good, solid, scientific studies that deal with cancer pain.

Bonica: Dr. Loeser, What can be done in the future to improve the area of neurosurgical approach to the management of cancer pain?

John Loeser

Department of Neurological Surgery, University of Washington, Seattle, Washington

I think that the primary problem in the use of neurosurgical procedures for the relief of cancer pain is careful selection of patients. Any surgeon who contemplates destructive or even stimulating neurosurgical procedure must know the process of the diseases that the patient has, must have the necessary technical skills, but most importantly, must have more than just a technical approach to human disease and human suffering. It is very difficult to evaluate the results of surgical procedures for pain-relief because there are much fewer of them done than nerve blocks, for example; and because all too often they are the last step in the treatment road, and the patient has already become a very different human being from what he or she was at the beginning of the illness.

Bonica: Dr. Loeser, Should all neurosurgeons be taught how to do all of the common techniques for cancer pain, or should we develop special centers where patients can be referred for particularly highly specialized techniques?

Loeser: Most of the stimulation techniques, and particularly the intracranial procedures, are experimental, and therefore their use should be restricted to major centers wherein surgeons will do enough cases to acquire extensive experience. However, I think that every neurosurgeon should be capable of performing cordotomies, dorsal rhizotomy, myelotomy, and the analogous procedures on the trigeminal and glossopharyngeal nerve. The number of centers needed is a function of the transportation and communication system that a community has. It is a lot cheaper to move patients to doctors than to try to put a neurosurgical center in every town.

Bonica: Dr. Bond, What needs to be done in the future regarding the role of psychiatrists and psychologists in the management of cancer pain?

Michael Bond

Department of Psychological Medicine, University of Glasgow, Glasgow, U.K.

My remarks must be interpreted against my background belief that cancer pain controlled by psychologic means is part of a psychosomatic attitude. That is one that takes account of psychologic, biological, and social aspects of the person's illness. I say this because in my view the balance is not right in medicine at the moment. The biomedical model or that part of medicine based on basic sciences far outweighs in terms of interest and resources the behavioral aspects of the disease. This needs to be corrected so that the two aspects can be brought into line with each other. Failure to treat cancer pain successfully is due in part to this tendency to use the unilateral (biomedical) approach to patients. The first goal or step to achieve this is to change the attitudes of graduate and postgraduate doctors and the general public towards illness in general and cancer in particular. Secondly, I believe it is clear to everyone here that no one person can deal with a cancer patient and his or her family. We have to have a team, the composition of which inevitably varies depending on the local resources. From a psychiatrist's point of view, and I think I speak for psychologists too, we need to extend our current methods of assessing the behavioral aspects of the pain of cancer and with that develop further contributions toward its control. One of the things we need to know a good deal more about is the pattern of psychologic changes which occur with different forms of cancer and with different treatments. We need to know not only what happens when the person is in pain, we need to know what happened before and what happens after treatment. Often people tend to be neglected in this phase. If we follow the model set by St.

Christopher's Hospice we can't go wrong. The reason for wanting to know more about the pattern of psychologic and social changes that occur is that this should enable us to identify people who are at risk in terms of their ultimate pain level and the behavior they exhibit when in pain. As psychiatrists and psychologists we are concerned not only with trying to lower the level of pain but we must also be involved in trying to help people come to terms with their disability, to cope with their pain if it cannot be completely relieved which is quite often the case. We need to look at these different age groups to find out what the patterns are.

In regard to the use of psychotropic drugs the literature is not sufficiently precise to allow their use with confidence. We need to be more precise about the indications for their use, and we also need to know more about the metabolism of these drugs in people who are in states of cachexia, or who are receiving potent drugs and who have a variety of physical problems including vomiting, and diarrhea, which may alter the normal metabolism of these drugs.

Finally, coming to psychologic treatments, my own view, like Dr. Saunders, is that psychiatrists usually are not there to treat cancer patients but are more likely to be involved in helping the doctors, nurses, and others who do the day-to-day treatments by counseling them and dealing with their own psychologic needs. One of the problems is that very few psychiatrists and psychologists will participate in this kind of work because the patients are very difficult to handle, and traditional training in psychiatry and psychology tends not to expose trainees to these types of problems. Therefore, we need to rectify this deficiency in our teaching program so that in the future psychiatrists and psychologists will play a more active role in managing patients with cancer pain. We also need to assess more extensively and precisely the therapies including individual psychotherapy, group therapy, family therapy, behavior modification, and biofeedback.

Bonica: Drs. Houde and Twycross, I would like you to discuss the proper use of systemic drugs for cancer pain, what new and better drugs might be developed and what else might be done for the better application of this general method of cancer pain control.

Raymond Houde

Department of Medicine, Memorial Sloan-Kettering Cancer Center, New York

I was glad to hear what Dr. Fink said about drugs, because most of the research that has been sponsored by the United States government has been supported by those agencies that have been concerned with drug abuse. In fact this is where we get most of our support. In terms of what we should do in the future, these fall into the three broad categories everyone has mentioned: education, training, and research. With respect to education it is quite obvious that there is a critical need to teach students and doctors how to use these drugs most effectively. Unfortunately, our international treaties have imposed a variety of constraints which have impaired the proper use of narcotics for cancer pain. The over-concern with the illicit traffic of drugs, for example, has had a serious impact on medical practice. We have to look at both sides of the coin: These drugs have particular pharmacologic properties which can be applied much more effectively to control pain in cancer. I agree with Dr. Saunders that we can control all pain of cancer with narcotics if we are willing to decrease consciousness. What we should be able to do is to achieve pain-relief but keep the patient as functional as possible within the capabilities of the consequences of their disease. This is what we should aim to do and this involves a lot more than just using analgesic drugs. Although our concern is with pain-relief, there are many other factors that impact on this, and the doctor must consider them in the total care of the patient. Narcotics don't just act on pain; they have other pharmacologic effects that must be considered. Moreover, the doctor may have to use adjuvant drugs in order to provide the patient with the most benefit.

Is there a need for new drugs? Obviously there is. We need new drugs that have different pharmacologic spectra. Not all patients are the same. There are some patients who tolerate one spectrum of pharmacologic activities of drugs and not another. For example, narcotic analgesics have many disadvantages in terms of some of their side effects; they produce constipation, but if the patient has diarrhea that is not a disadvantage but beneficial. In addition to their pain some cancer patients have intractable cough, which can be suppressed with narcotics. But then there are other patients who have different kinds of effects of their disease, and there you may need drugs of different spectra of activity.

Of the new drugs unrelated to narcotics, the new nonsteroidal anti-inflammatory drugs are extremely promising. What we do need to do is to look at them objectively. We have to design studies to look at them by methods scientifically acceptable and to make our decisions as to which drugs we wish to promote for the relief of pain on that kind of basis. Finally, we must acquire a better understanding of how drugs act in the body, of the physiology of pain, of drugs such as endorphins and to understand how best we can elaborate these endogenous antipain mechanisms.

Robert G. Twycross

The Churchill Hospital, Oxford, U.K.

I wish to discuss the problem of drugs for pain-relief under three headings: teaching, research, and political action. I will begin with political action. We are part of the International Association for the Study of Pain, which has helped us to come together and exchange information. We should help each other to make sure that in every country there are at least aspirin, codeine, and morphine available and the latter should be available for use both by mouth and by injection. Moreover, for patients who have some idiosyncratic disability we should have available at least one alternative to these three basic analgesics.

In regard to research, I agree with Dr. Houde. In teaching we must select the most important aspects of what we have been discussing. It is far more important that every nurse and every doctor should really understand that pain is a psychobiologic phenomenon or experience which is modulated by mood, meaning, culture, and many other factors. If the doctor and nurse appreciate these aspects of pain, he or she can do more for the patient in pain than if he or she is familiar with the latest information about A-delta and C-fibers, or the latest information about prostaglandins and endorphins. I am not against science, but we must give priority to those aspects that enable the doctor or nurse to help the patient most. The other point that should come out about teaching is that we cannot wait for all the clinical trials to be completed before we begin to use drugs. We know and can agree that certain drugs are better than others. We are agreed, for example, that partial agonists, like pentazozine, have little or no place in advanced cancer pain-relief. Broader aspects of teaching should also include that it is just as much a medical success to help a patient die in comfort as it is to cure him and see him walk out through the hospital door. The medical ethic, as I understand it, is not to preserve life at all costs but to sustain life when, from a biologic point of view, it is sustainable and worthwhile. Therefore the application of acute medical support systems and interventions with radical palliative methods that prolong the distress of dying rather than adding useful, worthwhile life should not be considered.

Bonica: Now I call upon Dr. Pannuti to comment about future needs and goals in oncology with emphasis on pain control.

F. Pannuti

Division of Oncology, Marcello Malpighi Hospital, Bologna, Italy

I am an oncologist, so I would like to give my point of view about some essential facts. First, what does the oncologist want in the future from society? We oncologists are looking for structures in which there are also present centers specializing in pain therapy. I want to make myself clear: I believe that in Pain Centers the oncologist is as important as the pain therapist in the management of pain of cancer. Oncologic structures mean a greater financial support from the government and society as a whole. We have to build schools for oncologists and pain therapists, and the wealthier nations have, in my opinion, to give this cultural heritage and make available the information presented at this conference and similar types of meetings, to underdeveloped countries.

Secondly, also we should want something new at the nurses' level. I believe that nurses should be good interpreters of the medical act, but to do this they must also develop their own role in their relationship with the patient. In this regard, I believe Rogers' description of the role of nurse is useful and I agree with it. Indeed we have already carried it out in Bologna, where nurses have become more cognizant of what they are doing and more autonomous toward the individual patient.

Another area where we oncologists can develop something new is in pharmacology. We must realize the difference between the pharmacology of analgesic drugs and the pharmacology of antitumoral drugs. I believe we should promote more extensive studies in stage 3, i.e., a precise check on new analgesic drugs compared with the traditional ones, in order to eliminate all those drugs that are not useful and to identify which new drugs are better than the traditional aspirin, codeine, and morphine. New and old antitumoral drugs constitute another important topic. As for the new ones, we oncologists should again require them to be studied preclinically, i.e., on animals not only to see whether or not they reduce tumor mass, but also to study their effectiveness in relieving pain. For example, currently we are testing MAP and comparing it with prostaglandins. We agree with Bonica that in addition to evaluating their anticancer efficacy the oncologic therapist should also monitor the signal symptoms such as pain and anorexia.

Still another level where something new can be foreseen is the one concerning the physician, but here the job is more complex. The physician should work in close relationship with the psychologist in order to be advised about the patient. After the oncologist has been at his job for many years he needs psychologic support for reasons given by Drs. Saunders and Bond. I believe the psychologist is important for modulating the physician-patient relationship. In regard to the patient-physician relationship we can act at two different levels: The first one is to ask ourselves whether or not we should tell the patient the truth about his or her disease. This will be determined by many considerations including the patient's personality, culture, traditional and social conditions. In my opinion, we must inform the patient whenever these considerations suggest it is to the best interest of the patient and family. The second important level is that physicians together with nurses must more and more keep the patient informed of what is happening. The last important point is that the physician must devise a therapeutic approach based on a comparison of other patients in a controlled way, i.e., by means of protocols and a data bank. In closing, I propose that Bonica and Ventafridda repeat this type of conference regularly every 2 or 3 years. Moreover, between each conference a permanent multidisciplinary commission should operate to get the proceedings published and to establish guidelines for interdisciplinary and international programs intended to improve the care of patients with cancer pain.

Leandro Gennari

Istituto Nazionale per lo Studio e la Cura Tumori, Milan, Italy

What can we do for the future? As regards the traditional therapies, I would say we cannot do more than what has been done already. Surgery has achieved its highest possibilities, if you take into account that to treat cancer and to avoid recurrence of the disease and pain, operations such as "hemicorporectomy" have been done. As for radiotherapy, we still have chances for the future. There is a lead that should be followed, which is further and more extensive radioimmunologic studies. The investigation of those antigenic substances, which are secreted by the tumor and found in the organism, are capable of giving signs that will make possible a very early diagnosis of the disease. This means that an early diagnosis allows not only a more appropriate and earlier surgical or radiation therapy, but equally important it means discovering the recurrence of the neoplastic process several months earlier than has been possible heretofore. Therefore, we can intervene with other methods to avoid the pain of advanced cancer.

As for chemotherapy, we are confronted by a great obstacle: that the lack of selectivity of the drugs at our disposal does not allow us to destroy the diseased cells and save the healthy tissue. We hope we can find a drug that has this selectivity or more drugs, so that we can study the best combination of drugs. Finally, I must say that chemotherapy can make a significant contribution not only in pain therapy but also in avoiding the development of pain when it is administered prophylactically after surgical removal of the tumor. There are documented cases of prolonged survival and of longer periods free from disease after surgical treatment of breast cancer or amputation of a limb for osteosarcoma followed by complementary chemotherapy.

Vittorio Ventafridda

Istituto Nazionale per lo Studio e la Cura Tumori, Milan, Italy

The struggle against pain can be carried out successfully provided that the oncologist also becomes involved in the treatment of pain. He or she becomes appropriately involved when he or she appreciates that pain is one of the most important aspects of cancer and assesses and collects it as one of the kinds of data that must be kept in the therapeutic files. I have seen dozens of protocols in the treatment of cancer, but pain is never taken into account or included in the protocol. Only when he or she has a quantitative dimension of the pain can he or she improve the strategy for its effective control.

Qualified persons must be trained for this task. The neurooncologists are among the most qualified persons to diagnose the pain and to help develop the most appropriate therapeutic strategy. Foley is a neurooncologist in a large cancer center, and she has shown us in a simple way the possibilities of achieving results. Those who work in pain therapy, whether anesthesiologists, neurosurgeons, or pharmacologists, must also be oncologists. There cannot be an anesthesiologist who does pain therapy in oncology, just because he does blocks. He must also know oncology!

Another important point is the development of rehabilitation programs: The physical disability is a very important factor which contributes to the patient's pain and suffering, and rehabilitation therapy gives wonderful results in these patients.

Clinical trials to evaluate analgesic agents must be controlled and carried out by well-established conditions and criteria. We also must develop pain-control departments or teams in cancer centers and institutes which are able to effectively treat all types of cancer pain. The team should include persons with experience and expertise to carry out the various therapeutic modalities which we have discussed here. In these centers, it should also be possible to administer narcotics to outpatients as well as inpatients under controlled conditions. This will require support from social workers and other health professionals.

Finally, such centers should carry out studies of new systemic analgesics which provide maximum relief with few or no side effects. There is a special need for the availability of an effective oral narcotic preparation in Italy.

John Bonica

Department of Anesthesiology, University of Washington, Seattle, Washington

It is clear that much needs to be done to improve the care of patients with pain of advanced cancer. I hope that the discussions and interactions of the past 4 days will help all of us to improve the care of these patients. Moreover, the publication of these proceedings should also help many other health professionals who could not attend and who have the serious responsibility of pain control and total management of patients with advanced cancer.

I hope I reflect the opinion of many, if not most of you, when I state that the goals and objectives of this symposium as enunciated at the beginning have been achieved. Indeed, the success of this conference is beyond my most optimistic expectations. For this I wish to express my sincerest thanks and appreciation, as well as those of the Scientific Program Committee, the Local Arrangements Committee, and the Floriani Foundation, to all the speakers and participants. Much of the success of the symposium has also been due to the interest, attentiveness, patience, and persistence of the audience. Despite the unique tourist attractions of Venice, most of the registrants have remained in attendance until the very end of each session.

I wish to thank again Cardinal Luciani and the various governmental officials for their moral support; special thanks are also due to the five agencies that auspiced this symposium.

Finally, I cannot adequately express the thanks and appreciation and indeed gratitude to the Floriani Foundation on behalf of all the participants and speakers and especially the millions of patients with cancer pain throughout the world who are suffering needlessly and hopefully will be helped by the information presented here. The foresight and generosity and warm friendship of Ing. and Mrs. Virgilio Floriani have made possible this highly successful symposium, this uniquely outstanding meeting facility, and the very elegant social activities that have been sponsored by Mr. and Mrs. Floriani. In this regard I thank them also on behalf of the wives of the speakers as well as others who took advantage of the opportunity to participate in these social activities.

Ing. and Mrs. Floriani have initiated what I believe will prove to be a long-range movement which will have a major impact on the care of patients with pain of advanced cancer. I hope that this highly successful international, multidisciplinary cancer pain symposium will be the first of many such meetings that will continue to provide a forum for the exchange of new information that eventually will have a beneficial effect on these patients.

I hope that in the near and remote future, federal, provincial, and municipal governmental agencies will support more research, better education, and better patient care. Moreover, we hope that this symposium will stimulate physicians and other health professionals, but especially oncologists to include the teaching of students and graduate doctors in providing optimal cancer pain control. The ultimate goal of these efforts is to provide people everywhere with better health care in the prevention and treatment of cancer and the associated pain.

I hope that the torch lighted by Ing. and Mrs. Floriani will be readily taken over and carried in the future not only by federal agencies but also private foundations in making possible this type of intense multidisciplinary international meeting on the subject of cancer pain.

Subject Index

A-delta fibers, 14, 17, 18, 305, 484, 673
  fast or slow, 478
Abdomen tumors in, 169
Ablation with alcohol of pituitary, 599
Ablative surgery, 180–181
Abnormalities, respiratory, 434
Abscess, 160
Acetylsalicylic acid, 147
Acidosis, metabolic, 203
ACS (American Cancer Society), 110
Actinomycin D, 142–143
Acupuncture, 228
  use of, 516
Addiction
  creation of, 663
  narcotic, 491
  and tolerance, 630-632
Adenopathies
  metastatic, 168–170
  retroperitoneal, 137
  supraclavicular, 137
Administration, efficient, 650-651
ADR, *see* Adriamycin
Adrenal
  cortex, 141
  glands, 149
  -hypothalamic axis, 156
Adrenalectomy, 150, 151, 153
  bilateral, 181
Adriamycin (ADR), 142, 143, 182, 183, 199, 205
Agents, anti-inflammatory, 514
Agitation, 217
Alanine aminotransferase (SGPT), 200
Alcohol, 362
  absolute, 364, 383
  block, 304
    technique of, 359-368
  blood levels of, 371
  neuroadenolysis, 153
Algogenic substances, 16, 17, 19
Allopurinol, 141, 200
Alpha-2-globuline, 211
American Cancer Society (ACS), 110
Amphetamine, 278
Amputation, rectal, 146
Anabolic effect, 160, 211

Analgesia
  behavioral, 487
  brain-stimulation, 487
  central nervous system mechanisms of, 20–26
  continuous, epidural, 334–335
  in cordotomy, open, 450
  electrical stimulation in, 31–32
  hypnotic, 227
  maximum, 665
  narcotic-like, 280
  obstetric, 334
  opioid and stimulation-induced, 33
  overview of, 619–635
  side effects of, 622
  stimulation-induced and opioid, similarities between, 33
Analgesics
  differences among, 267–268
  expectations in, 633–634
  league table, 299
  narcotic, 263–273, 627–630
    choice of, 265–267
    clinical pharmacology of, 264–265
    route of administration of, 268–269
  nonnarcotic, 255–262
    adverse effects of, 258
    efficacy of, 259
    site and mode of action of, 259
  and related drugs
    in chest and brachial plexus, 561–563
    in visceral and perineal pain, 593–595
  simple, 534
  systemic, 533
  tolerance, 269
  use of, 624–625
Anesthesia
  dolorosa, 407
  endotracheal, 454
  general, 518
  nitrous oxide-oxygen, 224
Anesthesiologists, 129
Anesthetic
  blocks, regional, 315
  local, 314, 360, 456, 457, 464, 586

SUBJECT INDEX

Androgen, 154, 560
Anger, 48–49
Anticancer modalities, 115
Antidepressant, tricyclic, 279–280, 491, 516
Antigen, CEA, 62
Antimetabolite, 143
Antimitotic drugs, 139
Antinociception
  biochemistry of, 31–41
  neuroanatomy and neurophysiology of, 31–41
Antipyrimidin, 142
Anxiety, 47–48
  chronic, 47
  overt, 216
Apex of chest, 566
Approach
  multidisciplinary, 664
  optimal integrator, 665
Architecture, imaginative use of, in hospices, 649–650
Arteriovenous shunts, 186
Arthralgia, 125
Ascites, 201
L-Asparaginase, 144
Aspartate aminotransferase (SGOT), 200
Aspirin, 625, 627
Atrophy, disuse
  of arm, 124
  of humerus, 70
Atropine, 197
Audio-biofeedback signal, 235
Autonomic
  arousal, 240
  responsivity, 239, 240

Bacillus prodigious, filtered extracts of, 195
Barbotage, 333
Behaviors, maladaptive, 231
Benzodiazepines, 219, 282
Beta-blocking agent(s), 186, 200
Beta-sympathetic blockade, 225
Biofeedback
  procedures, 235–236
  treatment, results of experimental, 239–240
Biomedical model of sickness, 45
Bleeding, intestinal, 175–176

Bleomycin, 142, 143, 169, 528
Block(s)
  axillary, 319
  brachial plexus, 572
  caudal, 318
  celiac plexus, 318, 357–371
  diagnostic, 537, 597–598
  epidural (lumbar or caudal), 598
  extradural, 571
  ganglion
    gasserian, 350, 537, 542
    stellate, 315–316
  intrathecal, 402
  nerve, *see* Nerve block(s)
  neurolytic, 306, 537
    extradural, 585
    in perineal pain, *see* Perineal pain, neurolytic block(s) in
  paravertebral, 571–572
  prognostic, 537, 579
  subarachnoid, 598–599
    and extradural, 325–337
    neurolytic, 569–571
  subdural, 571, 585
  sympathetic, 311–319, 572
    cervicothoracic, 561
    lumbar, 317–318, 598
    volume dependent, 316
  technique of caudal epidural, 603
  therapeutic, 598–599
  vagus, 573
Body chart, 298
Bone
  fractures, 137
  marrow, 143
    suppression, 134
  metastases, 140
  pain, diffuse, 137
  scan, 127
  tumor infiltration, 63–66
  tumors, 171
Brachial plexus, 168, 172
  blocks, 572
  compression of, 137
  fibrosis of, 125
    postradiation, 126
  pain, 571
Breast self-examination (BSE), 110–111
Brompton cocktail, 272, 291–300, 628
  formulation of, 295
  side effects of, 296
BSE (breast self-examination), 110–111

Bupivacaine, 315, 319

C-fibers, 14, 15, 17, 305, 478, 484
Cachexia, 178
Caevomepromazine, 301
Calcemia, 142
Calcitonin, 212–213
Cancer, *see also* Carcinoma
  advanced
    breast, 153–155, 160–161
    chemotherapy and whole body hyperthermia in treatment of, 195–213
    clear-cell kidney, 152
    hypnotherapy in, 223–229
    pain of, *see* Pain of advanced cancer
    percutaneous thermocoagulation of gasserian ganglion in treatment of, 463–468
    prostate, 150–151
  breast, 137, 199, 212, 381, 386
    bone metastases of, 142
    estrogens in, 148
    hormone dependency in, 141
    incidence of pain in, 145
    MAP in, 155
    remission in, 136
  bronchopulmonary, oat-cell type, 142, 559
  cost of, total, 111
  development of, personality in, 81–83
  emotion in, consequences of physical treatment upon, 85, 86
  emotional consequences, 216–218
    effects of, 82–83
  epidermoid, 142, 519
  esophageal, 568
  fear of, 224
  hospitalization, 111
  ovarian, 133, 141
  pain, 1–12, 465–466
    advanced, *see* Pain of advanced cancer
    behavioral aspects of, 45–56, 665
    beliefs of patients and, 51–53
    blocks with local anesthetics in treatment of, 311–322
    central gray stimulation for control of, 487–492
    chemotherapy in, *see* Chemotherapy in cancer pain
    of chest and brachial plexus, *see* Chest and brachial plexus, cancer pain of
    children with, 89–97
    compression of nerve roots and nerve trunks and plexuses and, 121
    compression of pain-sensitive structures in, 60
    control, current status of, 4
    cordotomy, open, in treatment of, 449–452
    current evaluation in, 668
    diagnosis, considerations for, 53–54
    diagnostic tools, use of appropriate, 62
    early treatment of, 63
    education, lack of, 8
    emotional aspects of, 81–87
    emotional changes in patients with, 84–85
    facial, 467
    follow-up in, 503
    of head and neck, *see* Head and neck, cancer pain of
    hypnotherapy for management of, 227–228
    implication for, 39–41
    importance of, 1–11
    incidence of, 2–3
    interest, lack of, 7–8
    local, 62
    magnitude of, 1–2
    management, recommendation for improvement of, 9–11
    mechanisms of, 121–129, 664
    mortality in, 1–2
    myelotomy in, 445
    narcotic analgesics in, 8–9
    necrosis of mucous membranes and other pain-sensitive structures and, 123
    nerve peripheral, and dorsal column stimulation for relief of, 499–507
    nerve block with neurolytic solutions for pelvic visceral, 597–600
    nursing aspects of, 103–112
    obstruction and, 122
    occlusion of blood vessels and, 122–123
    phenol subarachnoid rhizotomy for treatment of, 339–346

Cancer, pain *(contd.)*
    physiologic and psychologic effects of, 3–4
    postrhizotomy and, 440
    prevalence in, 59–60
    psychologic aspects of, 45–56, 81–87
    psychologic intervention in child, 93–97
    psychophysiologic control of, 231–243
    psychotropic drugs in treatment of, 285–289
    referred, 62
    relief, complete, 458
    relief, reasons for inadequate, 5–9
    research, lack of, 5–6
    severe, 453
    site, examination of, 62
    social effects of, 3–4, 99–102
    sociologic aspects of, 103–112
    spinal posterior rhizotomy and commissural myelotomy in treatment of, 439–447
    syndromes, 59–75
    systemic drugs for, 672
    therapy, considerations for, 53–54
    transcutaneous nerve stimulation in, 509–515
    tumefaction and swelling and, 123
    tumor infiltration of blood vessels and nervous structures, 121–122
    tumor invasion in, 60
    tumor invasion of bone and, 121
    unrelated to cancer or cancer therapy, 60
  patterns of, 670
  of prostate, 137, 141, 145
  rectal, 176
  recurrent, 490
  rehabilitation programs for, 247
  -related pain research, 670
  services for patients with, 658–661
  skeletal, 568
  stomach, 145
  terminal, 449, 591
  testicular, 133, 137
  therapy
    multi-step, 196
    pain syndromes associated with, 123–125
  thyroid advanced, 152
  type of, 330
Cancer Facts and Figures, 110
Cancer Nursing, 108
Cannabis, 277
  derivatives, 282
Carbamazepine, 464
Carcinoma, *see also* Cancer
  of biliary tract, 169
  of breast, 168, 181, 203, 375, 567, 575
  bronchial, oat cell, 142, 559
  bronchogenic, 133
  of colon, 203
  embryonal, 559
    of testicle, 133
  endometrial, 141, 155
    advanced, 151, 155
  epidermoid, 133
  epipharynx, 470
  gastric, 203
  gastrointestinal, 133, 199
  hormonodependent, 141
  intraperitoneal, 342, 345
  of large intestine, 175, 182
  of larynx, 470
  of lung, 567, 575
  pancreatic, 199
  prostate, 155, 171, 181
    hypophysectomy for relief of pain of, 393–403
  rectal, 182
  renal, 133, 155
  of sigmoid, 177
  of stomach, 175
  of thyroid, 133
  uterine, 182
Carcinomatosis, meningeal, 64, 69
Care
  community, 660
  home, program, 646
    schemes of, 662
    team of hospice, 647
  hospice, 637–652
    general principles of, 643–652
  immediate, 252
  inpatient, 646
  long-term, 649, 662
  methods of, 643
  primary, 662
  terminal, 589, 644, 652, 656, 661, 668–670

SUBJECT INDEX

teaching in all aspects of, 649
   from viewpoint of National Health
      Service, 655–663
Castration, 153, 181, 399
CAT (computerized transaxial
   tomography), 62, 208, 212, 577
Cauda equina, 171
Causalgia, 17
CDDP (cis-platinum), 143
CEA antigen, 62
Central gray stimulation, 517
   results in, 488–490
   technique of, 488–490
Central nervous system (CNS), 170
   subsystems of, 20
Centre median, 477, 478, 479
Cephalalgia, 170
Cerebral cortex in advanced cancer pain,
   77–80
Cerebrospinal fluid (CSF), 62
Chemotherapy, 674
   of chest and brachial plexus, 557–558
   cyclic, 134
   of head and neck, 526–531
   intra-arterial, 137
   local, intrapleural, 558
   regional, 558
   systemic, 528
Chest and brachial plexus, cancer pain of
   analgesics and related drugs in, 561–
      563
   bone metastasis, 556
   chemotherapy in, 557–558
   hormone therapy in, 559–560
   mediastinal compression in, 556
   in metastases, 555
   nerve blocks in, 565–574
   neurosurgery in, 575–584
   oncologic therapy in, 555–560
   radiation in, 556–557
Chest X-ray, 577
Children with cancer, pain in, 89–97
Chlorocresol, 326, 327, 329
Chlorpromazine, 219, 281
Cingulotomy, 418, 548
Cingulumotomy, 518, 616
Clergy, role of, 249
Clinical
   considerations in endocrine therapy for
      relief of pain, 145–148
   drug tolerance, 148

pharmacologists, 129
team, management by, 644
Clock watchers, 109, 269
CNS (central nervous system), 20, 170
CNV (contingent negative variation), 241
Coagulation, 431
   RF, 472
Cocaine, 294–295, 279
Codeine, 271
Coley's toxins, 195
Colic, renal, 139
Colostomy, 176
Commitment, cost of, 651–652
Complete remission (CR), 132, 133, 135,
   136, 158
Complications
   in celiac plexus block, 368–371
   in neurolytic blocks in perineal pain,
      605
   in subarachnoid neurolysis, 331–332
Compression
   brainstem, 65
   epidural spinal cord, 66, 69, 126
   mediastinal and chest and brachial
      plexus, 556
   nerve root, 65, 575
   radicular, 343
Concentration, tumoricidal (C), 134
Considerations, anatomic, in medullary
   tractotomy, 455
Constipation, 630
Contingent negative variation (CNV),
   241
Conurbations, 662
Coracoid process, 188
Cordotomy, 20–21, 58, 182, 328,
   613–615
   anterior percutaneous cervical, 433
   anterolateral, 169, 332, 409–412,
      579–580
   bilateral, 613
      percutaneous cervical, 433
   cervical, 411
   lateral percutaneous cervical, 428–432
   open, 409–411
      analgesia in, 450
      results in, 450
      in treatment of cancer pain, 449–452
   percutaneous, 411–412
      results in, 432–435
      side effects and complications in, 432

Cordotomy *(contd.)*
  stimulation technique, 430
  technique of puncture, 428
  percutaneous cervical, 425–437
    anatomic considerations in, 425–427
    conclusion in, 435–436
    technical considerations in, 427–428
  posterior percutaneous, 435
  spinothalamic, 342
Corticosteroids, 144, 553, 560, 625–627
Cortisol, 156
CR, *see* Complete remission
Creatinine, 200
Critical mass, 139
Cryodestruction, 153
Cryohypophysectomy, 397, 399
  indications for, 394
CSF (cerebrospinal fluid), 62, 127
CT scan, 62, 127, 208, 212, 577
Cultural comparison in pain manifestation, 52–53
Cure, 133
Cyanosis, intermittent, 187
Cyclophosphamide, 142–143, 212
Cyproterone acetate (CP), 150
Cystectomy, total, 170
Cystitis, 143
Cytology of CSF, 127

Deafferentation, 494–496
  chronic, 494
Death, peaceful, 650
Decarbazine, 142, 143
Deltopectoral groove, 188
Denervation, trigeminal, 544
Denial, mental mechanism of, 217
Dentate ligament, 429, 435, 580
Depression, 48, 251, 576, 624
  incidence of, 666
Deprivation, sensory, 418
Dermatomes, thoracic, 402
Desoxyribonucleic acid (DNA), 143
DES-P (di-ethylstilbestrol diphosphate), 148, 150, 151
Deterioration, mental, 548
Diabetes insipidus, 387, 599
Diagnostic
  blocks, 305, 308, 357
  tests, special, 127

Diamorphine (heroin), 268, 271, 291, 627, 631–632
  versus morphine, 292–294
Diathermy machine, Siemens 608
  Ultratherm, 197
DIC (disseminated intravascular coagulation), 201
Dietary aspects, 248
Di-ethylstilbestrol diphosphate (DES-P), 148, 150, 151
Digestive tract, 143
Disability, idiosyncratic, 672
Disarticulation, 178
Discharge
  neuronal unit, 475–478
  planning, 252
Discussion, frequent, 645
Disease,
  definition of, 49
  degenerative disc, 66
  epidural, 65
  terminal malignant, 662
Disseminated intravascular coagulation (DIC), 201
Disturbances, psychic, 416
DNA (desoxyribonucleic acid), 143
Doctor, family, 659
L-DOPA, 154
Dorsal column and peripheral nerve stimulation, 499–507
Dose-related toxicity, acute, 264
Doxorubicin, 142
Drugs
  adjuvant, 672
  anti-inflammatory, 625
  nonsteroidal anti-inflammatory, 625, 672
  psychotropic, 514, 671
DTT, 141
Duborimycin, 142
Dysesthesia, 124
  postoperative, 445
Dysfunction
  autonomic, 65
  bowel and bladder, 66
  cranial nerve, 64
  peripheral nociceptive, 124
  spinal-cord, 65
  visceral, 126
Dyspnea, 142
Dysrhythmias, cardiac, 200

SUBJECT INDEX

Dystrophy, sympathetic, 124, 126, 187, 312, 561

Ectopic beats, 200
　ventricular, 203
Edema, 187
　cerebral, 170
　peritumoral, 139
Ego-strength scores, 236
Electroanalgesia, 509
Electrode(s), 500–502, 510, 513
　migration of epidural, 505
　stability, 504
Electrolytes, serum, 198
EM (explanatory model), 51–52
Emotional
　aspects of cancer pain, 81–87
　changes in patients with cancer pain, 84–85
　disturbances and pain, treatment of, 218–222
　interactions, 221
Encoding and conduction, peripheral, 13–16
Endocrine therapy and pain relief, 150–161
Endomorphines, 228
Endoprosthesis, 187
　metallic, 191
α-Endorphin, 36
β-Endorphin, 36, 57, 378
Endorphins, 378, 665, 673
Enkephalins, 34, 36, 38, 503
Epidural
　continuous analgesia, 587
　neurolysis, 334
Epigastrium, 201
Epipharynx, carcinoma of, 470
Epithelium, digestive, 140
Erysipelas, 195
Estradiol, 156
Estrogen receptors, 181
Estrogens, 137, 148, 149, 154
Euphoria-withdrawal swings, 278
Euthenasia, active, 591–592
Evaluation, general, in commissural myelotomy, 444–446
　psychologic and psychosocial, 127
　of therapeutic modalities, 127
Ewing sarcoma, 212

Examination, 126–127
　electrophysiologic, 172
Explanatory model (EM), 51–52
Expression of despair, 217
Extracellular fluids, 198
Extralymphonodal component, 168

Fasciotomy, anterolateral, 186
Fear of death, 220, 225
Feedback
　combined, 232
　electroencephalographic (EEG), 232
　theta, 232
Femur, 125
Fibrillation, ventricular, 205
Fibrosarcoma
　recurrent, 203
　of thigh, 187
Fibrosis
　of lumbosacral plexus, 74, 125
　radiation, 169
　of brachial plexus, 73, 125–126
Flowmeter, 186
5-Fluorouracil, 142, 182, 183, 199
Follow-up, bereavement, 648
Foot drop, 186
Fracture(s)
　of bone, 137
　pathologic, 64
　of vertebra, 147
Frozen shoulder, 124
FSH, plasma levels of, 156

G_0 and G_1 phase, 134
Gamma-glutamyl-transpeptidase (gamma-GT), 200
Ganglion(s)
　dorsal, 3rd, 190
　gasserian, 168
　　percutaneous thermocoagulation of, in treatment of pain in advanced cancer, 463–468
　　technique of blocking, 350–352
　lumbar, 190
　stellate, 188, 190
　trigeminal, 471
Ganglionectomy, 615
GH, see Growth hormone
Glioma, recurrent malignant, 203

Glossopharyngeal nerve, *see* Nerve(s), glossopharyngeal
Goals
 future, 664
 and future needs in oncology, 673
Group and family therapy, 221–222
Group III fibers, 14, 17
Growth hormone (GH), 156, 396, 397
 assay, 397

Hallucinations, sensory, 430
Hartman's operation, 176
Head and neck
 cancer pain of
  adjuvant factors in, 521
  analgesics and related drugs in, 533–535
  bone invasion in, 520
  chemotherapy in, 526–531
  functional problems in, 521
  nerve blocks in, 537–542
  neurosurgery in, 543–552
  oncologic therapy in, 523–531
  pathogenesis of, 519–522
  problems in, 519–522
  psychological problems in, 521–522
  radiotherapy in, 523–524
  surgery in, 524–526
 tumors of, 145, 167–168
Health professionals, 245–247
Heart-lung machine, 185
Hematopoietic system, 143
Hematosarcoma, 142, 144
Hemorrhage
 acute, 203
 intratumoral, 212
Heparin, 143
Herpes
 labialis, 203
 zoster, 125
History of pain complaint, 126
Hodgkin's disease, 144
Hopelessness, 221
Hormone(s)
 assay, growth, 395
 dependence, 148, 149
 interference, 148–150
 pituitary trophic, 149
 sensitive tumors, 145
 sensitivity, 149
 sexual, 149
 synthetic, 141
 therapy, 148–150
Hospice, 588, 590
 care, 637–643
  general principles of, 643–652
  concept, nature and management of terminal pain and, 637–653
 development of, 643
 home, hospital or, 660–661
 home care team, 647
Hospital, district general, 658
Humerus, 125
 disuse atrophy of, 70
Hydroxyzine, 301
Hypercalcemia, 142, 213
Hyperesthesia, 124
Hypernephroma, 141
 metastasis, 180
Hypertonicity, 333
 of muscle, 562
Hypnosis, 127, 225
Hypnotic susceptibility, 234
Hypochondriasis, 85
Hypochondrium, 170
Hypogastrium, 169
Hypopharynx, 168
Hypophysectomy, 150, 151, 161, 171, 581–582, 586, 616
 chemical, 373–391
  material and methods of, 382–385
  mechanism of pain relief in, 376–380
  pain-relief in, 385–386
  results in, 374–375, 385–387
  side effects and complications of, 375–376, 386–387
  technical aspects of, 373–374
  technique of, 382–385
 clinical criteria for response in, 395
 radiologic, 181
 rationale, 393–394
 surgical, 181, 381
  technique in, 395–396
Hypophysis, 154
Hypotension, 199, 200
Hypothalamotomy, posteromedial, 481–485
Hypothalamus, 377, 497
 posterior, 481

Illness
 behaviors, abnormal, 3

definition of, 49
long-term, 643
Inadequacy, 216
Incontinence, urinary, 182
Indole anthranylic acid and phenyl propionic acid derivatives, 257–258
Infection, 520
Infiltration, meningeal, 137
Infusion
    endoarterial antiblastic, 187
    hepatic, 182
Inherent low susceptibility, 133
Intrathecal block, 402

17-Keto-steroid metabolites, endogenous, 156
Kidney, 143, 361
    puncture, 370

Lactate dehydrogenase (LDH), 200
Laetrile, 53
Laminectomy, 171
Laparotomy, 177
Large bowel, 169
Larynx, carcinoma of, 470
Learning, 329
Lethality, 134
Leukemia, 137, 144
    acute, 137, 142
    chronic myeloid, 144
Leukocytosis, 201
Leukotomy, unilateral extensive, 548
LH, plasma levels of, 156
Lidocaine, 200, 205
Life-expectancy, 576
    short, 582–583
Lifestyle, modification of, 633
Ligament, dentate, 429, 435, 580
β-Lipoprotein, 34–36
Lobotomy, saline, 582–583
LSD, 277
Lumbalgia, 139
Lumbosacral plexus, 170
    fibrosis, 125
Lymph node metastasis, 169, 520
Lymphedema, 125
    of arm, 137
Lymphomas, 132, 137, 519

McGill Pain Questionnaire (MPQ), 45–46, 237, 239
Management, pain and symptom, 661
Mania, serotonin, 517
Mannitol, 186
MAP, *see* Medroxyprogesterone acetate
Mastectomy, 124, 146
Maximum tolerable dose (MTD), 157
Meaning, search for, 651–652
Mechanisms
    endogenous anti-pain, 672
    sympathetic reflex, 315
Medication, adjuvant, 630
Medroxyprogesterone acetate (MAP), 145, 149–154, 211
    mechanism of action of, 156
    results
        with high doses, 157–161
        with low doses, 156–157
Melanoma, 142, 143, 187
    of limbs, 186
Melphalan, 142
Meningeal barrier, 141
Meningitis, 142
Menopause, 149
Mental state of patient, 255
Metastases, 597
    in arachnoid, 171
    to base of skull, 63–64
        bone, 62, 140, 142, 203, 212
        and chest and brachial plexus, 557
    to C_7-T_1, 65
    cerebral, 170
    to clivus, 64
    distant, 177
    epidural, 171
    extracerebral, 171
    hepatic, 142, 146, 169
    to L_1, 65
    to lung, 203
    lymph node, 520
        aortic, 169
        hypogastric, 169
        inguinal, 169
        neck, 525
        sacral, 169
    osseous, 132, 171
    osteoblastic, 171
    osteolytic, 132, 171
    pulmonary, 141, 178, 555
    sacral, 65–66
    skeletal, 136, 153

Metastases *(contd.)*
  sphenoid-sinus, 64
  to vertebral bodies, 64–65
Metencephalin, 378
Methods of relief, 645
Methotrexate, 142–143, 528
Methotrimeprazine, 594
Methyl-glyoxal, 144
Microscope, operating, 454, 455, 580
Micturition, 427
Minnesota Multiphasic Personality Inventory (MMPI), 246
Misulban, 144
Mithotane, 141
Mithramycin, 142
Mitomycin, 142, 182
Mitosis, 140, 143
Mitotic index, 140
MMPI (Minnesota Multiphasic Personality Inventory), 246
Molten paraffin, 205
Morbidity, 473, 537
  long, 648
Moricca's technique, 153, 373
Morphine, 278, 627, 631–632
  versus diamorphine, 292–294
  oral preparations, 589
  sulfate, 268
  suppositories, 628
Mortality, 544, 545
  rate, 186, 466, 517
MPQ (McGill Pain Questionnaire), 45–46, 237, 239
Mucositis, 125, 521
  intestinal, 135
  oral, 135
Mukuliecz's operation, 176
Multichannel monitoring system, 186
Multidisciplinary team management, 127–129
Multiple myeloma, 137
Muscle
  anterior scalene, 188
  biceps, 188
  external oblique, 190
  -hypertonicity, 562
  internal oblique, 190
  major pectoralis, 188
  omohyoid, 188
  pectoralis minor, tendinous insertion of, 188
  psoas, 190
  rectus, 190
  sternocleidomastoid, 188
  transversus abdominis, 190
  weakness of, 434
Myalgia, 125
Myelitis, transverse, 172
Myelogram, preoperative, 577
Myelopathy, radiation, 74, 125
Myelotomy(ies), 615
  commissural, 414–415, 443–446
    and spinal posterior rhizotomy, 439–447
  complete, 444
  conventional, 443–444
  stereotactic, 444
Myocardium, 143
Myodil, 428
Myography, cisternal and lumbar, 127

Nabilone, 282
Narcotic(s), 534, 576, 593–594
  agonists-antagonists, 270–271
  high-potency, 271
  low-potency, 271
  proper use of, 672
  side effects of, 588
National Cancer Institute (NCI), 6–7
National Health Service (NHS), 655–656
NCI (National Cancer Institute), 6–7
Neck, *see also* Head and neck
  dissection, radical, 124
  pain, 65
Necrosis of bone
  aseptic, 125
  radiation, 74
Needs, estimates of, in National Health Service, 656–658
Nefopam, 258
Neoplasms, endocrine-sensitive, 616
Nephropathy, 141
Nerve(s), *see also* Nerve block(s)
  endings, stimulation of mucosal and submucosal, 519
  glossopharyngeal, 349, 467, 516
    percutaneous differential radio-frequency rhizotomy of, 469–473
    thermorhizotomy of, 465
    and vagus blocking technique, 352–353
  intercostal, 572

mandibular, 350
    and maxillary blocking technique, 352
  peripheral, stimulation of, 500–502
  transections, 17
  trigeminal, 347, 349, 457, 516
  stimulation, transcutaneous, 509–515
    of peripheral and dorsal column, 499–507
Nerve block(s)
  of chest and brachial plexus, 565–574
  complications of, 309
  cranial, 347–355
    anatomic considerations in, 347–349
    clinical considerations in, 349–350
    neurolytic, 353
  epidural or lumbar somatic, 369
  in head and neck, 537–542
  historical perspective in, 303–304
  introduction to, 303–310
  with neurolytic solutions for pelvic and visceral cancer pain, 597–600
  requisites for optimal results in, 307–309
  side effects of, 309
  somatic, 318–320
  sympathetic, *see* Block(s), sympathetic
Nervous system, 143
Neuralgia
  glossopharyngeal, 469
  post-herpetic, 73, 135, 136, 513, 514 573
  pudendal, 441
  trigeminal, 469
    idiopathic, 463
Neuraxis, 124, 125
Neurectomy, 611–612
  or sensory rhizotomy, 578–579
Neuritis, carcinomatous, 311
Neuroleptic(s), 285
  threshold, 261
Neurolysis
  epidural, 334
  intrathecal, 328–331
  subarachnoid, 325–333
Neurolytic blocks, *see* Block(s), neurolytic
Neuroma, 17, 18
Neuromata, 124
Neurons, dorsal horn, 20–23
Neurooncologists, 674

Neuropathy(ies)
  peripheral, 72
  postsurgical, 124
Neurophysiologic map, 457
Neurosurgery
  in chest and brachial plexus, 575–584
  in visceral and perineal pain, 611–618
Neurotomy, extradural preganglionic, 466
Neurotransmitters, 32–33
NHS (National Health Service), 655–656
Nitrosourea(s), 137, 141
Nociception, neurophysiology of, 13–29
Nociceptive system, peripheral, 126
Nociceptors, 14–16
  chemical excitation and sensitization of, 16–17
  cutaneous, 15
  muscle, 15
  polymodal, 15
  visceral, 15–16
Non-parametric tests, 240
Numbness, 125
Nurse(s), role of, 250
  order sheet, 251–253
Nursing
  history, 251
  skilled and experienced team, 645
Nutritionists, 248

Objective improvement (OI), 132
Obstruction, intestinal, 175
Oncologist, 667
Oncology
  future needs and goals in, 673
  teams, 128
Operations, trigeminal, 543–544
Opiate(s), 203, 205, 264
  endogenous, 517
  system, 582
  withdrawal, 277
Opioids, 264
  endogenous, discovery of, 34–37
Opium, 627
Orchiectomy, 137–150
Oropharynx, 168
Orthostatic hypotension, 280
Osteomyelitis, 520
Osteoradionecrosis, 525
Osteosarcoma, 187

SUBJECT INDEX

Ovariectomy, 148, 149, 181, 212
Oxyprenolol, 200

PAG, see Periaqueductal gray
Pain, 368, 375, 405, 407, 562
  abdominal, lumbar, and inguinal, 342–343
  acupuncture for, 516
  of advanced cancer, 664; see also Cancer pain
  anticancer drugs in, 131–138
  cerebral cortex in, 77–80
  endocrine therapy for relief of, 145–165
  introduction to management of, 115–129
  oncologic chemotherapy in, 139–144
  percutaneous thermocoagulation of gasserian ganglion in, 463–468
  techniques of managing, 277–278
  anti-, endogenous, mechanisms, 672
  after anticancer therapy, 573
  assessment of, 620–623
  back, 137
  behavior, 20
    and drug dependence, 269–270
  behavioral aspects of, 671
  bilateral, 487
    lower limb, 451
  bone, 343, 567, 625
    diffuse, 137
  brachial plexus, 571
  breakthrough, 631
  burning, 124, 477, 538
  cancer, see Cancer pain
  in celiac plexus block, 369
  centers, 405
  central, 410
    mechanism of, 119
  central nervous system, mechanism of, 20–26
  cephalic, 413
    medullary tractotomy for, 453–462
  cervical, 413
  chest, severe, 565
  in chest and brachial plexus, see Chest and brachial plexus, cancer pain of
  in children with cancer, 89–97
  chronic, 128, 666, 668, 669
    general emotional effects of, 83–84
  mechanisms for, 16–20, 116–121
  peripheral mechanism in, 116–119
  psychologic mechanisms in, 119–121
  syndrome, 493, 513
  colicky, acute, 146
  complaints, 50, 126
    clarification of, 61
    fresh, of, 634
  complete relief of, 411
  consequences of staff-patient interactions and, 86–87
  contemporary theories of, 45
  control
    in cordotomy, 580
    in drug dependence, 631
    experience sharing in, 642
    methods for, 623
    theory, 509
  deafferentation, 517
  depersonalization, 228
  diagnostic and therapy team in, 129
  distancing, 288
  and drug tolerance, clinical, 148
  duration of, 657
  emotional, 466
  epicritic, 475, 495
  in esophageal cancer, 568
  fear of, 624
  fibers, 426, 427
  habit, 120
  heat, threshold of, 15
  and hormone therapy, 148–150
  incidence of, 639–642, 664–665
  information, peripheral encoding and conduction of, 13–16
  intensity of, 620
  intractable, 481
    relief of, 485
    stereotaxic thalamolaminectomy and posteromedial hypothalmotomy for relief of, 475–485
  lancinating, 124, 125
  lower limb, 343
  in lung carcinoma, 567
  magnitude of, 639–642, 664–665
  and MAP, 155–156
  mechanisms of, 669
  memory of, 416, 634
  mission of, 526
  modification of pathologic process, 623
  on movement, 633
  neck, 65

on neoplasms, effects of, 201
neurolytic blocks in perineal, 601–609
  complications of, 605–608
  material and methods in, 603–605
  results in, 605
neurophysiology of, 13–29
neurosurgery in visceral and perineal, 611–618
non-neoplastic, 147
organic, 91
palliative surgery for, 181
paroxysmal, 543
pathways, interruption of, 632–633
perineal, see Perineal pain
peripheral somatic, 344
persistent, 534, 631, 633
phantom-limb, 71–72, 513
pharmacodynamics and, 148–150
postamputation, 126
postchemotherapy, 72–73
postmastectomy, 71, 126
postoperative, 473
postradiation, 72–73, 135
postradical neck dissection, 71
postsurgery, 70–72, 124
postthoracotomy, 70–71, 126
problems, 663
profile questionnaire, 510
proprioceptive, 124
protopathic, 475, 495
psychogenic, 91
  mechanisms of, 120
psychologic mechanisms of, 92–93
radicular, 171
ratings, 237–238
  method of use of, 147–148
relief, reduction, relationship with, 240
  in advanced cancer, general principles, 298–299
  bilateral, 443–444
  in chemical hypophysectomy, 385–386
  depression and, 576
  duration of, 547
  endocrine therapy and, 150–161
  with hypophysectomy, 380, 387
  with nerve plexus block, 357
  with neurolysis, 332
  with peripheral nerve stimulation, 501
  with pituitary ablation, 599
  recording of, 251
  with rhizotomy, 544
research, 669
  cancer-related, 670
retro-orbital, 64
saddle, 342, 345
sciatic, 442
severe, 657
  intractable, 128
site of, 620
in skeletal cancer, 568
somatogenic, 120
spiral, 663
spontaneous, 477
stimulation-induced, 456
stimulation-response models of, 231
stump, 71, 124
subjective, 239
surgery for, 414
and symptom management, 661
syndromes
  associated with cancer therapy, 70–74, 123–125
  specific, in cancer pain of head and neck, 522
  specific, in patients with cancer, 63–71
terminal, 644
  management of, 651
  nature and management of, and hospice concept, 637–653
  results of comparative study in, 642–643
therapy, neurophysiology of, 13–29
thoracic segmental, 441
threshold in children, 95
  elevation of, 623–630
time characteristics of, 126
total, 638
trigeminal, 463, 465
uncontrolled, 619
unrelated to cancer, 75
  in children, 95
unrelieved, 658
upper chest and upper limb, 353
useless, 83
visceral
  analgesics and related drugs in, 593–595
  in children, 587
widespread, 490
Painful limb, 186
Palliative
  amputation, 178

Palliative *(contd.)*
    surgery, 175–183
        direct, 176–180
        indirect, 180–181
        mediate, 182–183
        necessary, 178–180
        for pain, 181
        reductive, 176–178
        urgent, 176
Palsy, VIth nerve, 64
Pancoast tumor, 137, 168
Pancreas, 169
Para-aminophenol derivatives, 257
Parametrium, 169
Paraplegia, 147
Parathormone, 171
Paresthesia, 124, 125
Partial
    remission (PR), 132, 133
    thromboplastin time (PTT), 201
Patient(s)
    with cancer, services for, 658–661
    care, 669
    longer-stay, 650
    mixed group of, 647
Pentazocine, 147, 270
Peptides, opioid, 394
Perforation, intestinal, 176
Perfusion
    hyperthermic-antiblastic, 195
    isolation, 185
Periaqueductal gray (PAG), 23, 481
Pericarditis, 172
Perineal pain, 442
    neurolytic blocks in, 601–609
        complications of, 605–608
        material and methods in, 603–605
        results in, 605
Period, terminal, 639
Perioperative care regimes, 247
Peripheral-central mechanisms, 124
Periventricular gray, stimulation of, 581
Periwinkle, 143, 144
Perspective
    patient's, 51
    physician's, 50
    rationale for behavior, 51
Phantom limb, 124
Pharmacodynamics, 148
    and pain, 148–150
Phelebepropane, 301
Phenergan, 281

Phenol, 329, 354, 364
    and alcohol, subarachnoid, 326–333
    hyperbaric, 304, 328
Phenothiazines, 280–281
Phosphates, alkaline, 200
Phrenic nerve, 188
Physical dependence, 269
Physician, managing, 668
Physiologic changes, 239–240
Pilot study, 151
Pituitary
    neuroadenolysis, 160
    -ovary axis, 156
Placebo, 127
Plasticity, 78
cis-Platinum (CDDP), 143
Pleura, 168
Plexuses
    location of, 597
    secondary, 359
Pneumonia, bronchial, 183
Podophyllotoxin, 141
Polychemotherapy, 526
Polyirradiation, 212
Polyneuropathy, symmetrical, 124
Postamputation pain, 126
Postchemotherapy syndromes, 124–125
Posteromedial hypothalamotomy, 475–485
Postradiation
    fibrosis, 169
        of brachial plexus, 126
    therapy pain, 73–74, 125
Postsurgical pain, 70–72, 124
Postthoracotomy pain, 70–71, 126
Posttreatment and outcome measures in biofeedback, 236
Potency, 267
    relative, 267
PR (partial remission), 136, 158
Pressure, central venous, 198, 200
Procedures
    neurosurgical, 670
    neurosurgical ablative, 405–423
    screening, 659
Progestational agents, 141
Progestins, 149, 151, 152, 154
Prognostic block(s), 305, 306, 308, 360
Programs, rehabilitation, 675
Progression of tumors, 132
Prolactin, 156
Promethazine, 197

SUBJECT INDEX

Prophine, 302
Prostaglandin, 625, 673
Prostaglandin E, 17
Prostate, tumors in, 137, 141, 170
Prothrombin time (PT), 201
Pseudo-rheumatism, steroid, 72, 124–125
Psychologic aspects of cancer pain, 81–87
  and demographic measures, 233
  and psychiatric techniques, 215–222
  and psychosocial evaluation, 127
  tests, 236–237
Psychologist, 674
Psychometric tests, 127
Psychophysiologic battery, 233–234, 237–240
Psychosocial and nursing technique, 245–253
Psychosurgery, 416–418
  for pain-relief, 547–548
Psychotherapy, 218, 220–221
Psychotomimetic reactions, 270
Psychotropic drugs, 219–220
  advantages of, 288
  ataractics and related drugs, 275–283
  dosage schedule of, 286
  mode of action of, 288
PT (prothrombin time), 201
PTT (partial thromboplastin time), 201
Puncture, 366
Pupil abnormalities, 384

Radiation
  of chest and brachial plexus, 556–557
  fibrosis
    of brachial plexus, 73
    of lumbar plexus, 74
  -induced peripheral tumors, 74
  ionizing, 167–168
  myelopathy, 74, 125
  skin changes, 125
Radicletomy, 409
Radicular symptomatology, 127
Radioactive
  indium, 169
  phosphorus, 171
  strontium, 425, 427
  yttrium, 171
Radiofrequency (RF), 454, 457, 469, 473
  coagulation, 472
  rhizotomy, technique of, 471–472
Radionecrosis, 521
Radiotherapy (RT), 73, 125, 137, 211
  interstitial, 525
  in oncologic therapy of head and neck, 523–524
  palliative, 137
  sequelae of, 172–173
Ratio, nurse-patient, 650
Rational-imaginative-process (R-I-P), 49
Reach to Recovery Programs, 247
Recalcification, partial, 132
Receiver, radio, 500–502
Receptors, opiate, 33–34
Recording, methodical, analysis and, 648–649
Rectum, 169
Recurrence, 132
Relationship, physician-patient, 674
Relaxation response, 239
Research, 652
Respiration, 427
Retention, bladder, 607
RF, *see* Radiofrequency
Rhabdomyosarcoma, 187
Rhizidiotomy, 409
  posterior, 442–443
Rhizotomy(ies), 586
  cervical, 440
  cervicobrachial, 440–441
  chemical, 603–605
  combined multiple, 466
  dorsal, 612
  multiple, 544, 545
  percutaneous differential radiofrequency of glossopharyngeal nerve, 469–473
  phenol, 339, 340, 342, 344
  RF, technique of, 471–472
  sacral, 441, 662
  sensory, or neurectomy, 578–579
  spinal, 439–442
    dorsal, 406–409
    posterior and commissural myelotomy, 407
    selective posterior, 409
  thoracic, 441
R-I-P (rational-imaginative-process), 49
Rorschach Test, 246
RT, *see* Radiotherapy

Rubidasone, 142

Sacral plexus, 172
Sagittal sinus, 171
Salicylates, 256–257
Saline
   hypertonic, 354, 402
   intrathecal, 333
   normal, 363
Sarcoma
   lymphoblastic, 142
   osteogenic, 186, 190
   soft-tissue, 187, 199
Satellitosis, 187
Scan, bone, 127
Schemes, home care, 662
Scintigraphy, 171
SCL-90 (Symptom Check List), 246
Section, frontothalamic, 418
Sector, private/charitable, 656
Sedative antihistamines, 281
Self-hypnosis, 233
Sensory deficits, 126
Serotonin
   mania, 517
   system, 488
Serum calcium and phosphate, 200
Services, community, 659
Signal
   -symptom, 146, 158, 213
   tumor, 213
Skin, arterial supply of, 313–315
Skull, base of, 168
   metastases to, 63–64
Social
   manipulation, 218
   setting, 248
   worker, 659
Solution(s)
   hyperbaric, 327
   hypertonic salt, 553
   local anesthetic, 365
   neurolytic, 362–364
Somatosensory system, 125
Spearman's rho, 237
Spindle poison, 143
Splanchnectomy, 615
Spread, lymphogenous, 312
Staff
   burn-out syndrome, 651
   full interdisciplinary, 645–646

hospice, 661–662
reception, 648
Stage of disease, 255
Stasis
   lymphatic, 139
   venous, 139
Stenosis, 176
Stimulation
   of central gray, 517
   intermittent, 581
   of mucosal and submucosal nerve
     endings, 519
   of peripheral nerve, 500–502
   of periventricular gray, 581
   of spinal cord, 502–506
     complications in, 502
Stimulator, 510, 513
   electrical, 499
   electrostatic, portable, 509
   external, 505
Streptococcus erysipelatis, filtered
   extracts of, 195
Streptozotocin, 141
Subarachnoid
   injection in celiac plexus block, 369
   neurolysis, 325–333
Subclavian artery, 188
Subjective assessment, 148
Survival, disease-free, 133
Sweat tests, 311
Sympathectomy, 406, 586, 615–616
Sympathetic
   block, *see* Block(s), sympathetic
   chain, 137
     paravertebral, 316
Sympathomimetic amines, 278–279
Symptom Check List (SCL-90), 246
Symptomatic desensitization, 226
Syndrome(s)
   Brown-Sequard, 431
   chronic pain, 493, 513
   Horner's, 64–65
   jugular-foramen, 63
   postchemotherapy, 124–125
   specific pain
     in cancer of head and neck, 522
     in patients with cancer, 63–70, 71
   staff burn-out, 651
Synergistic potency, 259

Tactile afferents, 16

SUBJECT INDEX

Tamoxifen, 154
Team
  domiciliary, 646
  hospice home care, 647
  symptom-control, 662
  work, 660
Technique(s)
  catheter, 320–321
  operative in medullary tractotomy, 454–458
Teratocarcinomas, 170
Terminal
  -cancer pain syndrome, 275
  phase, 127
Test, psychometric, 601
Testicle
  embryonal carcinoma of, 133
  tumors in, 170
Testosterone, 152
Thalamic and hypothalamic stimulation, 493–498
Thalamolaminotomy (intralaminar thalamotomy), 475–481
  results in, 479
  stereotaxic, 475–485
  therapeutic application of, 479
Thalamotomy, stereotactic, 415–416, 546–547, 580, 616
Theologians, 129
Therapeutic
  blocks, 306
  modalities, 125
    evaluation of, 127
Therapy
  anticancer, pain after, 573
  endocrine, 137
  estrogen, 399
  hormone, in cancer pain, 148–150
    of chest and brachial plexus, 559–560
  occupational, 639–641
  pain, 673, 675
  radiation, 125, 167–174
  radical curative, 169
  selection of, 125
Thermochemotherapy, 203
Thermocoagulation
  percutaneous controlled, 464
  of pituitary gland, 403
Thermorhizotomy of glossopharyngeal nerve, 465
Theta

  activity, 241
  range, 235
Thoracic inlet, 137
Thoracotomy, 124
Thought processes, 49
Thrombus, 171
Thymoleptics, 285
Thyroid, tumors in, 168
Time-distortion, 241
Tissue
  conjunctive, 140
  hematopoietic, 140
  hepatic, 142
Tolerance, 264
Tomography
  computerized transaxial, 62, 127, 208, 212, 577
  of skull, 64
Total parenteral nutrition (TPN), 177, 248
Toxicity, cumulative, 135
TPN (total parenteral nutrition), 177, 248
Tract, trigeminal, 457, 461
  spinal, 455, 458
Tractotomy
  medullary, 412
    anatomic considerations in, 455
    conclusions in, 459–461
    neurophysiologic considerations in, 455–457
    operative technique in, 454–458
    results in, 458–459
  mesencephalic, 413–414, 546
  trigeminal, 545
Transection, spinal cord, 587, 591
Trigeminal nerves, 168
Trigger zones, 138
Tropism, 141
Tumor(s)
  advanced
    anticancer drugs and their activity in, 131–138
  solid, 145
  of bones, 171
  burden, 135
  cell mass, 134
  cells, sensitivity of, 140
  of central nervous system, 141
  in chest, 168–169
  embryonal, 142–143
  endocrine, of adrenal, 141

Tumor(s) *(contd.)*
  of female genital system, 169
  glandular, 519
  of head and neck, 145, 167–168
  hormone sensitive, 145
  hyperacidity, 196
  hyperthermic perfusion with sympathectomy for, 185–194
  infiltration
    of brachial plexus, 67
    of lumbar plexus, 67–68
    of peripheral nerve or plexus or root or cord, 66–70
    of sacral plexus, 68
  intestinal, 145
  intracranial, 137
  of islets of Langerhans, 141
  kidney, 145
  lung, 145
  of male genital system, 170
  nasopharyngeal, 64
  in nervous system, 170–171
  ovarian, 142
  pediatric, 133
  primary, 496
    of lung, 168
  in prostate, 170
  in rhinopharynx, 167
  second primary, 62
  secondary, in chest wall, 168
  solid, 132, 135
  systemic, 171–172
  in testicle, 170
  in thyroid, 168
  of urinary apparatus, 170

Ulceration, 520
Units, special, 649
University of Washington Multidisciplinary Pain Clinic, 128
Uric acid, 200
  stones, 141

Verbal Rating Scale, 246
Vertebra, lumbar, 365
  first, 370
Vertebral bodies, metastases to, 64–65
Vincaleucoblastine sulphate, 143
Vincristine, 143, 199, 528
Vindesine, 1444
Visceral and perineal pain
  analgesics and related drugs in, 593–595
  neurosurgery in, 611–618
Visitors, 249
Visual Analogue Scale, 246
VM-26, 141, 199
VM-26-BCNU, 142
Volume-reduction of tumor masses, 150
Volunteers, role of, 249, 648
Von Norden technique, 212

Walking-impairment, 158
Wilm's tumor, 133

X-ray of chest, 577